Manipal Manual of
Clinical Anatomy
Volume 1

General Anatomy

General Embryology

Upper Limb

Lower Limb

Thorax

Manipal Manual of
Clinical Anatomy

Volume 1

Sampath Madhyastha PhD
Additional Professor
Department of Anatomy
Kasturba Medical College, Mangalore
Manipal University
India

Clinical Cases Editor
M Chakrapani MD
Professor of Medicine
Kasturba Medical College and Hospital
Mangalore, India

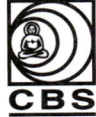

CBS Publishers & Distributors Pvt Ltd

New Delhi • Bengaluru • Chennai • Kochi • Kolkata • Mumbai • Pune
Hyderabad • Nagpur • Patna • Vijayawada

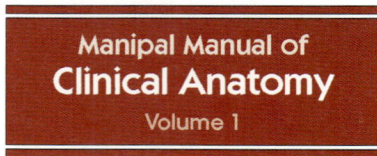

ISBN: 978-81-239-2477-9

First Edition: 2015
Reprint: 2016

Published by Satish Kumar Jain and produced by Varun Jain for
CBS Publishers & Distributors Pvt Ltd
4819/XI Prahlad Street, 24 Ansari Road, Daryaganj, New Delhi 110 002, India.
Ph: 23289259, 23266861, 23266867   Fax: 011-23243014   Website: www.cbspd.com
                                                                                            e-mail: delhi@cbspd.com; cbspubs@airtelmail.in.
Corporate Office: 204 FIE, Industrial Area, Patparganj, Delhi 110 092
Ph: 4934 4934   Fax: 4934 4935   e-mail: publishing@cbspd.com;   publicity@cbspd.com

Branches

- **Bengaluru:** Seema House 2975, 17th Cross, K.R. Road,
  Banasankari 2nd Stage, Bengaluru 560 070, Karnataka
  Ph: +91-80-26771678/79   Fax: +91-80-26771680   e-mail: bangalore@cbspd.com
- **Chennai:** 7, Subbaraya Street, Shenoy Nagar, Chennai 600 030, Tamil Nadu
  Ph: +91-44-42032115   Fax: +91-44-42032115   e-mail: chennai@cbspd.com
- **Kochi:** Ashana House, 39/1904, AM Thomas Road, Valanjambalam, Eranakulam 682 018, Kochi, Kerala
  Ph: +91-484-4059061-62-64-65   Fax: +91-484-4059065   e-mail: kochi@cbspd.com
- **Kolkata:** No. 6/B, Ground Floor, Rameswar Shaw Road, Kolkata 700 014, West Bengal
  Ph: +91-33-2289-1126, 1127, 1128,   e-mail: Kolkata@cbspd.com
- **Mumbai:** 83-C, Dr E Moses Road, Worli, Mumbai-400018, Maharashtra
  Ph: +91-22-24902340/41   Fax: +91-22-24902342   e-mail: mumbai@cbspd.com
- **Pune:** Bhuruk Prestige, Sr. No. 52/12/2+1+3/2 Narhe, Haveli
  (Near Katraj-Dehu Road Bypass), Pune 411 041, Maharashtra
  Ph: +91-20-64704058/59, 32392277   Fax: +91-20-24300160   e-mail: pune@cbspd.com

Representatives

- **Hyderabad**   0-9885175004   - **Nagpur**   0-9021734563
- **Patna**   0-9334159340   - **Vijayawada**   0-9000660880

Printed at: HT Media Ltd., Noida

It is a pleasure, delight and opportunity to write the Foreword to *Manipal Manual of Clinical Anatomy* authored by Dr Sampath Madhyastha. Among the several roles of a medical teacher, the role of a resource developer is one of the most exciting and challenging. To develop a resource for student learning as Dr Sampath has done with so much of passion, planning and perseverance requires the highest level of commitment from a teacher. To be able to put across content with clarity, conviction and clinical correlation is no easy task and Dr Sampath has accomplished this with verve. The hallmarks of the Manual are the clinical applications and the self-assessment opportunities.

Why another textbook in anatomy? When it comes from an anatomy teacher whose devotion and dedication to student learning is paramount, it deserves to be reckoned with much eagerness and expectation. One of the parameters by which scholarship in education is measured is publication of a book which will have wide acceptance in the student community. Dr Sampath's effort in this direction will go a long way in meeting a felt need for an anatomy book that captures the essentials without meandering into trivia. It is a commendable effort and I wish students and teachers of anatomy will find this Manual both indispensable and invaluable.

Dr K Ramnarayan
Vice Chancellor
Manipal University

The anatomy curriculum for the medical undergraduate students is a matter of debate in India since many years with medical education experts calling for restructuring/reframing of the same. Unfortunately, no substantial measures were implemented in the past in revising the syllabus and the student evaluation process. Most of the recommended books are loaded with excess of information for the undergraduate understanding with every new volume creating a 'curriculum hypertrophy'. At present, most of the standard recommended books for all branches of anatomy (general anatomy, gross anatomy, osteology, embryology, histology and neuroanatomy) accumulates to approximately 2500 pages with the students having to assimilate this 'information influx' in less than one academic year. Though opinions differ regarding the ideal duration of the study course in anatomy, the basic need is to tackle the 'curriculomegaly'. The *Manipal Manual of Clinical Anatomy* has embraced and matched this task to a great extent after continuous discussions with physicians, surgeons and senior anatomists. With exception of histology, all other branches of anatomy are succinctly covered in 1000 pages without any 'dilution' of the subject content, merely by omitting additional information that is not warranted at an undergraduate level.

The objectives that are clearly identified in each area after thorough discussion with experts will enable both teachers and students to focus on key issues of every topic. Currently, strong views are emerging that traditional methods of teaching anatomy as practiced by most medical schools have limitations in development of application skills of such knowledge in clinical practice. The teaching methodologies and student evaluations are mainly focused on memorizing and recalling the stringent course and relations of human body parts with no value-addition in development of application skills. *Manipal Manual of Clinical Anatomy* discusses the clinical relevance immediately after elaboration of the gross anatomy, which greatly aids the students in correlation of anatomy with the clinical application. Clinical case scenarios that are carefully designed to emphasise the importance of anatomy could be further elaborated for problem-based learning. These clinical case scenarios are placed immediately after clinical relevance boxes, so that the students can discuss the cases in groups where the teacher can act as a facilitator. Medical schools that follow the systemic rather than regional anatomy approach for integrated teaching will also be benefited by these case studies. Developmental events (embryology) are briefly summarized with more emphasis on birth defects and their embryological basis. Multiple choice questions are designed on the basis of clinical application of anatomy, which would help them in future competitive postgraduate entrance tests.

Manipal Manual of Clinical Anatomy is hereby offered as a genuine attempt to view human anatomy in a new dimension. Your suggestions and feedback are welcome to improve this Manual to meet the requirements of the students and make the learning of anatomy an enjoyable experience.

Sampath Madhyastha PhD
Additional Professor
Department of Anatomy
Kasturba Medical College, Mangalore
Manipal University
India 575001

Acknowledgements

Three years ago I had this audacious idea to reinvent my textbook 'Manipal Manual of Anatomy for Allied Health Sciences' into *Manipal Manual of Clinical Anatomy* for medical undergraduate students. It was a tough journey and I finally decided to put an end to the provoking ideas which were building up in me everyday to incorporate in this manual, as it has been never ending.

At the outset, I would like to acknowledge the Chancellor of Manipal University, Dr. Ramdas M Pai, who has been conducive for all of our academic accomplishments.

My heartfelt thanks and deepest gratitude to our Vice Chancellor, Dr. K. Ramnarayan for his excellent expression in the 'Foreword' of this book and for his tremendous encouragement.

My sincere thanks to Dr. M. Chakrapani, Professor of Medicine, KMC, Mangalore, for his ample assistance and editing of the clinical case scenarios. It was a great learning experience for me and I appreciate his consideration in devoting his time for the same.

My thanks to Dr. M.V. Prabhu, Dean, Kasturba Medical College, Mangalore, for his continuous encouragement. Acknowledgement and appreciation to Dr. Rajgopal Shenoy, Professor and Head, Dept. of Surgery, KMC, Manipal and Dr. Girish K.M., Professor and Head, Dept. of Medical Genetics, KMC, Manipal. Thanks to my friend Dr. Santhosh Rai, Associate Professor of Radiodiagnosis, KMC, Mangalore, for providing radiographic images.

I wish to acknowledge my teacher and mentor, Mr. Seetharam M. Bhat for his meticulous editing, suggestions and above all for boosting my confidence in writing this manual.

It is my duty to acknowledge my colleagues who have edited many chapters and shared their valuable thoughts with me. In this regard I would like to express my sincere thanks to Dr. Vasudha Saralaya, Professor and Head, Dr. Latha V. Prabhu, Professor of Anatomy, Dr. Chitra Prakash Rao, Professor and Head, AJ Institute of Medical Sciences, Mangalore, and Dr. Rajalakshmi Rai, Dept. of Anatomy, KMC, Mangalore.

I am indebted to my colleague, Dr. Rachana K who helped me in editing and compiling the chapters, thereby relieving me of a tremendous pressure. I offer my gratitude to my colleagues Dr. Mamatha, Dr. Prameela, Ms. Teresa who have contributed immensely to this manual.

I would also like to thank my colleagues Dr. Mangala M. Pai, Dr. Ashwin, Dr. Rajani, Dr. Ganesh, Dr. Murali Manju, Dr. Sujatha D'Costa, Ms. Jiji P.J. and Dr. Ashwin Rai, for their support.

I appreciate and thank my postgraduate student Dr. Divya Premchandran, for her incredible contribution to this manual. Special thanks to the students of KMC, Mangalore, who has been my source of inspiration.

I wish to express my gratitude to Dr. S.N. Somayaji, Dr. Ramachandra Bhat, Dr. A.S. D'Souza, Professor and Head of Anatomy, KMC, Manipal, Dr. Ramesh Rao, Dr. Kumar M.R., Dr. Mohandas Rao, Professor and Head of Anatomy, Manipal Melaka Medical College, Dr. Ullas Kamath, Dean, Manipal Melaka Medical College, Manipal, Dr. K.L. Bairy, Professor and Head of Pharmacology, KMC, Manipal, Dr. Shakunthala R. Pai, Professor and Head of Anatomy, Srinivas Institute of Medical Sciences, Mangalore, Dr. Prakash Shetty, Professor and Head, Dept. of Anatomy, Fr. Mullers Medical College, Mangalore and Dr. C.V. Raghuveer, Registrar, Yenopoya University, Mangalore.

I also wish to acknowledge the excellent illustrations rendered by Mr. Tilak and Mr. Steven and page making assistance by Mrs. Mamatha.

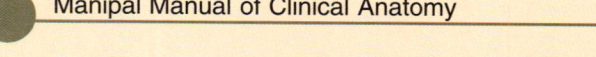

My sincere gratitude to Mr. Satish Kumar Jain, CMD, Mr. Y.N. Arjuna, Sr. Vice President, Deepak Rao, Vice President, CBSP&D.

I pay my sincere gratitude to my mother Mrs. Kamalakshi and my wife Mrs. Prashanthi for being my pillars of strength in bringing out this book successfully. Words are not enough to express gratitude to my in-laws, Professor. B.S. Ramananda and Mrs. Rajani Ramananda for giving me their valuable support and co-operation while writing this manual. Without them and their blessing this task could not have been achieved.

Last but not the least, my heart goes to my son, Pradhan whose innocent face gives me zest and energy. I dedicate this book to him.

Sampath Madhyastha

Dr. M. Chakrapani is a renowned physician with more than two decades of experience in both teaching and patient care. Currently he is a Professor of Medicine and Director of research at Kasturba Medical College and Hospital, Mangalore. Apart from his teaching and patient care commitment, he has immensely contributed to medical research by publishing original research articles in national and international reputed journals. He has many awards to his credit and to name a few are Gold medal for best out going medical graduate, Good teacher award, Distinguished Alumni awards. Above all his academic achievements he is a great human being.

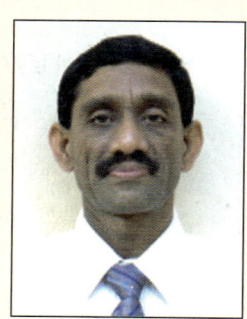

Contents

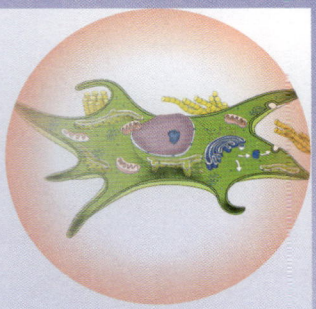

General Anatomy

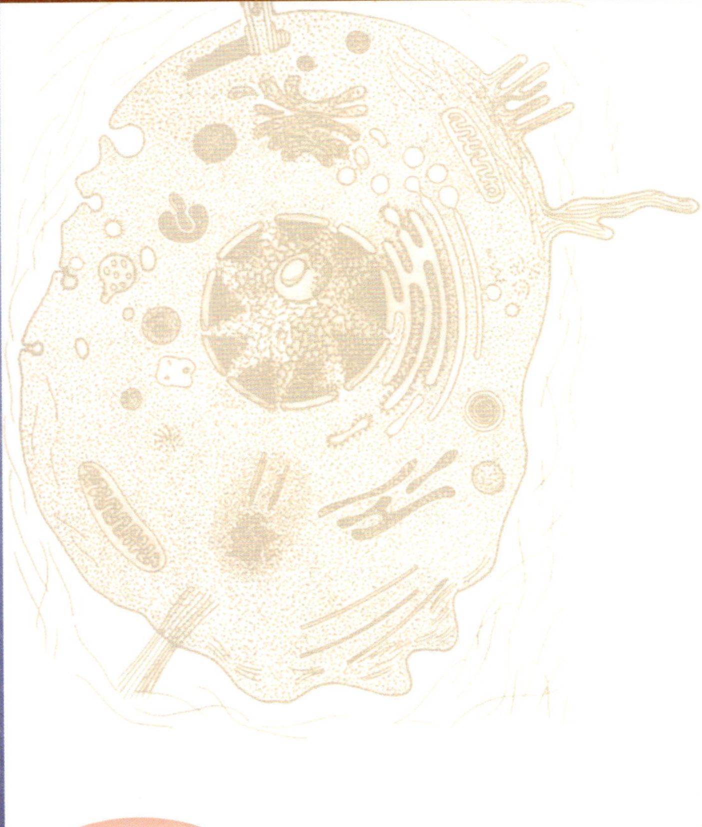

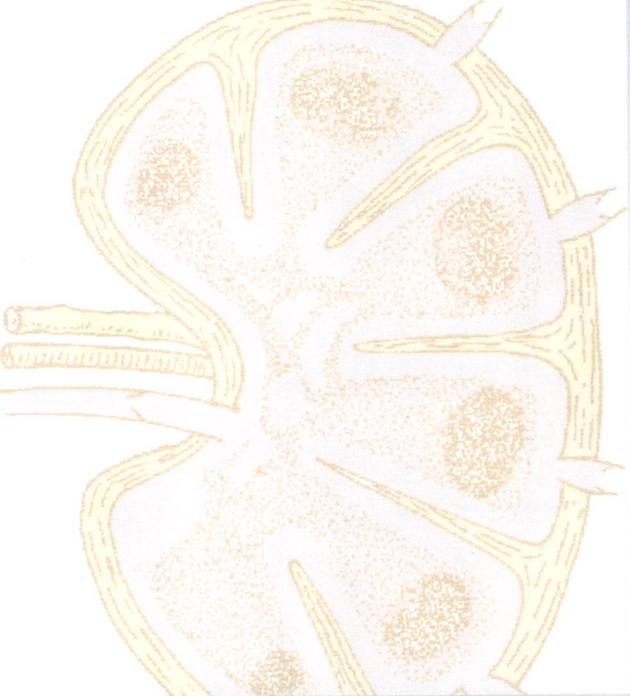

General Anatomy

- Introduction to Anatomy
- Cell and cell division
- Skin and fasciae
- Cartilage
- Muscle
- Blood vessels
- Nervous system
- Anatomical terms
- Tissues of the body
- Connective tissue
- Bone
- Joints
- Lymphatic system

Objectives

- To understand the anatomical terms and it's appropriate use in anatomical descriptions
- To understand the mechanism of cell division
- To explain the types of connective tissue fibres and cells and their functions
- To explain the structure and functions of skin, cartilage, muscles, blood vessels
- To classify the joints giving example to each variety and to explain the structure of a typical synovial joint
- To explain the functions of lymphatic system and to explain the primary and secondary lymphatic organs briefly
- To explain the structure and functions of neuron and glial cells

INTRODUCTION TO ANATOMY

Human anatomy is the science concerned with the structure of the human body. The term 'anatomy' is derived from the Greek word meaning "to cut up". The dissection of cadavers (dead bodies) has served as the basis for understanding the structure and function of the human body. Most of the terms that form the language of anatomy are of Greek or Latin derivations. In the past, human anatomy was an academic, descriptive science primarily concerned with identifying and naming body structures. Although dissection and description form the basis of anatomy, the importance of human anatomy is in its functional approach and clinical applications. Human anatomy is a practical, applied science that provides the foundation for understanding physical performance and body health.

Subdivisions of human anatomy

1. **Gross anatomy:** It is the study of the structures of a human body that can be observed with naked eye. Stringent courses in gross anatomy in professional schools provide the foundation for the students of entire medical or paramedical teaching.

2. **Surface anatomy:** It deals with the surface features of the body that can be observed or palpated (felt firmly).

3. **Microscopic anatomy:** It deals with the study of structures with the help of a microscope. The cytology (study of cells) and histology (study of tissues) are specialities of anatomy that have provided additional understanding of the structure and function of the human body. Certain cells/tissues can be stained by certain dyes (vital stains) which selectively colour the elements in the cell.

4. **Radiological anatomy:** It involves the study of anatomical structures as they are visualised by X-rays, ultrasound scans or other specialised procedures (CT/MRI scans) performed on living body. In contrast X-ray radiopaque substances is can be ingested or injected for visualising internal organs. Angiography involves taking a radiograph after injecting a dye into the blood stream. Since radiographs compress the body

image with an overlap of organs and tissues, diagnosis is often difficult.

The computerised axial tomography technique (CT or CAT scans) has greatly enhanced the versatility of X-rays, using a computer to display a cross-sectional image similar to that which could only be obtained in an actual section through the body. Magnetic resonance imaging (MRI) and positron emission tomography (PET) are the other techniques used to observe the structures of the body.

5. Surgical anatomy studies anatomical landmarks important for surgical procedures.

6. Developmental anatomy (embryology) examines the changes in form that occur during the period between conception and physical maturity. It is important in medicine because many structural abnormalities can result from errors in the development.

Anatomical terms

Though we are familiar with the common terms of many parts and regions of our body, it is essential that we use internationally accepted anatomical names/terms.

Body Positions

The following are the positions/postures of the human body during clinical examination/cadaver dissection/anatomical description.

Anatomical Position: All descriptions of the human body are based on the assumption that the person is:

- Standing erect
- Eyes look straight to the front
- Upper limbs are by the sides of the body, palms facing forward
- Lower limbs are together and digits (toes) pointing forward
- Supine position: Lying down on back with the face directed upwards.
- Prone Position: Lying down facing the ground.
- Lithotomy position: Lying down on your back with fully flexed (knees pointing to the roof) and abducted (widely spread) thighs.

Anatomical Planes

These are imaginary planes (lines) that cut through the body when it is in anatomical position. They help in identifying and studying the relative position of a structure/organs in relation to one another. They further help us in making precise surgical incisions (Fig. 1.1).

- **Median Plane:** Imaginary vertical plane passing longitudinally through the middle of the body from front to back, dividing it into two equal halves.

- **Sagittal Planes:** Imaginary vertical planes passing through the body along the median plane.

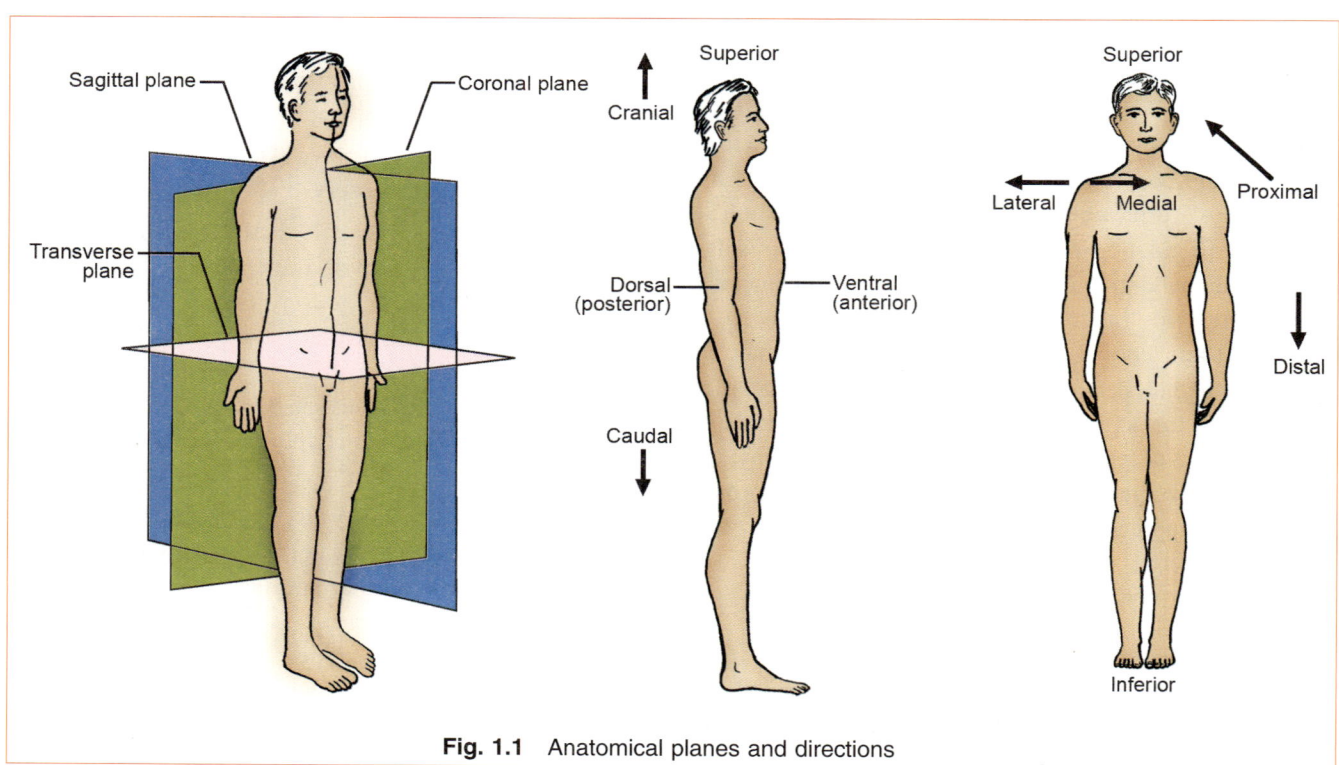

Fig. 1.1 Anatomical planes and directions

- **Coronal Planes:** These are imaginary planes passing through the body at right angle to the median plane, dividing it into anterior (front) and posterior (back) portions.
- **Horizontal Planes:** These are imaginary planes passing through the body at right angles to both the median and coronal planes. This plane is parallel to the ground. This plane divides the body into superior (upper) and inferior (lower) parts.
- **Oblique Planes:** Any plane other than those mentioned above, they slant or deviate from the other planes.

Terms of Relationship

Superior (cranial)   – Nearer to the head (Fig. 1.1)

Inferior (caudal)   – Nearer to the feet

Anterior (ventral)   – Nearer to the front

Posterior (dorsal)   – Nearer to the back

Medial   – Nearer to the median plane

Lateral   – Farther from the median plane

Terms of Comparison

Compare the relative positions of two structures with each other.

Proximal   – Nearer to the trunk/point of origin

Distal   – Away from the trunk/point of origin

Superficial   – Nearer to/on the surface

Deep   – Farther from the surface

External   – Towards/on the exterior

Internal   – Towards/in the interior

Central   – Nearer to/towards the center

Peripheral   – Away from the center

Parietal   – External wall of a body cavity

Visceral   – Pertaining to covering of an organ

Ipsilateral   – On the same side of the body

Contralateral – On the opposite side of the body

Evagination   – Outward bulging of the wall of a cavity

Invagination   – Inward bulging of the wall of a cavity.

Terms describing movements at joints

- Flexion: Bending/decreasing the angle between the bones or parts of the body. In this movement there is an approximation of flexor surfaces.
- Extension: Straightening of a bent part or making an increase in the angle between bones of the body. In this movement there is an approximation of extensor surfaces.

- Abduction: Moving away from the median plane.
- Adduction: Moving towards the median plane.
- Rotation: Moving around the long axis.
- Medial rotation: Inward rotation.
- Lateral rotation: Outward rotation.
- Circumduction: Circular movement combining flexion, abduction, extension and adduction.
- Eversion: Raising the lateral border of the foot.
- Inversion: Raising the medial border of the sole of the foot.
- Pronation: Rotation of the forearm so that the palm is turned backwards.
- Supination: Rotation of the forearm so that the palm is turned forwards.
- Protraction: Moving anteriorly (forward).
- Retraction: Moving posteriorly (backward).

Terms related to muscle

- Origin – is the end of the muscle, which is fixed and shows relatively less movement during contraction.
- Insertion – is the end of the muscle, which shows relatively more movement during contraction. The origin of the muscle is considered as proximal attachment and insertion as distal attachment.
- Belly – The fleshy and contractile part of a muscle.
- Tendon – The fibrous, non-contractile part of the muscle.
- Aponeurosis – The flattened sheet of dense connective tissue, which attaches the muscles to the bone/skin.
- Raphe – A fibrous band made up of interdigitating aponeurotic fibers of the muscles.

Terms related to vessels

- Arteries – Carry oxygenated blood away from the heart.
- Veins – Carry deoxygenated blood towards the heart.
- Arterioles – These are the smallest branches of the arteries within the tissue (with diameter 100 microns or less).
- Venules – These are the minute vessels in the tissue, which join to form vein.
- Capillaries – Microscopic vessels connecting arterioles to venules.

The umbilical artery and pulmonary artery are exceptions, they carry the deoxygenated blood.

The pulmonary vein and umbilical vein carry oxygenated blood.

Body organisation

Study of the human body will begin with an overview of microscopic anatomy and then proceed to the gross or macroscopic anatomy of each organ system. While considering events from the microscopic to macroscopic scales we will examine several interdependent levels of organisation.

To begin with, chemical or molecular level of organisation. The human body consists of over a dozen different elements, but four of them (hydrogen, oxygen, carbon and nitrogen) account for more than 99% of the total number of atoms (Fig. 1.2).

At the chemical level, atoms interact to form compounds with distinctive properties. The major classes of compounds in the human body are illustrated in (Fig. 1.3).

1. **Cellular level:** The cell is the basic structural and functional component of life. It is at the cellular level that such vital functions of life such as metabolism, growth, irritability and adaptability, repair and reproduction are carried out.

   Cells are composed of minute particles called atoms, which are bound together to form larger particles called molecules. Certain molecules are arranged into small functional sources called organelles. Each organelle carries out a specific function within the cell. The nucleus, mitochondria and endoplasmic reticulum are organelles.

   The human body contains of many distinct kinds of cells; each specialised to perform specific function, e.g. muscle cells, bone cells, fat cells, blood cells and nerve cells.

2. **Tissue level:** Tissues are groups of similar cells that perform specific functions. An example of a tissue is the muscle within the heart, which functions to contract and pump the blood through the body.

3. **Organ level:** An organ is an aggregate of two or more tissues, assigned to perform a particular function. Each organ usually has one or more primary tissues and several secondary tissues. In the stomach, for example, the inside lining epithelium is considered as primary tissue because it performs the basic functions like secretion and absorption. Secondary tissue of the stomach is the supporting connective tissue and vascular, nervous and muscular tissue.

4. **System level:** The system of the body constitutes the next level of structural organisation. A body system consists of various organs that have similar or related functions. Examples of systems are the circulatory system, endocrine system etc. Certain organs may serve several systems. All the systems of the body are interrelated and function together, constituting the total organism.

Body regions

The human body is divided into several regions that can be identified on the surface of the body. Learning the terminology used with reference to these regions now will make it easier to learn the names of underlying structures later. The major body regions are the head, neck, trunk, upper extremity and lower extremity. The trunk is further divided into the thorax and abdomen (Fig. 1.4).

Head

The head is divided into the facial region (which includes the eyes, nose and mouth) and the cranial region, which covers and supports the brain.

Neck

The neck is referred to as the cervix or cervical region. It supports the head and permits it to move.

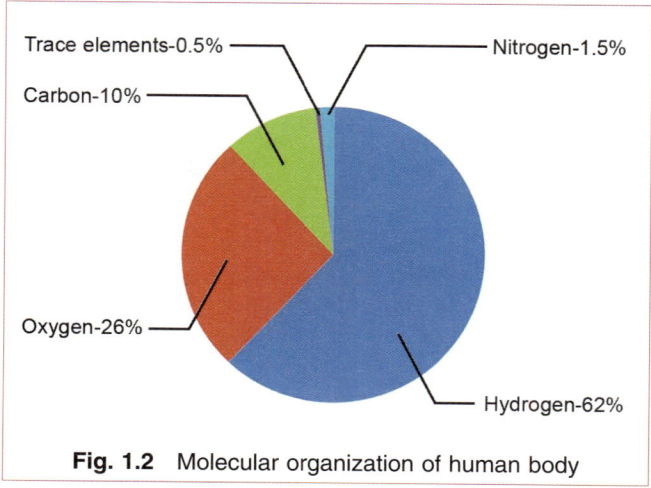

Fig. 1.2   Molecular organization of human body

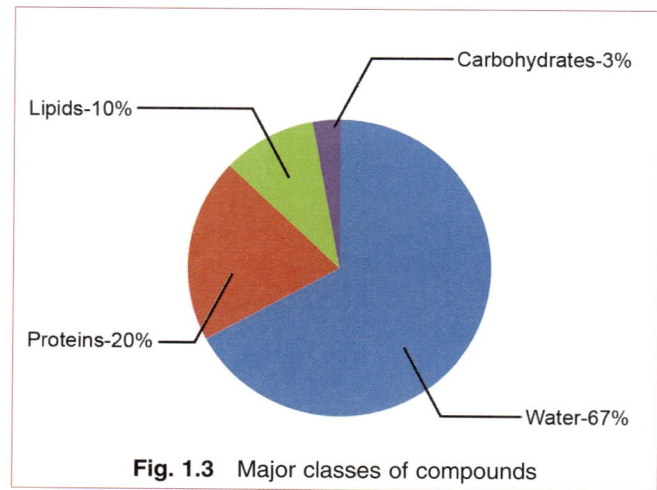

Fig. 1.3   Major classes of compounds

Thorax

The thoracic region is commonly referred as chest. The mammary region of the thorax surrounds the nipple and in sexually mature females it is enlarged as the breast. Between the mammary regions is the sternal region. The armpit is called axilla. The vertebral region, following the vertebral column extends through the length of the back.

Abdomen

The abdomen is located below the thorax. The umbilicus is a landmark on the front and center of the abdomen. The abdomen has been divided into nine regions in order to describe the location of internal organs (Fig. 1.4).

The pelvic region forms the lower portion of the abdomen. The perineum is the region containing the external sex organs and the anal opening. The center of the back of the abdomen is called lumbar region. The sacral region is located further down at the point where the vertebral column terminates. The large hip muscles forms the buttock or gluteal region.

Upper extremity (Upper limb)

The upper limb is anatomically divided into the shoulder, brachium (arm), ante brachium (forearm) and hand. The front of the hand is referred to as the palm and back of the hand is called dorsum. The fingers are referred to as digits.

Lower extremity (Lower limb)

The lower limb consists of thigh, knee, leg and foot. The sole of the foot is referred to as the plantar surface. The dorsum of the foot is the top surface.

Body cavities

Body cavities are confined spaces within the body. During development, the cavity within the trunk is called coelom, which is lined with a membrane that secretes a lubricating fluid. The coelom is portioned by the muscular diaphragm into an upper thoracic cavity, or chest cavity, and a lower abdominopelvic cavity. Organs within the coelom are collectively called viscera. The thoracic cavity is further divided into two pleural cavities by invagination of lungs on either side and a pericardial cavity in the middle by the heart. Similarly with invagination of some abdominal organs, the abdominal cavity is referred as peritoneal cavity. In addition to these large cavities, there are several small cavities like oral or buccal cavity, middle ear cavities and nasal cavities. The cranial cavity contains brain and its coverings.

CELL

The cell can be defined as "Structural and functional unit of all living organisms". Cells were first observed more than 300 years ago by the English Scientist Robert Hooke. With the advancement of microscope, more information was obtained. The cell theory was unified in 1838 and 1839 by two German biologists, Matthias Scleiden and Theodor Schwann. Their work laid the foundation for a new science called cytology, which is concerned with the study of structure and function of cells.

Knowledge of the cellular level of organization is important for understanding the basic body processes like cellular respiration, protein synthesis, mitosis and meiosis. An understanding of cellular structure gives meaning to the concept of tissue, organs and system levels of functional body organization. Further, many body dysfunctions and diseases originate in the cells. Although cellular structure and function have been investigated for many years, we still have much to learn about cells. The etiologies or causes of a number of complex diseases are yet not known. Scientists are seeking answers to why and how the body ages. The answer will come only through a better understanding of cellular structure and functions.

Some of the cells and their specific functions are listed below:

1. Movement — muscle cell
2. Conductivity — nerve cell
3. Synthesis of enzymes — e.g. pancreatic acinar cells
4. Secretion of mucous — mucous gland cells
5. Secretion of steroids — cells of adrenals, testes, ovaries
6. Ion transport — cells of kidney, ducts of salivary glands
7. Intracellular digestion — macrophages

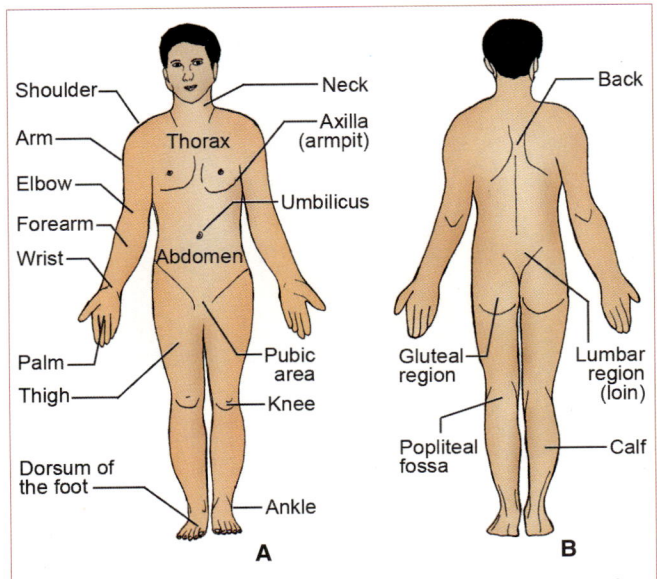

Fig. 1.4 Body regions: **A** - Anterior view; **B** - Posterior view

8. Transformation of physical and chemical stimuli into nervous impulses — receptors.

9. Metabolic absorption — cells of intestine.

Each cell has a cell membrane enclosing cellular organelles, cytoplasm and nucleus (Fig. 1.5).

Cell Membrane/Plasma Membrane/Plasmalemma

The outermost part of the cell is covered by a membrane called the cell membrane/plasma membrane/plasmalemma. It separates the cell from the "extracellular substance" (the material which lies between the cells). It is an extremely thin and delicate membrane and its thickness ranges from 6 to 10nm.

Structure of cell membrane

Under the electron microscope the membrane appears as a trilaminar structure, with outer and inner dark layers and a light layer in between them. Chemically they are made up of phospholipid and protein molecules, externally covered by a coat of glycocalyx (sugar + protein). Each phospholipid molecule has a 'head' and a 'tail'. The head contains phosphate and is water soluble (hydrophilic). The tail consists of two fatty acids and is water insoluble (hydrophobic). Phospholipid molecules line in two rows with their heads lying on the surface and tails pointing at each other (Fig. 1.6).

The permeability of a membrane is a property that determines its effectiveness as a barrier. When substances cannot cross a membrane, it is described as impermeable.

When substances can cross the membrane without difficulty, the membrane is freely permeable. Most of the cell membranes fall in-between and are thus said to be selectively permeable. Passage across the membrane may be passive or active. In a passive process ions or molecules move across the cell membrane without any energy expenditure by the cell, e.g. diffusion, osmosis and filtration. The active transport across the cell membrane requires energy in the form of ATP, e.g. pinocytosis and phagocytosis.

In many places, the cell membrane becomes modified to form microvilli and cilia for special functions.

• The microvilli increase the surface area for absorption e.g. cells lining the intestine.

• The cilia propel the fluid/particles in one direction. They are motile and larger than microvilli, e.g. cells lining the nasal cavity.

• Flagellum is a single hair-like projection from the cell surface. It is present in sperms and is commonly called sperm tail.

Cell junctions or contacts

In tissues like epithelium where cells are closely packed, the following types of cell contacts can occur:

i. Zonula occludens

ii. Zonula adherens

iii. Desmosome

iv. Gap junction

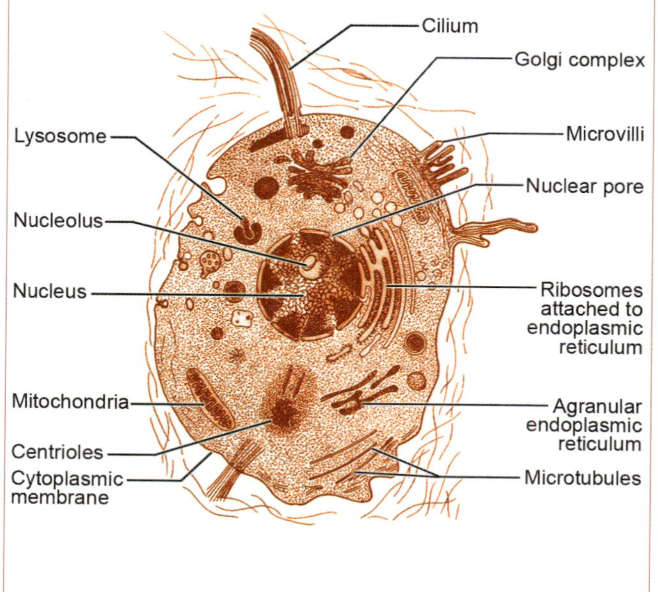

Fig. 1.5 Cell and its constituents

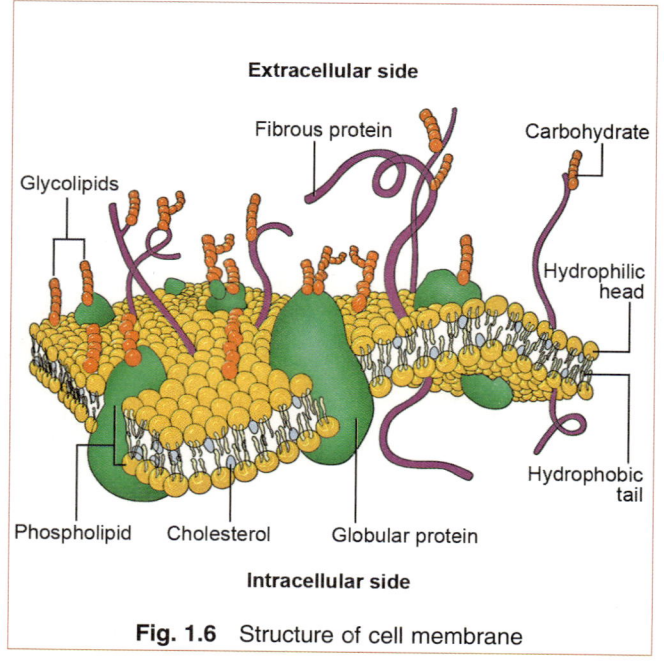

Fig. 1.6 Structure of cell membrane

Functions of cell membrane are –

- Maintaining the integrity of the cell
- The semipermeable membrane is involved in endocytosis (phagocytosis) and exocytosis
- Cell membrane bears receptors for specific hormones, enzymes and neurotransmitters.
- They serve as identification tags.

Cytoplasm

The cytoplasm contains the structures concerned with the metabolic processes and products of metabolism. The cytoplasmic bodies are mainly of two types:

1. Organelles (Living structural component)
2. Inclusions (Non-living accumulations of cell products)

The cytoplasmic organelles are ribosomes, endoplasmic reticulum, golgi apparatus, centrosomes, mitochondria, lysosomes, microbodies (Peroxisomes), microtubules and microfilaments. The chemical composition of the cytoplasm is water (75%), proteins (10–20%), lipids (2–3%), carbohydrates (1%), sodium, potassium, magnesium, phosphates, bicarbonates and vitamins.

The cytoplasmic inclusions are classified into organic and inorganic compounds. Organic compounds contain carbon and are formed by living organisms. Proteins, carbohydrates (glycogen granules) and lipids are organic compounds. Inorganic compounds generally lack carbon and are not formed by living organisms. Water and electrolytes (acids, bases and salts) are examples of inorganic compounds.

Endoplasmic reticulum (ER)

Endoplasmic reticulum is a network of intracellular membranes. It can be present in the form of hollow tubes, flattened sheets or round chambers. It synthesises proteins, carbohydrates and lipids. It is also involved in its storage and transport. There are two types of endoplasmic reticulum. (Fig. 1.7A)

Rough endoplasmic reticulum (granular)

The membranes of these endoplasmic reticulum are associated with minute particles of RNA called ribosomes. The presence of ribosomes gives the membrane a rough appearance. They synthesize proteins.

Smooth endoplasmic reticulum (Agranular)

The membranes are devoid of ribosomes. These endoplasmic reticulum are involved in lipid cholesterol and carbohydrate metabolism. They are also concerned with steroid hormone synthesis in testes and adrenals.

Golgi apparatus

- It consists of flattened membrane discs called saccules. A typical Golgi apparatus consists of five to six saccules. (Fig. 1.7B).
- They lie near the nucleus of the cell.
- They show microvesicles (secretory granules) on their surface.
- They are involved in the process of receiving, concentrating and storing of secretory products (proteins).
- They also secrete polysaccharides.

Ribosomes

- They are small dense granules roughly 25 nm in diameter (10–20 nm).
- Each ribosome consists of roughly 60% RNA and 40% proteins.

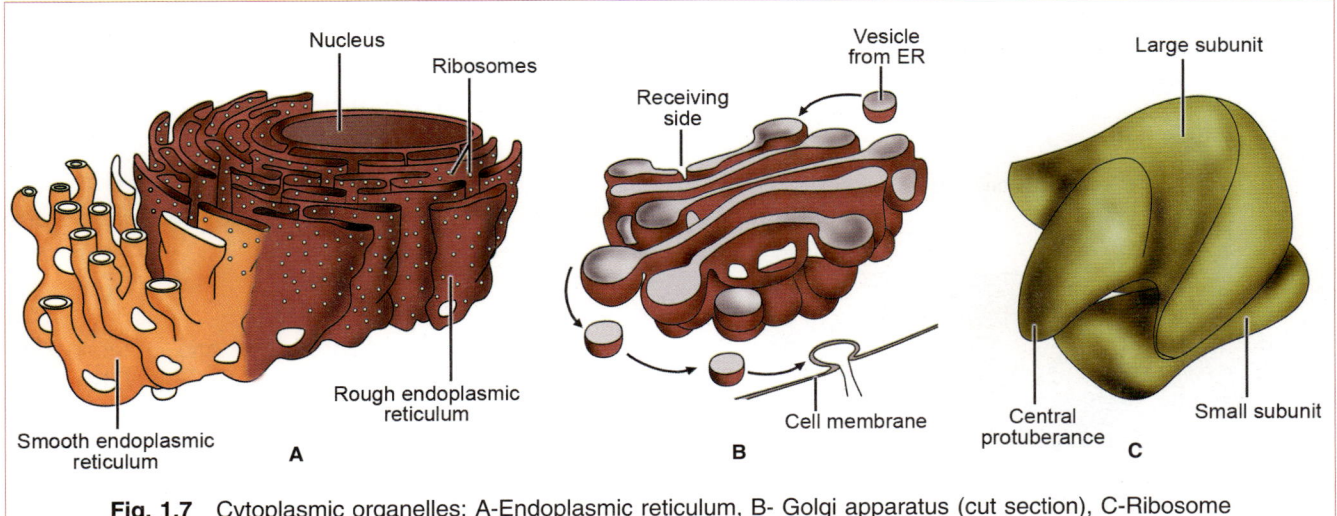

Fig. 1.7   Cytoplasmic organelles: A-Endoplasmic reticulum, B- Golgi apparatus (cut section), C-Ribosome

- They manufacture proteins using information provided by the DNA of the nucleus.
- There are two types of ribosomes – free and fixed. Free ribosomes are scattered throughout the cytoplasm while fixed ribosomes are attached to the endoplasmic reticulum (Fig. 1.7C).

Lysosomes

- They are membrane bound bodies, contains various hydrolytic enzymes (e.g., acid phosphatase).
- They are responsible for intracellular digestive processes and in the breakdown of materials ingested by them.
- They are found in large numbers in macrophages and cells of the reticuloendothelial system. They are often termed as "suicide bags".
- The painful inflammation of rheumatoid arthritis occurs when enzymes from lysosomes are released into the joint cavity and initiates digestion of the surrounding tissue

Mitochondria (Power house of cells)

- They are found in cells with higher metabolic rates.
- They are sausage shaped structures, enclosed by two membranes. The inner membrane is thrown into folds called "cristae", which divides the interior into compartments.
- Mitochondria are the sites of production of high-energy compounds (ATP, GTP).
- The dehydrogenase enzyme present in them is responsible for Kreb's citric acid cycle, protein and lipid synthesis (Fig. 1.8).

Centrosome

- All cells capable of division contain a pair of structures called "Centrioles".
- Centriole is a cylindrical structure composed of short microtubules. There are nine groups of microtubules, with three in each group.

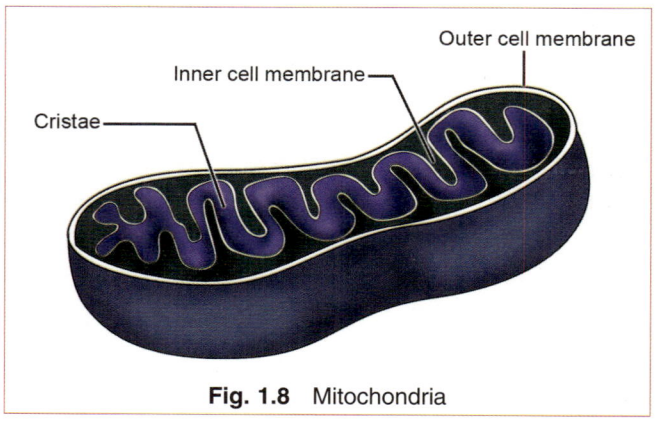

Fig. 1.8 Mitochondria

- Mature red blood cells and skeletal muscle cells lack centrioles. Centrosome is the cytoplasm surrounding this pair.
- Centrioles direct the movement of chromosomes during cell division. They are said to be absent in nerve cells.

Microtubules

- They are tubular structures made up of proteins.
- They act as cytoskeleton to maintain cell shape.
- In mitosis, they form the spindle along which the chromosomes move.

Nucleus

- Nucleus is found in all cells except mature erythrocytes (RBCs) and platelets of the blood.
- The shape is normally rounded and placed centrally.
- Nucleus contains the genetic material and influences the metabolic activities of the cells.

Normally each cell has a single nucleus. But some cells have two or more nuclei, e.g., osteoclasts, skeletal muscle.

Structure of the nucleus

In a resting cell the nucleus is surrounded by a nuclear membrane. The outer part of the nuclear membrane is continuous with endoplasmic reticulum while its inner surface provides attachment to the ends of the chromatids. The membrane has many gaps called nuclear pores, through which substances can pass from the nucleus to the cytoplasm and vice-versa. The cytoplasm of the nucleus (nucleoplasm) contains –

a) Chromatin material (carriers of genes)

b) Nucleolus – They are rich in RNA and concerned with protein synthesis.

Chromatin: It is made up of a substance called deoxyribonucleic acid (DNA) and proteins

Heterochromatin: The chromatin fibres are tightly coiled on themselves forming solid mass (inactive)

Euchromatin: The coiling of chromatin is not so marked (active). During cell division, the chromatin within the condensed nucleus becomes tightly coiled to form structures called chromosomes.

Chromosomes

Chromosomes are made up of DNA and proteins. The number of chromosomes in each somatic cell is fixed for a given species and in human it is 46. This is referred as the diploid number (diploid = double). However, spermatozoa and ova have 23 chromosomes. This is called haploid number (haploid = half).

Among the 46 chromosomes in a cell 44 are autosomes and two are sex chromosomes. In males the sex chromosomes are X and Y whereas in females it is X and X.

Structure of the chromosome

- Each chromosome consists of two parallel rod-like structures called 'chromatids' (Fig. 1.9)

- The two chromatids are joined to each other at a narrow area, which is called 'centromere' (or kinetochore). The chromosomes appear to be constricted in this region and is called 'primary constriction'

- Each chromatid has a long arm (q-arm) and a short arm (p-arm) (centromere is not exactly in the middle of the length of the chromosome).

Classification of Human chromosomes

On the basis of the location of centromere the chromosomes are classified into –

Metacentric chromosome: The two arms of the chromatid are of equal length (Fig. 1.10).

Submetacentric chromosome: One arm of the chromatid is somewhat shorter than the other.

Acrocentric chromosome: One arm is much shorter than the other.

Telocentric chromosome: Each chromatid has only one arm. The centromere is at one end of the chromosome.

The chromatids of some chromosomes show secondary constrictions. Such constrictions are found nearer to one end of the chromatid. The part of the chromatid 'distal' to the constriction is called '**satellite body**'. Secondary constrictions are concerned with the formation of nucleoli

Groups	Chromosomes	Description
A	1–3	Largest;1,3 is metacentric and 2 is submetacentric
B	4–5	Large;submetacentric with two arms of different size
C	6–12 and X	Medium size; submetacentric
D	13–15	Medium size; acrocentric with satellites
E	16–18	Small; 16 is metacentric but 17 and18 are submetacentric
F	19–20	Small; submetacentric
G	21–22 and Y	Small; acrocentric with satellite on 21 and 22 but not on Y

and are therefore called nucleolar organising regions (NORs).

Based upon size, position of the centromere and presence or absence of satellites, chromosomes are divided into 7 groups.

Each chromosome bears on itself a very large number of functional segments that are called **genes**.

Chromosomes are made up of nucleic acids called deoxyribonucleic acid (DNA) and ribonucleic acid (RNA).

DNA in a chromosome is in the form of very fine fibres. Each fibre consists of two parallel strands that are together twisted spirally to form 'double helix'. The two strands are linked to each other at regular intervals. Each strand of the

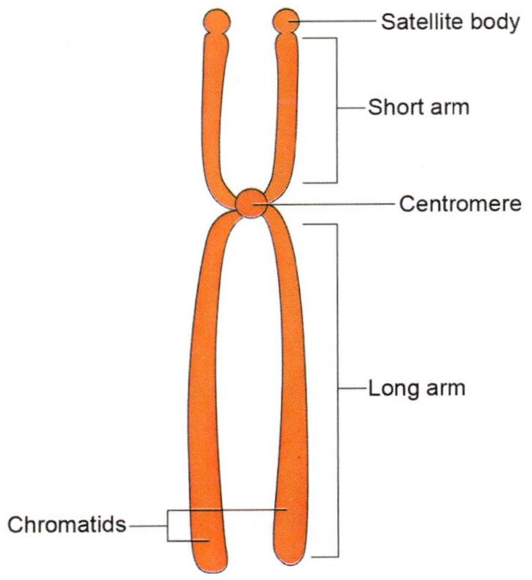

Fig. 1.9 A typical submetacentric chromosome

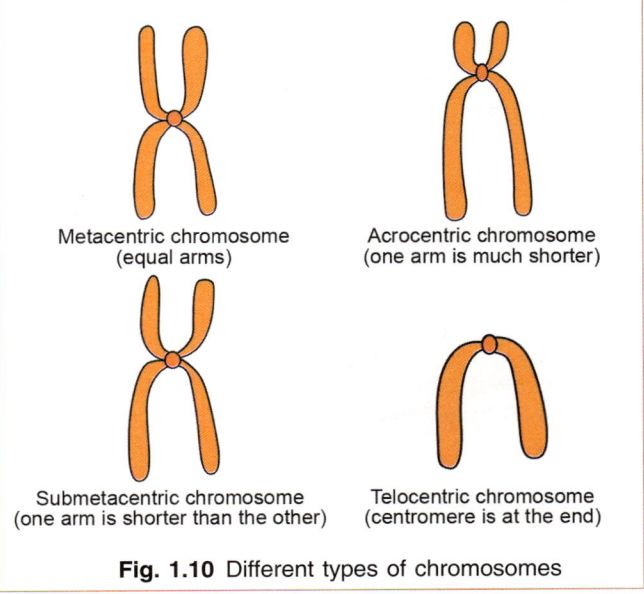

Metacentric chromosome
(equal arms)

Acrocentric chromosome
(one arm is much shorter)

Submetacentric chromosome
(one arm is shorter than the other)

Telocentric chromosome
(centromere is at the end)

Fig. 1.10 Different types of chromosomes

DNA fibre consists of a chain of nucleotides. Each nucleotide consists of a sugar-deoxyribose, a molecule of phosphate and a base. The phosphate of one nucleotide is linked to the sugar of the next nucleotide. The base, which is attached to the sugar molecule, may be adenine, guanine, cytosine or thymine.

RNA resembles close to one strand of DNA except for the sugar ribose instead of deoxyribose. Instead of the base thymine, RNA contains uracil.

Genes

Genes are the units of heredity. They are arranged in linear series within the chromosomes. The genes cannot be seen under microscope. A typical gene is composed of a strand of DNA that includes a transcription unit and regulatory sequence (promoter region). Genes are responsible for the synthesis of proteins through transcription from DNA to RNA and translation from RNA to proteins. It is estimated that the human DNA consists about **23,000 genes.**

Genetic diseases occur due to abnormal genes. Abnormal genes are due to mutation. A change of a base pair of the DNA molecule is known as **gene mutation**.

Human genomic project

The Human genomic project (HGP) was coordinated by US. Department of Energy and National Institutes of Health. The project mainly focused on identifying approximately 20,000–25,000 genes in human DNA, and determining the sequences of the 3 billion chemical base pairs that make up human DNA. The HGP concluded in 2003, but analyses of the data still continues for many years. The sequence of the DNA is stored in databases and is available to anyone on the Internet.

Chromosomal abnormalities and karyotyping is discussed in general embryology chapter.

Barr bodies (sex chromatin)

- It is observed beneath the nuclear membrane during interphase stage in normal female.

- It is one of the X-chromosomes of females, which is highly coiled. It helps in nuclear sexing of the tissues.

- Female with two X-chromosomes will have only one Barr body. However, in triple X-syndrome, there are two Barr bodies.

Cell Division

All nucleated cells can undergo division except highly differentiated cells, e.g. nerve cells.

Cell multiplication is an essential feature of embryonic development, which is necessary after birth for growth and replacement of dead cells. Common type of cell division is mitosis (indirect cell division), in which a parent cell will divide into two daughter cells. The daughter cells will have same number of chromosomes and genetic content as that of the parent cell.

A special type of cell division called meiosis occurs during the formation of gametes (sex cells). In this division, the daughter cell will have half the number of chromosomes. Hence mature sex cells (both male and female) will have haploid (half) number of chromosomes, so that when they fuse (fertilization) the diploid number of chromosomes is restored.

Mitosis

For descriptive purpose, this is divided into four phases. The resting phase during which the cell does not divide is described as interphase. During interphase there is synthesis of proteins (Fig. 1.11).

1. Prophase

- Chromosomes are long, thin and show spiralization. It produces primary and secondary coils, convert the chromosome into a helical structure.

- Increase in the chromosome diameter and decrease in the chromosome length is observed. Chromosome is double stranded (chromatids) and held together by centromeres.

- Nucleolus is prominent in early prophase but later disappears.

- Nuclear membrane breaks down releasing chromosome.

- Centrioles separate and move towards opposite poles of the cells. Centrioles give rise to microtubules. Central microtubules form 'spindle' and others radiate to form 'astral rays'.

2. Metaphase

- Relatively of short duration.

- Chromosomes are sharply defined.

- Chromosome moves towards equator.

- Centromeres of chromosome are attached to the spindle fibre.

3. Anaphase

- Active and shortest stage of mitotic division.

- Centromere of each chromosome, containing a pair of chromatids splits longitudinally. Original chromosome now splits into two new chromosomes.

- Separated chromosomes move towards each pole of the cell.

- Anaphase chromosome shows different shape, based on position of centromeres, e.g. metacentric, sub-metacentric, acrocentric and telocentric.

4. Telophase

- Stage of reconstruction giving rise to two daughter cells.
- Chromosomes become grouped at each pole of the cell, both groups now having diploid number (46).
- Nuclear membrane and nucleoli reappear.
- Spindle and aster disappear.
- Cytoplasm becomes divided into 'two' either by constriction or by new cell membrane formation.
- Each daughter cell receives its compliment of cytoplasmic organelles.

Meiosis

Meiosis consists of two cell divisions - Meiotic division first and meiotic division second (Fig. 1.12).

First Meiotic Division

This is also called the reduction division (chromosome numbers are reduced to half).

1. Prophase: This division is prolonged and divided into a number of stages as follows.

A. Leptotene:

- Chromosomes are long, slender and thread like. Each appears like a string of beads (as in mitosis).
- Individual threads are attached to the nuclear envelope by one end.
- Nucleolus is large and X-chromosome is clear.

B. Zygotene:

- There is a recognition and alignment of homologous chromosomes, so that they become paired. Pairing begins from nuclear envelope. This process is called 'synapsis' (conjugation).
- Each pair of chromosomes is called 'bivalent'.
- Nucleolus and X-chromosomes are clearly visible.

C. Pachytene:

- Chromosomes are shorter and still thicker.
- Each chromosome is formed of two chromatids joined at the centromere. Each 'bivalent pair' consists of four chromatids (tetrads).

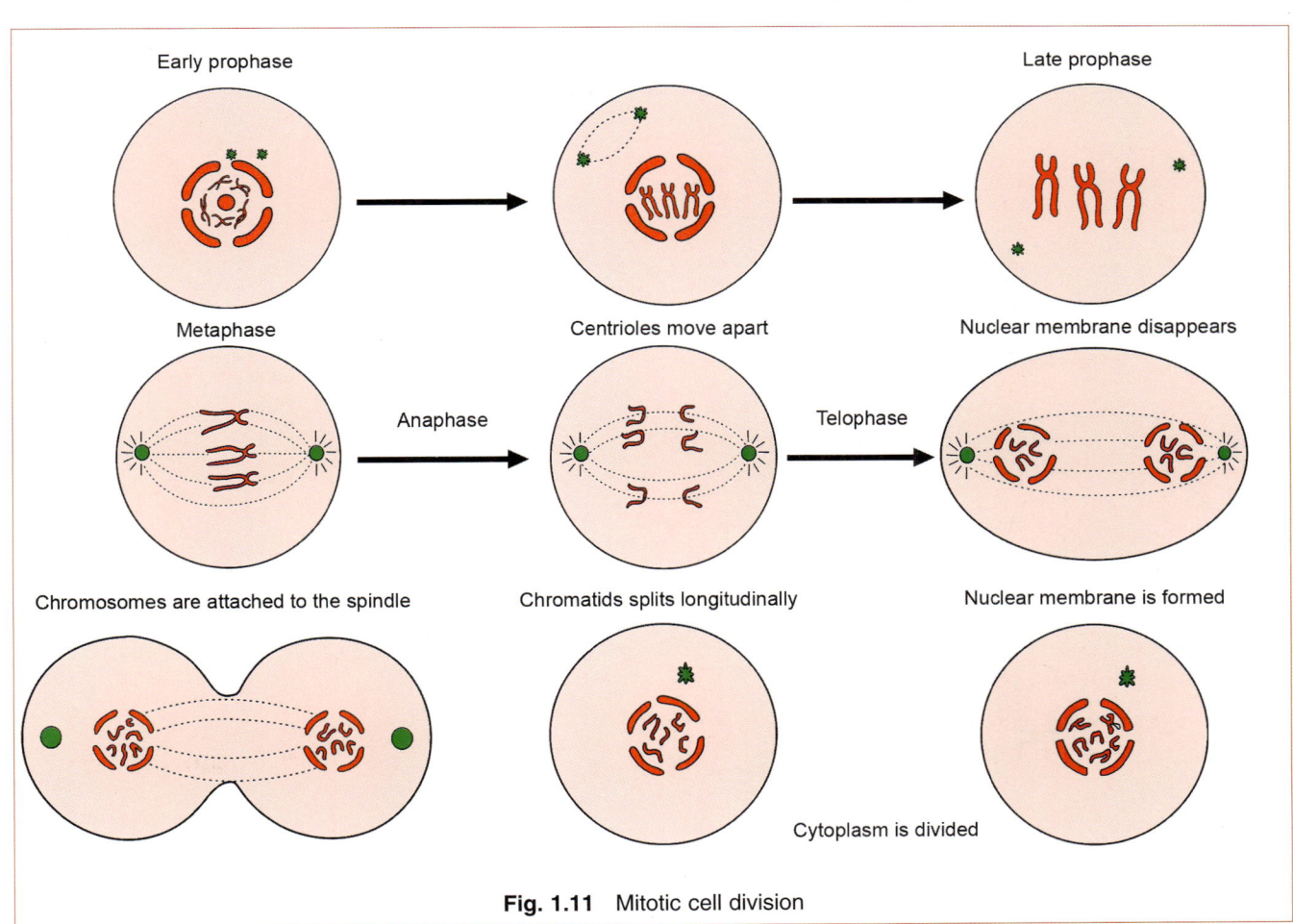

Fig. 1.11 Mitotic cell division

- Each chromosome becomes partially coiled around each other.
- Crossing over (exchange of DNA): A segment of the one of the chromatids (of one chromosome) and a segment of another chromatid (of other chromosome) exchange their places. Since each segment of chromatid carries specific genes, some of the genes are transferred from one chromosome to the other.

D. Diplotene:
- Cross-shaped configuration is prominent at the point of crossing-over. They are called 'chiasmata'.
- Chromosome surface is still freezy.

E. Diakinesis:
- Freezy appearance of diplotene is lost.
- Bivalent pairs move away from each other and spread out against the nuclear membrane.

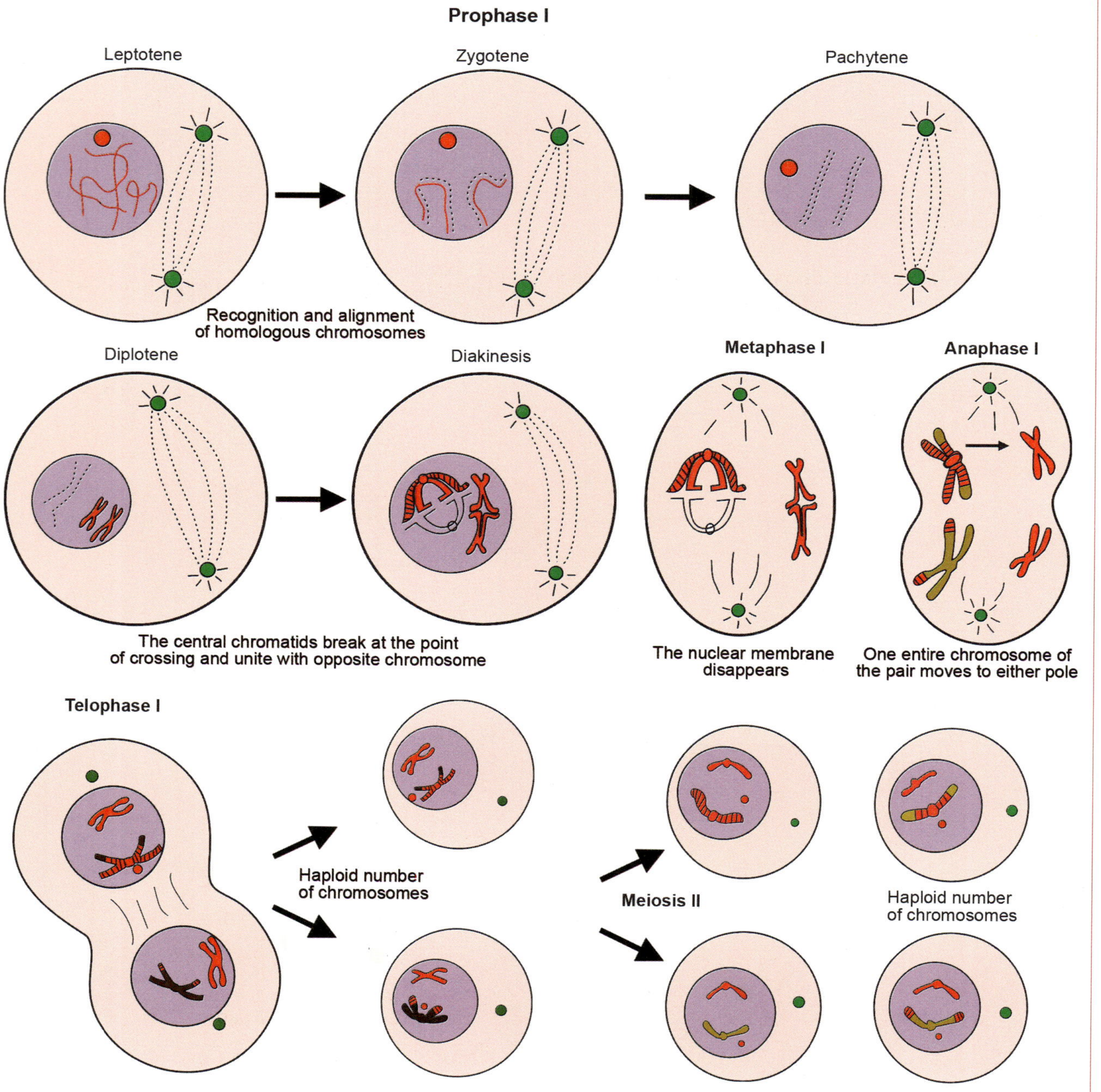

Prophase I

Leptotene Zygotene Pachytene

Recognition and alignment of homologous chromosomes

Diplotene Diakinesis **Metaphase I** **Anaphase I**

The central chromatids break at the point of crossing and unite with opposite chromosome

The nuclear membrane disappears

One entire chromosome of the pair moves to either pole

Telophase I

Haploid number of chromosomes

Meiosis II

Haploid number of chromosomes

Fig. 1.12 Meiotic cell division

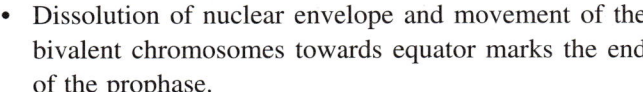

- Dissolution of nuclear envelope and movement of the bivalent chromosomes towards equator marks the end of the prophase.

Metaphase I

- Chromosomes are attached on equator (arms of the chromosomes are on equator and centromeres face the poles).
- Spindle is fully formed and spindle fibres establish connections with centromeres.

Anaphase I

- Chromosomes migrate with centromere (they do not split like in mitosis). Hence double stranded chromosomes move towards the pole.
- All chiasmata are lost.

Telophase I

- Double stranded chromosomes reach poles.
- Their identity is lost and they appear like mass.
- When the first meiotic division is complete, each daughter cell contains haploid number of chromosomes (23).

Second Meiotic Division

- This division is same as mitosis.
- The 23 double structured chromosomes divide at the centromere.
- Each daughter cell receives 23 chromosomes.

Advancements in microscopic technology have had a tremendous impact on the science of cytology. In a new process called microtomography, the capabilities of electron microscopy are combined with those of CT scanning to produce highly magnified, three dimensional, micrographic images of living cells. With this technology, living cells can be observed as they move, grow and divide. The clinical applications are immense, as scientists can observe living and diseased (including cancerous) cells and their response to various drug treatment.

Aging: Although, there are obvious external indicators of aging (graying and loss of hair, wrinkling of skin, loss of teeth and decreased muscle mass) changes due to aging within the cells are not as apparent and not well understood. The mitochondria may change in structure and number and Golgi apparatus may fragment. Also, lipid vacuoles tend to accumulate in the cytoplasm. Extracellular substances also change with age. Collagen and elastic fibres change in quality and numbers. Elastic fibres deterioration in the wall of the blood vessels causes arteriosclerosis in aged persons.

Cancer: Mitotic rates are usually well controlled and in normal tissue the rate of cell division balances cell loss or destruction. When that balance breaks down, the tissue begins to enlarge. A tumour or neoplasm is a mass or swelling produced by abnormal cell growth and mitosis. In a benign tumour the cells remain within the connective tissue capsule. Such tumour seldom threatens an individual life. Surgery can usually remove the tumour if its size or position disturbs tissue function.

Cells in a malignant tumour are no longer responding to normal control mechanisms. These cells divide rapidly, spreading into the surrounding tissues and they may also spread to other tissues and organs. This spread is called **metastasis**. The term cancer refers to an illness characterised by malignant cells. Cancer cells gradually lose their resemblance to normal cells. They change size and shape. Organ function begins to deteriorate as the number of cancer cells increases. Cancer cells compete for space and nutrients with normal cells.

TISSUES OF THE BODY

A group of cells having similar origin, structure and function is called a tissue.

Types: There are four types of basic tissues in the body:

1. Epithelial tissue
2. Connective tissue
3. Muscular tissue
4. Nervous tissue

Cartilage and bone are specialized connective tissues.

Epithelial tissue

It is a layer of cells, which covers the external surface (skin) or lines the internal surface of gastrointestinal, respiratory and urogenital tract.

Functions

- Protection: It protects the body surface from drying or bacterial invasion.
- Transport: Mucous and particulate matters are carried to epithelial surface. Fluid may pass through the cell.
- Secretion: The cells secrete the product synthesized, either to the lumen or blood.
- Excretion: May excrete metabolic waste products.

- Absorption: It absorbs essential substances from the lumen of the GIT and kidney tubules (where it is called reabsorption).
- Lubrication: Peritoneum, pleura and pericardial epithelium serve this function.
- Sensory: In the skin (touch sensation), nasal mucosa (smell sensation) and tongue (taste sensation), it serves as sensory organ.

Types of epithelium

Epithelium is classified into simple, pseudostratified and stratified varieties.

Simple epithelium

It consists of single layer of cells resting on a basement membrane (Fig. 1.13).

1. **Simple squamous:** Irregular flat cells with height less than width.

- Distribution: Alveoli of the lungs, bowman's capsule and loop of Henle of kidney, mesothelium lining the peritoneum, pleura and pericardial cavities, endothelium lining blood vessels.

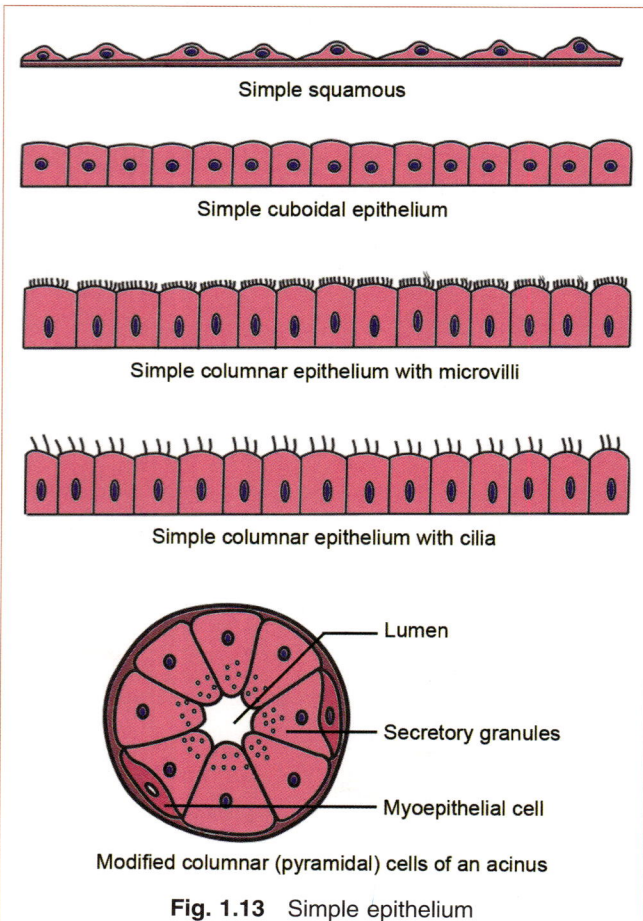

Fig. 1.13 Simple epithelium

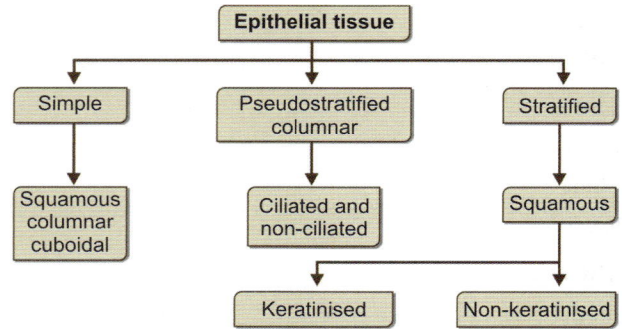

2. **Simple cuboidal:** Height and width are nearly equal and nuclei are central in position.

- Distribution: Thyroid follicles, ducts of many glands and surface of the ovary (germinal epithelium)

3. **Simple columnar:** Height of the cells is greater than width. Nuclei are elongated and placed towards the base.

- Distribution: Small bronchi and bronchioles, uterine tube, ependymal lining the cavities of the brain, efferent ductules of the testis.

4. **Non-ciliated simple columnar:** Distribution: Lining of gastro-intestinal tract from stomach to rectum and gall bladder (with brush border).

Pseudostratified columnar epithelium

- Single layer of epithelial cells resting on a basement membrane.
- Some cells are shorter and do not reach the lumen, while tall cells reach the lumen.
- The nuclei of the cells therefore lie at different levels. This gives the impression of stratification (false stratification).

A. **Pseudostratified non-ciliated**

   Distribution: Male urethra (membranous and penile part), auditory tube and vas deferens.

B. **Pseudostratified ciliated**

Distribution: Upper part of the respiratory tract (trachea and larger bronchi).

Stratified epithelium

Epithelium is made up of many layers of cells. They are found in areas which are subjected to friction.

A. **Stratified squamous non-keratinised**

Epithelium is made up of many layers of cells. Basal cells resting on the basement membrane are columnar or low cuboidal.

- Superficial cells are squamous and flat, hence are called stratified squamous epithelium (Fig. 1.14).

- Distribution: Epithelium lining mouth, pharynx and oesophagus, anal canal, vagina and cornea.

B. Stratified squamous keratinised epithelium

The superficial layer consists of non-living cells with keratin in their cytoplasm. They are tough and water-resistant.

Distribution: Epidermis of the skin.

C. Stratified cuboidal epithelium

It consists of few layers of cuboidal cells.

Distribution: Ducts of sweat glands.

D. Stratified columnar epithelium

It consists of two or more layers of cells.

Basal cells are polyhedral, while superficial cells are columnar.

Distribution: Male urethra (membranous part).

Transitional epithelium (urothelium)

This is a stratified epithelium with three to four layers of cells. The deepest cells are columnar or cuboidal.

The middle layers are made up of polyhedral or pear-shaped cells. The cells of the surface are large and are shaped like an umbrella (Fig. 1.15).

Distribution: Renal pelvis, ureter, urinary bladder and proximal part of the urethra.

Transitional epithelium can be stretched considerably without being damaged. When stretched the cells become flattened. Presence of a glycoprotein membrane on the surface cells is believed to protect the underlying tissue from toxic substances present in the urine.

Glandular epithelium

The epithelial cells are specialized to perform secretory function. Such epithelial cell in-groups constitute glands (single epithelial cell can also be a gland (unicellular).

There are two main types of glands:

A. Exocrine glands: When the secretion from the gland is poured through duct system, they are called exocrine glands. E.g. salivary gland.

The secretory part of the gland may be in the form of rounded sac (or acini) or flask shaped tube (alveoli). Exocrine glands may be in the form of (Fig. 1.16):

- Unicellular gland—e.g. Goblet cells.
- Simple tubular gland—e.g. Intestinal glands.
- Simple alveolar gland—e.g. It represents a stage in the development of simple branched glands.
- Compound tubular gland—e.g. Mucous glands.
- Compound alveolar gland—e.g. Mammary gland.
- Compound tubulo-alveolar gland—e.g. Salivary gland.

Depending upon the nature of secretion, the exocrine glands may be classified into mucous glands and serous glands. The mucous glands secrete 'mucopolysaccharide' and secretions of serous glands are watery in nature rich in proteins.

Glands are also classified into:

Apocrine gland: The luminal part of the cell disintegrates as a part of secretion. The basal part will regenerate. E.g. Mammary gland.

Holocrine gland: The cell itself will be disintegrated as a part of secretion. E.g. Sebaceous gland.

Merocrine gland (epicrine gland): The secretion is discharged without disintegrating the cell. Most of the glands belong to this type.

B. Endocrine glands: These glands are 'ductless' and pour their secretion directly into the blood stream. Their secretion is called 'hormone'. The cells of the endocrine glands are

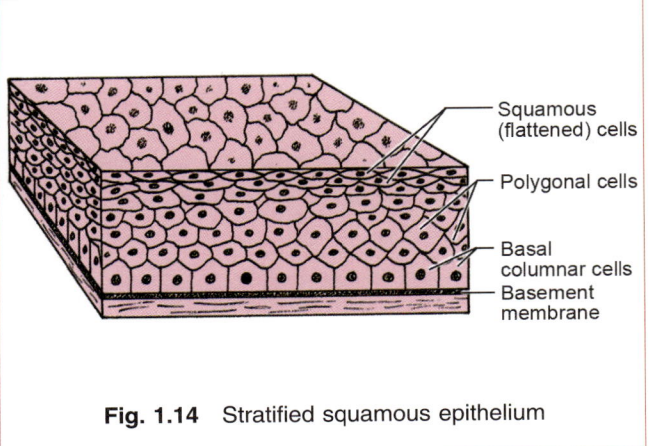

Fig. 1.14 Stratified squamous epithelium

Squamous (flattened) cells

Polygonal cells

Basal columnar cells

Basement membrane

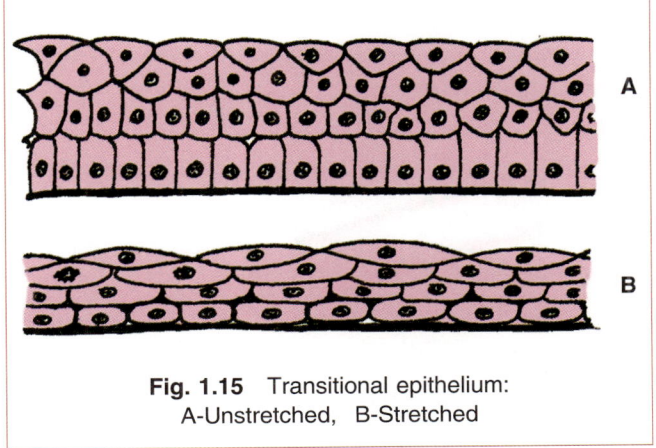

Fig. 1.15 Transitional epithelium:
A-Unstretched, B-Stretched

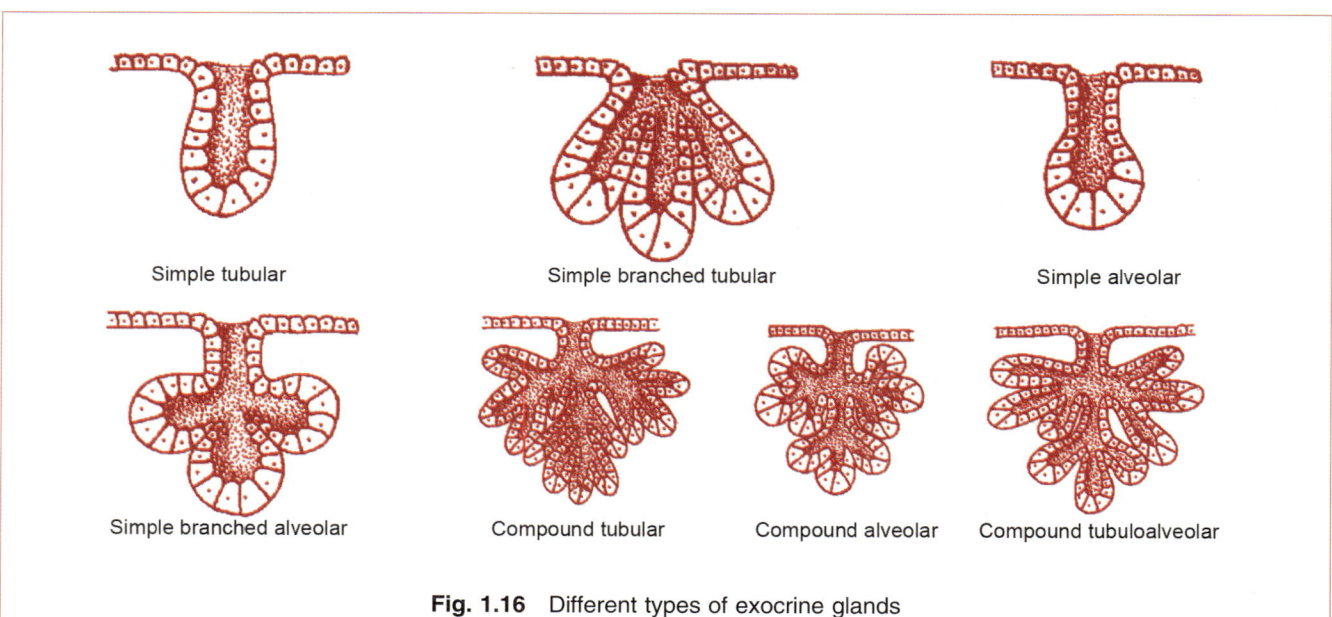

Simple tubular   Simple branched tubular   Simple alveolar

Simple branched alveolar   Compound tubular   Compound alveolar   Compound tubuloalveolar

Fig. 1.16 Different types of exocrine glands

usually arranged in cords or in clumps with rich network of blood capillaries around them.

CONNECTIVE TISSUE

- Connective tissue comprises of formed elements (fibres and cells) and amorphous substance (ground substance).
- This tissue binds various other tissues of the body.
- Components of the connective tissue: Connective tissue has two components – Cells and Matrix, which has fibres and ground substance.
- Cells – Seven types of cells are found in the connective tissue.
- Fibres – The connective tissue fibres are of three types, collagen, elastic and reticular fibres (Fig. 1.17).

Collagen fibres

- In fresh state, they appear white and therefore are also called white fibres.
- It contains a protein called 'collagen', which is derived from tropocollagen.
- Collagen fibres run in straight or wavy bundles. The individual fibres do not branch but bundles themselves can branch.
- The fibres are soft but strong and flexible, but they are not elastic.
- Collagen fibres are formed and maintained by 'fibroblasts'.
- They are found in all types of connective tissues.
- The individual collagen fibres are 1–12 μm in diameter.

- Depending upon their diameter, they are classified into four types.

Types and distribution

- Type I (diameter of about 250 nm) They are found in tendons, ligaments, aponeurosis, bone and meninges.
- Type II (diameter of about 20 to 100 nm): This variety is found in cartilages.
- Type III: They are also called 'reticular fibres', which is discussed below.
- Type IV: They form the basement membrane of the epithelium.

Reticular fibres

- These are similar to collagen fibres (type-III) in chemical composition.
- They are thin fibres showing branching and hence form a network or a reticulum.
- They do not run in bundles.
- These fibres form the skeletal framework of the lymphatic organs.

Distribution

- Basement membrane of the epithelial tissue.
- Walls of the blood vessels.
- Lymphatic organs.

Elastic fibres

- Elastic fibres are thin and highly elastic.
- These fibres branch and anastomose with each other but do not form bundles.

- In bulk they appear yellow, hence are also called yellow elastic fibres.
- Elastic fibres can be stretched (like a rubber band) and return to their original length when tension is released. The cut ends of the fibres show spiraling and kinking.
- Elastic fibres are made up of proteins called 'elastin'. They are digested by the enzyme elastase. Elastin contains amino acid valine and is also rich in 'glycine' and 'proline'.

Distribution

- Loose connective tissue.
- Walls of the blood vessels.
- Ligamentum flava.
- Capsules of the glands.

Ground substance (Intercellular substance)

The ground substance consists of water, carbohydrates, lipids and proteins. They together constitute matrix. The carbohydrates are in the form of mucopolysaccharides, which may be either sulfated or non-sulfated, in combination with hyaluronic acid.

- Chondroitin 4 – sulphate in cartilage matrix
- Chondroitin 6 – sulphate in cartilage matrix
- Chondroitin sulphate B in skin and cornea
- Hyaluronic acid in synovial fluid, soft connective tissue, vitreous humor.

Cell Types

1. **Fibroblasts:** Each cell is flattened or fusiform in shape with centrally placed nucleus. The cell shows numerous processes. They are responsible for the formation of collagen, reticular and elastic fibres. They help in healing of wounds (Fig. 1.18A).

2. **Macrophages (Histiocytes or Clasmatocytes):** These cells are less numerous than the fibroblasts. Their cytoplasm has 4 hydrolytic enzymes. These cells are phagocytic in function. They phagocytose bacteria and other foreign bodies. Macrophages are classified into fixed and wandering varieties. The fixed type is attached to the reticular fibres of the connective tissue. They are irregular in shape. The wandering type is free and become ovoid (Fig. 1.18B).

3. **Plasma Cells:** These cells are numerous in mucous and submucous coats of the gut. The cells are rounded in shape with eccentrically placed nucleus. These cells produce antibodies to counteract the actions of antigens in defense mechanism of the body. The antibodies may be stored within the cell itself in the form of Russell's body (Fig. 1.18C).

4. **Mast Cells:** Each cell is rounded in shape with a centrally placed nucleus. They are present in the fibrous capsule of the liver, along the blood vessels, beneath the mucosa of alimentary and respiratory tracts. They secrete heparin, which is an anticoagulant. They also produce histamine, which causes allergic reactions.

5. **Pigment Cells:** They are present in the iris and choroid of the eye.

6. **Reticular Cells:** These are present in the reticular connective tissue. They produce reticular fibres. They are also phagocytic in function.

7. **Fat Cells (Adipocytes):** These cells are polygonal in shape with eccentrically placed nucleus. The cytoplasm contains large amount of fat. They are numerous in adipose tissue.

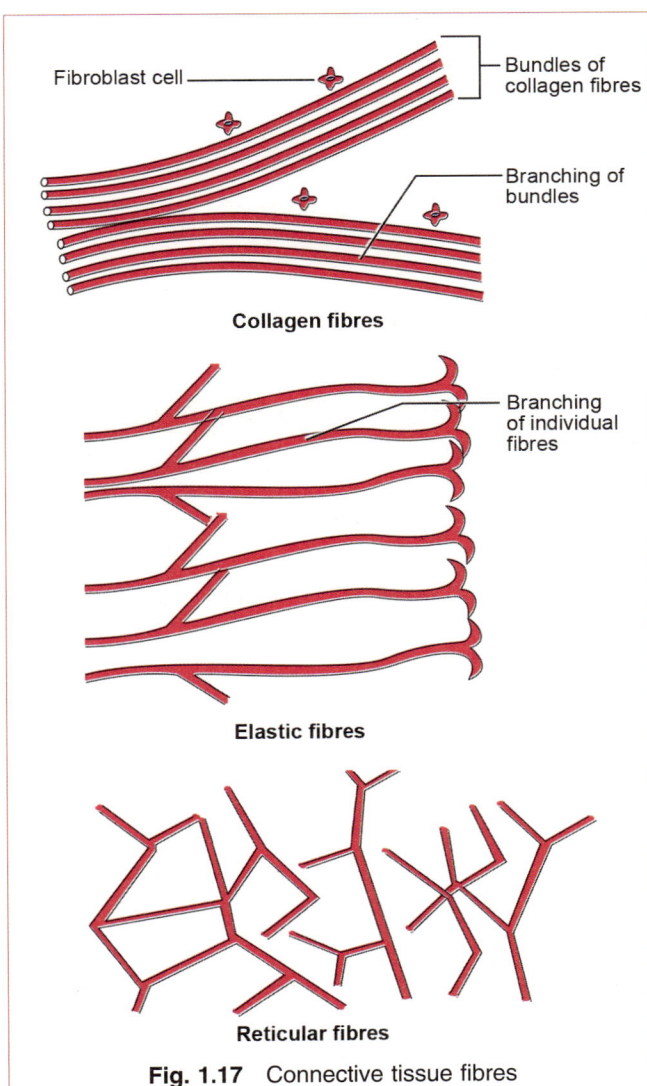

Fibroblast cell

Bundles of collagen fibres

Branching of bundles

Collagen fibres

Branching of individual fibres

Elastic fibres

Reticular fibres

Fig. 1.17   Connective tissue fibres

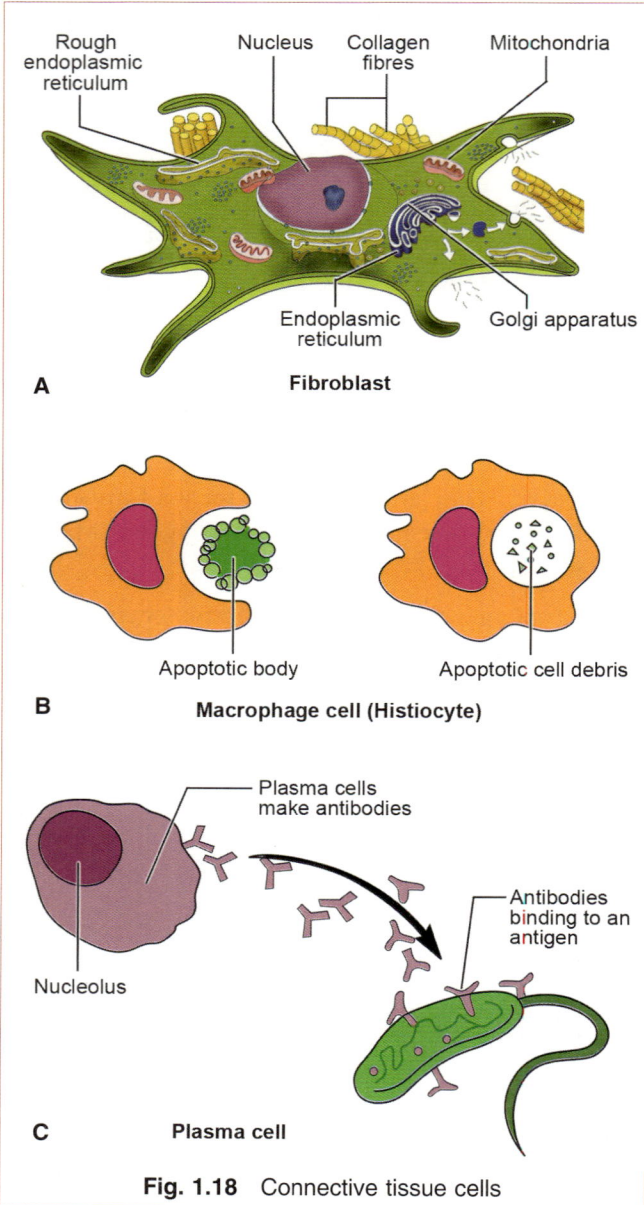

Fig. 1.18 Connective tissue cells

Adipose tissue

- This is an aggregation of fat cells.
- It serves as insulating material to conserve body heat, as storage depot for food, as protective pad around organs.
- It is abundant in females (under the hormone influence) especially in pectoral region and gluteal region.

Distribution:

- Subcutaneous tissue
- Mesenteries and omenta
- Bone marrow
- Ischiorectal fossa, axilla, bony orbit.

Myxomatous tissue

The matrix consists of mucoid substances with few collagen fibres. It also shows star shaped fibroblasts. This type of tissue is present in the umbilical cord (Wharton's jelly) and vitreous body of the eye.

Reticular tissue

- It consists of network of reticular fibres.
- These fibres are associated with specialized fibroblasts called 'reticulocytes'.
- This type of tissue is present in lymphatic organs and bone marrow.
- Connective tissues form the internal framework of the body. It is the main constituent of fascia.

SKIN (INTEGUMENT)

Skin covers the entire external surface of the body including external auditory meatus and lateral aspect of tympanic membrane.

Structurally skin is complex and highly specialized lamina having an area between 1.2 and 2.2 m^2. The thickness ranges from about 1.5 to 4.0 mm.

Skin provides protection against microorganisms, toxic substances, dehydration, ultraviolet radiation and friction. It acts as a sensory receptor and has a role in excretion, vitamin D metabolism, and the regulation of blood pressure and body temperature.

The outer surface of the skin presents various markings which are referred to as 'skin lines'. They include:

1. Flexure lines- Externally visible grooves of the epidermis near or opposite the joints.

2. Tension lines over the surface of hairy skin.

Areolar tissue

It is the most common connective tissue where collagen and elastic fibres are loosely arranged. The ground substance is semifluid in nature. They have plenty of fibroblasts and macrophages. They are traversed by nerves and vessels.

Distribution:

- Subcutaneous tissue
- Submucous coat in the gastrointestinal tract
- Between muscles, vessels and nerves
- Space between the organs
- Inside the organ between lobes and lobules

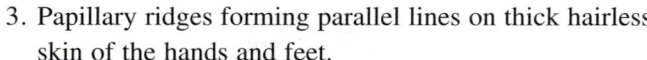

3. Papillary ridges forming parallel lines on thick hairless skin of the hands and feet.

4. Striae gravidarum bands appear after rapid local expansion of underlying structure (after pregnancy/ Linea albicantes)

5. Voight lines are boundary lines between darker and lighter areas on the upper limbs.

6. Mongolian spots - blue grey patches on trunk.

7. Naevi (moles) - accumulation of pigment cells in the epidermis.

Lines of cleavage (Langer's line)

Skin is normally under tension. In the dermis of the skin there are collagen fibres arranged in parallel rows. This direction of rows of collagen is known as Langer's line.

These Langer's lines tend to run longitudinally in limbs, horizontally in the neck and trunk.

A surgical incision along the rows of collagen fibres causes minimum disruption of collagen and leaves minimum amount of scar.

Types of skin

The fundamental structure of skin of the entire body is similar, but there are local variations like degree of keratinization, size and texture of hair, pigmentation, vascularity, innervation and others. On this basis skin is classified into 2 types.

1. Thin hairy skin (Hirsute) constitutes great majority of body's covering

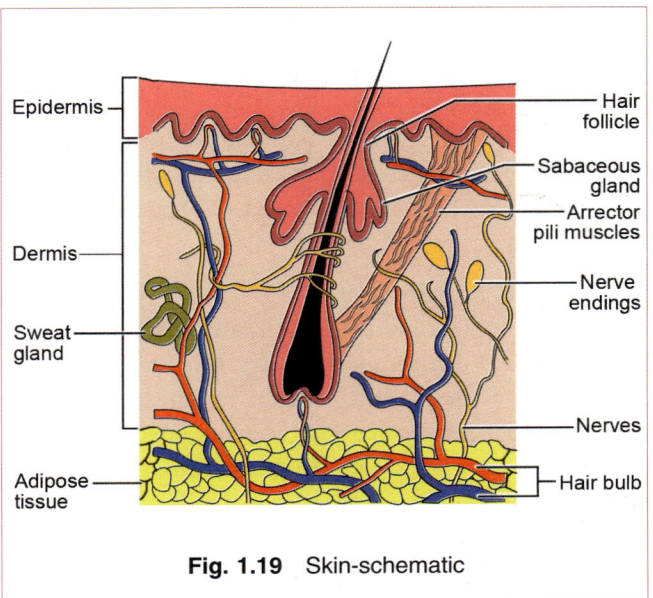

Fig. 1.19 Skin-schematic

2. Thick hairless skin (Glabrous) forming the surfaces of palm of hand, sole of feet and flexor surface of digits.

Microscopic structure of the skin

Skin is made up of two distinct layers (Fig. 1.19)

1. Epidermis: It is the outer layer of the skin made of stratified squamous keratinized epithelium. Developmentally it is from surface ectoderm and is avascular. It receives its nutrition by diffusion from dermis

2. Dermis: It is deeper connective tissue layer. Developmentally it is mesodermal in origin and is vascular.

Epidermis: In this layer, there is a continuous replacement of cells. The cells are arranged in many layers. The living cells from the basal layer are transferred to the surface as dead cells with accumulation of 'Keratin' in their cytoplasm. These cells are called **"Keratinocytes"**. But there are other cell types in epidermis which are not engaged in this replacement. These include pigment forming melanocytes, phagocytic Langerhans' cells and neurally associated cells like Merkel cells (Meissner corpuscles, Pacinian corpuscles in dermis). The cell layers from deep to superficial are as follows—stratum basale, stratum spinosum, stratum granulosum, stratum lucidum and stratum corneum. The width of these layers differs in thick and thin skin.

The junction between the epidermis and the dermis presents zigzagging inter-digitations between upward projection of dermis (dermal papillae) and downward projection of the epidermis (epidermal ridges).

Epidermis mainly consists of keratinocytes. The different layers of the epidermis represent process of keratinization (a living cell from stratum basale getting transformed to a dead cell). The process involves 4 overlapping stages: cell renewal (mitosis), cell differentiation (keratinization), cell death (apoptosis), and the sloughing of dead cells from the surface (exfoliation). The entire process takes 15 to 30 days.

1. Stratum Basale

A single layer of columnar (mostly) and cuboidal cells attached to basement membrane (basal lamina). These cells give rise to the keratinocytes in all other superficial layers.

2. Stratum spinosum (Prickle cell layer)

It contains more mature keratinocytes with several layers. The polygonal cells are placed closely and it gives spiny appearance and is called prickle cell layer. Mitotic division occur only at stratum basale and spinosum and is referred to as malpighian layer.

3. Stratum granulosum

In this layer, drastic changes in keratinocyte structure occur. The cells become flattened and accumulate basophilic granules called keratohyalin. Their pyknotic nuclei begin to disintergrate and other cellular organelles degenerate.

4. Stratum lucidum

The layer is found only in thick skin. It stains strongly with acidic stains than stratum corneum. It appears as translucent band of flattened keratinocytes whose nuclei and intercellular borders are not visible.

5. Stratum corneum

It consists of closely packed layers of flattened dead cells with keratin filaments in their cytoplasm. Dead cells are continuously exfoliated from the surface and replaced by cells from the deeper layers.

Other cell types in epidermis

1. Langerhans' cells

These cells are derived from bone marrow. The 'star' shaped cell bodies of Langerhans' cells are situated in stratum spinosum and their branched dendrites are insinuated between the surrounding cells.

The function of Langerhans' cell is cellular defense. They are particular in detecting, binding and presenting antigens to local lymphocytes. It is a part of immune mechanism of skin. This is important in cell mediated immunity to epidermal viral infection, in elimination of epidermal cancers etc.

2. Epidermal melanocytes

These cells lie in stratum basale in contact with basal lamina. They are derived from the neural crest cells. They provide a pigment shield against ultraviolate light from sun. Melanocytes are more in face, mucosal orifices, external genitalia nipple and areola.

In amphibia, these cells are abundant and are responsible for quick changes in the colour of the skin.

3. Merkel's cells

These cells are present is the stratum spinosum. It acts as a mechanoreceptors and nerve fibres terminate in them.

Dermis: Mechanically dermis provides strength to skin by its collagen fibres and elastin content. The dermis can be divided into 2 zones, a narrow superficial papillary layer and deeper reticular layer.

Papillary layer lies immediately deep to epidermis, consists of extensive network of capillaries. It provides mechanical anchorage, metabolic support and trophic maintenance to the overlying tissue. The superficial surface of this layer is marked by numerous papillae which interdigitate with recess in the base of epidermis. The papillae are few and small in thin skin whereas larger and closely aggregated in thick skin. The reticular layer consists of many arterio-venous anastomoses that help to regulate the blood pressure and body temperature

Meissner's corpuscular nerve endings: They are present in papillary layer of the dermis. These corpuscles are believed to be responsible for touch.

Reticular layer is rich in strong collagen fibres and also elastic fibres. The layer also contains adipose tissues and capillaries.

Appendages of the skin

Hair

- Hair is filamentous, keratinized structures which assist thermoregulation, provide some protection and have sensory function.

- The distribution of hair differs in different parts of the body and also differs in two sexes.

- The length varies from less than a millimeter to a meter.

- The structures that form hair and maintain their growth are called as hair follicles. The hair follicle consists of shaft and root. The visible part on the surface is called shaft and embedded part is called root.

Hair shaft: It is made of keratin filaments. It shows 3 concentric zones—the cuticle, cortex and medulla.

Hair root: It is covered by several layers which includes Outermost connective tissue sheath, external root sheath and internal root sheath composed of Henle's layer and Huxley's layer.

Arrector pili muscles (Fig. 1.19)

These are non-striated (smooth) muscles which link between hair follicles and papillary layer of the dermis. Contraction of these muscles tends to pull the hair more vertically and skin in the region of its attachments gets elevated while neighboring region which gives attachment to this muscle is depressed to give rise to 'goose skin'. The muscle is supplied by sympathetic nerves. The Arrector pili contract and hair stand erect in response to cold, fear and anger.

Sebaceous glands

- Sebaceous glands are present in dermis of almost whole body except palms and sole.
- The gland secretes an oily substance called sebum to skin surface and hair.
- The gland consists of clusters of acini. The duct of the gland opens at the apical portion of hair follicle (Fig. 1.19).
- Wherever hair follicle is absent, the duct opens directly into skin surface (e.g.: lips, corners of mouth, nipple).
- Sebaceous glands are numerous over face, which cause 'acne' in adult with retention of secretion.
- The sebaceous gland assists in water proofing of epidermis, discourages blood sucking ectoparasites and contributes to the characteristic body odour.

Sudorific glands (Sweat glands)

Eccrine sweat gland (Typical): It is present in dermis. The gland is long unbranched tubular structure with highly coiled secretory part called fundus.

The wall of the duct fuses with base of the epidermal papillae and lumen passes between keratinocytes. The duct opens into the skin surface.

Apocrine sweat gland: These are large sweat gland, unlike endocrine glands they discharge their secretion into apical regions of hair follicles.

These glands are present only in few parts of the body like axilla and perineal region.

Cyanosis

When blood is poorly oxygenated, the skin appear blue, this condition is called as cyanosis. Skin often becomes cyanotic during heart failure or severe respiratory disorders. In black people, the skin is too dark to reveal the colour of the underlying vessels, but cyanosis is apparent in the mucous membranes and nail beds.

Erythema: Infection, inflammation or allergic reaction of the skin causes superficial capillary engorgement. This makes skin abnormally red. This sign is called erythema. In jaundice yellowish pigment called bilirubin builds up in the blood, giving yellowish appearance to the skin and white of the eye.

Albinism

It is a genetic disorder causing specific trait. The enzyme responsible for conversion of tyrosine to melanin (DOPA pathway) is deficient. These individuals are more prone to dermal cancers.

Lacerations (skin cuts or tears) can be superficial or deep. Superficial cuts do not interrupt the continuity of the dermis. Deep cuts penetrate the deep layers of the dermis and require approximation of the cut edges of the dermis by suturing or stitches.

Wound healing: Lacerations (cuts), abrasions, and burns cause structural damage to the skin. In the process of healing the fibroblasts initially proliferate to secrete mainly type III collagen fibres. Subsequently most of these fibres are replaced by type-I collagen. Small, shallow wounds are typically recovered by keratinocytes arising from the stratum basale. In wounds that remove the epidermis from a larger area, keratinocytes in the external root sheath of hair follicles divide and migrate to replace the epidermal tissue. Eventually normal epidermal and dermal architecture may be restored. Larger and deeper wounds, in which the hair follicles are lost are destroyed, may never be completely recovered by normal epidermis, thus may leave a scar at the site.

Fasciae

It is a connective tissue layer present deep to the skin. It is further divided into superficial fascia and deep fascia. The superficial fascia is mainly composed of adipose tissue, which provides insulation and padding and lets the skin or underlying structure move independently.

The deep fascia is mainly made up of connective tissue fibres. They also surround the muscle groups, blood vessels, nerves binding some structure together or allowing the structures to glide smoothly over each other. In the limbs the deep fascia form compartments between flexor and extensor group of muscles. The deep fascia also provide thick protective coat for arteries like carotid sheath, axillary sheath and femoral sheath. In few places the deep fascia gives attachment to the underlying muscles.

Understanding of the arrangement of the fascial planes, their extent and attachments are important for surgeons

CARTILAGE

Cartilage is a specialised dense connective tissue. It is hard but not rigid like bone. It can be bent and also brought back into its original form when bending force is withdrawn. This cartilage forms the 'skeletal' basis of some parts of the body (auricle of the ear, external nose).

At the time of birth, many parts of the skeletal framework of the newborn are made up of cartilage. Later this cartilage gets converted into bones by a process called 'ossification'.

However, depending on the functional need, some of them remain as cartilages even in adults.

General Features

- They are rigid structures, hence provide protection and support the organs. They can withstand the effects of pressure, pull or torsion.
- They are present in the body where elasticity and rigidity is required.
- They are avascular structures, nourished by diffusion from adjacent tissues.
- Repair of cartilage is slow and takes time due to its avascularity.
- There are three types of cartilages: Hyaline, elastic and fibrocartilage.

Cartilage consists of

1. Cells called chondrocytes
2. Fibres
3. Ground substance

Based on the type of fibres present in the matrix, the cartilages are classified into three types – Hyaline, Elastic and White fibrocartilage.

1. Hyaline Cartilage

- It appears transparent glass like in fresh condition.
- It is covered by a vascular fibrous membrane called 'perichondrium'. This perichondrium has an outer fibrous layer and inner cellular layer. The cellular layer consists of chondroblasts (immature chondrocytes).
- It has a homogeneous matrix, which is glassy and transparent in appearance (Figs 1.20 and 1.21A).
- The matrix contains collagen fibres (type-II) which run in parallel bundles.
- The chondrocytes are placed in 'lacunae' of the matrix.
- They are arranged in-groups of two, four and six (isogenous group). This arrangement is called the 'cell nest condition'.
- The ground substance is made up of carbohydrates and proteins. The carbohydrates are glycosaminoglycans. It includes chondroitin 4-sulphate and hyaluronic acid.
- The fibres cannot be seen under light microscope because the refractive index of the fibres and ground substance is same and hence it is homogeneous.

Distribution

1. Costal cartilages of the ribs.
2. Cartilage covering the articulating surfaces of the bones.

3. Cartilages of the larynx – thyroid and cricoid cartilage.
4. The tracheal rings.

2. Elastic Cartilage

Structurally the elastic cartilage is mainly made up of elastic fibres and the chondrocytes. The chondrocytes are not arranged in groups (Fig. 1.21B). The surface of the elastic cartilage is covered by 'perichondrium'.

Elastic cartilage is more flexible than hyaline cartilage.

Distribution

- Pinna of the external ear
- Epiglottis, corniculate and cuneiform cartilages of the larynx.
- Medial part of the auditory tube

3. Fibrocartilage (white fibrocartilage)

- Structurally the white fibrocartilage contains mainly thick bundles of collagen fibres (type I) and a few chondrocytes (Fig. 1.21C).
- It has no perichondrium.
- It is very tough and strong but resilient.
- It has great tensile strength and considerable elasticity.

Distribution

- Articular disc of the temporomandibular joint and sternoclavicular joint.
- Intervertebral discs present between the bodies of vertebrae.
- Glenoidal labrum of shoulder joint.
- Acetabular labrum of hip joint.
- Menisci of the knee joint.

Growth of the cartilages

Cartilages grow by two mechanisms.

In appositional growth, cells of the perichondrium (chondroblasts) undergo repeated division. These cells produce cartilaginous matrix and are transformed into chondrocytes. This differentiation gradually increases the size of the cartilage. Chondrocytes within the cartilage matrix also undergo division, and the daughter cells produce additional matrix. This cycle enlarges the cartilage rather as a balloon is inflated; the process is called interstitial growth. Neither interstitial nor appositional growth occurs in adult cartilages and they cannot repair themselves after a severe injury.

The cartilage tissue grows rapidly during youth, but has little capacity for regeneration and healing in adults. Adult cartilage regenerates poorly because chondrocytes have lost

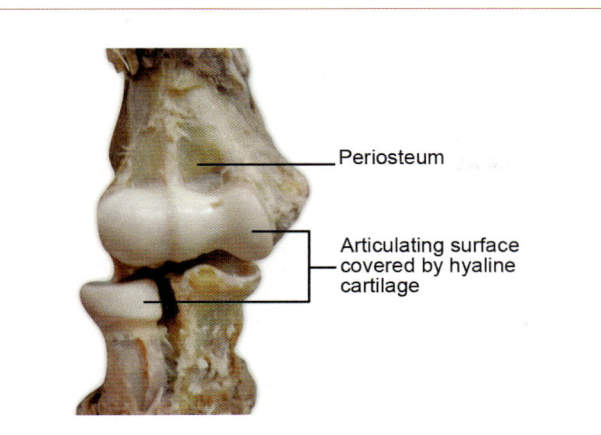

Fig. 1.20 Articular cartilage

capacity for division. The little healing that occurs within adult cartilage is due to the ability of the surviving chondrocytes to secrete more extracellular matrix.

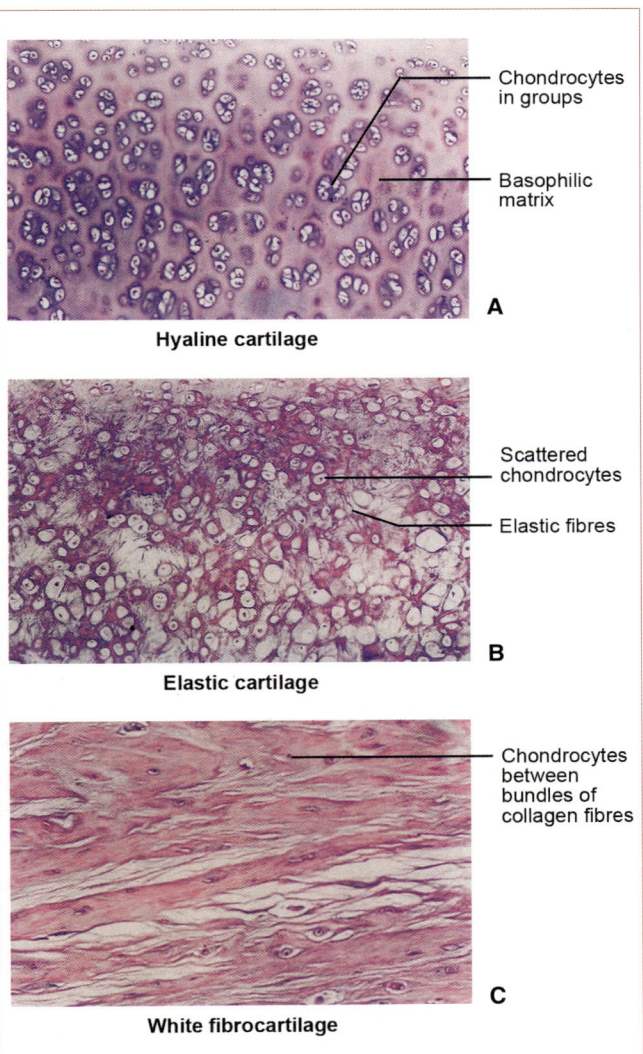

Hyaline cartilage

Elastic cartilage

White fibrocartilage

Fig. 1.21 Types of cartilage (H & E stained)

BONE

Bone is a highly vascular living connective tissue in which the matrix is calcified by the deposition of calcium phosphate.

The human skeleton consists of **206 bones**.

Functions of the bone

- Bone provides supporting framework and shape for the body.
- It protects vital organs of the body (e.g. heart and brain).
- They help in transmission of the body weight.
- They provide attachment to the muscles and act as levers of the joints helping in locomotion.
- Bone is the storehouse of calcium salts.
- Involved in erythropoiesis.
- They provide attachment to the muscles and act as levers of the joints helping in locomotion.
- Bone is the storehouse of calcium salts.
- Involved in erythropoiesis.

Classification of the bone

According to their position

1. **Axial:** Bones forming the axis of the body, e.g. skull, ribs, vertebrae.
2. **Appendicular:** Bones of the limbs.

According to the shape

1. **Long bones:** They have three parts: upper end, lower end and a middle shaft. The ends of these bones take part in forming the joint (articulates with other bone), e.g. bones of limbs (humerus, ulna, radius, femur, tibia, fibula).
2. **Short bones:** These bones are small and generally cuboidal in shape, e.g. carpal and tarsal bones.
3. **Flat bones:** These bones are expanded and are flat, e.g. sternum, scapula, ribs, and parietal bone.
4. **Irregular bone:** The shape is irregular without any proper outline, e.g. vertebrae, sphenoid, temporal bones etc.

According to gross structure

1. **Compact (lamellar bone):** Structurally it is made up of bony plates (lamellae) which are arranged compactly, e.g. outer cortical part of the long bone.
2. **Spongy bone (cancellous):** Structurally it is made up of bony plates, which are arranged irregularly leaving spaces in between them. It gives a spongy appearance, e.g. flat bones; irregular bones, ends of the long bone.

3. **Diploic bones:** It consists of inner and outer tables of compact bone with an interval, which is occupied by bone marrow and diploic veins, e.g. most of the cranial bones (parietal, frontal, occipital).

According to the development

All the bones are developed from the mesoderm.

1. **Membranous bones:** The mesenchymal tissue (mesoderm) is directly transformed into a bone, e.g. clavicle, bones of the face and cranial vault.

2. **Cartilaginous bones:** The mesenchymal tissue is first transformed into a 'cartilage'. Later cartilage undergoes ossification to form bones, e.g. majority of the limb bones and bones at the base of the skull.

Special types of bones

1. **Pneumatic bone:** These are flat or irregular bones with hollow spaces in their body. These spaces contain air, e.g. ethmoid, maxilla, and mastoid part of temporal bone.

2. **Sesamoid bone** (Sesamoid = seed like): These bones develop within the tendon of some muscles.

- They do not possess periosteum and Haversian system.
- They ossify after birth.
- They minimise the friction and also change the direction of the pull of a muscle.

E.g. Pisiform bone (in the tendon of flexor carpi ulnaris muscle), patella (in the tendon of quadriceps femoris muscle), fabella (in the tendon of lateral head of gastrocnemius muscle).

Macroscopic structure of a bone

- The long bone consists of two ends (epiphysis) and a shaft (diaphysis).

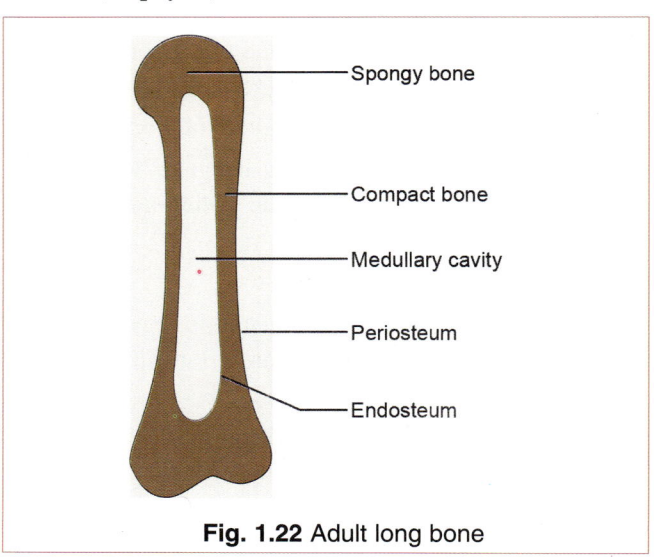

Fig. 1.22 Adult long bone

- Spongy bone
- Compact bone
- Medullary cavity
- Periosteum
- Endosteum

- The shaft consists of a cylindrical cavity inside called 'medullary cavity', which is filled with bone marrow. The outer (cortical) part of the shaft is made up of compact bone (Fig.1.22).

- The two ends of the long bone are filled with tiny plates of bone containing numerous spaces. This is referred as 'spongy bone' to which the medullary cavity does not extend.

- The outer surface of the bone is covered by a highly vascular connective tissue membrane called 'periosteum' except at the articular surfaces. This articular surface is covered by articular cartilage, usually hyaline type.

- The medullary cavity is lined by another connective tissue membrane called 'endosteum'.

Bone marrow

It is the vascular connective tissue present in the medullary cavity of the bone. The bone marrow differs in composition in different bones and at different ages. It occurs in two forms, yellow marrow and red marrow. The red marrow is actively engaged in the production of blood cells. The yellow marrow derives its colour from the large quantity of fat cells it contains. At birth the red marrow is present throughout the skeleton. After about five years of postnatal life, the red marrow is gradually replaced by yellow bone marrow in the long bones.

Microscopic structure

An adult long bone consists of the following components: Bone cells and Matrix

Compact bone (Figs 1.23 and 1.24)

- The compact bone is made up of 'lamellae'.
- Lamellae are thin plates of bone consisting of collagen fibres embedded in ground substance.
- Lamellae are placed one over another.
- The spaces between the lamellae are called 'lacunae'.
- Lacunae are occupied by osteocytes.
- The adjacent lacunae are connected through canaliculi, which are occupied by cytoplasmic processes of osteocytes.
- Most of the lamellae are arranged in the form of concentric rings that surround a 'Haversian canal', which is present at the center of each ring.
- Haversian canals are placed parallel to medullary cavity and they are occupied by blood vessels and nerve fibres.
- Adjacent Haversian canals are connected by Volkmann's canal.

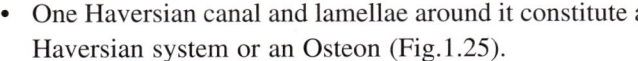

- One Haversian canal and lamellae around it constitute a Haversian system or an Osteon (Fig.1.25).

Matrix (ground substance)

The matrix of the bone consists of both organic and inorganic constituents.

a) Organic constituent (25% of the matrix)

- It is mainly made up of collagen fibres.
- These collagen fibres are embedded in proteins, carbohydrates and water.
- The collagen fibres are responsible for toughness and resilience of bone. These fibres are synthesized by osteoblasts.
- Chondroitin sulphate is another important organic constituent of the bone.

b) Inorganic constituent (75% of the matrix)

- Following mineral salts are present:
- Calcium phosphate (85%)
- Calcium carbonate (10%)
- Small amount of calcium fluoride and magnesium phosphate.
- Most of the calcium, phosphate and hydroxyl ions are in the form of needle shaped crystals called 'hydroxyapatite crystals'
- These crystals lie parallel to collagen fibres.

Bone cells

Osteoblasts

- These are bone forming cells.
- They are more numerous in periosteum.
- The cells are ovoid, triangular or cuboidal in shape with oval nucleus.
- These cells are responsible for laying down the organic matrix of bone including the collagen fibres.
- They are responsible for calcification of the matrix.

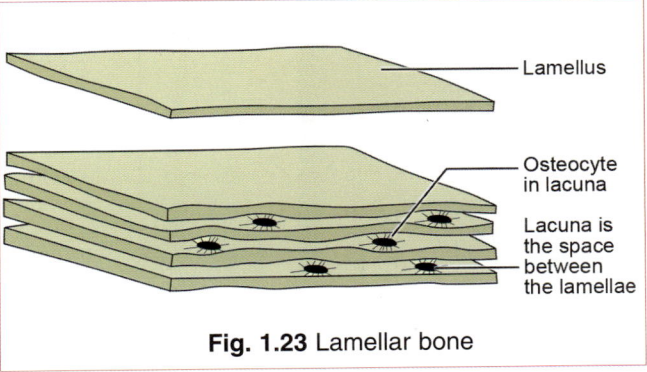

Fig. 1.23 Lamellar bone

Osteocytes

- These are mature bone cells.
- They are derived from osteoblasts after they have laid down the matrix.
- They are present in the 'lacunae' of the bone between the lamellae.
- Osteocytes show many cytoplasmic processes, which establish connections with other osteocytes.
- Osteocytes maintain the integrity of the lacunae and thus keep open the channels for diffusion of nutrients.

Osteoclasts

- These are bone removing cells and found in relation to the surfaces of the bone.
- Osteoclasts are multinucleated large cells (diameter varies from 20 to 100 μm).
- The lysosomes present in their cytoplasm contain 'acid phosphatase'.
- Osteoclasts are involved in demineralization and removal of bone matrix.
- Osteoclasts are stimulated by parathyroid hormone.

Periosteum

The external surface of the bone is covered by a connective tissue membrane called 'periosteum' except the articular surface.

The periosteum consists of outer fibrous layer and inner cellular layer consisting of osteoblasts.

Parts of the developing long bones

1. **Epiphysis** is the part of the bone, which develops from the secondary center of ossification, e.g. ends of the long bones (Fig.1.25).

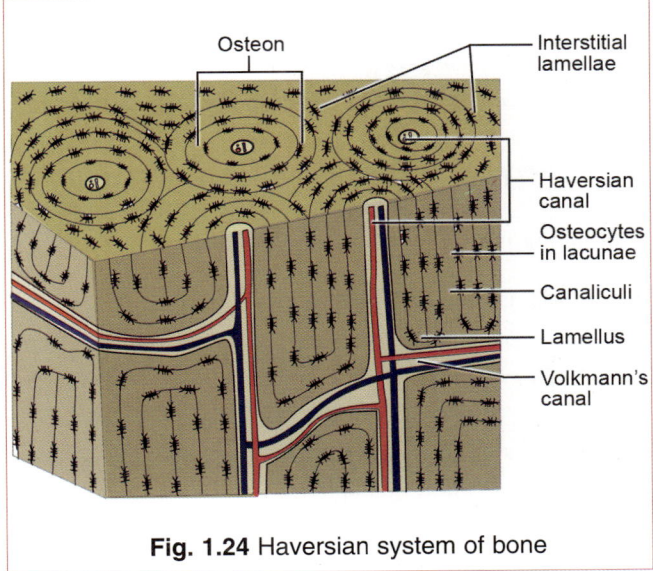

Fig. 1.24 Haversian system of bone

Types of epiphysis:

a) Pressure epiphysis: They ossify from centers exposed to pressure at the joints, e.g. epiphysis of the head of the femur.

b) Traction epiphysis: They ossify from centers subjected to tension by the pull of the muscle, e.g. greater and lesser trochanters of the femur.

c) Atavistic epiphysis: These epiphysis are formed by centers of ossification which are believed to represent the skeletal elements which were separate in some lower vertebrates. e.g. coracoid process of scapula.

2. Diaphysis is the part of the bone, which develops from the primary center of ossification. E.g. Shaft of the long bones.

3. Metaphysis is the zone of the bone where active growth is seen. It is present at the junction of the epiphysis and diaphysis of the long bones.

Ossification

The process of bone formation is called 'ossification'. All the bones are developed from the mesenchymal tissue of the embryo. There are two types of ossification.

1. Membranous ossification: The embryonic mesenchymal tissue will directly form the bone. E.g. bones of the cranial vault, mandible and clavicle.

2. Cartilaginous ossification: The mesenchymal tissue is first transformed into a 'cartilage'. Later this cartilage is ossified to form a bone.

Ossification of a long bone

The ossification begins in one or more areas of future bone model. These areas are called centers of ossification.

Primary center of ossification

The ossification starts in the central part of the cartilaginous model (i.e. at the center of the future shaft). The portion of the long bone developed from this primary center of ossification is called 'diaphysis'. The primary center of ossification normally appears before birth.

Secondary center of ossification

These centers appear at the two ends of the long bone usually after birth. The portion of the long bone developed from secondary center of ossification is called 'epiphysis'.

The two ends of the diaphysis, which are actively involved in growth, are called 'metaphysis'.

In a long bone between epiphysis and diaphysis is a part of the cartilage that remains unossified until epiphysis fuses

with diaphysis and it is called 'epiphyseal plate'. They also undergo ossification at puberty.

Laws of ossification

1. The epiphysis which ossifies first (or appears first) unites (fuses) with the diaphysis last and the epiphysis which ossifies last fuses first. Exception: lower end of the fibula.

2. The end of a long bone where epiphysis appears first and fuses last is called the 'growing end' of the bone.

3. The direction of nutrient artery is always away from the growing end.

4. In the long bones, growing ends fuse with the shaft at about 20 years and the opposite ends at about 18 years.

Intramembranous ossification (dermal ossification)

This type of ossification normally occurs in the deeper layers of the dermis, and the bones that result are often called dermal bones. E.g. clavicle. It involves following steps:

Step-1

Osteoblasts first cluster together and start to secrete the organic components of the matrix.

The matrix consists of collagen fibres then mineralised through crystalization of calcium salts.

The location in a bone where ossification first occurs is called primary ossification center. As ossification proceeds, it traps some osteoblasts inside bony pockets; these cells differentiate into osteocytes.

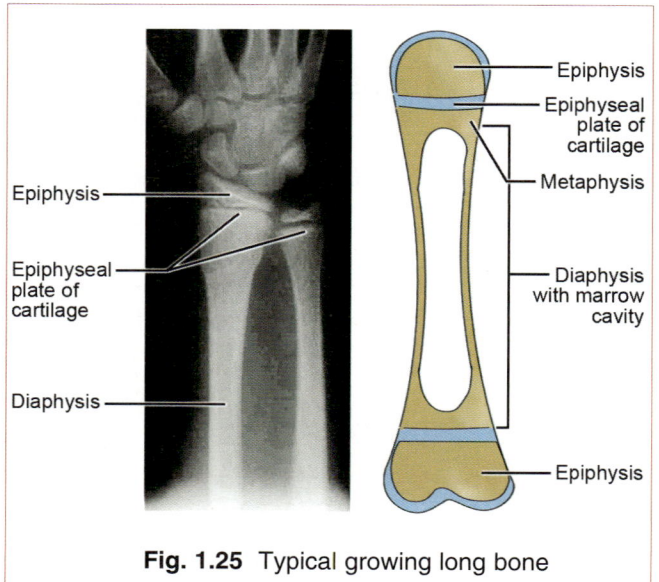

Fig. 1.25 Typical growing long bone

Step-2

The developing bone grows outward from the ossification center in small struts called spicules. Although, osteoblasts are still being trapped in the expanding bone, mesenchymal cell division continues to produce additional osteoblasts.

Bone growth is an active process and osteoblasts require oxygen and a supply of nutrients. Blood vessels that branch between the spicules meet these demands.

Step-3

Over the time, the bone assumes the structure of spongy bone. Although, initially the intramembranous bone resembles spongy bone, subsequent remodeling around the trapped blood vessels can produce compact bone.

Cartilaginous ossification (Endochondral ossification)

It begins with the formation of a hyaline cartilaginous model. It involves the following steps.

Step-1

As the cartilage enlarges, chondrocytes near the center of the shaft increase greatly in size and surrounding matrix begin to calcify. Deprived of nutrients these chondrocytes die and disintegrate.

Step-2

Cells of the perichondrium surrounding this region of the cartilage develop into osteoblasts. The perichondrium has now been converted into a periosteum and the inner organic layer soon produces a thin layer of bone around the shaft of the cartilage.

Step-3

While these changes are under way, the blood supply to the periosteum increases. Capillaries and osteoblasts

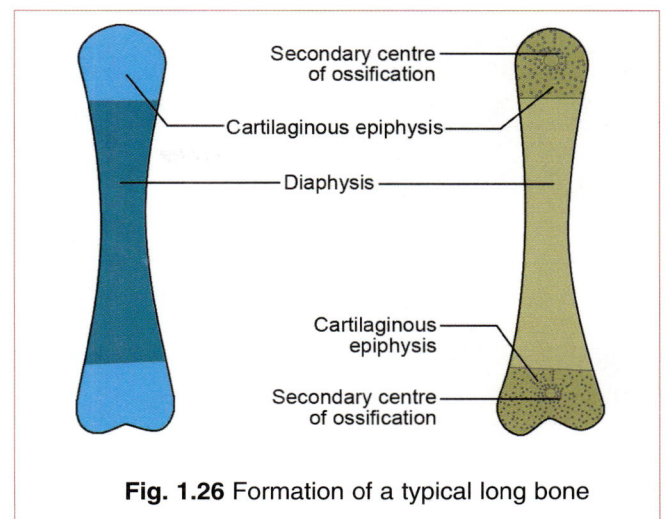

Fig. 1.26 Formation of a typical long bone

migrate into the cartilage invading the space left by the disintegrating chondrocytes. The calcified cartilaginous matrix breaks down and osteoblasts replace it with spongy bone. Bone development proceeds from this primary center of ossification located in the shaft towards the ends of the cartilaginous model.

Step-4

While the diameter is small, the entire diaphysis is filled with spongy bone but as it enlarges osteoblasts erode the central portion and create a bone marrow cavity. Further growth involves two distinct processes, an enlargement in diameter and an increase in size.

Bone development and growth

The growth of the skeleton determines the size and proportions of our body. The bony skeleton begins to form

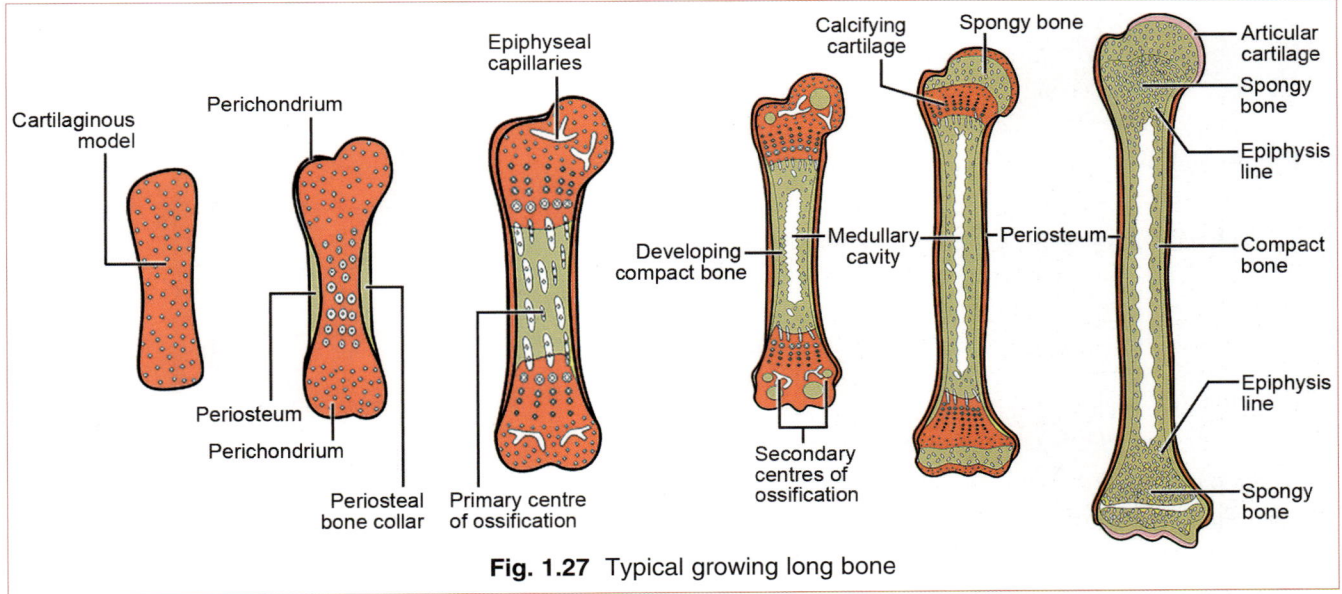

Fig. 1.27 Typical growing long bone

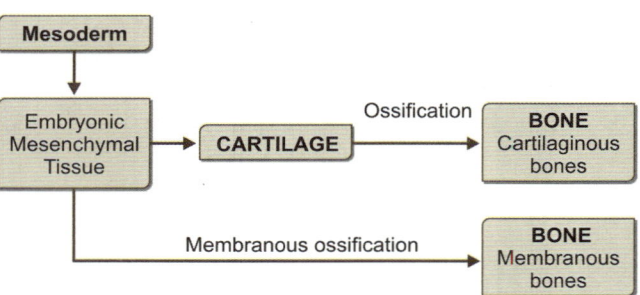

about six weeks after fertilization. Bone growth continues through adolescence.

Factors regulating the bone growth

- Normal bone growth requires constant dietary source of **calcium and phosphate** salts.
- **Vitamin A and C** are essential for normal bone growth and remodelling. These vitamins are obtained from the diet.
- **Vitamin D** plays an important role in normal calcium metabolism by stimulating the absorption and transport of calcium and phosphate ions into the blood.
- The thyroid gland secretes the hormone calcitonin which stimulates osteoblasts to produce new matrix.
- The secretion of parathyroid indirectly stimulates osteoclastic activity.
- Growth hormone produced by the pituitary and thyroxine from the thyroid gland stimulate the bone growth.

Blood supply to a long bone

1. **Nutrient artery:** It enters the shaft through a nutrient foramen with one or two veins. On reaching the bone marrow cavity they divide into ascending and descending branches. They proceed towards each end, supplying the bone marrow, spongy bone and deeper portion of the compact bone (Fig. 1.29).

2. **Epiphyseal arteries:** They are several in number and enter the bone near the ends.

3. **Metaphyseal arteries:** They enter the bone along the line of attachment of capsular ligament (near the articular end). The metaphyseal and epiphyseal arteries are mainly from the arteries supplying the joint. The metaphyseal arteries in children (before epiphyseal union) form hairpin bends. The bacteria or infective emboli get trapped in these bends causing osteomyelitis.

4. **Periosteal arteries:** They are numerous and enter the bone along the muscular attachment. These branches are responsible for nourishment of most of the compact bone.

Branches of all these arteries form a rich sinusoidal plexus in bone marrow. Many branches from the plexus enter Haversian canal.

These vessels provide blood to the superficial osteons of the shaft. During endochondral ossification, these vessels also enter the epiphysis providing blood to the secondary ossification centers. Following the closure of epiphysis all these sets of vessels become extensively interconnected.

Nerve supply to the bone: Bones are innervated by sensory nerves and injuries to the bone can be very painful.

A long bone that is taken from a fresh cadaver and soaked in a solution of weak acid for several weeks will maintain its original form but will look leathery and can be easily tied into a knot. The acid dissolves away the bone's mineral, leaving only the organic component (mainly collagen). The fact that a demineralised bone can be knotted demonstrates the great flexibility provided by collagen fibres within the bone. This fact also confirms that without its mineral content, bone bends too easily to support weight.

Bone remodelling: Bone remodelling may involve a change in the shape or internal architecture of a bone or a change in the total amount of minerals deposited in the skeleton. Osteoblasts and osteoclasts remain active even after the epiphyseal plates have closed. As one osteon forms through the activity of osteoblasts, another is destroyed by osteoclasts. The turnover rate for the bone is quite high. Each year almost one fifth of the adult skeleton is demolished and is rebuilt or replaced.

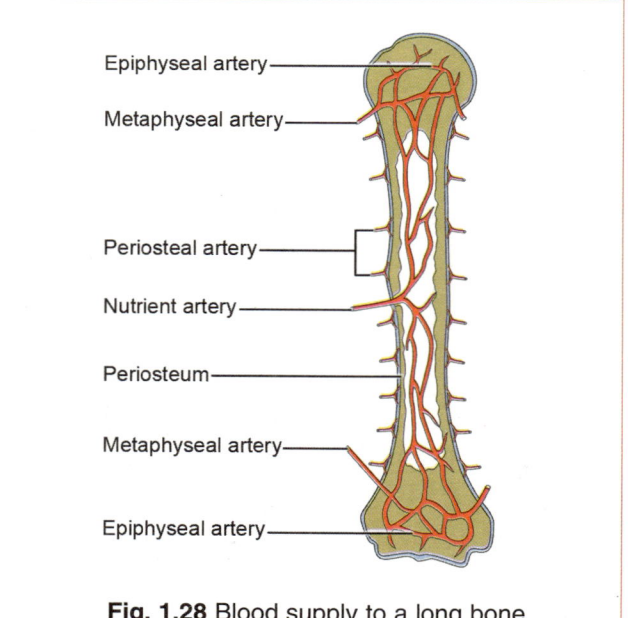

Fig. 1.28 Blood supply to a long bone

Injury and repair: Despite its mineral strength, bone may crack or even break if subjected to extreme loads or stresses from unusual directions. The damage produced constitutes a fracture. Healing of a fracture usually occurs even after severe damage, provided the blood supply and the cellular components of the endosteum and periosteum survive.

A fracture is the loss of continuity of a bone as a result of cracking or breaking. Radiographs (X-rays) are often used to diagnose the position and extent of fracture. Most fractures are caused by injuries and few result from diseases that weakens the bones. The following is the description of several kinds of traumatic fractures.

1. Simple or closed: The fracture bone does not break through the skin.

2. Compound or open: The fractured bone is exposed to the outside through an opening in the skin.

3. Partial (fissured): A fracture extending from the surface to deep, but not completely.

4. Complete: The fracture has separated the bone into two pieces

5. Capillary: A hair like crack occurs within the bone

6. Comminuted: The bone is broken into small fragments

7. Spiral: The fracture line is twisted as it is broken

8. Avulsion: A portion of the bone is torn off.

9. Greenstick: In this there is an incomplete break, one side of the bone is broken and the other side is bowed.

When a bone fractures, medical treatment involves realigning the broken ends and then immobilising them, until new bone tissue is formed and the fracture is healed. The methods of immobilisation include tape, splints, casts, straps, wires and steel pins.

When bone is fractured the surrounding periosteum is usually torn and blood vessels in both tissues are ruptured. A blood clot called a fracture hematoma forms at the damaged area. During healing of fracture a cartilaginous mass called a 'bony callus' fills the gap within the fragmented bone.

Assessment of Bone age: The knowledge of ossification of each bone is important in forensic science and anthropology. The sites where ossification appears, the rate at which they grow and time of fusion epiphyses with diaphysis for every bone is important even in clinical medicine. This knowledge is also important because the epiphyseal plates (cartilaginous structures) appear radiolucent (dark) which could be mistaken for a fracture. The age of a young person can be determined from X-ray by assessing the ossification centres.

Loss of arterial supply to an epiphysis or other parts of a bone results in avascular necrosis of bone tissue. In children the disorders of epiphysis due to avascular necrosis is referred as 'osteochondroses'.

Osteoporosis: A reduction in organic and inorganic components of bone to a degree that compromises normal function. The bone becomes brittle, lose their elasticity and fracture easily. Bone scanning will reveal the reduction of bone mass.

Achondroplasia: A condition resulting from abnormal epiphyseal activity. The epiphyseal plate grows unusually slow and the individual develops short, stocky limbs. The trunk is normal in size while sexual and mental development remains unaffected..

Rickets: A disorder that reduces the amount of calcium salts in the skeleton seen in children. It is characterised by 'bowlegged' appearance.

Osteomalacia: A softening of bone due to a decrease in the mineral content.

MUSCLE

Muscle is a contractile tissue, which brings movement of the body.

Types: There are three types of muscles – skeletal, cardiac and smooth (Fig. 1.29).

Smooth muscle (Non-striated/Involuntary)

1. Each muscle fibre is an elongated spindle shaped cell with a single nucleus placed centrally.

2. The length of the smooth muscle is highly variable (15–500 μm).

3. They often aggregate to form bundles and fascicles.

4. They are found in the walls of gastrointestinal tract, respiratory tract, urogenital tract, blood vessels and few muscles of the eye. They are arranged circularly inside and longitudinally outside in the walls of the gastro-intestinal tract, urogenital tract etc.

5. They do not exhibit cross striations and are smooth in form, supplied by autonomic nerves, hence involuntary.

6. They are made up of actin and myosin filaments.

7. These muscles respond slowly to stimuli, being capable of sustained contractions, therefore do not fatigue easily.

8. There are two types of smooth muscles - multi unit and unitary.

a. Multi unit smooth muscles: Nerve fibres establish direct contact with several myocytes. Muscles contract under nervous stimulus, e.g. smooth muscles of iris and large arteries.

b. Unitary smooth muscles: They have their own rhythmic contractility that is independent of nerve supply. Contraction of muscle is stimulated by stretch. However, the nerve supplying them can alter the rate of contraction, e.g. smooth muscles of the stomach, intestine, uterus and ureter.

Cardiac muscle (Striated/Involuntary)

1. It forms the myocardium of the heart, shows striations but is involuntary. It is meant for automatic and rhythmic contractions.

2. Each muscle fibre has a single rounded nucleus placed centrally.

3. Each muscle fibre branches and anastomoses with the neighboring fibres at intercalated discs.

4. Myocytes are about 80 μm long and 15 μm broad.

5. Their sarcoplasm contains more number of mitochondria and less number of myofibrils and sarcoplasmic reticulum when compared to skeletal muscle (Fig. 1.29).

Skeletal muscle (Striated/Voluntary)

1. These are most abundant, found attached to the skeletal system.

2. They exhibit cross striations under the microscope.

3. They are supplied by somatic (cerebrospinal) nerves, hence under voluntary control.

4. Each muscle fibre is a multinucleated cylindrical cell containing a group of muscle fibrils, e.g. muscles of the limb and body wall.

Arrangement of the muscle fibres

The arrangement of muscle fibres varies according to the direction, force and range of movement at a particular joint. The force of contraction is directly proportional to the number and size of muscle fibres, and the range of movement is proportional to the length of the fibre.

The fascicles of the muscle can be parallel or oblique. When fascicles are obliquely set to the line of pull, the power of contraction is more, but range of movement is less (Fig. 1.30)

Unipennate: e.g. palmar interossei of hand

Bipennate: e.g. rectus femoris

Multipennate: e.g. middle fibres of deltoid

Lubricating mechanisms for the muscles

Synovial bursa: Bursa is a lubricating device to minimise the friction. Structurally, it is a closed sac of synovial membrane with synovial fluid. Bursa is often present around the joint but it can be subcutaneous. Bursa can communicate with joint cavity.

Synovial sheaths: The tendinous part of the muscle while passing deep to fibrous bands is surrounded by synovial sheath.

Blood supply: The blood vessels and nerves enter the muscle at a point called neurovascular hilum. The arteries branch repeatedly to form arteriole and capillaries in the muscle.

Connective tissue support to the muscle

A connective tissue membrane called endomysium surrounds each muscle fibre. Similar membrane covering each bundle of muscle fibres (fascicles) is called

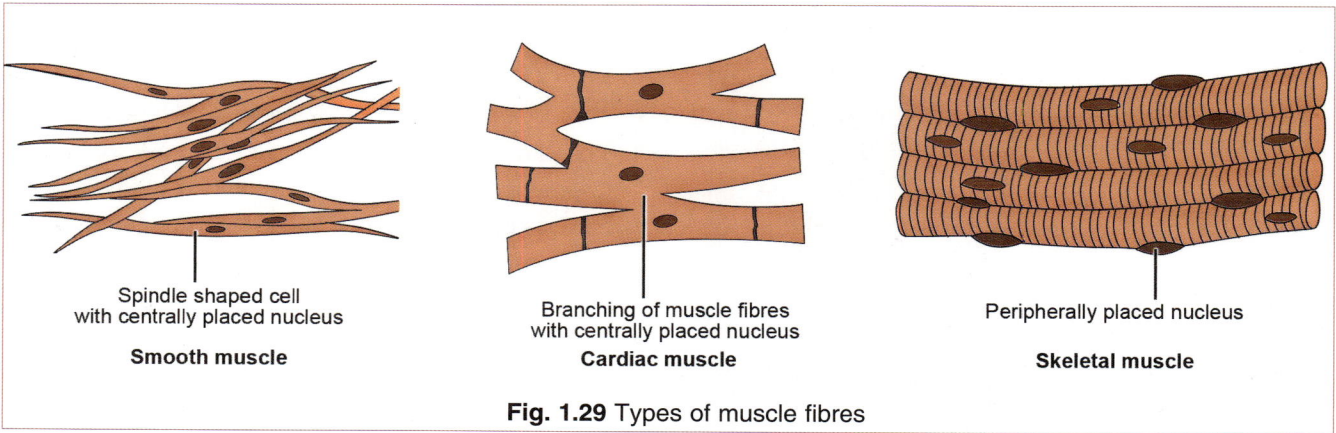

Spindle shaped cell with centrally placed nucleus
Smooth muscle

Branching of muscle fibres with centrally placed nucleus
Cardiac muscle

Peripherally placed nucleus
Skeletal muscle

Fig. 1.29 Types of muscle fibres

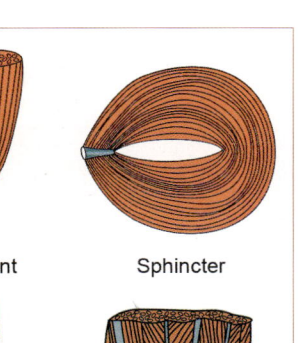

Parallel　　　　Convergent　　　　Sphincter

Unipennate　　　Bipennate　　　Multipennate

Fig. 1.30 Arrangement of fasciculi of skeletal muscle

perimysium. Epimysium surrounds the entire muscle (Fig. 1.31).

Microscopic structure of the skeletal muscle

Each muscle is made up of a number of muscle fibres.

- Each muscle fibre is multinucleated and shows striations. They are also called myocytes and their length varies from 1–300 mm.
- The outer membrane of the muscle fibre is called sarcolemma and its cytoplasm is called sarcoplasm (Fig. 1.32).
- The sarcoplasm shows many peripherally placed nuclei and large number of myofibrils.
- Each myofibril shows alternate dark and light bands.
- Dark bands are known as A bands (anisotropic) and the light bands as I bands (isotropic).

- Each myofibril has two protein filaments (myofilaments).
- They are called actin (thin) and myosin (thick) filaments.
- The dark band (A-band) is the area where the actin and myosin filaments overlap each other (Fig. 1.33).
- Only actin filaments occupy the light band (I-band).
- This arrangement of actin and myosin filament is responsible for striations in skeletal muscle (Fig. 1.34).
- In the middle of the dark band there is a light H band where there are no actin filaments.
- In the middle of the I band there is a dark Z line.
- The part of the myofibril between two Z lines is called sarcomere.

Nerve supply to a skeletal muscle

- The nerve supplying the muscle is called motor nerve. However, this motor nerve has 60% motor fibres, 40% sensory fibres and also autonomic fibres.
- The motor fibres are axons of the ventral horn cells of the spinal cord. On stimulation, the muscle contracts.
- The sensory fibres arise from muscle spindles (stretch receptors present in the muscle) which give information about the position of the muscle (proprioceptive sensation).
- Autonomic fibres innervate the smooth muscles present in the wall of the blood vessels inside the skeletal muscles.

Neuromuscular Junction

A nerve supplying a muscle is composed of both motor and sensory components. As the motor portion of the nerve penetrates a muscle, it plays into a number of branching neuron processes called axons. The terminal ends of axons contact the sarcolemma of muscle fibres by means of motor

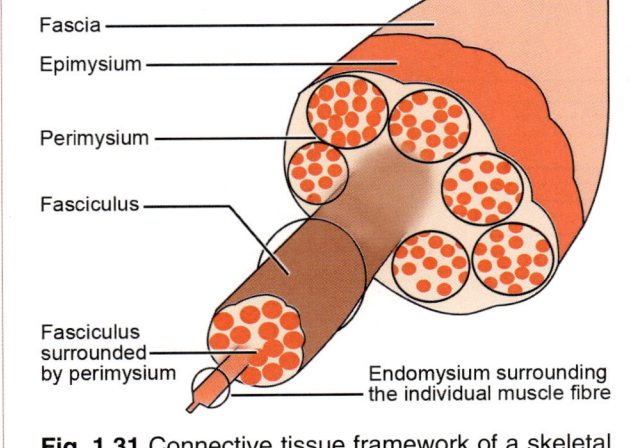

Fascia
Epimysium
Perimysium
Fasciculus
Fasciculus surrounded by perimysium
Endomysium surrounding the individual muscle fibre

Fig. 1.31 Connective tissue framework of a skeletal muscle (transverse section)

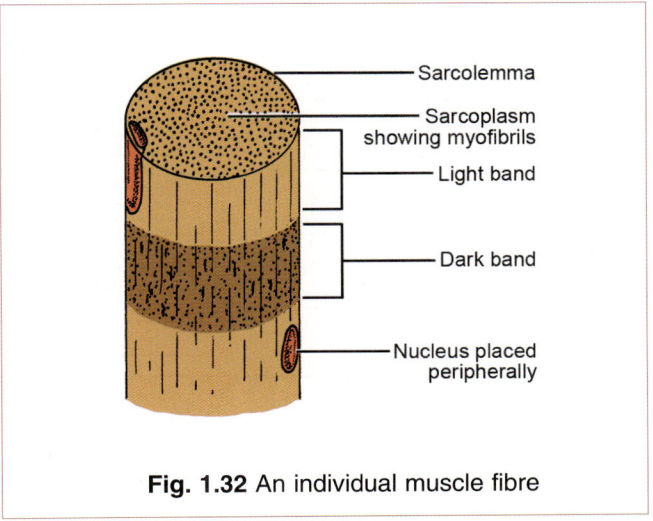

Sarcolemma
Sarcoplasm showing myofibrils
Light band
Dark band
Nucleus placed peripherally

Fig. 1.32 An individual muscle fibre

31

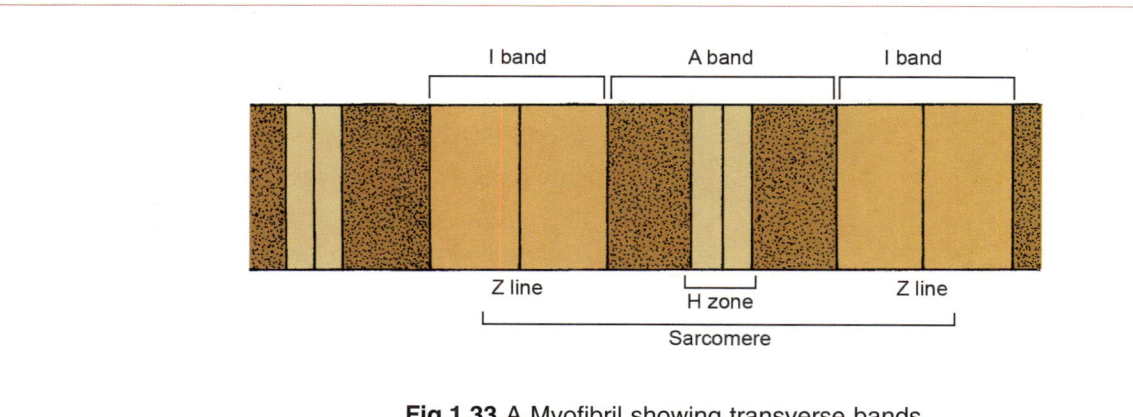

Fig.1.33 A Myofibril showing transverse bands

end plates. Each axon may split into numerous branches to serve dozens of muscle fibres. The area consisting of the motor end plate and the sarcolemma of the muscle fibre is known as the neuromuscular junction. Acetylcholine is a neurotransmitter chemical stored in synaptic vesicles at the terminal end of the axons. A nerve impulse reaching the terminal end of an axon causes the release of acetylcholine into the neuromuscular cleft of the neuromuscular junction. As this chemical mediator contacts the sarcolemma, it initiates physiological activity within the muscle fibre, resulting in contraction.

Motor unit

A motor unit consists of a single motor neuron and the aggregation of muscle fibres innervated by that motor neuron. When a nerve impulse travels through a motor unit, all of the fibres served by it contract simultaneously to their maximum. Most muscles have an innervation ratio of one

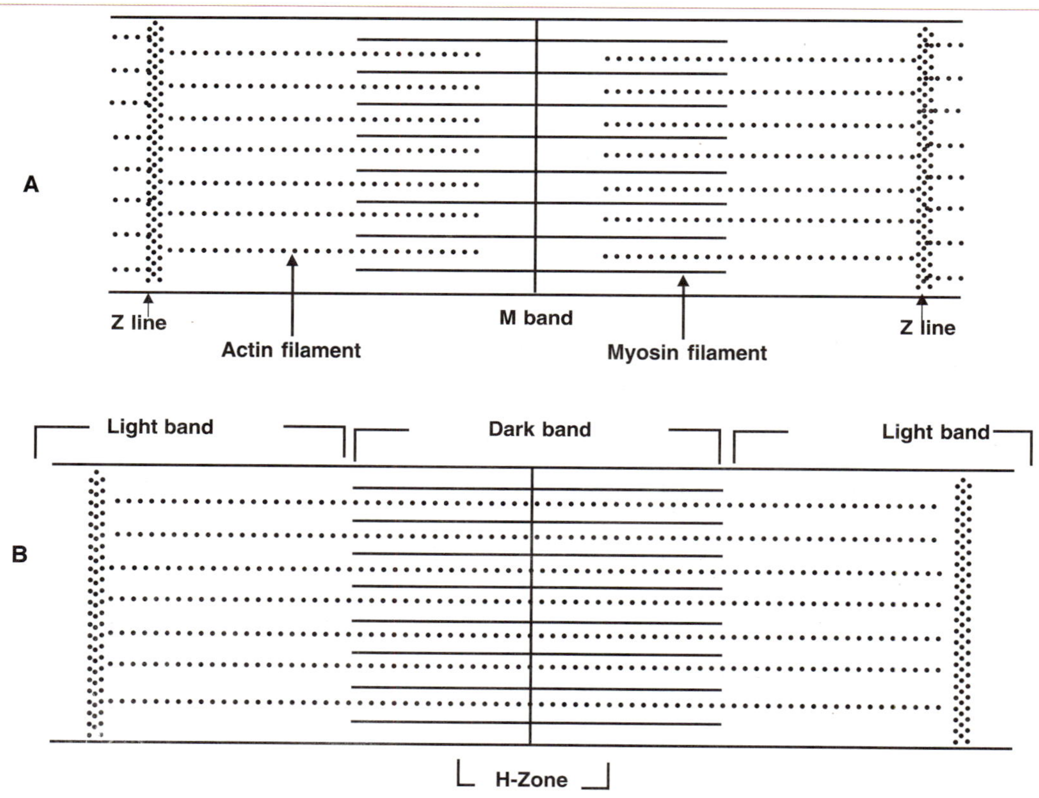

Fig. 1.34 Structure of skeletal muscle

motor neuron per 100–150 muscle fibre. Muscle capable of precise movements, such as an eye muscle, may have an innervation ratio of 1:10. Massive muscles that are responsible for gross body movements, such as those of the thigh may have an innervation ratio exceeding 1:500.

Action of muscle

When a muscle contracts, it shortens by 30% of its original length (length of fleshy part) and brings about a movement.

Agonists (prime movers): They bring the desired movement. When a prime mover helps opposite action by active controlled lengthening against gravity, then this action is called action of paradox, e.g. keeping an empty glass back on the table after drinking is assisted by gravity but controlled by a gradual active lengthening of biceps brachii.

Antagonists (opponents): They are opposite to the prime movers, but they help prime movers by active controlled relaxation so that the desired movement is smooth and precise.

Synergists: When prime movers cross more than one joint, the undesired actions at the proximal joint is prevented by certain muscles called synergists, e.g. when making a tight fist by long flexors, the wrist is kept fixed in extension by the synergists (extensors of wrist).

Muscle pull: Skeletal muscles are limited in their ability to lengthen. Muscle cannot elongate beyond 1/3rd of its resting length with its bony attachments, beyond which the muscle sustain damage, which is often referred as muscle pull.

Rigor Mortis: When death occurs, circulation ceases and the skeletal muscles are deprived of nutrients and oxygen. The calcium ions accumulate inside the sarcoplasm, which results in locking of the muscles in contracted position. All the skeletal muscles of the body are involved. This condition is called rigor mortis.

Muscle hypertrophy: Excessive increase in the activity of muscle results in increase in number of myofibrils. This causes enlargement of the muscles/ hypertrophy. Hypertrophy occurs in muscles that have been repeatedly stimulated. A weight lifter or body builder is an excellent example of hypertrophied muscular development.

Muscle atrophy: When a skeletal muscle is not stimulated by a motor neuron on a regular basis, it losses muscle tone and mass. The muscle becomes flaccid and the muscle fibre becomes smaller and weaker. This reduction in muscle size, tone and power is called atrophy.

Paralysis: The loss of contraction power of muscle is called paralysis. It may be due to an injury to the nerve supplying it or the disease of the muscle itself. It is characterized by sudden and involuntary tightening of muscle fibres.

Polio: Progressive paralysis of muscles due to destruction of CNS motor neurons (ventral horn cells of the spinal cord) by the polio virus.

Fibrosis: A process in which excess amount of connective tissues develops, making muscles less flexible.

JOINTS

The articulation between two or more bones is called a joint.

Joints are classified into two types on the basis of presence or absence of joint cavity. They are:

1. Synarthroses (without joint cavity): which is further divided into fibrous and cartilaginous varieties.
2. Diarthroses (with joint cavity): which are mobile that includes the synovial joints.

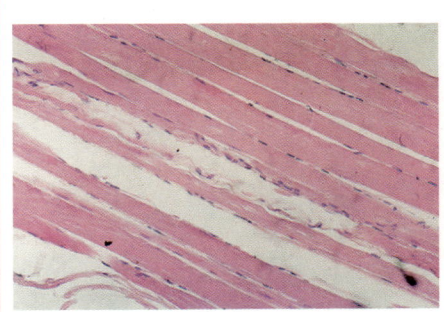

Skeletal muscle LS   Cardiac muscle LS   Smooth muscles

Fig. 1.35 Microscopic structure of muscles-H& E staining

Fibrous Joints

In this type of joint the articulating surfaces of the bones are connected by fibrous tissue, and thus very little movement is possible. Following are the types of fibrous joints:

1. **Sutures:** Sutural ligament (fibrous connective tissue) connects the bones without allowing movement, e.g. many skull bones are held together by sutures (Fig. 1.36).

2. **Syndesmosis:** The articulating parts of the bones are connected by interosseus ligament, e.g. inferior tibiofibular joint.

3. **Gomphosis** (Peg and socket): e.g. tooth in its bony socket.

Cartilaginous joints

In these joints articulating surfaces are connected by a cartilage. There are two types of cartilaginous joints:

1. **Primary cartilaginous joint (synchondrosis):** The articulating ends of the bones are connected by a plate of hyaline cartilage. These joints are temporary because after certain age the cartilaginous plate is replaced by bone (it will ossify into a bone). These joints are immovable (Fig. 1.36), e.g. (i) Joint between the epiphysis and diaphysis of a growing long bone (ii) Joint between the body of the sphenoid and basilar part of the occipital bone.

2. **Secondary cartilaginous joint (Symphysis):** The articulating surface is covered by hyaline cartilage. However, an articular disc is present between the articulating surfaces. This articular disc is a white fibrocartilage. These joints are permanent (except symphysis menti). These joints allow a limited movement (Fig. 1.36), e.g. pubic symphysis, manubriosternal joint, intervertebral joints between the bodies of vertebrae.

Synovial joint

In a synovial joint the articular surfaces of the bones are separated by a joint cavity filled with synovial fluid. Synovial joints are highly mobile.

Structure of a typical synovial joint (Fig. 1.37)

1. **Articular surface**: The articulating surface is smooth and is covered by hyaline cartilage (in some cases by white fibrocartilage, e.g. temporomandibular joint). Periosteum being highly vascular, joint movement can cause rupture of capillaries, hence articulating surfaces are covered by cartilages which are avascular. This articular cartilage is nourished by synovial fluid. These articular cartilages provide slippery surface for the free movement.

2. **Joint cavity:** The space between the articulating surfaces is called joint cavity, which is filled with synovial fluid. In some joints, the cavity is divided into two compartments by the presence of an articular disc or meniscus (complex joint). A fibrous capsule externally closes the joint cavity.

3. **Fibrous capsule:** Structurally, it is made up of collagen and elastic fibres, which provide strength and elasticity respectively. Functionally, it holds the two bones and prevents their dislocation. It is attached to the margins of the articulating surfaces. It has stretch receptors, which are innervated by nerve fibres. They carry the information from the joint (proprioceptive information) and also execute reflexes to protect the joint from sprain. Fibrous capsule has rich vascular plexus.

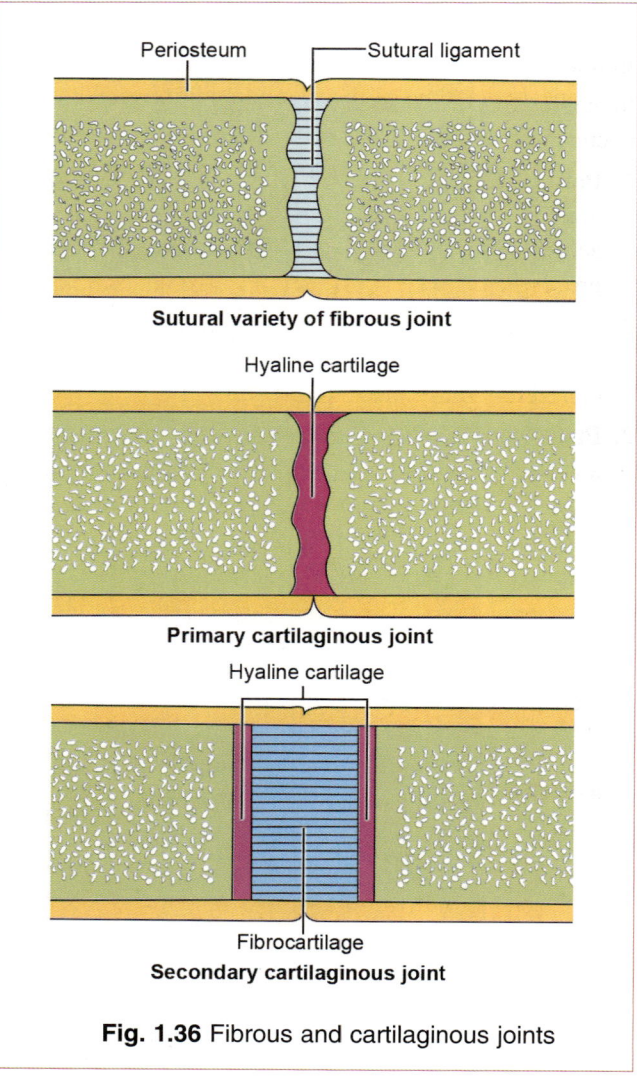

Sutural variety of fibrous joint

Periosteum — Sutural ligament

Hyaline cartilage

Primary cartilaginous joint

Hyaline cartilage

Fibrocartilage

Secondary cartilaginous joint

Fig. 1.36 Fibrous and cartilaginous joints

4. **Synovial membrane:** The fibrous capsule is lined by synovial membrane on its inner aspect. It is a highly vascular and cellular connective tissue membrane. They secrete synovial fluid and also hyaluronic acid, which maintains viscosity of the fluid.

5. **Synovial fluid:** It is a viscous fluid present in the joint cavity. It contains hyaluronic acid, monocytes, lymphocytes, macrophages and traces of protein. It provides nutrition to the articular cartilage and also lubrication to the joint.

6. **Ligaments**: The synovial joint is stabilized by ligaments outside or inside by the fibrous capsule. They may be thickened portions of the fibrous capsule or separate structures. These ligaments permit desirable movements and prevent undesirable ones. Their main function is to maintain stability of the joint. The tone of the muscles around the joint is an important factor in maintaining the stability.

Types of synovial joint

Synovial joints are classified into many subtypes according to the shape of the articular surfaces and types of movement occurring in them.

1. **Plane joints:** In these joints, the articular surfaces are flat permitting only sliding movement, e.g. acromioclavicular joint and joints between the articular processes of the vertebrae.

2. **Hinge joints:** These joints resemble the hinge on a door. Only flexion and extension movements are possible, e.g. elbow joint, knee joint (modified hinge), ankle joint.

3. **Pivot joints:** In these joints, there is a central pivot or an axis surrounded by a bony or ligamentous ring. In this joint either the pivot or the ring rotates. Rotation is the only movement possible, e.g. Atlanto-axial joint, superior radioulnar joint.

4. **Condylar joints:** A condylar articulation is structured so that an oval, convex articular surface of one bone fits into an elliptical, concave depression on another bone. This permits angular movement in two directions as in an up-and-down and side-to-side movements, e.g. temporomandibular joint, knee joint.

5. **Ellipsoid joints:** In these joints, there is an elliptical convex articular surface that fits into an elliptical concave articular surface. The movements are flexion, extension, abduction and adduction, but rotation is not possible, e.g. wrist joint.

6. **Saddle joints:** In these joints, the articular surfaces are reciprocally concavo-convex and resemble a saddle on a horse's back. This joint permits flexion, extension, abduction and rotation, e.g. carpometacarpal joint of the thumb.

7. **Ball and socket joints:** In these joints, a ball-shaped head of one bone fits into a socket-like concavity of another. This arrangement permits very free movements, including flexion, extension, abduction, adduction, medial and lateral rotation and circumduction, e.g. shoulder joint, hip joint.

Blood supply to a synovial joint

The epiphyseal branches of the artery supplying the bone form a periarticular plexus close to the attachment of fibrous capsule. Numerous minute vessels arising from this plexus pierce the fibrous capsule and form a rich vascular plexus on the outer surface of the synovial membrane. The blood vessels of the synovial membrane supply capsule, synovial membrane and the epiphysis. Before the fusion of epiphysis with metaphysis these vessels do not anastomose with metaphyseal arteries. However, after fusion, the communications between epiphyseal and metaphyseal arteries are established.

Nerve supply to a synovial joint

The nerve supplying the joint contains sensory and autonomic fibres. The sensory fibres are proprioceptive in function. They provide the information regarding position and movement of the joint. They are concerned with reflex control of posture and locomotion. They also convey pain sensation from the joint. The autonomic fibres provide motor fibres to the blood vessels. The capsule and ligaments possess a rich nerve supply and specialised receptors (golgi tendon end organs).

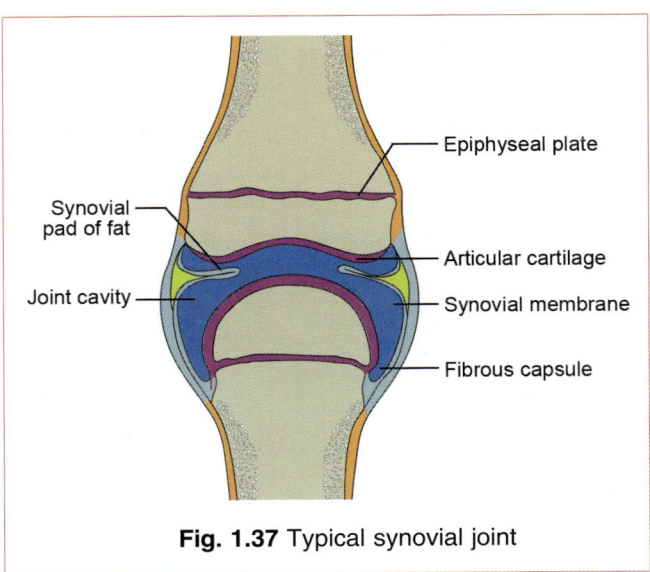

Fig. 1.37 Typical synovial joint

Labels: Epiphyseal plate; Synovial pad of fat; Joint cavity; Articular cartilage; Synovial membrane; Fibrous capsule

S E C T I O N   1

Hilton's law: It claims that, a motor nerve supplying a muscle which acts on a joint also supplies the skin covering that particular joint.

Movements at synovial joints

Movements at synovial joints are produced by the contraction of skeletal muscles that span the joints and attached to the bones articulating. In these actions, the bones act as levers, the muscles provide the force, and the joints are the fulcra or pivots (Figs 1.38 and 1.39).

The range of movement at a synovial joint is determined by the structure of the individual joint and the arrangement of the associated muscle and the bone. The movement at hinge joint, e.g. occurs in only one plane, whereas the structure of a ball and socket joint permits movements around many axes. Joint movements are broadly classified as angular and circular.

Angular movements

Angular movements increase or decrease the joint angle produced by the articulating bones. Following are the types of angular movements:

1. **Flexion:** Flexion is a movement that decreases the joint angle on an antero-posterior plane. Examples of flexion are the bending of the elbow or knee. Flexion of the elbow joint is a forward movement, whereas flexion of the knee is a backward movement. Flexion in most joints is simple to understand, such as flexion of the neck as the head is bowed. In the ankle joint the flexion occurs as the dorsum of the foot is elevated. This movement is frequently called dorsiflexion. Pressing the foot forwards is plantar flexion.

2. **Extension:** In extension, which is the reverse of flexion, the joint angle is increased. Extension returns the body to the anatomical position. In an extended joint the angle

between the articulating bones is 180°. The exception to this is the ankle joint, in which there is a 90° angle between the foot and leg in the anatomical position. Examples of extension are the straightening of the elbow or knee joints from flexed positions. Hyperextension occurs when a part of the body is extended beyond the anatomical position so that the joint angle is greater than 180°. An example of hyperextension is bending the head backwards.

3. **Abduction:** Abduction is the movement of a body part away from the main axis of the body or away from the midsagittal plane, in a lateral direction. Examples of abduction is moving the arms sideward and away from the body or spreading the fingers apart.

4. **Adduction:** Adduction, the opposite of abduction is the movement of a body part towards the main axis of the body. In the anatomical position the arms and legs have been adducted towards the midplane of the body.

Circular movements

Joints that permit circular movement are composed of a bone with a rounded or oval surface that articulates with a corresponding cup or depression on another bone. The two basic types of circular movements are rotation and circumduction.

1. Rotation: Rotation is the movement of the body part around its own axis. There is no lateral displacement during this movement. Examples are turning the head from side to side as in 'no' motion.

   Supination (rotation of the forearm in which the palm of the hand being turned anteriorly) and pronation (rotation of the forearm in which the palm being turned posteriorly) are the specialised rotations of forearm.

2. Circumduction: Circumduction is the circular, cone like movement of a body segment. The distal extremity forms

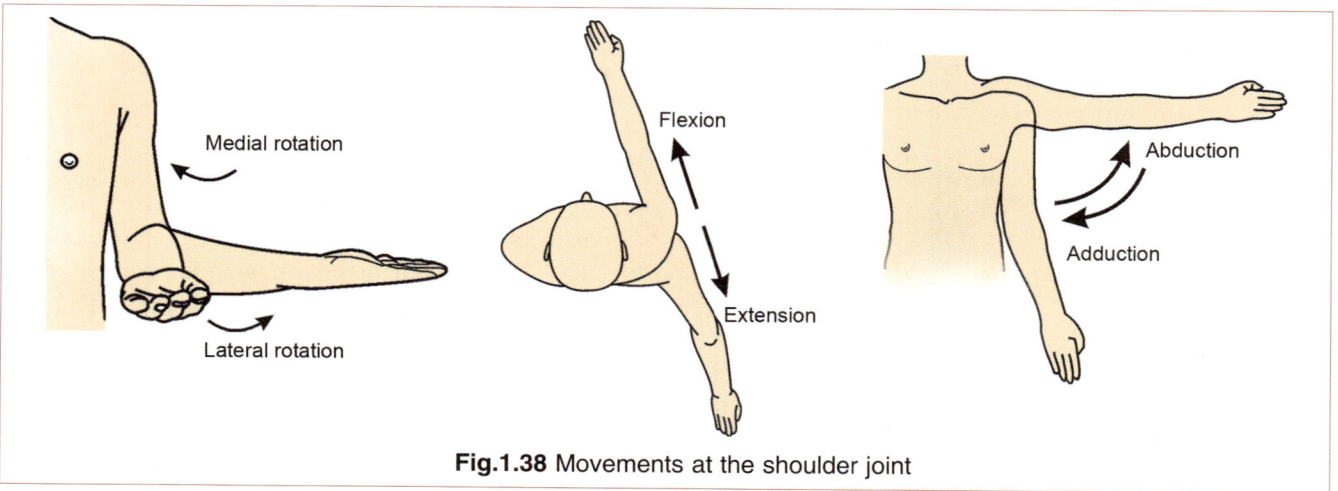

Fig.1.38 Movements at the shoulder joint

the circular movement and proximal attachment forms the pivot. The example for circumduction is the bowling action (in cricket) at shoulder joint.

Eversion, inversion, protraction, retraction, elevation and depression are the special movements described in certain joints.

Dislocation (luxation): The articulating surfaces of the bones are forced out of position. This displacement can damage the articular cartilages, tear ligaments or distort the joint capsule. The capsule and ligaments are innervated by nerves and hence dislocation is very painful. The damage accompanying a partial dislocation or subluxation is less severe.

Sprain: Ligament tear causing severe pain in the joint.

Age related structural changes in the articular cartilages is one of the chief causes of joint problems in elderly people often affecting the weight bearing joints like knee and hip. As a result the articular cartilage becomes less effective shock absorber and becomes vulnerable to repeated friction that occurs during joint movement. This can cause severe pain.

Arthritis: It is the inflammation of the joint(s). It can be caused by a variety of causes. The joint is swollen and the movements are restricted and painful (e.g. rheumatic arthritis, rheumatoid arthritis). Osteoarthritis is a degenerative joint disease in elderly people characterized by stiffness, discomfort and pain. It usually affects the weight bearing joints like hip and knee.

Arthroscopy: It is a procedure by which the joint cavity can be visualised through an arthroscope. This procedure not only helps in identifying joint abnormalities (such as torn menisci), but some surgical procedures can also be performed during this procedure.

BLOOD VESSELS

Blood vessels and lymphatic vessels are tubular channels, which carry nutrients to the tissue and bring back the metabolites from the tissues into circulation (Fig. 1.41).

Heart acts as a pumping organ which pumps oxygenated blood (arterial blood) to all the parts of the body through arteries. The deoxygenated blood (venous blood) is brought back to the heart by veins, which is later carried to the lungs for oxygenation.

Arteries

- They carry blood away from the heart.
- They branch like trees on their way to different parts of the body.
- The tiny branches of arteries are called 'arterioles' with diameter greater than 0.3 mm.

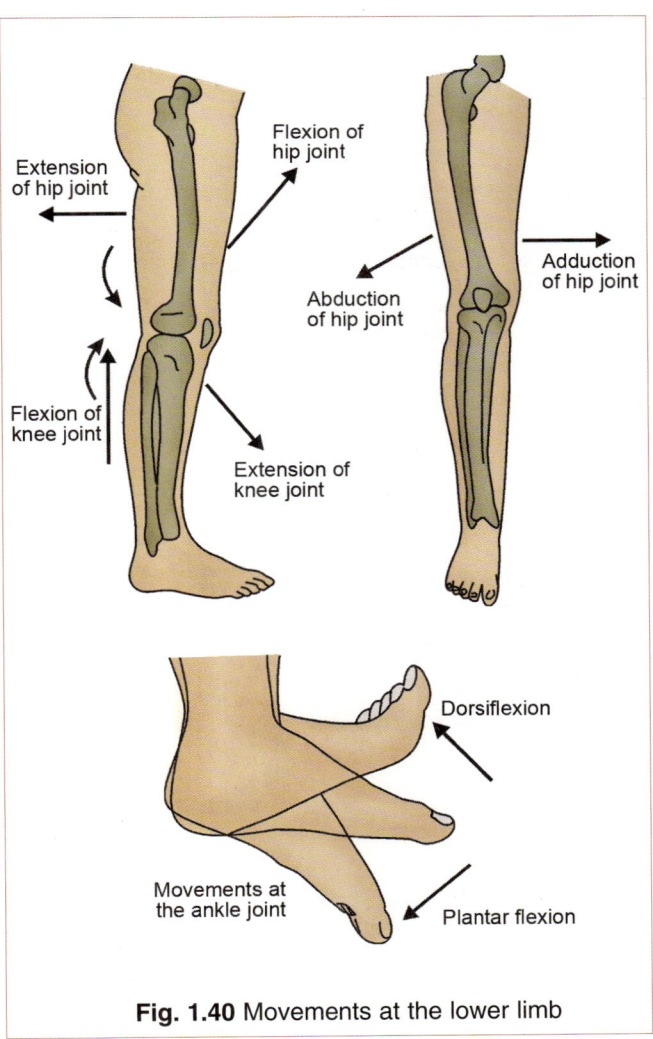

Fig. 1.40 Movements at the lower limb

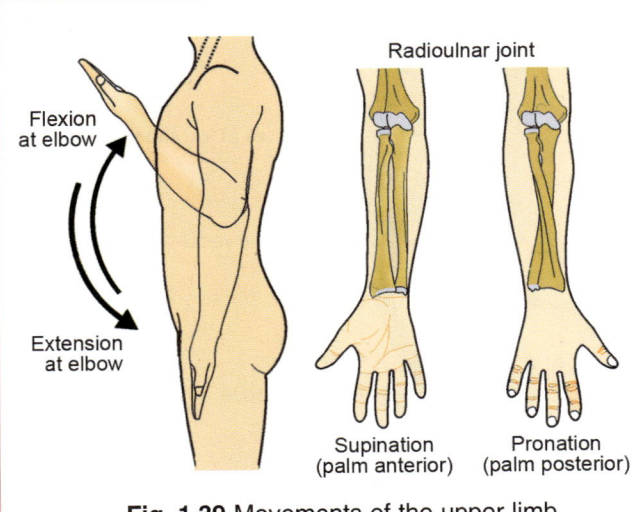

Fig. 1.39 Movements of the upper limb

- Arteries are thick walled, being uniformly thicker than the accompanying veins.
- The lumen is smaller than that of the veins accompanying it.
- Arteries do not have valves.

Structure of an artery

The basic structure of the artery and the vein is almost the same with few differences. Fig. 1.42 shows the different layers forming the wall of the blood vessels.

- The wall of the artery is made up of three layers, tunica intima, media and adventitia (from inside to outside).
- Endothelium is the lining epithelium and is part of the tunica intima.
- Tunica media is the thickest of all the three coats, which is made up of elastic fibres and smooth muscles.
- The large arteries contain more elastic fibres and medium sized artery has more smooth muscles.
- Small arteries called 'vasa vasorum' that nourishes the wall of the large artery.
- Internal elastic lamina is a membrane formed by elastic fibres deep to the endothelium of the tunica intima. It is better defined in a medium sized arteries (Fig. 1.44).

Veins

- They bring blood from various tissues of the body back into the heart
- The veins are formed by the union of many tributaries (like a river)

  The small veins are called 'venules', they join to form veins, which further form large veins and finally forms vena cavae before entering the heart.

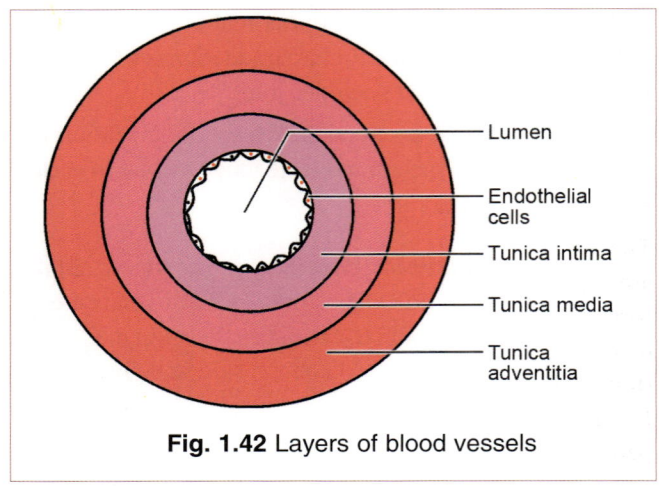

Fig. 1.42 Layers of blood vessels

- Veins are thin walled, than the arteries.
- Their lumen is larger.
- Veins have 'valves' which are reduplications of endothelium. They maintain the unidirectional flow of blood against gravity (Fig.1.43). However, some of the veins do not have valves, e.g. emissary veins and veins of the vertebral column.

Structure of a vein

- The wall of the veins is made up of three layers like arteries – tunica intima, media and adventitia (from inside to outside). Endothelium is the lining epithelium and is part of the tunica intima. Tunica media has a mixture of connective tissue and few smooth muscle fibres.
- Tunica adventitia is the thickest and best developed in large veins. Tunica adventitia has large amount of smooth muscle fibres along with collagen and elastic fibres.

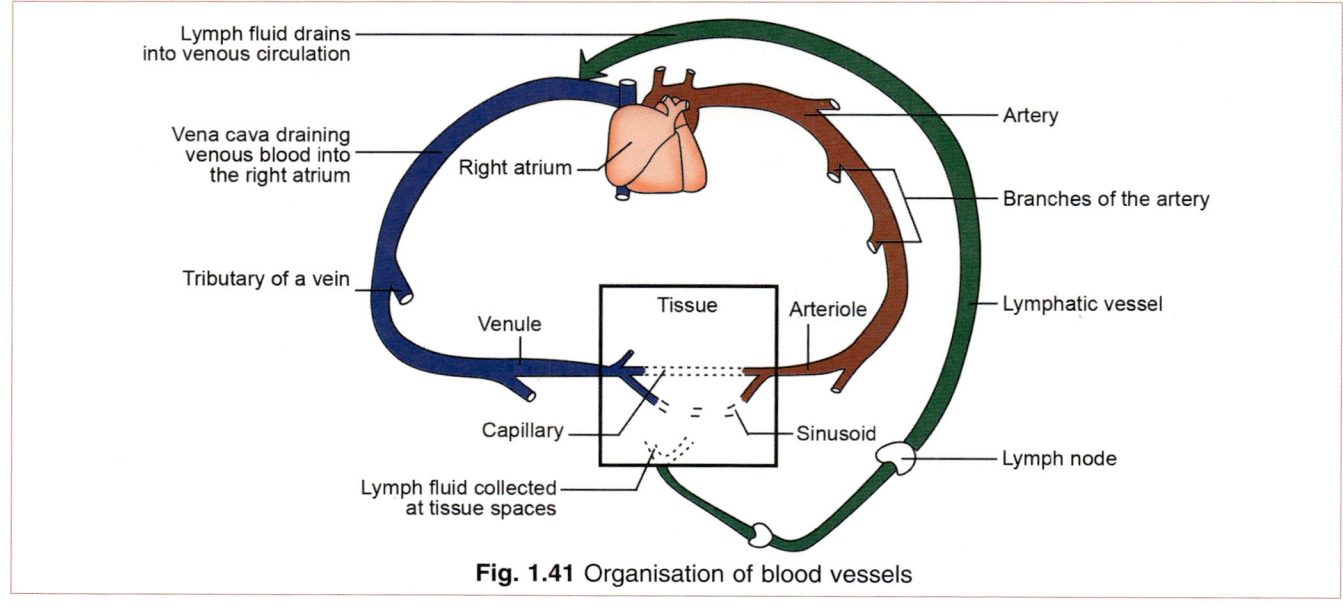

Fig. 1.41 Organisation of blood vessels

- The muscular and elastic tissue content of the venous wall is much less than that of the arteries.
- The walls of the larger veins are supplied by nutrient vessels called 'vasa vasorum', which may penetrate up to the tunica intima.

Blood supply to the wall of the blood vessels

The large arteries (of more than 1 mm diameter) and veins are supplied by nutrient vessels called vasa vasorum. They form a capillary network in tunica adventitia and outer part of the tunica media. The inner portion of the vessel wall (tunica intima) is nourished directly by diffusion from the luminal blood. However, in the veins the vasa vasorum may penetrate up to the intima, probably because of the low venous pressure. Minute veins accompanying the arteries drain the blood from the outer part of the arterial wall. Lymphatics are also present in the adventitia.

Nerve supply to the blood vessels

They are supplied by non-myelinated sympathetic fibres, which are vasoconstrictor in function (with few exceptions). Myelinated nerve fibres are believed to be sensory in function.

Capillaries (capillus = hair)

These are microscopic blood vessels within the tissue. They have single layer of endothelial cells resting on a basement membrane, without any outer coats (Fig. 1.45)

- Capillaries have arterial and venous ends.
- The diameter of a capillary is 6–8 microns. However the capillaries of skin and bone marrow have larger diameter.

Types of capillaries:

1. Continuous capillaries: In muscle and brain (Fig. 1.45A)
2. Fenestrated capillaries: In kidney, intestine and endocrine glands
3. Sinusoids: In lymphoid organs (Fig. 1.45B)

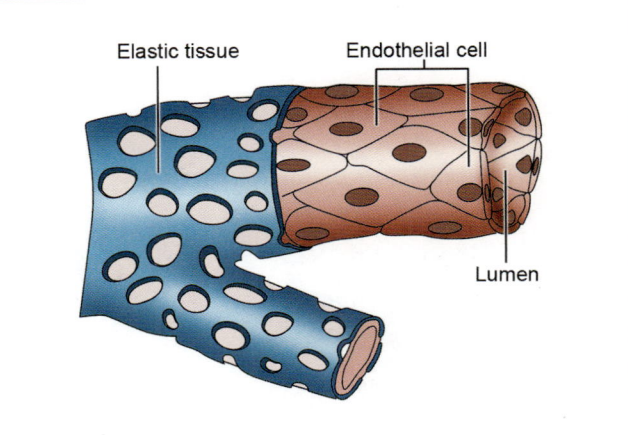

Fig. 1.44 Schematic representation of tunica intima

Transport across capillary walls:

1. Fenestrae: penetrate endothelium, passive diffusion
2. Intercellular clefts: Spaces between the neighboring endothelial cells
3. Pinocytosis: Plasma or tissue fluid is endocytosed followed by transport of pinocytic vesicles in either diameter
4. Diapedesis: Some leukocytes pass into tissue from blood through openings in junctional complexes (Histamine-increases vascular permeability)

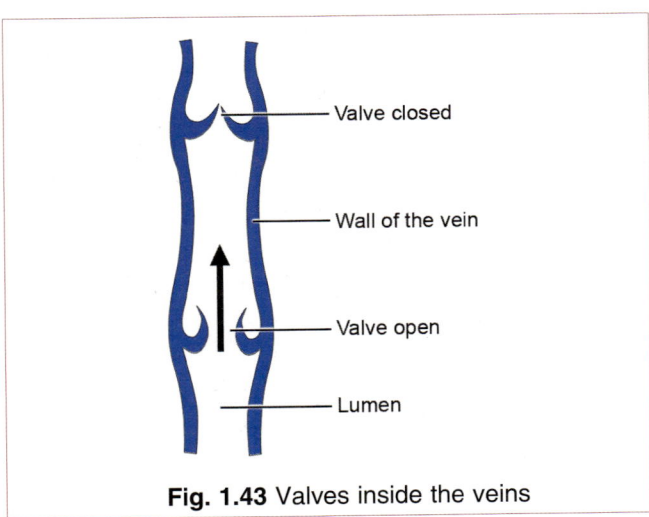

Fig. 1.43 Valves inside the veins

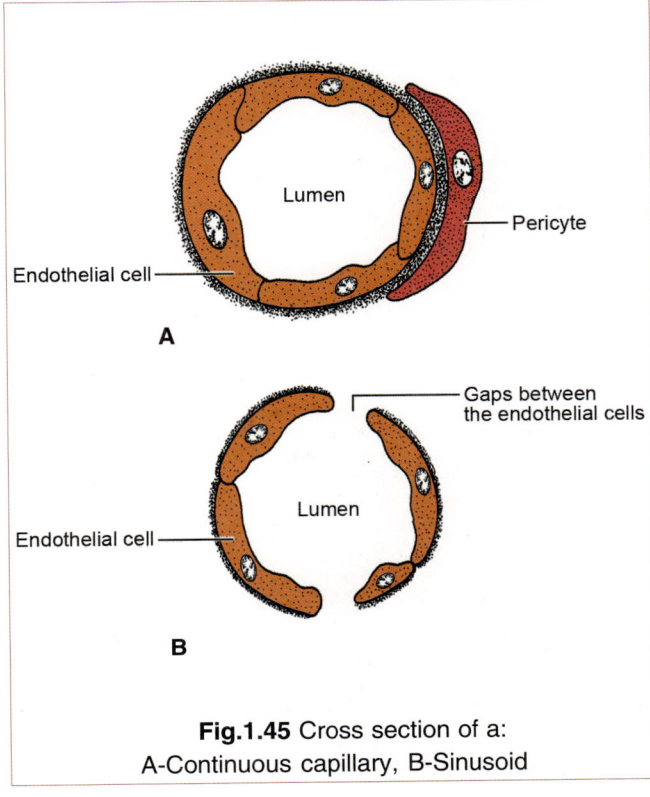

Fig.1.45 Cross section of a:
A-Continuous capillary, B-Sinusoid

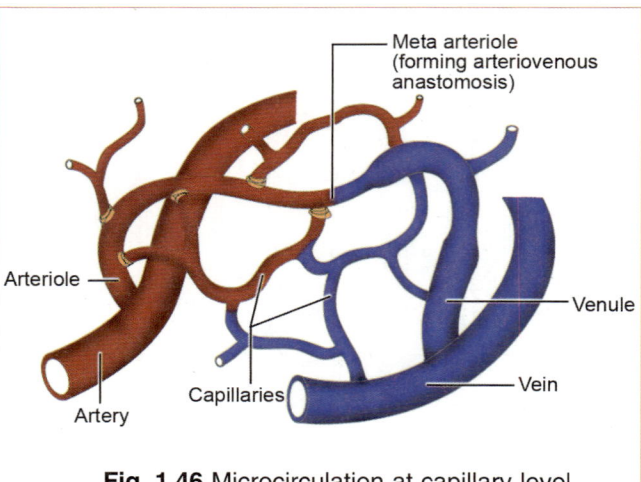

Fig. 1.46 Microcirculation at capillary level

Sinusoids

- Sinusoids replace capillaries in certain organs like liver, spleen, bone marrow and endocrine glands.
- The lumen of the sinusoid is large and irregular.
- Their wall is thinner and incomplete with spaces between endothelial cells.
- The basal lamina of endothelial cells is replaced by fine reticular fibres (Fig. 1.45B)

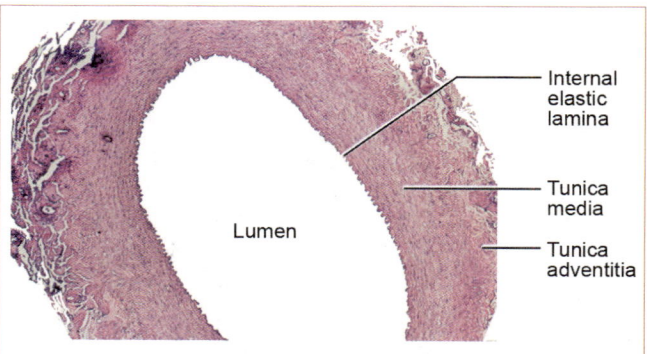

Fig. 1.47 Cross section of a medium sized (muscular) artery (H & E staining)

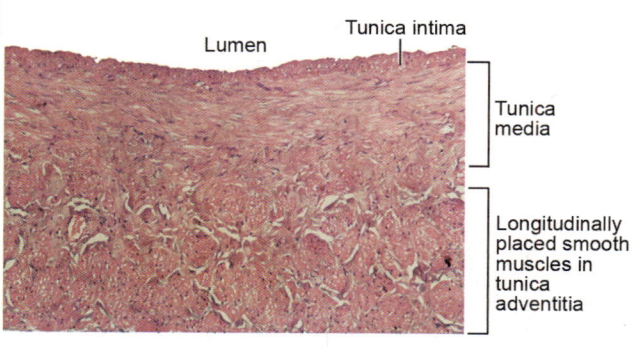

Fig. 1.48 Cross section of a large vein (H & E staining)

Anastomosis

A precapillary or postcapillary communication between the neighbouring vessels is called anastomosis.

Types

1. **Arterial anastomosis:** The terminal branches of arteries or arterioles join with each other to form anastomosis, e.g. palmar arch, plantar arch, circle of willis, intestinal arcades. On sudden occlusion of a main artery, the anastomosis may facilitate a collateral circulation.

2. **Venous anastomosis:** It is the communication between the veins or tributaries of the vein, e.g. dorsal venous arch of hand and foot.

3. **Arteriovenous anastomosis:** It is the direct communication between the arteries and veins. There is a network of capillaries between the arteriole and venule. When the organ is at rest the blood bypasses these capillaries. The arteriovenous anastomosis is observed in skin, nasal cavity, lips, mucous membrane of the alimentary canal, erectile tissue, tongue, thyroid gland etc.

End-arteries

Arteries which do not anastomose with their adjacent arteries are called end arteries. Occlusion of an end artery causes severe ischemia resulting in death of the tissue. Occlusion of central artery of retina results in permanent blindness.

Examples: (i) central artery of retina (ii) central branches of cerebral arteries (iii) vasa rectae of the mesenteric arteries.

Endothelial cell structure

- Nucleus causes each cell to bulge out and cells thins out towards periphery
- Pinocytic vesicles throughout cytoplasm
- Organelles and filament collect near nucleus
- Pericytes (Adventitial cells): It is contractile and can differentiate into other variety

Key functions:

1. Converting Angiotensin I to II (It regulates the blood pressure by smooth muscle contraction)
2. Inactivating bioactive compounds, thus regulating their effect (bradykinin, serotonin, prostaglandins, Norepinephrine, Thrombin)
3. Breaking down of lipoprotein (lipolysis) to yield triglycerides, cholesterol (for energy metabolism)
4. Preventing thrombus (clot) formation. Release prostacyclin inhibitor of platelet aggregation
5. Participates in capillary transport.

Haemorrhage (bleeding) is a flow of blood out of vessel wall. Arterial haemorrhage causes spurting of bright red blood and venous haemorrhage cause oozing (steady stream) of dark blood.

Arteriosclerosis: In old age the arteries become stiff. It is a thickening and toughening of arterial wall. The amount of blood flow through these arteries is reduced which can rise the systolic blood pressure.

Atherosclerosis is a type of arteriosclerosis characterised by changes in the endothelial lining. A fatty mass of tissue is deposited in the lumina of the vessels.

Ischemia: It refers to reduction of blood supply to an organ or region as a consequences of atherosclerosis, thrombus formation or occlusion of a vessel by adjacent structure. Arterial occlusion resulting in ischemia is characterized by **5 Ps – pallor (pale), pain, puffiness, pulselesness and paralysis** (involving muscles).

Infarction: It refers to death or necrosis of an area of tissue or an organ resulting from reduced blood supply. Such infarction in heart causes heart attack, stroke in brain and gangrene in distal parts of the limbs.

Arteritis: An inflammation of an artery is called arteritis. Inflammation of a vein is called 'phlebitis'.

Thrombosis: It is the coagulation of blood in the vessels. The clot thus formed is termed as thrombus.

Embolism: An obstruction of blood vessel, usually an artery by a detached thrombus, fat cells, air etc.

Aneurysm: A permanent dilatation of an artery usually with rupture of the internal and middle coats. The thoracic aorta and the innominate artery (brachiocephalic trunk) are usually affected.

Varicose veins: This refers to abnormally dilated and twisted superficial veins, which more frequently affects the limbs. The walls of the vein become weak and do not withstand the pressure resulting in its dilation. The valves becomes incompetent, thus the blood flow towards the heart is broken causing more pressure to the valves. Varicose vein can also occur due to inflammation of valves.

LYMPHATIC SYSTEM

Lymphatic system is a drainage system, which removes larger particles from the tissue fluid.

The lymphatic system consists of

- Lymph vessels
- Lymphoid organs
- Circulating lymphocytes

The nutrients to the tissue are given by artery, arteriole and finally capillaries at tissues. The fluid from the tissue is taken up by venous end of the capillaries and then circulates through venules and veins. However, lymphatic vessels absorb about 10–20% of the tissue fluid, which begins at the tissue spaces. The tissue fluid flowing through these vessels is called "lymph". This lymph fluid finally drains into larger veins through lymphatic vessels (Fig. 1.42).

Lymphatic vessels

- The lymphatic capillaries begin blindly in the tissue spaces.
- Lymphatic vessels are connected to each other forming a network.
- The superficial lymphatic vessels accompany veins while deep lymphatic vessels accompany arteries.
- Larger lymphatic vessels are named; for example thoracic duct.
- Lymph nodes are present in relation to the lymphatic vessels.
- The caliber of lymphatic capillary is greater and less regular than blood capillaries.
- Lymph fluid is colourless but in the intestine it is milk-white due to absorption of fat. It is called chyle.
- Lymphatic capillaries are absent in brain, spinal cord, bone marrow and other avascular structures.

Lymphoid organs

Lymphatic organs are classified into central and peripheral parts.

a) **Central lymphatic organs** are bone marrow and thymus.

- The lymphoid stem cells are produced by bone marrow except during early fetal life (produced by spleen and liver).
- The stem cell undergoes differentiation in these central lymphatic organs and becomes competent.
- Bone marrow differentiates the B-lymphocytes, which are capable of synthesizing antibodies.
- Thymus differentiates immunologically competent but uncommitted T-lymphocytes.

b) **Peripheral lymphatic organs** include lymph nodes, spleen, tonsil and lymphoid tissue present in the wall of the gastrointestinal and respiratory tracts.

• The B- and T-lymphocytes reach peripheral lymphatic organs where they proliferate and mature into immuno competent cells.

Lymph nodes

• Lymph nodes are oval or bean shaped structures present in the course of small lymphatic vessels.

• They filter the lymph and multiply lymphocytes.

• Lymph nodes are present in-groups. The superficial lymph nodes are arranged along the veins and the deep nodes along the arteries.

• Each lymph node has a hilum. The artery enters the node and vein and one efferent lymphatic vessel emerges at this place. However, afferent lymphatic vessels are many in number, which enter the lymph node at many points along its periphery.

Structure of a lymph node

1. Outer covering of the lymph node is made up of connective tissue fibres (collagen and few elastic fibres) which form capsule of the lymph node.

• Number of trabeculae extends from the capsule into the substance of lymph node, which provides a media for the passage of blood vessels.

• The substance of the lymph node shows reticular fibres forming irregular network on which lymphocytes are placed.

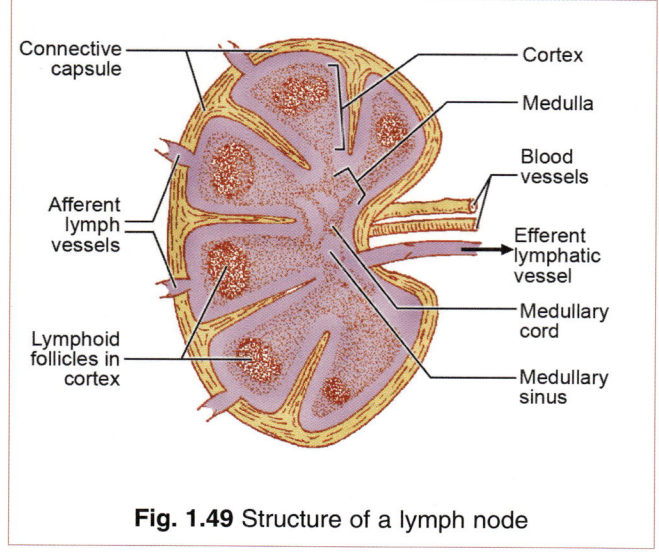

Fig. 1.49 Structure of a lymph node

2. The substance of the lymph node is divided into outer cortex and inner medulla (Fig. 1.49).

• The cortex is absent at the hilum.

• Lymphocytes are arranged in the form of follicles (or nodules) in the cortex. Each lymphatic follicle consists of densely packed lymphocytes outside and large lymphocytes (lymphoblasts) called germinal center in the center.

3. The medulla shows medullary cords where lymphocytes are arranged in irregular masses with spaces in between them called medullary sinuses. These medullary sinuses contain lymph fluid.

4. Apart from the lymphocytes, the lymph node also has macrophages, plasma cells and reticulocytes.

5. The afferent lymphatic vessel entering the lymph node at multiple sites opens into a subcapsular sinus. The

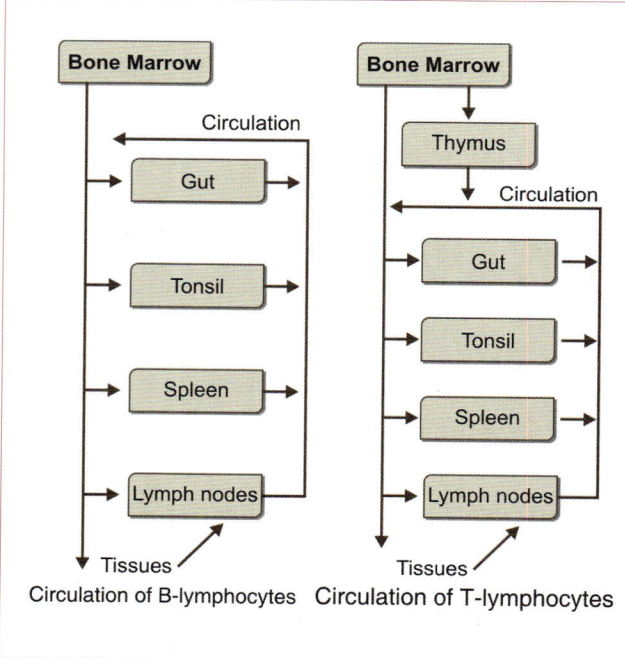

Circulation of B-lymphocytes   Circulation of T-lymphocytes

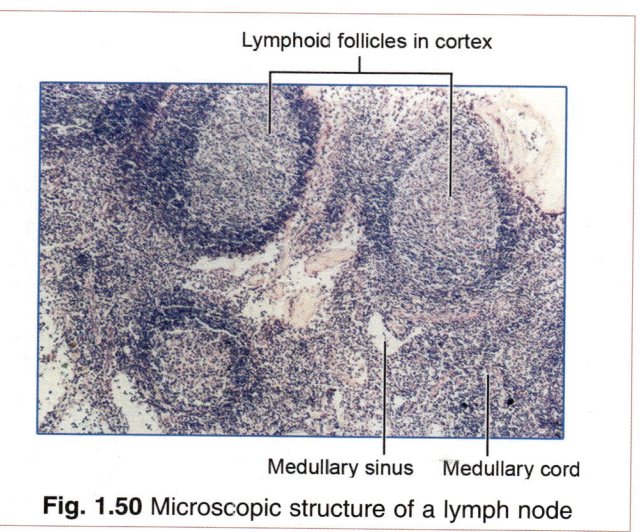

Fig. 1.50 Microscopic structure of a lymph node

subcapsular sinuses are connected with medullary sinuses through radiating cortical sinuses. The lymph collected in the medullary sinuses is drained out from the lymph node by efferent lymphatic vessel (Fig. 1.50).

Functions of the lymphoid system

1. Lymphatic vessels drain large protein molecules from the tissue places. Thus cellular debris and foreign particles (dust particles inhaled into the lungs, bacteria and other micro-organisms) are drained by this system.

2. Lymphatic vessels help in transportation of fat from the gut.

3. Lymph node serves the following functions:

•   They filter the lymph and prevent the foreign particles entering into the blood stream.

•   The foreign particles are phagocytosed by macrophages.

•   They lymphocytes multiply in the lymph nodes.

•   These lymphocytes provide both humoral and cellular immunity against the antigens.

Lymphadenopathy: It refers to enlargement of lymph nodes.

Lymphomas: A malignant cancer consisting of abnormal lymphocytes or lymphocytic stem cells.

Autoimmune disorder: A disorder that develops when the immune response mistakenly targets normal body cells and tissues.

Lymphangitis: Inflammation of the lymphatic vessels can occur while draining an infected area. The lymphangitis are marked on the skin as painful red lines and swollen lymph nodes.

Elephantiasis: The filarial parasites in the lymphatic vessel may block it and this results in oedema at the peripheral area of the drainage.

Cancer spread through lymphatic vessels: Cancer can invade the adjacent tissue by direct contact and spread into distant sites (metastasis) by lymphatic vessels or blood vessels. Lymphatic route is the most common way of metastasis. Hence lymphatic drainage of those organs which are commonly involved in cancer should be studied in greater detail which will help in the diagnosis of the primary site of the cancer. From the affected organ the cancer spread in the direction of lymph from that organ, hence it is important to know proximal and distal sets of lymph nodes for each organ. Understanding of lymphatic drainage of an organ helps

1. To know what nodes are likely to be affected when a tumour is identified in an organ or a tissue.

2. To be able to locate the likely primary cancerous sites, when enlarged node is detected.

NERVOUS SYSTEM

The human nervous system is the most complex physical system known to mankind. At present our understanding of this complex system seems to be very rudimentary. This system provides a complex mechanism by which the living organism can react to the ever changing external and internal environment and thus has enabled the survival of human species.

Nervous tissue: The nervous tissue consists of two types of cells: Neurons and Neuroglial cells.

Neurons

•   Neurons are basic structural and functional units of the nervous system

•   They respond to physical and chemical stimuli

•   They conduct impulses and release specific chemical regulators

•   Neurons cannot divide mitotically, but some neurons can regenerate

Microscopic structure of a neuron

The principal components of the neurons are (Fig. 1.51)

1. Cell body

2. Dendrites

3. Axon

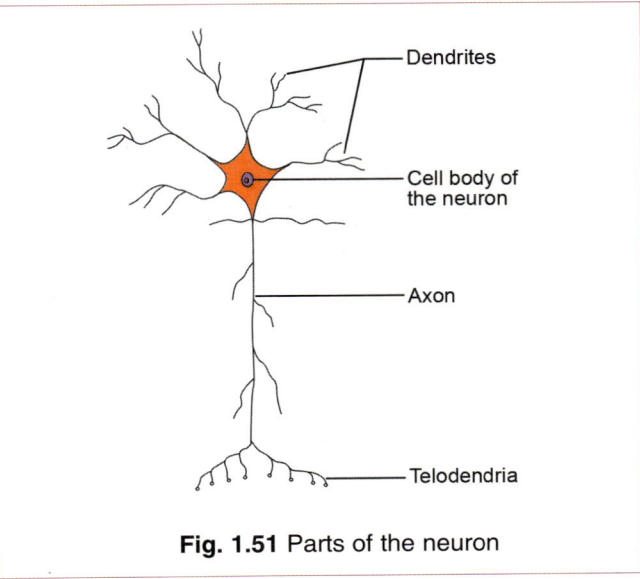

Fig. 1.51 Parts of the neuron

Cell body:

- The cytoplasm of the cell body is covered by a cell membrane with centrally placed nucleus

- The cytoplasm presents numerous mitochondria, Golgi complex, ribosomes and lysosomes

- It is said that centrioles are absent in neurons, however, recent electron microscopic studies have confirmed the presence of centriole.

- The characteristic feature of the cytoplasm of the nerve cell body is presence of granular material called 'Nissl substance' (Nissl bodies/granules). This Nissl substance is composed of rough endoplasmic reticulum.

- The cytoplasm of also shows 'neurofibrils' which consist of microfilaments and microtubules.

- The cytoplasmic processes are of two types: dendrites and axons.

Dendrites:

- These are branched processes that extend from the cytoplasm of the cell body.

- Their function is to receive stimuli and conduct impulses to the cell body.

- Some dendrites present minute 'spines' that increase their surface area.

- The dendrites contain 'Nissl substance' which is absent in the axons. The Nissl-free zone extends partly to the cell body and is called axon hillock.

Axon:

- Axon is the long cytoplasmic extension from the cell body.

- The term 'nerve fibre' is commonly used with reference to either an axon or an elongated dendrite.

- Axons conduct impulses away from the cell body.

- Their length varies from few millimeters in the CNS to over a meter in the PNS.

- Side branches called collateral branches extend for a short distance from the axons.

Types of neurons

According to the number of cytoplasmic processes they may be classified into (Fig. 1.53):

- **Unipolar neurons/Pseudo unipolar neurons: One** process arising from cell body dividing into two—one central process (axon) and the other peripheral process (dendrite), e.g. mesencephalic nucleus of trigeminal nerve and dorsal root ganglia of spinal nerves.

- **Bipolar neurons:** Two processes arises from the cell body one acting as axon and the other as dendrite, e.g. spiral and vestibular ganglion of the internal ear.

- **Multipolar neuron:** The cell body presents many cytoplasmic processes, one acting as axon and the rest as dendrites. Majority of the neurons are multipolar.

According to the length of axon, the neurons are classified into:

Golgi type-I - with long axons.

Golgi type-II - with short or no axons.

Neuroglia (Glial cells)

- These are non-excitable supporting cells of the nervous tissue (Fig. 1.54)

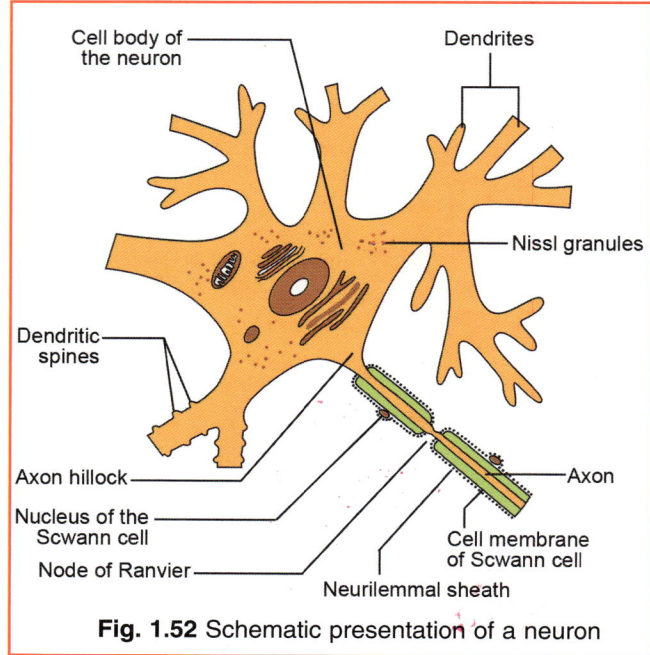

Fig. 1.52 Schematic presentation of a neuron

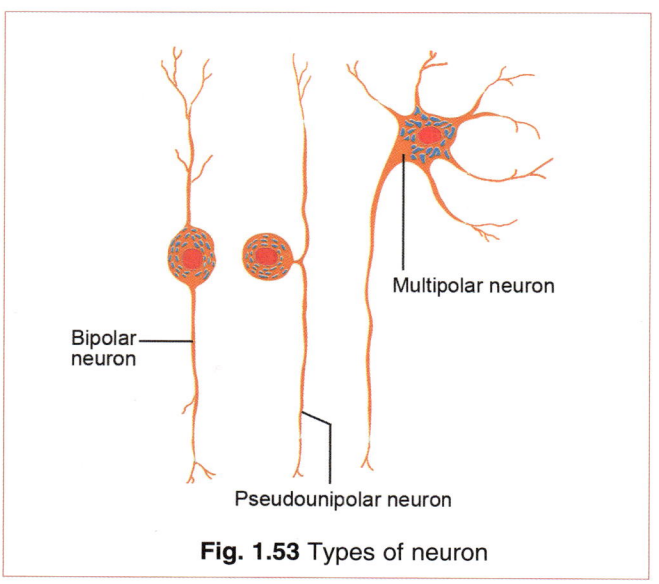

Fig. 1.53 Types of neuron

- They are numerous than the neurons and have limited mitotic capacity.
- There are many varieties of neuroglial cells.

1. Astrocytes

- These cells are stellate in appearance.
- They are present at the site of blood brain barrier.
- Astrocytes are the most abundant neuroglia in the CNS.
- They regulate the passage of molecules from the blood to brain.
- Astrocytes are the primary glycogen stores in the central nervous system (CNS).

2. Oligodendrocytes

- These cells form myelin sheath around the axons in CNS.

3. Microglial cells

- They are derived from mesoderm.
- These are small cells with flat cell body and few short cellular processes.
- They are found along the perivascular coat of blood vessels in CNS.
- They are phagocytic in function and act as macrophage cells of the CNS.

4. Ependyma

- These are simple columnar cells with non-motile cilia, lining the cavities of the brain (ventricles) and central canal of the spinal cord.

5. Schwann cells

- These cells provide myelin sheath for the axons of PNS.

Blood brain barrier:

The vascular processes (cytoplasmic extensions) of the astrocytes surround most of the outer surface of the capillaries. Before molecules in the blood can enter neurons in the CNS, they may have to pass through both the endothelial cells and the astrocytes. Astrocytes, therefore, contribute to the blood brain barrier, which is highly selective; some molecules are permitted to pass, whereas closely related molecules may not be allowed to the cross the barrier.

The blood brain barrier presents difficulties in the chemotherapy in brain diseases as the drug may not be able to enter the brain. For example, in the treatment of Parkinson's disease ,patients who need dopamine in the brain must be given a precursor molecule called levodopa (L-dopa). This is because dopamine cannot cross the blood brain barrier, whereas L-dopa can enter neurons and is converted to dopamine in the brain.

Synapse

The junction between the neurons is called synapse. Synapses may be of various types depending on the parts of neurons that come in contact.

1. Axodendritic synapse: It is the most common type where axon terminals contact with dendrites.

2. Axosomatic synapse: Axon terminal synapses with cell body of another neuron.

The impulses are transmitted across a synapse by specific neurotransmitters like acetylcholine, noradrenaline, dopamine, serotonin, histamine, glycine, GABA (Gamma-aminobutyric acid) and certain polypeptides.

Synaptic transmission may be affected by various drugs or diseases. Caffeine is a stimulant that increases the rate of transmission across the synapse. Aspirin causes a moderate decrease in the transmission rate.

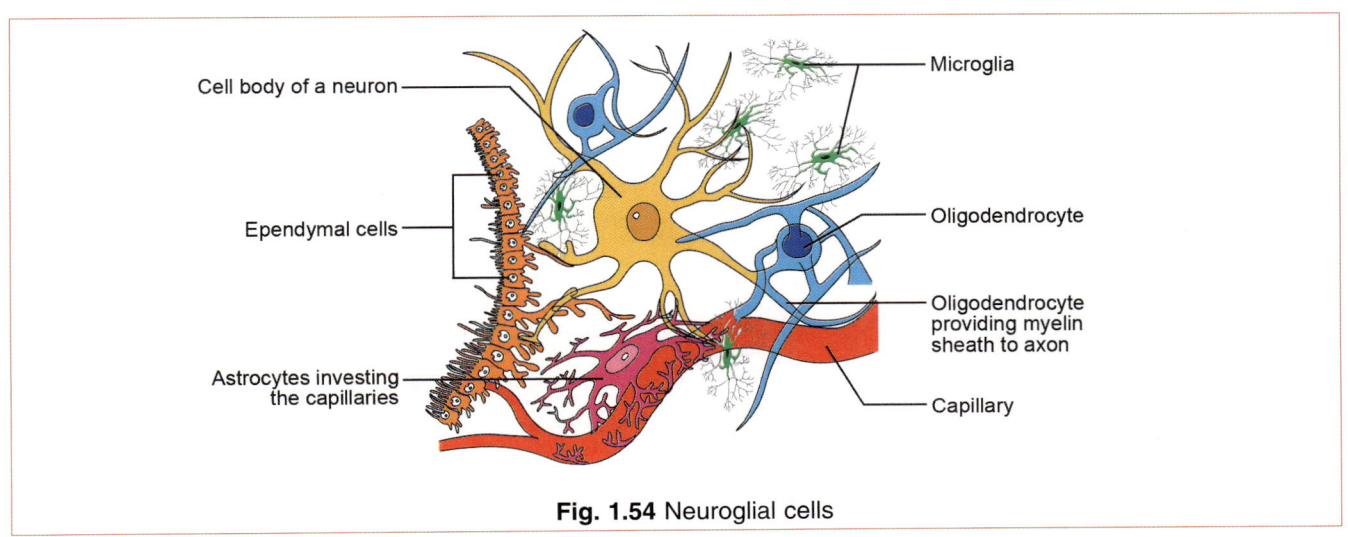

Fig. 1.54 Neuroglial cells

SECTION 1

Nerve fibre

A nerve fibre or a nerve can be defined as 'collection of cytoplasmic processes (mainly axons) of neurons'.

Myelination

- Myelination is a process in which a neuroglial cell surrounds a portion of the axons or dendrite to provide support and to facilitate the conduction of impulses.

- If the axons are covered with a myelin sheath, then the nerve is myelinated. Myelinated nerve fibres are found in peripheral nerves and in the white matter of the CNS. The grey matter of the brain and spinal cord is mostly composed of non-myelinated fibres (Fig. 1.55).

Structure of myelinated peripheral nerve fibre (inside to outside)

- **Axoplasm:** The cytoplasm of the axon, which contains neurofibrils and mitochondria.

- **Axolemma:** It is a semi permeable membrane covering the axoplasm.

- **Myelin sheath (Medullary sheath):** Myelin sheath is formed by Schwann cells in peripheral nervous system, which are arranged in linear manner along the axon. The Schwann cells undergo spiraling around the axon and deposit concentric layers of lipids and proteins. The sheath is interrupted at intervals by 'node of Ranvier' where adjacent Schwann cells meet.

- **Neurilemmal sheath:** It is the outer cell membrane of the Schwann cells. Neurilemmal sheath is absent in the nerves of central nervous system. Peripheral nerves, if damaged, may regenerate. Nerves within the CNS cannot regenerate after injury due to the absence of neurilemmal sheath and endoneurium.

- **Endoneurium:** It is the outermost connective tissue covering of the nerve fibre. The nerve fibres are grouped in fasciculi and connective tissue covering them is called 'perineurium'. A nerve consists of numerous fasciculi, which are enclosed by connective tissue membrane called 'epineurium'.

Functionally, nerves resembles electric wires. Like the electric current flowing though the wires, the impulses (sensory and motor) are conducted through the nerves.

The myelin sheath act as an insulator of nerve fibre and reduce the loss of electrical activity into the surrounding tissue by dispersion. The node of Ranvier helps in faster conduction of impulses.

Spinal nerves

- These nerves arise directly from the spinal cord.

- There are 31 pairs of spinal nerves.

- It includes 8 cervical, 12 thoracic, 5 lumbar, 5 sacral and 1 coccygeal nerves.

Formation of a typical spinal nerve

- Each spinal nerve arises from the spinal cord by two roots.

- Ventral root is motor, which arises from the anterior grey horn of the spinal cord. Dorsal root is sensory which presents a ganglion called 'dorsal root ganglion'.

- The ventral and dorsal roots join to form mixed spinal nerve trunk, which again divides into ventral and dorsal rami.

- At certain places, ventral ramus of the spinal nerves join together and branch to form nerve plexus, e.g. cervical plexus, brachial plexus, lumbar plexus, sacral plexus of nerves (Fig. 1.56).

Reflex arc

It is a neuronal pathway that controls the action reflex. A simple monosynaptic reflex pathway consists of only two

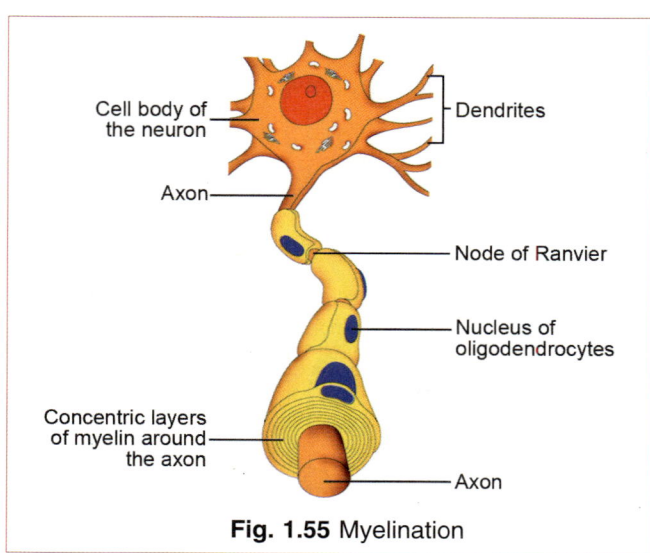

Cell body of the neuron

Dendrites

Axon

Node of Ranvier

Nucleus of oligodendrocytes

Concentric layers of myelin around the axon

Axon

Fig. 1.55 Myelination

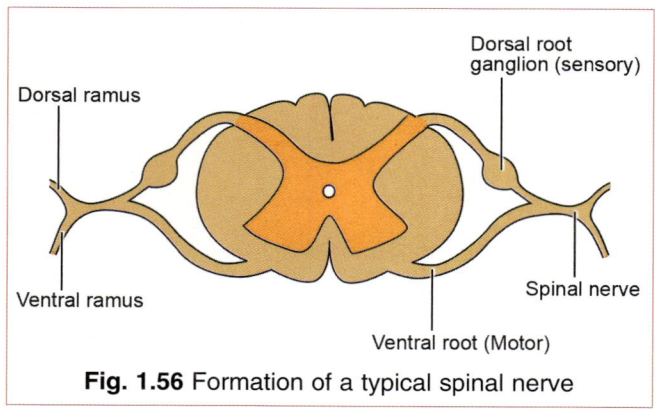

Dorsal ramus

Dorsal root ganglion (sensory)

Ventral ramus

Spinal nerve

Ventral root (Motor)

Fig. 1.56 Formation of a typical spinal nerve

neurons. For example, touching fire and reflex withdrawal of the hand. The pain fibres from the receptors in the skin is carried by neurons present in the dorsal root ganglion (afferent pathway) to the spinal cord, where it stimulates the motor neurons. The impulses from the motor neurons pass through the nerve fibres (efferent pathway) and ends in the muscle (effector organ) required to act for withdrawal of the hand. These reflex pathway do not involve brain but are mediated through the spinal cord for relatively quicker action. Hence a reflex arc has afferent and a efferent limb (Fig. 1.57).

If the reflex arc consists of more than two neurons, it is referred as polysynaptic reflex arc, e.g. light reflex.

Patellar reflex (knee jerk): When the ligamentum patellae is tapped just below the knee, the patellar reflex is initiated and the leg kicks forward (via contraction of the quadriceps). The impulses from the muscle spindle present in the quadriceps femoris muscle travels to the spinal cord via a sensory axon which chemically communicates by releasing glutamate onto the neuronal junction. These motor neurons innervates the quadriceps femoris muscle and causes its contraction, leading to extension of the leg at the knee. The sensory input from the quadriceps also activates local interneurons that release the inhibitory neurotransmitter glycine onto motor neurons, blocking the innervation of the antagonistic (hamstring) flexor muscles. The relaxation of the opposing muscle facilitates extension of the lower leg (Fig.1.59).

Some of the important terminologies used in the nervous system

1. **Nerve** is a collection of nerve fibres outside the central nervous system.

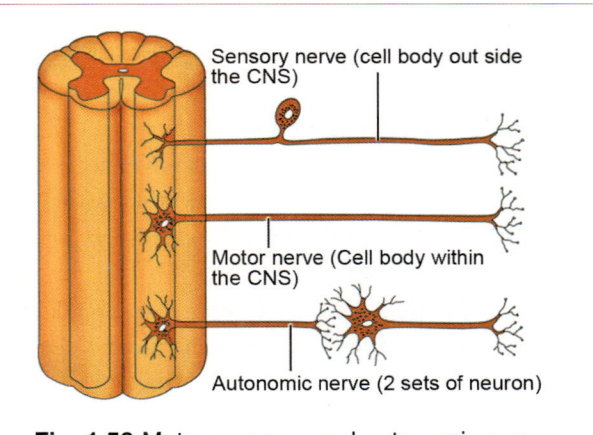

Fig. 1.58 Motor, sensory and autonomic nerves

2. **Sensory nerves** carry information from the peripheral part to the CNS, e.g. cutaneous nerve, optic nerve, vestibulo-cochlear nerve.

3. **Motor nerve** is the nerve which carries impulses from the CNS to the target structure (Fig.1.58).

4. **Grey matter** is the collection of cell bodies of neurons within the central nervous system. Such aggregation, when it is smaller in size is referred as 'nucleus' (not to be confused with nucleus of a cell).

5. **White matter** is mainly collection of nerve fibres with few supporting glial cells in the central nervous system.

6. **Ganglia** are a collection of cell bodies of neurons outside the central nervous system.

7. **Root value:** The root value of a nerve refers to its segmental origin from the spinal cord. For example, the root value of axillary nerve is C5 and C6. It means the axillary nerve is derived from fifth and sixth cervical segments of the spinal cord.

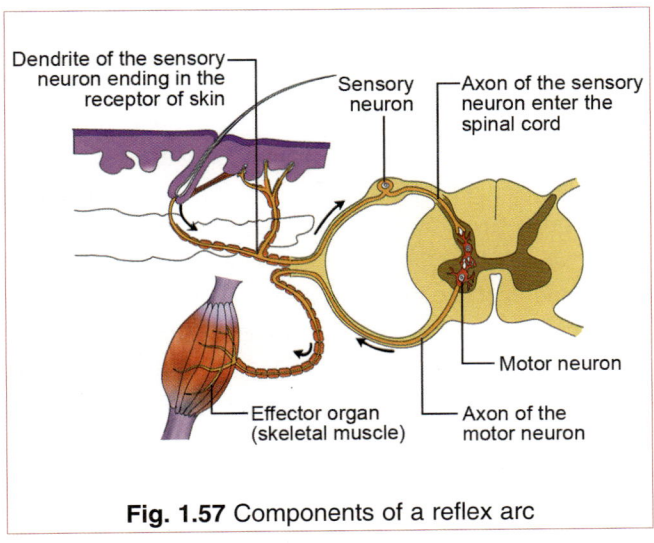

Fig. 1.57 Components of a reflex arc

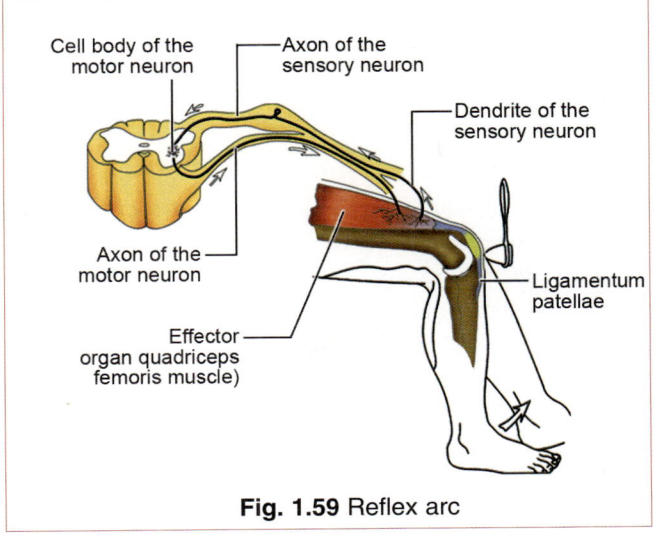

Fig. 1.59 Reflex arc

Cranial nerves

There are 12 pairs of cranial nerves that arises directly from the brain.

Following are the cranial nerves:

1. **Olfactory:** It is the first cranial nerve concerned with carrying smell sensation from the nasal cavity.

2. **Optic:** It is the second cranial nerve carrying visual impulses from retina.

3. **Occulomotor:** It is a motor nerve that supplies many extraocular muscles (muscles, which move the globe of the eye).

4. **Trochlear:** It is the fourth cranial nerve that supplies superior oblique muscle of the globe of the eye.

5. **Trigeminal:** It is the fifth cranial nerve having 3 divisions namely; ophthalmic, maxillary and mandibular. Through these branches it supplies head and neck region, having both sensory and motor distribution.

6. **Abducent:** It is the sixth cranial nerve, supplies lateral rectus muscle of the globe of the eye.

7. **Facial:** It is the seventh cranial nerve, supplies mainly the facial muscles.

8. **Vestibulocochlear:** It is the eight cranial nerve having 2 components. The vestibular component concerned with maintaining body balance and a cocchlear component which is concerned with hearing.

9. **Glossopharyngeal:** It is the ninth cranial nerve supplies sensory fibres to tongue and pharynx and also a muscle of the pharynx and parotid salivary gland.

10. **Vagus**: It is the tenth cranial nerve. Its parasympathetic fibres supply heart, lung and abdominal organs.

11. **Accessory:** It is the eleventh cranial nerve. Its fibres are distributed through vagus to supply muscles of palate, pharynx.

12. **Hypoglossal:** It is the twelfth cranial nerve, supplies muscles of the tongue.

Autonomic nervous system

Autonomic nervous system along with endocrine glands maintains the constant internal environment (both of them are under the influence of hypothalamus). The maintenance of the constant internal environment (homeostasis) is performed by regulating the body temperature, blood pressure, cardio-respiratory rate, gastro-intestinal motility and glandular secretion. They supply cardiac and smooth muscles (e.g. smooth muscles of the viscera, blood vessels, erector pylorum muscle and intrinsic muscles of the eye and many glands).

Autonomic nervous system has two components.

    a. Sympathetic

    b. Parasympathetic

Sympathetic system

Functionally this system is 'sympathetic' to the body and its nerve is considered as 'nerve of emergency'. It prepares the body for fight or flight.

The pre-ganglionic sympathetic neurons are derived from intermediate (or lateral) horn cells of all thoracic and upper two lumbar segments of the spinal cord. This is often referred as 'thoraco-lumbar outflow'.

The fibres from these neurons pass through ventral motor root of the spinal nerve, then into the mixed spinal nerve. They leave the spinal nerve and reach sympathetic ganglion by white rami communicans (pre-ganglionic) and relay in the sympathetic ganglion. It is referred white because they are slightly myelinated.

Neurons of sympathetic ganglion act as post-ganglionic neurons.

Postganglionic fibres from the sympathetic ganglion

a. Joins the spinal nerve again through grey rami communicans (post-ganglionic). This is unmyelinated.

b. Post ganglionic sympathetic fibre semerge as 'splanchnic nerves' from the ganglia. They finally reach the target structures by forming plexus around the blood vessels.

The sympathetic fibres also carry visceral pain sensation to the spinal cord through dorsal root ganglia.

Ganglionated sympathetic chain

- There are two sympathetic chains (right and left), which lie in front of the vertebral bodies (Fig. 1.60).

- They extend from the base of the skull to the first piece of coccygeal vertebra where both chains unite to form a median ganglion called 'ganglion impar'.

- Each chain presents about 22 ganglia (3 cervical, 11 thoracic, 4 lumbar and 4 sacral).

- All the thoracic and upper two lumbar sympathetic ganglia are connected with corresponding spinal nerves by both pre and post ganglionic communicants. However, other ganglia send only postganglionic communicans to the corresponding spinal nerve (hence 31 pairs of grey rami communicantes but only 14 pairs of white rami communicantes).

- Structurally the ganglia consist of multipolar neurons with supporting cells.

- Sympathetic system secretes non-adrenaline at the post-ganglionic endings.

Sensory component of the sympathetic system conveys visceral pain sensation.

Parasympathetic system

The pre-ganglionic parasympathetic neurons are located mainly in few cranial nerve nuclei and also in sacral segments of the spinal cord (**Craniosacral outflow**).

Parasympathetic fibres are distributed through third, seventh, ninth and tenth cranial nerves. The parasympathetic system liberates acetylcholine at the post-ganglionic endings.

The preganglionic parasympathetic fibres end in a ganglion (peripheral parasympathetic ganglion), which are located close to the target structure.

The preganglionic parasympathetic fibres in the occulomotor nerve relays in ciliary ganglion, of the facial nerve relays in pterygopalatine and submandibular ganglia, of the glosspharyngeal nerve relays in otic ganglion and of the vagus nerve in many unnamed ganglia located near the viscera.

The pelvic splanchnic nerve carries fibres from ventral horn cells of second to fourth sacral segments of the spinal cord. These parasympathetic fibres supply pelvic organs like urinary bladder, uterus, uterine tubes, rectum, anal canal etc.

Neurotransmitters in ANS

- Acetylcholine is liberated at all preganglionic endings of both sympathetic and parasympathetic nerves.

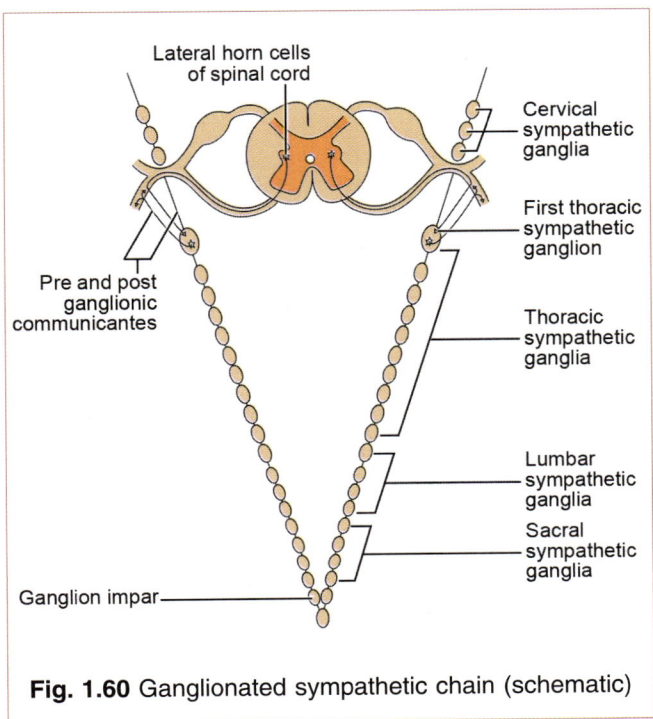

Fig. 1.60 Ganglionated sympathetic chain (schematic)

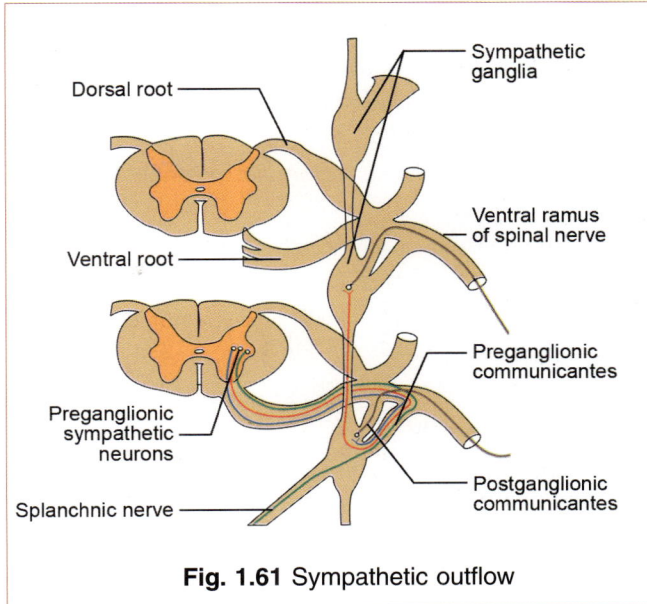

Fig. 1.61 Sympathetic outflow

- Acetylcholine is liberated at all postganglionic endings of parasympathetic nerves.

- Norepinephrine, a catecholamine, is the neurotransmitter at most sympathetic postganglionic endings. EXCEPT: sympathetic postganglionic neurons to eccrine sweat glands, and sympathetic vasodilator neurons to blood vessels in skeletal muscle which like parasympathetic secretes acetylcholine.

- Nitric oxide as their neurotransmitter in parasympathetic system for penile erection.

- Sympathetic cholinergic activation releases acetylcholine that binds to muscarinic receptors, which stimulates sweating and dilates arteries in some tissues, most notably in the skin and skeletal muscle.

Sympathetic system	Parasympathetic system
• Increase the heart rate	• Decrease the heart rate
• Bronchodilator	• Bronchoconstriction
• Generally vasoconstriction (In coronary vessels, the vessels of the skeletal muscles and external genitalia, it causes vasodilation	• Vasodilatation
• Inhibitory to GIT motility and secretion	• Stimulate the GIT motility and secretion
• Motor to sphincter of GIT	• Inhibitor to the sphincter GIT
• Dilates the pupil	• Constrict the pupil

SECTION 1

Irritation of a nerve or nerve injury

- Irritating lesions (compression) of sensory nerve result in reduced sensation (hypesthesia) or altered sensation (paresthesia).
- Destructive lesions of sensory nerve result in a loss of sensory modality.
- Irritating lesions of motor nerve result in weakness of skeletal muscle (paresis).
- Destructive lesions of motor nerve result in paralysis of skeletal muscle.

When nerves are stretched, severed or crushed, their axons degenerate distal to the lesion because they depend on the cell bodies for survival. If the axon is damaged with intact cell body, regeneration and restoration of function is possible. In crushing type of injury the connective tissue coverings of the nerve is intact, which guides the cut ends of the axons to grow to their destination. But a cutting nerve injury requires surgical intervention because regeneration of axons requires apposition of the cut ends by suture through epineurium. Compression of blood vessels supplying the nerve can also cause nerve degeneration.

CNX axons with myelin sheath formed by oligodendrocytes do not regenerate if cut. Myelinated axons in the PNS have the capacity to regenerate due to neurolemmal sheath of Schwann cells.

Demyelination: The progressive destruction of myelin sheath in the CNS and PNS, leading to a loss of sensation and motor control. Demyelination is associated with heavy metal poisoning, diphtheria and multiple sclerosis.

Neuralgia: A severe pain along the distribution of a nerve.

Neuritis is an inflammation of a nerve with neuralgia and is also associated with the loss of sensory and motor functions.

Why are neurons amitotic?

With the exception of the sensory neurons of the olfactory epithelium, human neurons in the adult brain are amitotic (do not divide), though new neurons are generated in restricted brain regions. Exactly why this is true is not known but it is generally agreed that neurons cannot divide because they have switched off much of the machinery that allows cells to divide. Cell division is a complex process that requires the precise orchestration of many cellular components. These components are largely under the control of specialized cell cycle proteins. Other proteins that are required for the full differentiation and maturation of neurons may bind and inactivate these cell cycle proteins, so perhaps a differentiated neuron cannot divide because the proteins required for cell division are "tied up" in the maintenance of a differentiated state. Why is this case? Lack of neuronal division is an evolutionarily conserved trait, so it must exist for good reasons.

One possibility is that neuronal division is logistically difficult. Neurons have many long processes that contact thousands of other neurons. Division would require complex cytoskeletal rearrangements and navigation through brain tissue that is densely packed with processes. Usually, mitotic cells have a simple shape to avoid these issues.

Another possible reason that neurons are amitotic is the need for relative stability of networks in the brain. The output of the brain can be modified by changing the way the neurons are connected, a process known as plasticity. Plasticity tends to be high early in life but low later in life; for example, learning a language is quick and effortless when you are young but slow and difficult later. If neurons divided, the brain might be too plastic and the resulting instability could interfere with important behaviors.

MCQs

1. Which of the following processes requires energy (ATP) for movement across the cell membrane?
   A. Osmosis
   B. Phagocytosis
   C. Diffusion
   D. None of the above

2. Which of the following is/are not a cell junction/s?
   A. Zonula occludens
   B. Desmosome
   C. Zonula adherens
   D. Centrosomes

3. Which of the following structures is known to maintain the shape of a cell?
   A. Nucleus
   B. Mitochondria
   C. Microtubules
   D. Ribosomes

4. When the two arms of the chromatid are in equal length, the chromosome is called
   A. Metacentric chromosome

B. Acrocentric chromosome
C. Telocentric chromosome
D. None of the above

5. Which of the following syndromes is associated with presence of an extra X- chromosome?

    A. Cri-du-chat syndrome
    B. Down's syndrome
    C. Klinefelter's syndrome
    D. Turner's syndrome

6. Which of the following stages of mitosis involves splitting of chromosomes?

    A. Telophase
    B. Anaphase
    C. Metaphase
    D. Prophase

7. The shortest stage of mitotic cell division is

    A. Anaphase
    B. Prophase
    C. Telophase
    D. Metaphase

8. In karyotyping, chromosomes are identified in

    A. Telophase stage
    B. Prophase stage
    C. Anaphase stage
    D. Metaphase stage

9. In which of the following stages of the meiotic division does "crossing over" of the chromosome occur?

    A. Leptotene
    B. Zygotene
    C. Pachytene
    D. Diplotene

10. Alveoli of the lungs are lined by

    A. Simple squamous epithelium
    B. Simple cuboidal epithelium
    C. Simple columnar epithelium
    D. Pseudostratified columnar epithelium

11. Transitional epithelium lines

    A. Mucous membrane of the stomach
    B. Epidermis of the skin
    C. Mucous membrane of the trachea
    D. Mucosa of the urinary bladder

12. The secretory unit of the mammary gland is an example for

    A. Compound tubulo-alveolar gland
    B. Compound alveolar gland
    C. Compound tubular gland
    D. Simple alveolar gland

13. The gland in which the entire cell is discharged during secretion is called

    A. Merocrine gland
    B. Holocrine gland
    C. Apocrine gland
    D. None of the above

14. Which of the following cells are responsible for synthesis of collagen fibres?

    A. Fibroblasts
    B. Lymphocytes
    C. Plasma cells
    D. Macrophages

15. Which of the following sentences is incorrect regarding the collagen fibres?

    A. They are formed by fibroblasts
    B. They consist of a protein called 'collagen'
    C. The individual fibres branch and anastamose
    D. Tendon of the muscle is made up of collagen fibres

16. Which of the following cells are involved in phagocytosis?

    A. Reticular cells
    B. Mast cells
    C. Histiocytes
    D. Plasma cells

17. Mast cells are involved in

    A. Production of antibodies
    B. Production of histamine
    C. Phagocytosis
    D. Wound healing

18. Myxomatous tissue is found in

    A. Vitreous body of the eye
    B. Lymphatic organs
    C. Bone marrow
    D. Mesenteries

19. Which of the following structures is made up of elastic cartilage?

    A. Costal cartilage
    B. Thyroid cartilage
    C. Tracheal rings
    D. Pinna of the external ear

20. Which of the following statements is incorrect regarding hyaline cartilage?

    A. It is highly vascular
    B. It is made up of collagen fibres
    C. It can ossify to form a bone
    D. Its matrix is homogenous

21. Intervertebral disc is an example for
    A. Hyaline cartilage
    B. Spongy bone
    C. Elastic cartilage
    D. Fibrocartilage

22. Following are the examples for fibrocartilage except
    A. Glenoidal labrum
    B. Epiglottis
    C. Menisci of the knee joint
    D. Intervertebral discs

23. Which of the following bones is an example for pneumatic bone?
    A. Parietal bone
    B. Mandible
    C. Hyoid bone
    D. Maxilla

24. Following are the sesamoid bones except
    A. Malleus
    B. Fabella
    C. Pisiform
    D. Patella

25. The part of the long bone developed from secondary center of ossification is called
    A. Epiphysis
    B. Diaphysis
    C. Metaphysis
    D. None of the above

26. Which of the following statements is incorrect regarding the compact bone?
    A. Lamellae are made up of collagen fibres
    B. Osteocytes are present between the lamellae
    C. Lamellae with Haversian canal constitute an osteon
    D. Volkmann's canals are placed parallel to the medullary cavity

27. Which of the following bones is an example for dermal bone?
    A. Femur
    B. Hip bone
    C. Clavicle
    D. Humerus

28. Which of the following bones violates the laws of ossification?
    A. Tibia
    B. Fibula
    C. Radius
    D. Ulna

29. Which of the following statements is incorrect regarding the structure of a skeletal muscle?
    A. The dark band is the area where the actin and myosin filaments overlap each other.
    B. Only myosin filaments occupy the light band
    C. The H band traverse the middle of the dark band
    D. The Z line is in the middle of light band

30. Which of the following muscles is an example for bipennate muscle?
    A. Middle fibres of deltoid
    B. Rectus femoris
    C. Palmar interossei
    D. Flexor carpi ulnaris

31. The inferior tibiofibular joint is an example for
    A. Primary cartilaginous joint
    B. Syndesmosis
    C. Gomphosis
    D. Secondary cartilaginous joint

32. Which of the following joints is an example for pivot variety of synovial joint?
    A. Atlanto-occipital joint
    B. Elbow joint
    C. Ankle joint
    D. None of the above

33. Which of the following arteries is an example of an end artery?
    A. Superficial palmar arch
    B. Mesenteric artery
    C. Central artery of retina
    D. None of the above

34. Which of the following structures is an example for a lymphatic vessel?
    A. Thoracic duct
    B. Bile duct
    C. Cystic duct
    D. Parotid duct

35. Following are the lymphatic organs except
    A. Spleen
    B. Thymus
    C. Thyroid gland
    D. Palatine tonsil

36. The internal elastic lamina is well defined in
    A. Medium sized vein
    B. Large vein
    C. Medium sized artery
    D. Large sized artery

37. The wall of the large artery mainly consists of
    A. Collagen fibres
    B. Elastic fibres
    C. Smooth muscles
    D. Reticular tissue

38. Unipolar neurons are found in
    A. Mesencephalic nucleus
    B. Spiral ganglion
    C. Sympathetic ganglion
    D. Vestibular ganglion

39. Which of the following cells in CNS are phagocytic in function?
    A. Oligodendrocytes
    B. Astrocytes
    C. Schwann cells
    D. Microglial cells

40. Collection of cell bodies of the neurons outside the central nervous system is called
    A. Nucleus
    B. Ganglion
    C. Grey matter
    D. White matter

41. The neuroglial cells that form myelin sheaths in the peripheral nervous system are
    A. Astrocytes
    B. Schwann cells
    C. Microglial cells
    D. Oligodendrocytes

42. Neurotransmitters are stored in synaptic vesicles within the
    A. Sarcolemma
    B. Motor units
    C. Axon terminals
    D. Myofibrils

43. Muscles capable of highly dexterous movements contain
    A. One motor unit per muscle fibre
    B. Many muscle fibres per motor unit
    C. Few muscle fibers per motor unit
    D. Many motor units per muscle fibre

44. The site at which a nerve impulse is transmitted from the motor nerve ending to the skeletal muscle is the
    A. Sarcomere
    B. Neuromuscular junction
    C. Myofilament
    D. Z line

45. An interosseus ligament is characteristic of
    A. Suture
    B. Synchondrosis
    C. Symphysis
    D. Syndesmosis

46. Specialised bone cells that reabsorb bone tissue are
    A. Osteoblasts
    B. Osteocytes
    C. Osteons
    D. Osteoclasts

47. Cardiac muscle fibre does not have
    A. Striations
    B. Intercalated discs
    C. Property of rhythmical contractions
    D. Peripheral nucleus

48. Cartilage is slow in healing following an injury because
    A. It is non-living
    B. It is avascular
    C. Its chondrocytes cannot reproduce
    D. It has a semisolid matrix

49. The organelle that combines proteins and carbohydrates and stores them for secretion is the
    A. Golgi apparatus
    B. Rough endoplasmic reticulum
    C. Smooth endoplasmic reticulum
    D. Ribosomes

50. The phase of mitosis in which the chromosomes line up at the equator of the cell is called
    A. Prophase
    B. Metaphase
    C. Anaphase
    D. Telophase

51. Which of these organelles contains strong hydrolytic enzymes?
    A. Lysosome
    B. Golgi apparatus
    C. Ribosome
    D. Mitochondria

52. Layers or aggregations of similar cells that perform specific functions are called
    A. Organelle
    B. Tissue
    C. Organ
    D. Gland

53. The abdominal region superior to the umbilical region is called
    A. Hypochondriac region
    B. Epigastric region
    C. Pelvic region
    D. Inguinal region

SECTION 1

54. Most of the arteries in the body contain oxygen-rich blood with the exception of
    A. Aorta
    B. Renal arteries
    C. Pulmonary arteries
    D. Coronary arteries

55. Nissl bodies corresponds to which of the following cytoplasmic organelles?
    A. Golgi apparatus
    B. Mitochondria
    C. Nucleoli
    D. Rough endoplasmic reticulum
    E. Smooth endoplasmic reticulum

Answers to MCQs

1. B
2. D
3. C
4. A
5. C
6. B
7. A
8. D
9. C
10. A
11. D
12. B
13. B
14. A
15. C
16. C
17. B
18. A
19. D
20. A
21. D
22. B
23. D
24. A
25. A
26. D
27. C
28. B
29. B
30. B
31. B
32. D
33. C
34. A
35. C
36. C
37. B
38. A
39. D
40. B
41. B
42. C
43. C
44. B
45. D
46. D
47. D
48. B
49. A
50. B
51. A
52. B
53. B
54. C
55. D

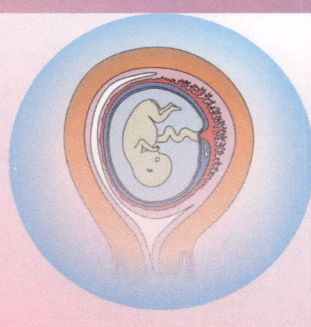

General Embryology

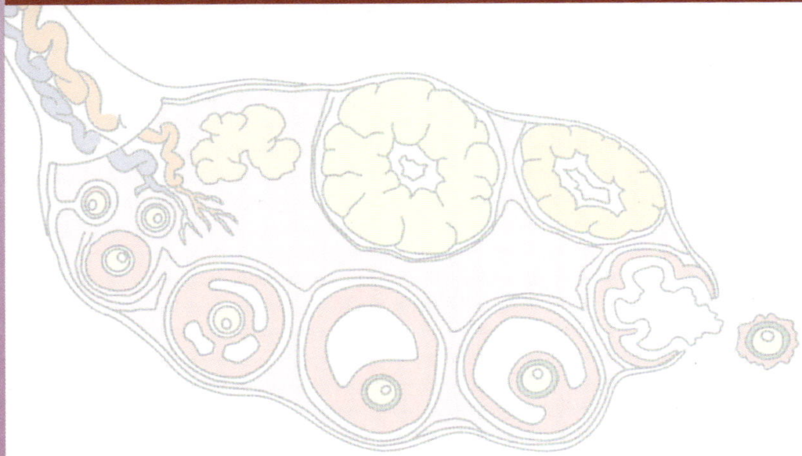

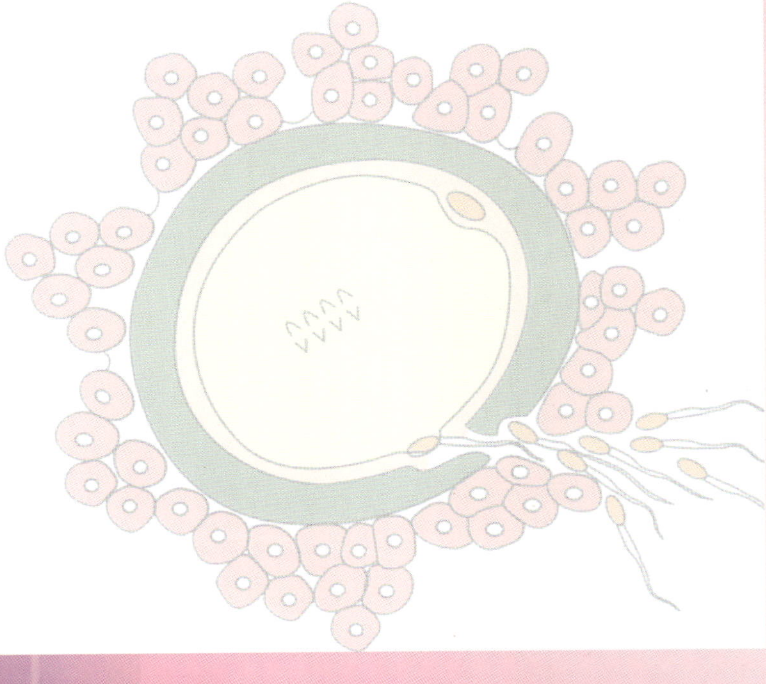

General Embryology

2

- Gametogenesis
- Fertilization
- Development during 2nd week
- Development during 3rd and 4th week
- Formation of neural tube
- Placenta
- Teratology and prenatal diagnosis
- MCQs

Objectives

- To explain the formation, maturation of germ cells and to understand the cyclical changes taking place in the ovary and the uterus
- To explain the steps involved in fertilization, transport of zygote, its cleavage division and implantation
- To list the important events taking place during second week of development
- To explain the process of gastrulation, neurulation and their defects
- To explain the formation, structure and functions of placenta
- To list the major teratogenic agents and their effect on embryo and to know the prenatal diagnosis available to detect birth defects.

What is embryology?

It deals with the study of prenatal stages of development. The series of dynamic events unfolding from the time of fertilization to the birth of a new individual is very interesting.

The time of prenatal development or the time of pregnancy is called 'gestation' period. The human gestation period is usually 266 days or 280 days from the beginning of the last menstrual period to parturition or childbirth. The transformation of a zygote (fertilized product) into a multicellular organism involves series of events that includes cell division, growth, differentiation, cell migration and also folding of embryo.

Students must be familiar with some of the terminologies used in embryology, which includes

Embryo – First 2 months of development

Foetus – From 3rd month to birth

Infant – After birth upto 1 year

Neonatal period: It extends from birth to the end of four weeks.

Period of embryogenesis: First 8 weeks of human development.

Foetal period: From 8 weeks of intrauterine development to birth.

Infancy: The period of infancy begins from the end of the neonatal period at 4 weeks until 2 years of age.

Childhood: Childhood is the period of growth and development extending from infancy to adolescence, at which time puberty begins.

Scope and relevance of learning embryology

- It is helpful in understanding the adult anatomy and congenital anomalies.
- Understanding of human development resulted in development of new techniques for prenatal diagnosis and treatments.
- It has opened new avenues of therapeutic procedures to problems of infertility.
- The research in the field of embryology has developed many tools to prevent birth defects

GAMETOGENESIS

Anatomy of the male genital tract

The male gonads are testes, which are suspended in the scrotum. The mature male gametes are called spermatozoa (sperms) which are formed inside the seminiferous tubules of the testes after puberty. These sperms move into the efferent ductules (about 15 to 20) which emerge from the upper pole of the testes. These efferent ductules join to form the duct of the epididymis which is about 6 meters in length. The tail of the epididymis continues as vas deferens. The vas deferens is about 45 cm in length, which ascends along the posterior border of the testis, inguinal canal, and then lateral pelvic wall. The terminal end of the vas deferens joins with duct of the seminal vesicle to form ejaculatory duct, which opens into the prostatic urethra (Fig. 2.1).

Spermatogenesis

This is a process of formation of sperms within the seminiferous tubules of the testes. At birth, the seminiferous tubules are lined by primordial germ cells and supporting cells. At puberty, they acquire a lumen and primordial germ cells gives rise to spermatogonial stem cells (Fig. 2.2).

- The primordial germ cells divide by mitosis to give spermatogonia, which again undergo repeated mitotic divisions to give more spermatogonia.

- After four generations of division, the spermatogonia gives rise to primary spermatocytes, which has 46 chromosomes (44 autosomes + XY sex chromosomes)

- The primary spermatocytes undergo 1st meiotic division to produce 2 daughter cells called 'secondary spermatocytes' each having 23 chromosomes (haploid number). One secondary spermatocyte having 22 autosomes and an X chromosome, and the other having 22 autosomes and a Y chromosome.

- The secondary spermatocytes immediately complete the 2nd meiotic division to produce spermatids. Therefore each primary spermatocytes produces 4 spermatids, two of them having X chromosomes and two of them having Y chromosomes.

- The spermatids are then metamorphosed into spermatozoa, which does not involve any further cell division. This part of the spermatogenesis is called 'spermiogenesis'.

Spermiogenesis: This is a process by which a spermatid gets transformed into a spermatozoon (Fig. 2.3).

- The Golgi apparatus join together to form a cap over the nucleus called 'acrosomal cap', which covers the 2/3rd of the nucleus.

- The nucleus having all the chromosomes forms the 'Head' of the spermatozoon.

- The proximal centriole gives axial filaments of the body and tail of the spermatozoon.

- The distal centriole forms the ring centriole (annulus) at the junction of body and tail.

- All the mitochondria arrange spirally around the body (middle piece).

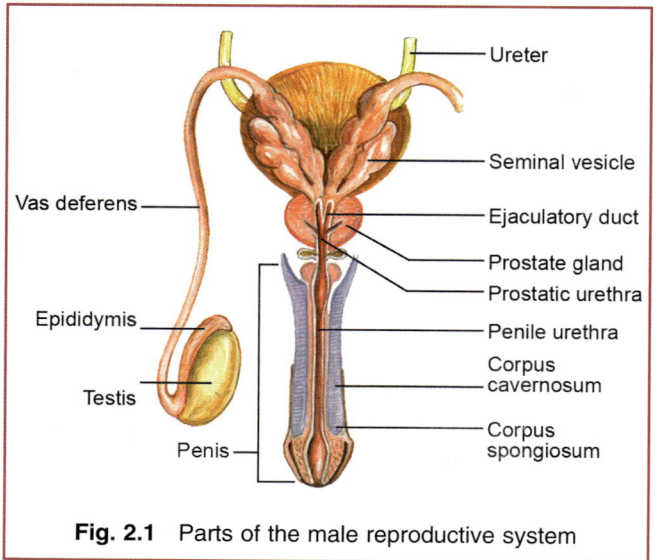

Fig. 2.1 Parts of the male reproductive system

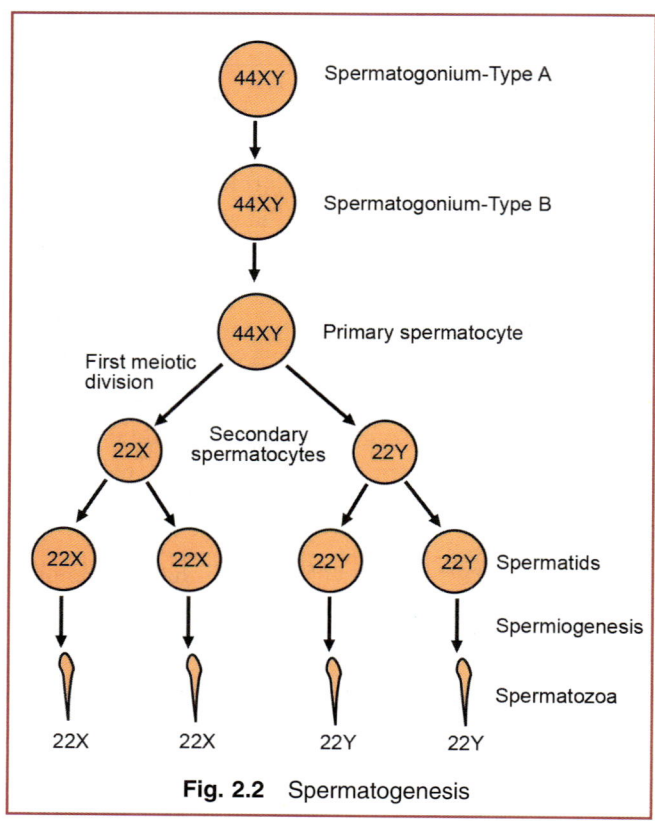

Fig. 2.2 Spermatogenesis

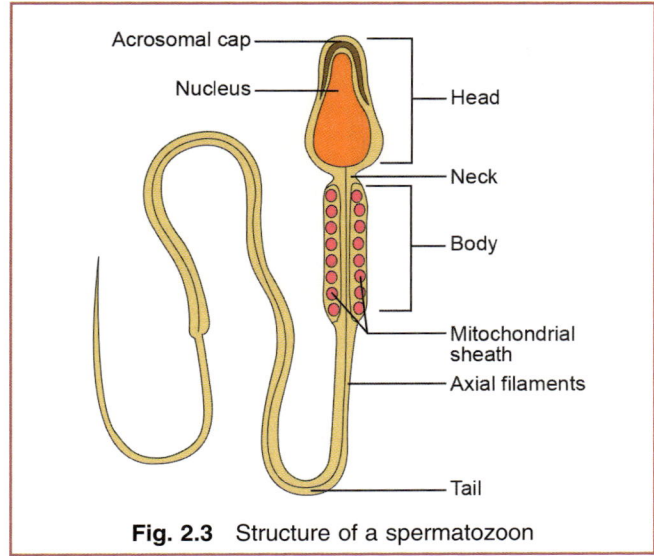

Fig. 2.3   Structure of a spermatozoon

The process of conversion of type A spermatogonia to the spermatozoa requires approximately 74 days under the influence of LH and testosterone.

Structure of Spermatozoan

A mature spermatozoon measures about 50 microns in total length. It has a head, neck, body (middle piece) and a tail (principal piece) (Fig. 2.3).

Head: The head is formed from nucleus and measures about 4 microns in length and has 23 chromosomes. Only the anterior 2/3rd is covered by acrosomal cap, but entire head is covered by a cell membrane.

Neck: The neck is about 0.3 microns in length. It connects the head with the body.

Body: The body is cylindrical shaped measuring about 4 microns in length. It consists of axial filaments in the centre, surrounded by a spirally arranged sheath of mitochondria and outside by a cell membrane.

Tail: The tail is about 40 micron in length having axial filaments in the centre surrounded by a fibrous sheath and further outside by a cell membrane. The terminal portion of the tail where the fibrous sheath is absent is known as 'end piece'.

Semen: It is a whitish or grey coloured liquid excreted from male urethra during ejaculation. The seminal fluid contains spermatozoa, secretion from seminal vesicle, prostate and bulbourethral glands. About 2 to 5 ml of semen ejaculated consists of 200 to 300 million sperms.

The seminal vesicles produce a yellowish viscous fluid rich in fructose and other substances that make up about 70% of human semen. Seminal vesicle fluid is alkaline, resulting in human semen having a mild alkaline pH prolonging the life span of sperms. The alkalinity of semen helps to neutralize the acidity of the vaginal tract.

The prostatic secretion, influenced by dihydrotestosterone, is a whitish (sometimes clear), thin fluid containing proteolytic enzymes, citric acid, zinc, acid phosphatase and lipids. The bulbourethral glands secrete a clear secretion into the lumen of the urethra to lubricate it.

The fertilizing capacity of the sperms persists up to 24 to 48 hours after ejaculation in the female genital tract.

If the concentration of spermatozoa in the semen is less than 20 million, the individual is usually infertile.

Oligospermia: The normal sperm count is 20 to 120 million/milliliter. Oligospermia is a term referring to very few live sperms (less than 20 million sperms per milliliter/ejaculation).

Azoospermia: It is a condition where there is absence of any measurable level of sperms in the semen. It is characterized by very low levels of fertility or even sterility. In humans, azoospermia affects about 1% of the male population and may be seen in 20% of male infertility cases.

Anatomy of the female genital tract

Female gonads are called ovaries, which are placed in the pelvic cavity. The mature female gametes are called 'Ova'. In every ovarian cycle (cyclical changes occurring inside the ovary), an ovum is shed from the ovary and this process is called 'ovulation'. The ovum which is shed into the peritoneal cavity is received by the uterine tube. The ovum traverses the uterine tube. The fertilization normally occurs at the ampulla of the uterine tube. The fertilized product proceeds medially in the uterine tube towards the uterus. The implantation of the fertilized product occurs in the uterus where it grows till parturition.

Primitive sex cells

There are interesting differences between the number and maturation of primitive sex cells in males and females. In females at 5th month of intrauterine life, there are about 6 to 7 millions of oogonia in the ovary. Their number is reduced to 2 millions at birth. At the time of birth, the primary oocytes have started prophase of meiosis-I and enter the **diplotene stage**. The size of the primary oocyte at birth is about 135 μ in diameter. The primary oocytes remain arrested in **prophase** and do not finish their first meiotic division until puberty is reached. At puberty the number is further reduced to 40,000 oocytes. During reproductive period (about 30 years from puberty to menopause) about 400 oocytes will be liberated alternatively from the right and left ovaries respectively.

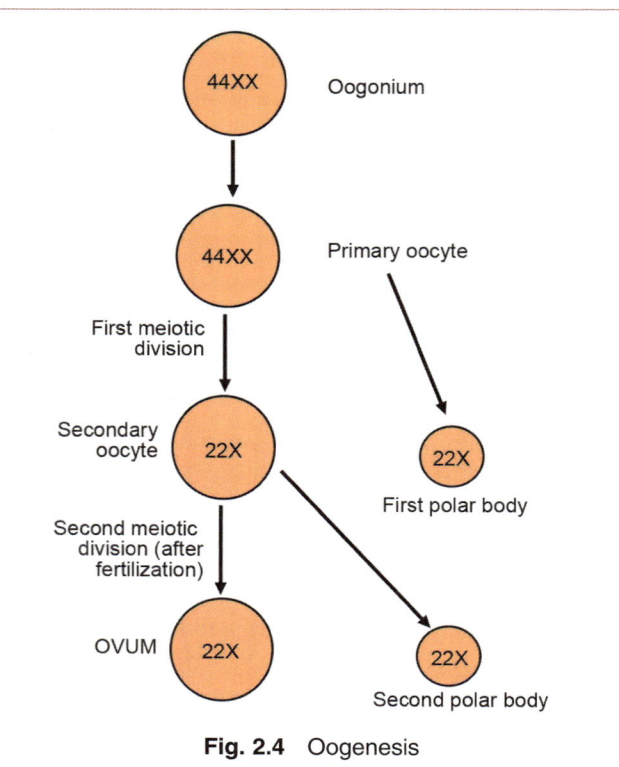

Fig. 2.4 Oogenesis

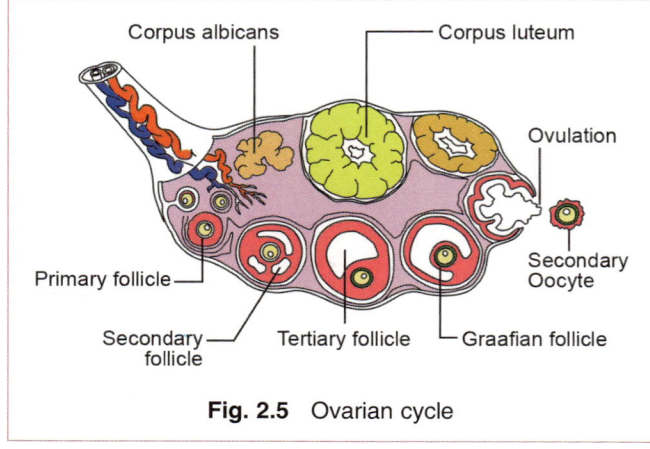

Fig. 2.5 Ovarian cycle

Oogenesis

• It is the process of maturation of primary oocyte to mature ovum by a process of meiotic cell division (Fig. 2.4)

• The primary oocyte undergoes first meiotic division (reduction of chromosome number to half) to form secondary oocyte which has 22X chromosomes and a first polar body.

• This division is unequal so that greater volume of cytoplasm passes into secondary oocyte (Fig. 2.4).

• This secondary oocyte further undergoes second meiotic division to give rise to 'mature ovum' which is having 22X chromosomes and second polar body. Hence one primary oocyte will produce only one ovum.

• During ovulation the secondary oocyte is shed from the ovary. The second meiotic division is completed only if fertilization takes place.

Ovarian cycle

The cyclical changes occurring in the ovary, which involves maturation of primordial follicle to Graafian follicle, ovulation and also formation of corpus luteum is referred as 'ovarian follicle (Fig. 2.5).

Formation of Ovarian follicle

1. Primordial follicle: These follicles are more numerous before puberty. Each consists of a primary oocyte (most

in deplotene stage of meiosis I prophase) surrounded by one layer of squamous cells.

2. During maturation of female germ cells (primary oocyte to ova) the stromal cells of the ovary provide a protective coat outside them.

3. Growing follicles: During follicle growth (under the influence of FSH from pituitary), the oocyte enlarges to a diameter of 125 to 150 μm.

a. Primary follicles: It consists of primary oocyte surrounded by single or multiple layers of cuboidal follicle cells. They have no antrum. A glycoprotein rich layer called '**Zona pellucida**' is formed between oocyte and follicular cells.

b. Secondary follicles: During this stage cavities filled with fluid (liquor folliculi) appear between the follicle cells. These cavities gradually join each other to form a large cavity, or antrum. The follicular cells differentiate to form inner cellular layer called 'theca interna' and an outer fibrous layer called 'theca externa'. The cells of the theca interna secrete 'oestrogen'.

4. Mature follicle (Graafian follicle): It differs from secondary follicle by its large diameter (2.5 cm). At this stage the primary oocyte completes 1st meiotic division. The oocyte then enters meiosis II but arrests in metaphase approximately 3 hours before ovulation.

5. Atretic follicles: Of the 400,000 follicles present at birth, approximately 450 develop to maturity during entire reproductive life. More than 99% become atretic at various stages. Atresia of the primary follicle does not leave any space and is filled with stroma. Autolytic remnants of larger primary and secondary follicles are removed by macrophages and are replaced by wavy collagenous scar, which is also gradually replaced by stromal cells. Some thecal cells from the atretic follicles may remain, becoming interstitial cells that secrete steroids specially androgens.

6. **Corpus luteum:** It is formed by the remnant of the graafian follicle after ovulation. The cells of the Graafian follicle enlarge and accumulate yellow pigments called 'lutein'. Corpus luteum is formed under the influence of LH from anterior pituitary. It secretes 'PROGESTERONE' and small amount of oestrogen, which is required for maintenance of integrity of uterine endometrium. and prepare the uterus for the reception and nourishment of fertilized ovum.

Corpus luteum of menstruation: In the absence of fertilization, the corpus luteum persists for only 12 to 14 days and gets transformed into 'corpus albicans'. The degeneration of corpus luteum results in sudden withdrawal of progesterone from circulating blood. This results in loss of integrity of uterine endometrium and initiates the menstrual bleeding.

Corpus luteum of pregnancy: In case of pregnancy, the corpus luteum persists for 6 months. In addition to oestrogen and progesterone, the corpus luteum, also produces 'relaxin' a polypeptide hormone, which relaxes pubic symphysis, allowing the birth canal to enlarge during parturition.

Ovulation

It is the process of rupture of the Graafian follicle with the liberation of secondary oocyte from ovary. It occurs approximately 14 days before the onset of next menstrual bleeding. It is due to the increased secretion of LH from the anterior pituitary. During ovulation some women feel a slight pain, known as middle pain (it normally occurs near the middle of the menstrual cycle). Ovulation is generally characterized by a rise in basal body temperature. Some women fail to ovulate because of low concentration of gonadotropins. Administration of agents stimulating gonadotropin release would help but can cause multiple ovulation

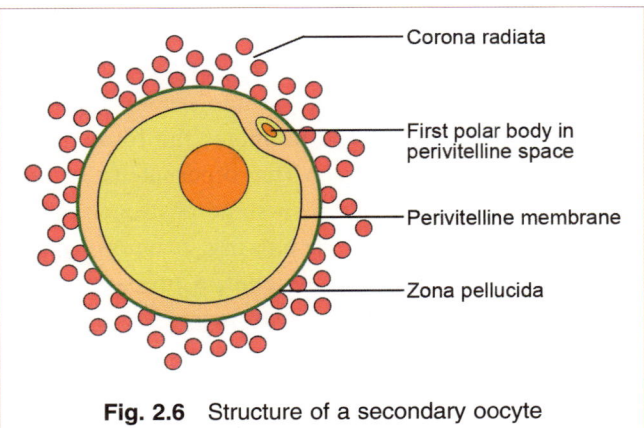

Fig. 2.6   Structure of a secondary oocyte

Primordial germ cells are formed from epiblast during 2nd week and migrate to the wall of the yolk sac. From here, they migrate to the gonadal ridge during 4th week. Abnormal migration of germ cells during embryogenesis can cause extragonadal germ cell tumours (example: **germ cell tumours of the mediastinum**)

Structure of the Secondary Oocyte

• It is about 140 micron in diameter (Fig. 2.6)
• The cell membrane is known as the vitelline membrane, which is enveloped by zona pellucida.
• The perivitelline space accommodates the first polar body.
• The nucleus is eccentric in position and contains 23 chromosomes.
• The cytoplasm of the oocyte is known as yolk (deutoplasm).
• Granulosa cells radiates from the zona pellucida.

Uterine/Menstrual Cycle

The periodic structural change of the endometrium of uterus during the reproductive life is known as uterine or menstrual cycle. The cycle is counted from 1st day of menstrual bleeding to the first day of next menstrual bleeding, on an average the cycle is repeated at an interval of 28 days. Hormones liberated from the ovary during ovarian cycle regulate the various phases of menstrual cycle. The menstrual cycle is divided into the following phases (Fig. 2.7).

1. **Proliferative phase (day 4 to 13):** In this phase the thickness of the endometrium is about 1–2 mm. The lining epithelium is low cuboidal. The uterine glands are straight and narrow, lined by low columnar cells. The stroma is dense with lymphocytes. During day 11 and 12 of proliferative phase, under the influence of increased oestrogen level, cells multiply (in stroma as well as uterine glands)

2. **Secretory phase (day 14 to 28):** It corresponds with luteal phase of ovarian cycle, hence is under the influence of progesterone and oestrogen of corpus luteum. During early secretory phase, glycogen masses accumulate in cells of uterine glands and lining epithelium. By the mid-secretory phase the endometrium may be up to 6 mm deep. There is a notable stromal oedema and a corresponding decrease in the density of collagen fibres. In the late secretory phase, the glandular secretory activity declines. The endometrium of mid and late secretory phase can be divided into

i. Stratum compactum, where uterine glands are slightly expanded

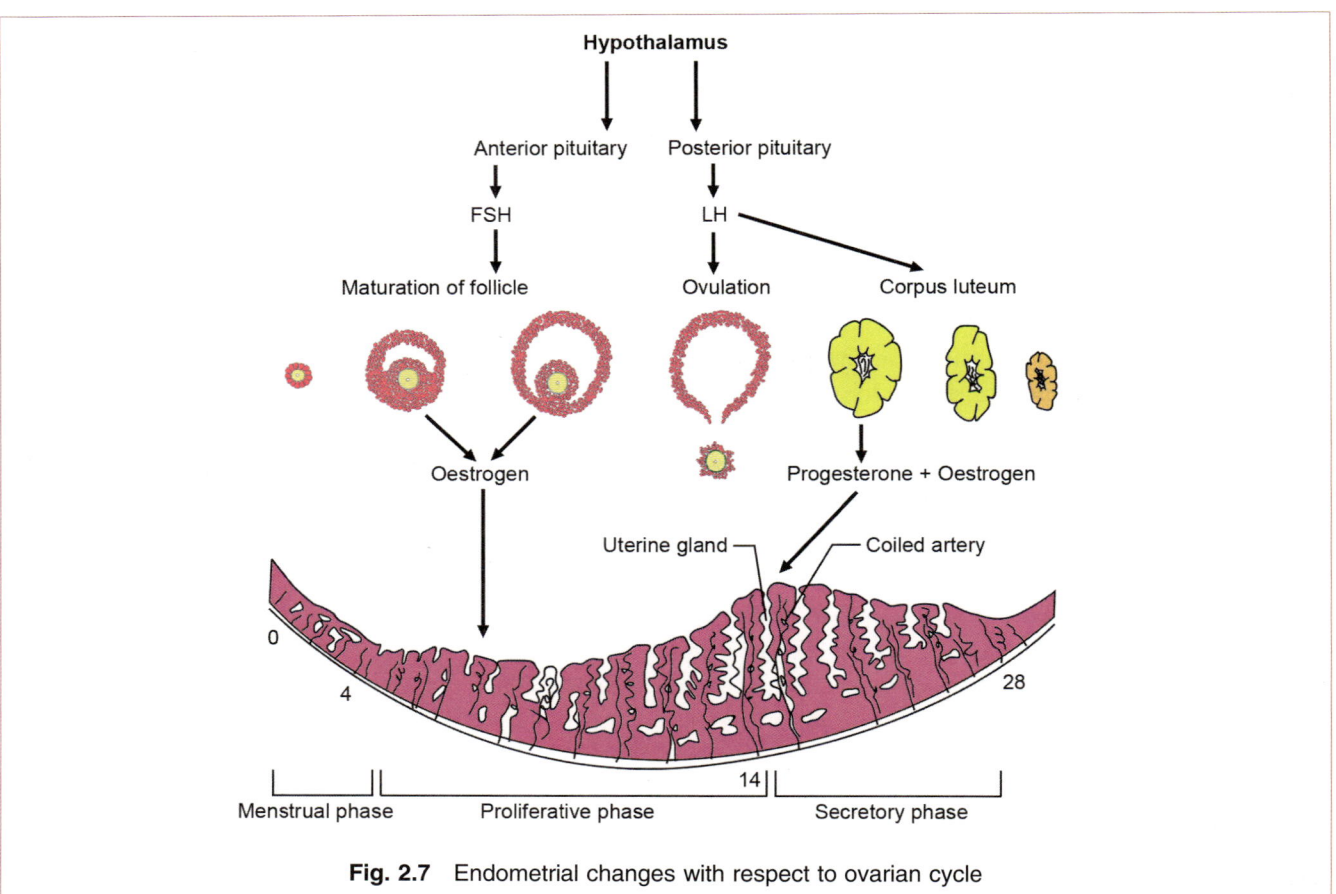

Fig. 2.7 Endometrial changes with respect to ovarian cycle

ii. Stratum spongiosum, where uterine glands are tortuous and dilated

iii. Stratum basale consists of unaltered stroma

The secretory phase of uterine cycle is mainly characterized by thick endometrium (5–7 mm in thickness), **saw-toothed appearance of uterine glands and spiral arteries**.

3. **Menstrual phase:** With the regression of corpus luteum, stratum compactum and stratum spongiosum undergo degenerative changes and endometrium diminishes in thickness. The spiral arteries become more coiled and the circulation through them diminishes. Vasoconstriction affects the spiral arteries, one by one, so that endometrium is blanched. This is followed by dilatation of the arteries and the blood escapes through the damaged capillaries with detachment of small pieces of endometrium (Stratum compactum and spongiosum). The blood escaped from the capillaries form haematoma beneath the epithelia. Stratum functionalis is shed in piecemeal, leaving stratum basale intact. The blood usually does not clot because of fibrinolytic enzymes which prevents coagulation. The average amount of blood loss is about 50 to 60 ml/cycle.

Hormonal control in ovarian and menstrual cycle

The cyclic changes occurring inside the ovary and the endometrium of the uterus is under the influence of hormones secreted from the anterior pituitary. The follicular stimulating hormone (FSH) promotes the maturation of the ovarian follicles inside the ovary. The growing and matured follicles within the ovary secrete oestrogen and progesterone. Prior to ovulation, the oestrogen level of blood is increased, which inhibits the secretion of FSH from the pituitary. At the same time oestrogen stimulates the secretion of luteinizing hormone (LH) from the anterior pituitary. The LH surge is important for conversion of primary oocyte into secondary oocyte and also ovulation. The LH promotes the formation of corpus luteum inside the ovary. The corpus luteum secretes progesterone hormone and also some oestrogen. These hormones intensify the repairing process of the endometrium by making it thicker, a preparation for bedding the fertilized ovum. With regression of corpus luteum, the progesterone level in circulating blood is reduced, which causes disintegration of uterine endometrium in the form of menstrual bleeding.

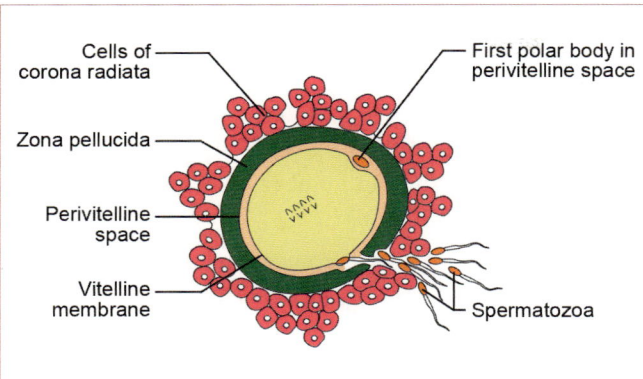

Fig. 2.8   Barriers for sperm around the secondary oocyte

The contraceptive pill prevents the release of FSH and LH from anterior pituitary. The pills are taken for 21 days and then stopped for menstruation to occur. This is called as withdrawl bleeding.

FERTILIZATION

It is a process by which male and female gametes fuse, which normally occur at the ampulla of the uterine tube.

The mechanism of fertilization can be studied under three headings.

1. **Approximation of gametes:** The sperm deposited in the vagina enter the cervix and then into the uterine tube by its own propulsion, which is assisted by movements of fluids created by cilia. It is also said that prostaglandin of the semen and oxytocin released during coitus in female partner induces contraction of uterine musculature. The vacuum created in the uterine cavity in between the successive contraction aspirates the sperms to uterine tube along with the secretion of uterine glands. It requires 2 to 7 hours for sperms to reach the uterine tube. Only 300 to 500 sperms will reach the site of fertilization out of 200 to 300 million sperms ejaculated.

   The transport of secondary oocyte from the ovary to uterine tube is assisted by fimbriae of the uterine tube and further its movement towards ampulla of the tube by ciliary beats of uterine tube epithelium and also rhythmical contraction of musculature of uterine tube. The chemoattractants produced by the cumulus cells surrounding the oocyte also helps in approximation of the male and female gametes.

   Out of 200 to 300 sperms present at the site of fertilization, only one sperm unites with the oocyte. The remaining sperms are involved in disintegrating the

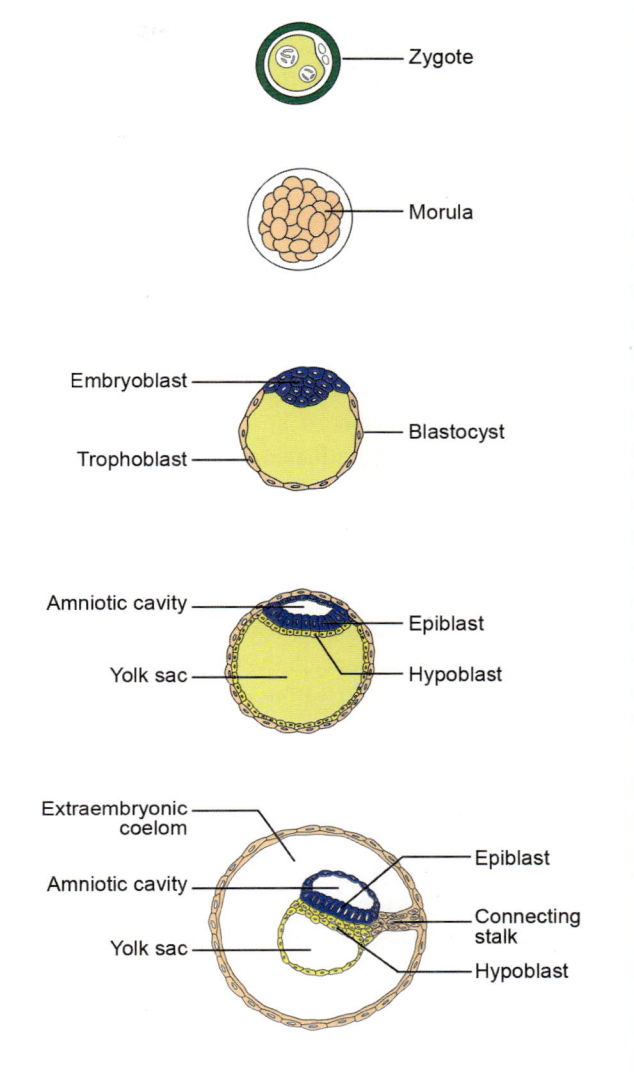

Fig. 2.9   Cleavage and formation of bilaminar germ disc

corona radiata by an enzyme 'hyaluronidase' secreted by the acrosomal cap of sperms. After disintegrating the corona radiata, the sperm has to break two more barriers, the zona pellucida and the vitelline membrane of the secondary oocyte. Before breaking these barriers the sperms undergo a process of capacitation.

2. **Capacitation:** It is a period of conditioning of sperms in female genital tract and lasts for about 7 hrs. The secretion of the uterine glands causes removal of glycoprotein coat and seminal plasma proteins from the acrosomal region of the spermatozoa. Only capacitated sperms can cross the barriers around the secondary oocyte. In vitro fertilization study, however suggests that the human sperms do not require capacitate.

3. **Acrosome reaction:** Acrosome forms a bilaminar membrane which covers the anterior 2/3rd of nucleus

of spermatozoa (deep to the plasma membrane). When spermatozoa approaches close to the oocyte, fusion between plasma membrane and outer acrosomal membrane takes place at multiple points. It liberates the acrosomal contents (acrosin) for the penetration of the barriers around secondary oocyte. The corona radiata is dispersed by 'hyaluronidase' enzyme from acrosomal cap. The zona pellucida is penetrated by sperm head with release of trypsin like substances. Permeability of zona pellucida changes when the head of the sperm comes in contact with the oocyte surface. Only one sperm is able to penetrate. Fertilizin secreted by zona pellucida helps in agglutination of sperms and antifertilizin secreted by sperm agglutinates the ova. The two plasma membranes (vitelline membrane of oocyte and cell membrane covering the posterior region of the sperm head) fuse and the head and neck of the spermatozoon is incorporated in the cytoplasm of oocyte. The cytoplasmic granules of the oocyte having lysosomal enzymes accumulate beneath the vitelline membrane and prevent penetration of other spermatozoa (vitelline block). The oocyte finishes second meiotic division immediately after entry of spermatozoon into the oocyte. The zona pellucida still persists and it prevents abnormal implantation of the fertilized product (Fig. 2.8).

The nucleus of the spermatozoon becomes swollen and forms male pronucleus and its tail detaches and degenerates. The male and female pronuclei come into close contact and lose their nuclear envelope. Each pronucleus replicate its DNA and the chromosomes get arranged in the spindle in preparation of normal mitotic division. The 23 paternal and 23 maternal chromosomes split longitudinally at the centromere, and sister chromatids move to opposite poles, providing each cell

of the zygote with the normal diploid number of chromosomes.

Results of fertilization

1. Completion of 2nd meiotic division of female gamete
2. Restoration of diploid number of chromosome in the zygote (44 X, X OR Y)
3. Determination of the chromosomal sex: If X-bearing spermatozoon fertilizes an ovum, the zygote contains 2 X chromosomes + 44 autosomes and female embryo is formed. If the ovum is fertilized by Y bearing spermatozoon, the sex of the embryo will be male.

The nucleus of the zygote contains equal shares of chromosomes and hereditary materials from both parents, but amount of cytoplasm contributed to the zygote is exclusively derived from the mother (Fig. 2.10).

Y chromosome determines sex: Testis determining factor (TDF), located in the short arm of the Y chromosome is referred to as sex-determining region of Y chromosome (SRY-gene). Action of SRY gene in the early indifferent embryo in the male develops into a testis, in the absence of this gene, the gonad becomes an ovary. However the presence of Y chromosome or SRY gene will not ensure that the embryo will become a normal male fetus. There are many other factors that determine the gonadal sex and phenotypic sex of the embryo. These factors will be discussed in the chapter 'Development of genital system'.

Mutations of SRY gene give rise to XY females with gonadal dysgenesis (Swyer syndrome) and translocation of part of the Y chromosome containing this gene to the X chromosome causes XX male syndrome.

Infertility: The infertility rate is steadily increasing in India and is especially affecting male population. There are many factors like anatomical, genetic, hormonal and environmental causing male and female infertility. Male infertility is mainly due to reduced sperm count and sub-optimal sperm quality. Female infertility can be due to blockage in the uterine tube as a result of pelvic inflammatory diseases, abnormal mucous projections in cervix, absence of ovulation, immunity to spermatozoa. A Robertsonian translocation in either partner may cause recurrent spontaneous abortions and permanent infertility. Diabetes, maternal age and thyroid disorders can also contribute to infertility.

Assisted reproductive technology: It is a term referring to methods used to achieve pregnancy by artificial or partial artificial means.

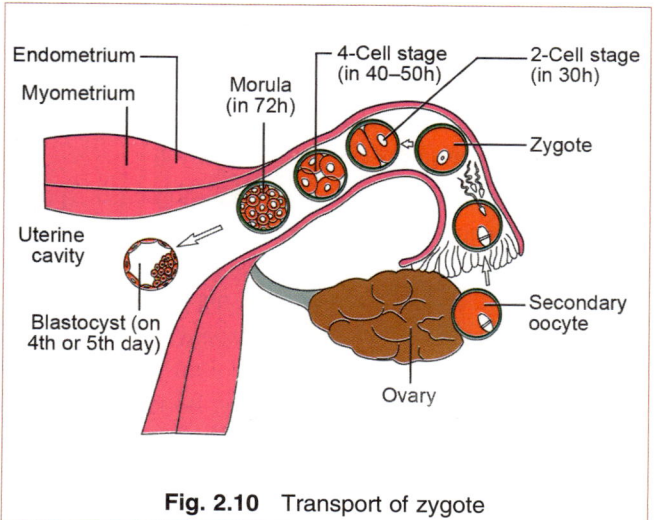

Fig. 2.10 Transport of zygote

Endometrium
Myometrium
Morula (in 72h)
4-Cell stage (in 40–50h)
2-Cell stage (in 30h)
Zygote
Uterine cavity
Blastocyst (on 4th or 5th day)
Secondary oocyte
Ovary

In vitro fertilization (IVF): In this method sperms and ova are fertilized outside the female body. The oocytes are collected from the ovary in the late stages of first meiotic division by a laparoscopic procedure and then treated in a culture medium to which sperms are added. Fertilized oocytes are monitored and placed in the uterine endometrium at eight cell stage. Though in vitro fertilization results in low birth defects, its success rate is very low (20%). To increase the chances of successful pregnancy, usually four to five oocytes are fertilized and then implanted, which leads to multiple births.

Gamete intra fallopian transfer (GIFT): It is a method of assisted reproductive technology in which oocytes are collected from the ovary and then placed in the ampulla of the uterine tube with sperms, allowing the fertilization to take place.

Zygote intra fallopian transfer (ZIFT): In this method, the oocyte and the sperm are collected and then allowed to fertilize in the laboratory to form the zygote. The zygote is transferred into the uterine tube.

Intracytoplasmic sperm injection (ICSI): This procedure involves injection of single sperm into the cytoplasm of the oocyte to cause fertilization. It is beneficial in the case of male factor infertility with low sperm count. This method is also sometimes employed when donor sperm is used.

DEVELOPMENT DURING 2ND WEEK

- Implantation of the blastocyst is completed by 12th day of fertilization.
- Trophoblast differentiation – on 8th day
- Embryoblast differentiates into bilaminar germ disc
- Formation of yolk sac and amniotic cavities (Fig. 2.9)

Cleavage division

It is a process of repeated segmentation of the zygote within the zona pellucida by mitotic divisions in rapid succession. The cells which become smaller in each division are known as blastomeres. The cell division follows in this way

2 cell stage – 30 hrs after fertilization

4 cell stage – 40 to 50 hrs after fertilization

12 cell stage – about 72 hrs after fertilization

16 cell stage – 96 hrs after fertilization

It takes approximately 72 hrs (3 days) for the zygote to reach uterine cavity at 12 to 16 cell stage.

Morula: Approximately 3 days after fertilization, about 12 to 16 cell stage of the fertilized mass is called morula (resembles a mulberry). The cells differentiate into an inner cell mass and outer cell mass. The inner cell mass gives rise to tissue of the embryo proper.

Blastocyst: Formation of the blastocyst takes place between the 4th and 5th day of development. Uterine fluid begins to penetrate through the zona pellucida into the intercellular spaces of the inner cell mass. Gradually, the intercellular spaces join each other to form a single cavity called blastocele. The embryo at this stage is called blastocyst. Out of 107 cells composing of blastocyst on the 5th day of development only 8 cells form the embryoblast and remaining cell forms trophoblasts.

Implantation of Blastocyst

The implantation of blastocyst occurs on 6th or 7th day after fertilization. The Zona pellucida disappears at the end of 5th day of fertilization. Proteolytic action of trophoblasts

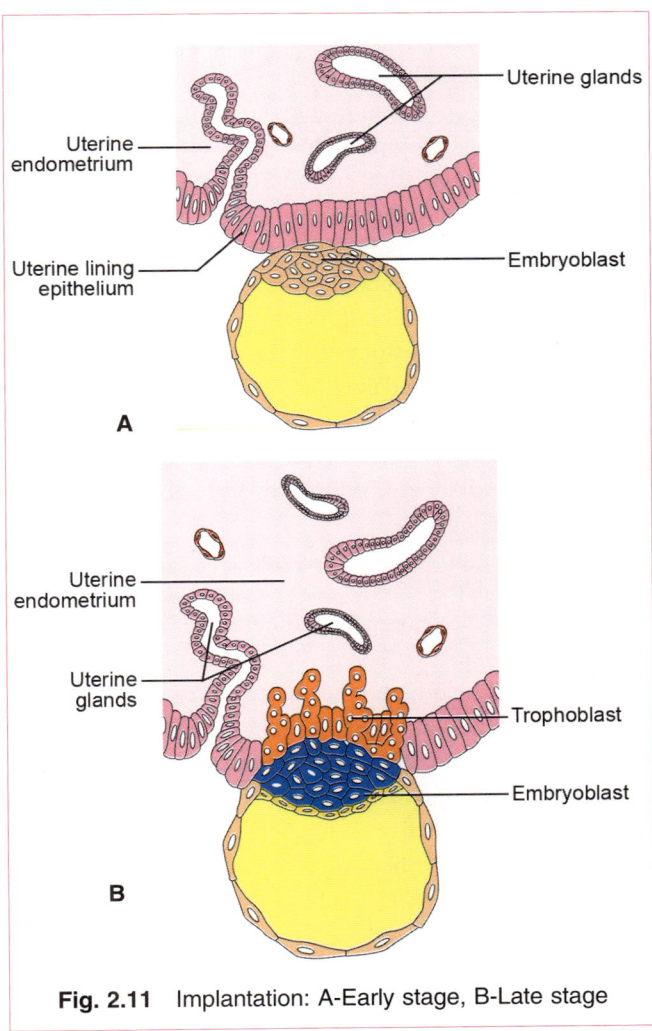

Fig. 2.11 Implantation: A-Early stage, B-Late stage

erodes the uterine endometrium (Fig. 2.11). Implantation normally occurs at the anterior or posterior wall of the fundus of the uterus. The blastocyst is completely embedded in endometrium by the 12th day of development (Fig. 2.11).

Abnormal implantation (ectopic pregnancy) may occur in the uterine tube, abdominal cavity or in the ovary. However, 90% of the ectopic pregnancy occurs in the ampullary part of the uterine tube. It can also get implanted in recto-uterine pouch. Most ectopic pregnancy terminates by second month of gestation causing severe bleeding and abdominal pain in the mother.

Sometimes the blastocyst grows with normal trophoblast but with little or no embryonic tissue. The trophoblast cells continue to secrete HCG and this blastocyst is called hydatidiform mole.

Subdivision of the trophoblast

On further development on day 8, the trophoblast cells differentiate into inner cytotrophoblast and outer syncytiotrophoblast. The cytotrophoblast cells retain their cell membrane while the syncytiotrophoblast lose their cell membrane to form a continuous layer of cytoplasm with many nuclei (syncytium). The syncytiotrophoblast cells divide rapidly in relation to the uterine endometrium. In subsequent development, number of spaces (lacunae) appear within the syncytiotrophoblast, which join each other. The syncytiotrophoblast cells present between the lacunar spaces are called trabeculae. The lacunae enlarge around the entire blastocyst. The endometrial veins and arteries break down and the blood fills these lacunar spaces to begin uteroplacental circulation. Further changes in the trophoblastic layer forms the chorionic villi and subsequently placenta, which will be discussed under separate heading.

Embryoblast and its fate

On 8th day of development the cells of the embryoblast differentiates into two layers. At first the cells lining the inner aspect (towards the blastocyst cavity) differentiates to form flattened or cuboidal cells known as **hypoblast** (Fig. 2.12). The remaining cells of the embryoblast which are present in relation to the trophoblast form **epiblast**. Thus a **bilaminar germ disc** is formed with an extracellular basement membrane between the hypoblast and epiblast (Fig. 2.13).

Decidua: The endometrium of the uterus after implantation is called 'decidua'. The changes taking place in the endometrium is referred to as decidual reaction. The stromal

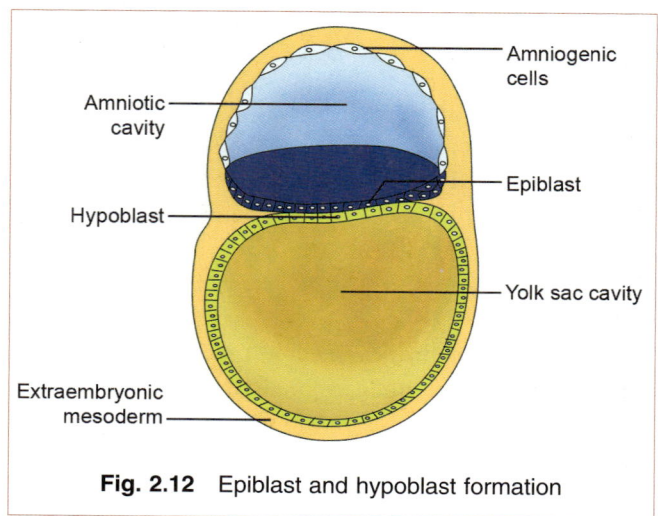

Fig. 2.12   Epiblast and hypoblast formation

cell gets accumulated with glycogen and lipid droplets. The portion of the decidua where the placenta is to be formed is called decidua basalis. The part of the decidua that separates the embryo from the uterine lumen is called decidua capsularis and remaining part of the decidua lining the uterine cavity is called decidua parietalis (Fig. 2.31).

Amniotic cavity formation

On day 8 of development a small cavity appears within the epiblast which enlarges to form amniotic cavity (space appearing between epiblast below and trophoblast above). Thus the floor of the amniotic cavity is formed by epiblast and the roof by flattened cells called amnioblasts.

Primary Yolk sac formation

On day 9 of development flattened cells arising from the hypoblast line the inside of the blastocyst cavity. This thin membrane is referred as Heuser's membrane. This membrane continues with hypoblast layer at the periphery of the disc. The blastocyst cavity now lined by hypoblasts and Heuser's membrane is called as primary yolk sac.

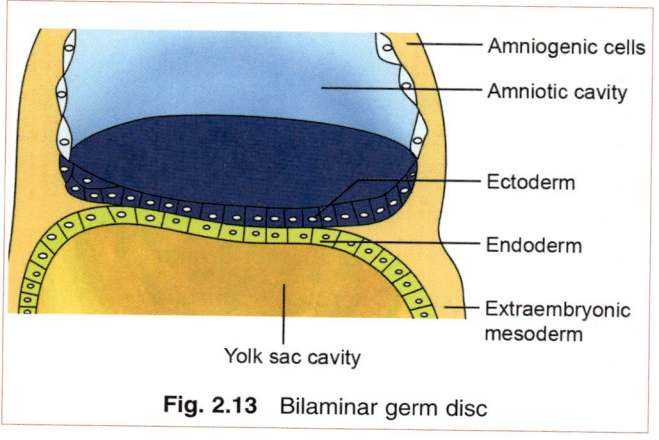

Fig. 2.13   Bilaminar germ disc

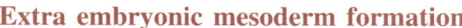

Extra embryonic mesoderm formation

On day 11 and 12 of development a network of tissues appears between inner surface of the cytotrophoblast (externally) and the outer surface of the primary yolk sac (internally) (Fig. 2.14). This fine, loose connective tissue is called extra embryonic mesoderm. Eventually this tissue fills all of the space between trophoblast externally, amniotic cavity and yolk sac internally.

Extra embryonic coelom formation

Soon large cavities appear within the extra embryonic mesoderm which joins each other to form the extra embryonic coelom except at the caudal end. This cavity is also referred to as chorionic cavity. With the formation of this cavity the extra embryonic mesoderm is divisible into two layers (Fig. 2.14).

1. Somatopleuric (parietal)—lining inside the trophoblast and outside the amniotic cavity.
2. Splanchnopleuric (visceral)—lining outside the primary yolk's.

Connecting stalk

The unsplit extra embryonic mesoderm through which embryo along with amniotic cavity and yolk sac is attached to the trophoblast (at the caudal end) is called '**connecting stalk**'. It forms the umbilical cord with the development of blood vessels in it.

Chorion

The trophoblast with somatopleuric extra embryonic mesoderm forms a membrane called chorion. These two cellular layer sends finger like projections to the endometrium to form the chorionic villi all around the blastocyst on day 13 of the development. The chorionic villi formed in relation to the deciduous capsularis are transitory and they degenerate. This part of the chorionic membrane becomes smooth and is called '**chorion laevae**'. The chorionic villi developed in relation to deciduas basalis undergoes considerable development to form the placenta. This part of the chorion that is involved in development of placenta is called '**chorion frondosum**'. With the expansion of amniotic cavity the extra embryonic coelom gets obliterated causing fusion of amnion and chorion membranes. At the time of child birth the amnion, chorion membranes with outer thin decidua capsularis layer forms 'membranes' which ruptures with increased pressure of the amniotic fluid.

On day 13 of development the hypoblast produces additional cells which lines the primary yolk sac. These cells proliferate to form a new generation of cells and the primary yolk sac is now called '**secondary yolk sac**' or '**definitive**

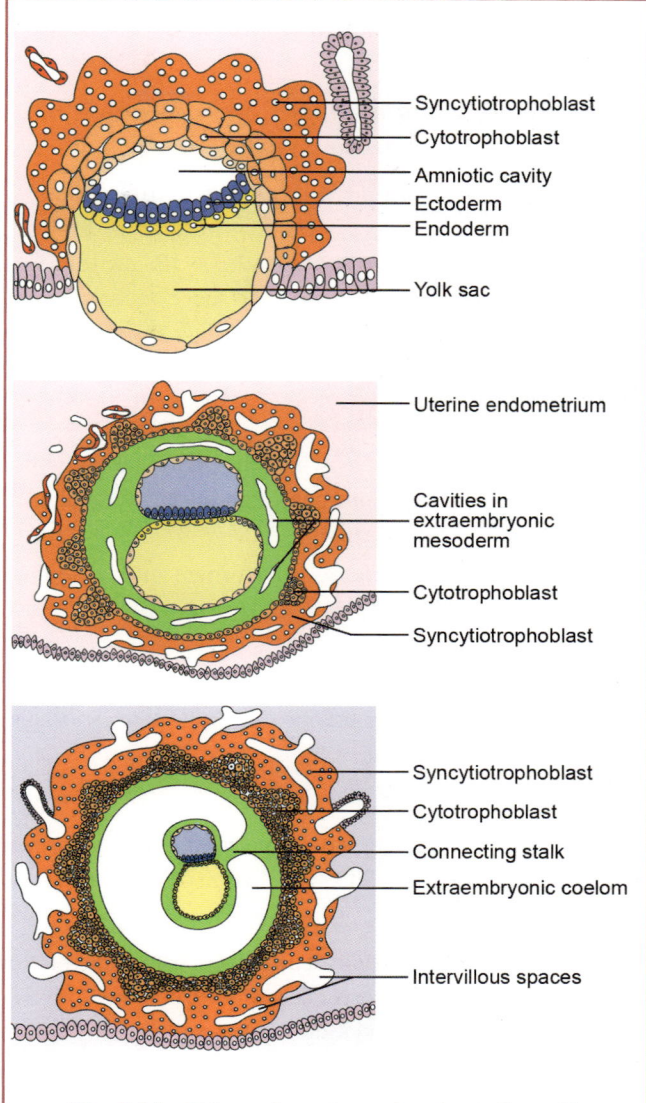

Fig. 2.14 Extraembryonic coelom formation with connecting stalk and implantation

yolk sac'. This yolk sac is smaller than the primary yolk sac. During its formation, a small portion of the primary yolk sac is pinched off to form 'exocoelomic cyst' which are often found in the chorionic cavity.

Human Chorionic Gonadotropin (hCG):

It is produced by trophoblast cells and excreted in the urine of the mother as early as 8 days after the first missed period. The presence of this hormone in urine is an indication of pregnancy. It maintains the growth of corpus luteum upto the 3rd month, which is required to produce 'progesterone'. The level of HCG in maternal blood decreases after the 16th week. Sometime in an abnormal blastocyst, the trophoblast develops placental membranes and is called hydatidiform mole (molar pregnancy), which continues to secrete HCG.

Why the fertilized product (conceptus) does not get rejected by maternal system?

Production of immunosuppressive cytokines and proteins and the expression of an unusual major histocompatibility complex class IB molecule (HLA-G) blocks recognition of the conceptus as foreign tissue.

DEVELOPMENT DURING 3rd AND 4th WEEK

- Gastrulation: An event by which the bilaminar germ disc is converted into trilaminar (formation of ectoderm, endoderm and mesoderm)

- Primary chorionic villi are transformed into secondary and tertiary villi

  The beginning of the 3rd week of development is highly sensitive stage for teratogenic insult. Maternal alcohol at this stage can cause holoprosencephaly (craniofacial defects).

Gastrulation

It is a process by which bilaminar germ disc is transformed to trilaminar germ disc with the formation of intraembryonic mesoderm.

Primitive streak formation: It appears at the caudal part of the germ disc in epiblast layer at mid-line at about 15th day of development. It appears as a narrow groove with slightly bulging on either sides. The cephalic part of the streak is enlarged to form primitive node (Hensen's node) with a small primitive pit within it. The primitive streak induces the differentiation of the notochord and intra embryonic mesodem. Hence called as primary organiser (Fig. 2.15).

Cells of the epiblast migrate towards the primitive streak. These cells detach from the epiblast and slip beneath it. This inward movement is known as invagination and is controlled by fibroblast growth factor (FGF-8). These invaginated cells displace the hypoblast cells also to form embryonic **endoderm** which lines the secondary yolk sac. The invaginated cells trapped between the epiblast and newly formed endoderm forms the intra embryonic **mesoderm**. The remaining cells form the **ectoderm**. Thus the epiblast forms all the three germ layers by a process called gastrulation. Further, formation and migration of more intraembryonic mesodermal cells migrate laterally and cranially. These cells are continuous with extraembryonic mesoderm at the margin of the disc.

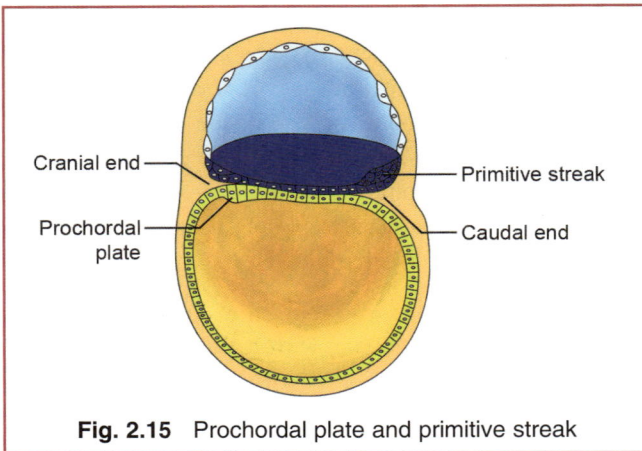

Fig. 2.15 Prochordal plate and primitive streak

Prochordal plate (prechordal plate): It is a thickening of the endodermal cells near the cephalic end of the embryo. This plate consists of columnar cells that is tightly adherent to the overlying ectodermal layer. The prochordal plate is important for the induction of forebrain (Fig. 2.15).

Notochord

It is visible on 17th or 18th day of development. It extends from primitive node to prochordal plate. It is a midline structure that develops from the upper end of the primitive streak to the lower end of the prochordal plate. Notochord is considered as secondary organizer. It induces the formation of neural tube.

Functions: Notochord induces the formation of neural tube.

Formation of notochord:

- Notochordal process: Cells multiply from the primitive streak in the midline between ectoderm and endoderm and extends in cephalic direction towards prochordal plate. This cellular cord is referred as notochordal process (Fig. 2.16).

- Notochordal canal: Primitive pit extends into the notochordal process, converting it into a canal.

- The cells lining floor of the notochordal canal break down, hence the notochordal canal communicates with yolk sac and also with amniotic cavity through primitive pit. This communication is referred to as neurenteric canal, which temporarily communicates the fluid of the yolk sac with amniotic cavity.

- Notochordal plate: The cells of the notochordal canal become flattened to obliterate the canal.

- Definitive notochord: The notochordal plate again becomes curved to assume the shape of the tube. Further proliferation of cells from solid rod cells constitutes definitive notochord which gets completely separated from the endoderm.

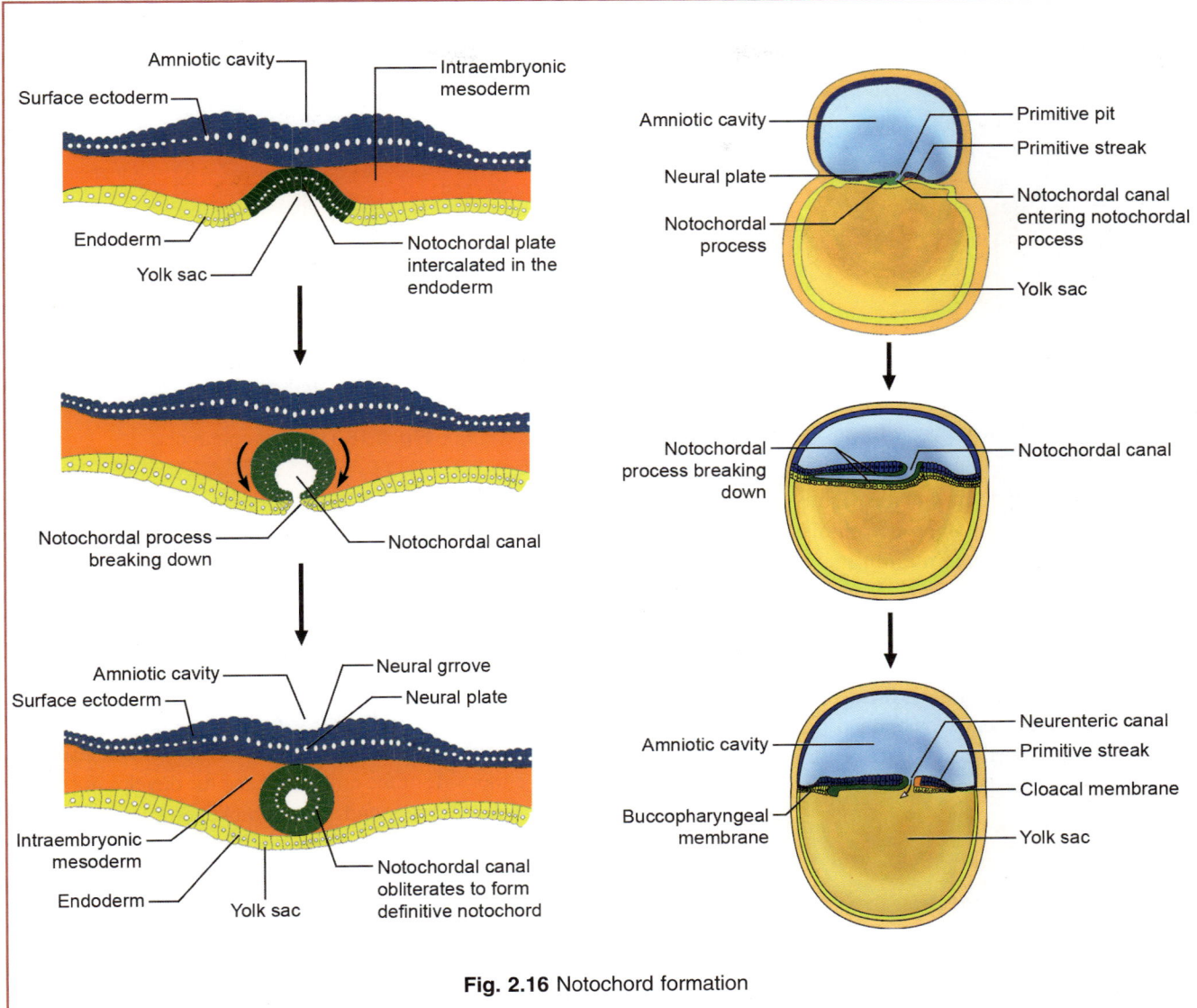

Fig. 2.16 Notochord formation

The major part of the notochord disappears and its position is occupied by the vertebral column, however it does not form vertebral column. Notochordal cells persists in the first decade of life as nucleus pulposus of the intervertebral disc, apical ligament of the dens.

Craniopharyngeoma: Occasionally traces of cranial end of the notochord attached to the foregut remains and transforms into a cartilaginous tumour in the roof of the nasopharynx

Intra embryonic mesoderm formation

During 17th and 18th day of development cells proliferate from primitive streak, pass sideways beneath the epiblast as intraembryonic mesoderm which is now placed between ectoderm and endoderm. The intra embryonic mesoderm spreads between ectoderm and endoderm except at three regions - prochordal plate, area behind the primitive streak and in the midline where notochord occupies. Cranial to the prochordal plate the mesoderm of the two sides meet in the midline and is referred as 'pericardial bar'. At the edges of the embryonic disc, the intra embryonic mesoderm is continuous with extra embryonic mesoderm.

Buccopharyngeal membrane: At the prochordal plate (near the cephalic end of the embryo) the ectoderm and endoderm remains tightly adherent to each other, as intraembryonic mesoderm fails to extend into this region. This oval shaped bilaminar membrane is called 'buccopharyngeal membrane' or 'oral membrane'. The area cranial to the buccopharyngeal membrane forms 'stomodeum' or 'primitive oral cavity'.

Cloacal membrane: At the chordal end of the embryo between the primitive streak and the connecting stalk the

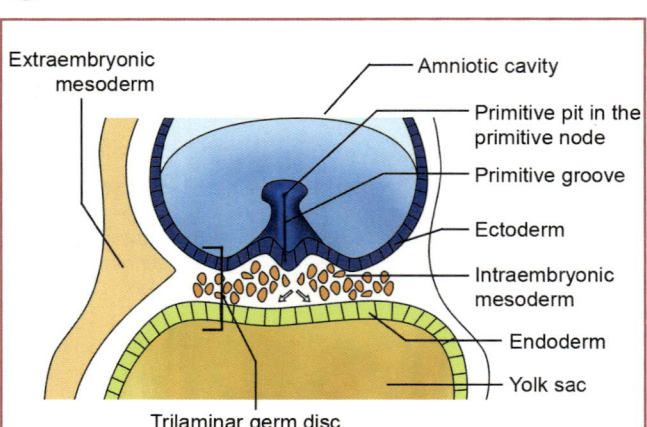

Fig. 2.17 Intraembryonic mesoderm formation

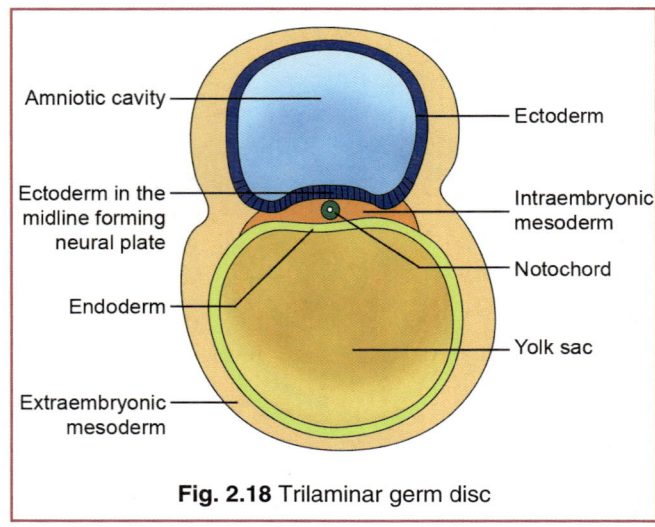

Fig. 2.18 Trilaminar germ disc

ectoderm and endoderm remains tightly adherent to each other as intraembryonic mesoderm fails to extend into this region. This bilaminar membrane is called **'cloacal membrane'**. This membrane later occupies the bottom of endodermal cloaca. The area caudal to this membrane forms **'proctodeum'** which later forms anal canal.

When the cloacal membrane is formed, a small diverticulum from the yolk sac extends to connecting stalk. This is called 'allantoenteric diverticulum' or 'allantois', which appears around 16th day of development.

The primitive streak regresses at the end of third week of development and disappears by 26th day of development.

Sacrococcygeal teratoma: It is the most common tumour present in newborns. It is derived from the remnants of the primitive streak. The clusters of pluripotent cells that persist in the sacrococcygeal region proliferate and forms tumours known as sacrococcygeal teratoma. It commonly contains tissues derived from all the three germ layers (Fig. 2.19).

Another important event taking place during third week is transformation of primary chorionic villi to tertiary chorionic villi. This is explained in the chapter on placenta.

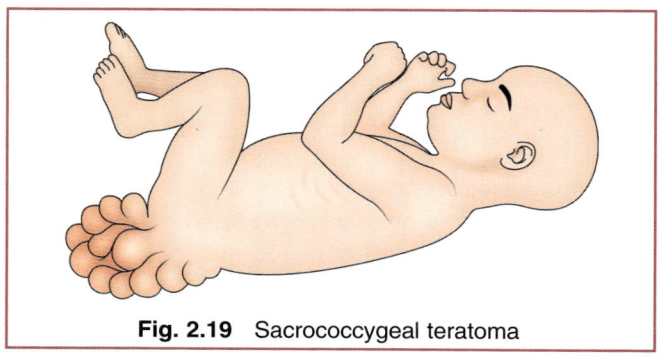

Fig. 2.19   Sacrococcygeal teratoma

The fourth week of development is mainly characterized by differentiation of germ layers and formation of folds of embryo (Fig. 2.18).

Differentiation of intra embryonic mesoderm

The intra embryonic mesoderm is subdivided into three parts namely paraxial, intermediate and lateral plate mesoderms (Figs 2.17 and 2.20).

1. **Paraxial mesoderm:** The intra embryonic mesoderm on either side of the notochord and the developing neural tube proliferates and forms thickened plates of tissue know as paraxial mesoderm. This event begins approximately on 17th day of development.

Somites

These paraxial mesoderms are organized into segments which are called **'somitomeres'**, which first appear in the cephalic region of the embryo. The process of segmentation extends in cephalo-caudal direction. In the head region the somatomeres form neuromeres which contributes to mesenchyme in the head region. The somatomere formed in the occipital region (just caudal to the tip of the notochord) constitutes first pair of **somites** which appears approximately on 20th day of development (Figs 2.21 and 2.22).

New somites are formed in craniocaudal direction at the rate of approximately 3 pairs per day. At the end of the fifth week 42 to 44 pairs of somites are formed. There are 4 occipital, 8 cervical, 12 thoracic, 5 lumbar, 5 sacral and 8–10 coccygeal pairs. The first occipital and last five to seven coccygeal somites later disappear, while the remaining somites form the axial skeleton. The fourth week of development is referred to as the somite period. The age of the embryo may be assessed by the number of somites, which is shown in next page (Fig. 2.21).

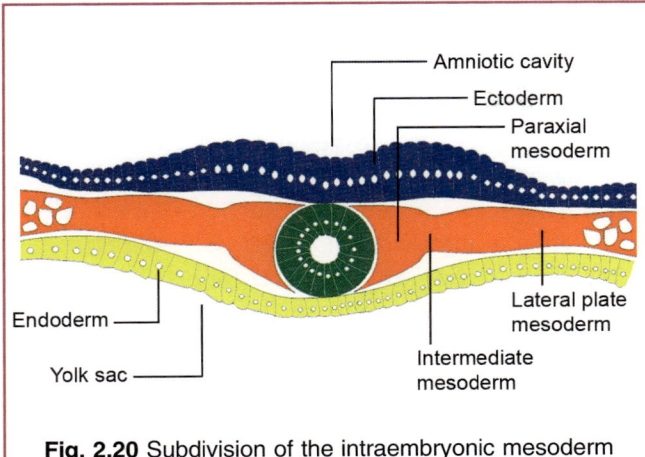

Fig. 2.20 Subdivision of the intraembryonic mesoderm

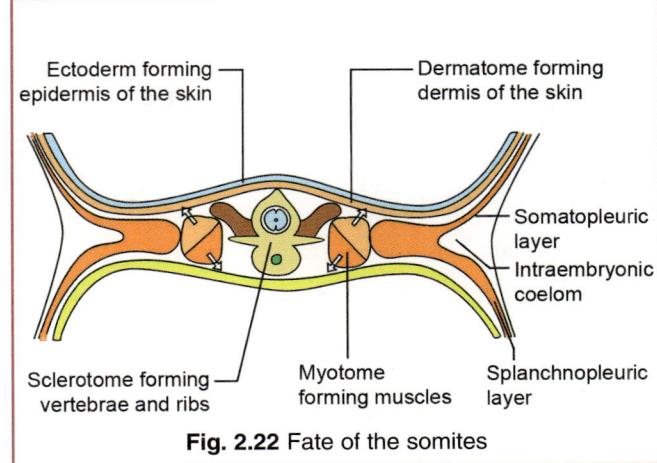

Fig. 2.22 Fate of the somites

The occipital somites forms muscles of tongue and preotic somites give rise to muscles of eyeball. On cross section, somite is triangular in shape and has a cavity which gets obliterated later. Each somite is divisible into three parts namely sclerotome, dermatome and myotome.

Sclerotome: The cells forming the ventral and medial wall of somite become polymorphs and shift their position to surrounding notochord. This part of the somite is called sclerotome. These mesenchymal tissues present around the notochord and the spinal cord form the vertebral column.

The cells of the dorsolateral part of the somites is referred to as dermo-mytome, which is further divided into dermatome and myotome

Dermatome: These cells migrate to the under surface of the ectoderm and give rise to dermis of the skin and subcutaneous tissue

Myotome: They give rise to striated muscles. Each myotome is segmentally arranged and invaded by a spinal nerve arising from the spinal cord. Each myotome and dermatome retains its innervation from its segment of origin, no matter where the cells migrate. For example, diaphragm present between thorax and abdomen is supplied by C3, 4 (phrenic) nerves indicating migration of myotome from cervical region retaining its original nerve supply.

2. **Intermediate mesoderm:** It is present between paraxial and lateral plate mesoderm. It give rise to urogenital organs. It produces a bulging to the coelomic cavity which is called as nephrogenic cord.

3. **Lateral plate mesoderm:** This is the lateral part of the intraembryonic mesoderm, which continues with extraembryonic mesoderm at the periphery of the embryonic disc. During fourth week of development small cavities appear in the lateral plate mesoderm, which

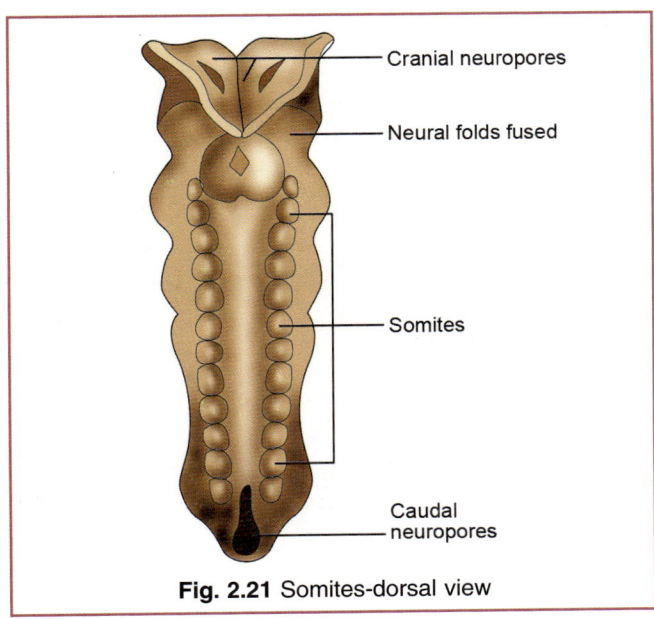

Fig. 2.21 Somites-dorsal view

Number of somites	Approximate age (in days)
1–4	20
4–7	21
7–10	22
10–13	23
13–17	24
17–20	25
20–23	26
23–26	27
26–29	28
34–35	30

join each other to form a single cavity called intra-embryonic coelom. A pericardial sac develops in relation to the pericardial bar present cranial to the prochordal plate. The pericardial sac also communicates with intra embryonic coelom. The intra embryonic coelom gives rise to pericardial, pleural and peritoneal cavities. With the formation of the intra embryonic coelom the lateral plate mesoderm is divisible into

- **Somatopleuric layer** – which is in contact with the ectoderm.
- **Splanchnopleuric layer** – which is in contact with the endoderm.

The somatopleuric layer gives rise to parietal layer of the peritoneum, dermis and subcutaneous tissue of the body wall and probably skeletal and muscle elements of the limb buds. The splanchnopleuric layer forms the visceral layer of the peritoneum, musculature of the gut and the heart.

The cavity formation (intraembryonic coelom) does not affect the cephalic part of the embryo cranial to the pericardial sac. This unsplit intraembryonic mesoderm is called 'septum transversum'. It contributes to the formation of fibrous pericardium of the heart, central tendon of the diaphragm and capsule of the liver. The splanchnopleuric layer of lateral plate mesoderm in the midline cranial to the prochordal plate is called 'cardiogenic area'. The heart develops in relation to this area.

Anomalies related to gastrulation:

Holoprosencephaly: Beginning of the third week of development is highly sensitive stage for teratogens. Maternal alcohol during this period is known to cause a 'holoprosencephaly', a severe birth defect involving

midline craniofacial structures. It is characterized by small forebrain, single midline lateral ventricle, closely placed eyes (hypotelorism).

Caudal dysgenesis (Sirenomelia): It is a defect during gastrulation by genetic abnormalities or toxic insults, in which there is insufficient mesoderm formation in the caudal most regions of the embryo. These mesoderms are responsible for development of lower limb and urogenital organs. The birth defects includes hypoplasia of the lower limbs, vertebral anomalies, absence of kidney, anomalies of the genital organs, imperforate anus. In humans, this condition is associated with maternal diabetes.

Situs inversus: It is a condition in which transposition of thoracic and abdominal organs occur. For example the appendix developing on the right side is now placed on the left side.

Folding of the embryo

At the end of the third week of development there is a progressive growth in the central part of the embryonic disc. This results in formation of head fold, tail fold and two lateral folds in the embryo which gives cylindrical contour to the embryo. The head and tail folds are formed mainly due to longitudinal growth of the neural tube and lateral folds are formed by rapid growth of somites. During this process of fold formation the growth of the yolk sac is restricted. The amniotic cavity enlarges and surrounds the outer surface of the embryo. The head, tail and two lateral folds now converge on the ventral surface of the embryo (Fig. 2.23). The amniotic membrane provides tubular investment to the connecting stalk, which now forms the umbilical cord.

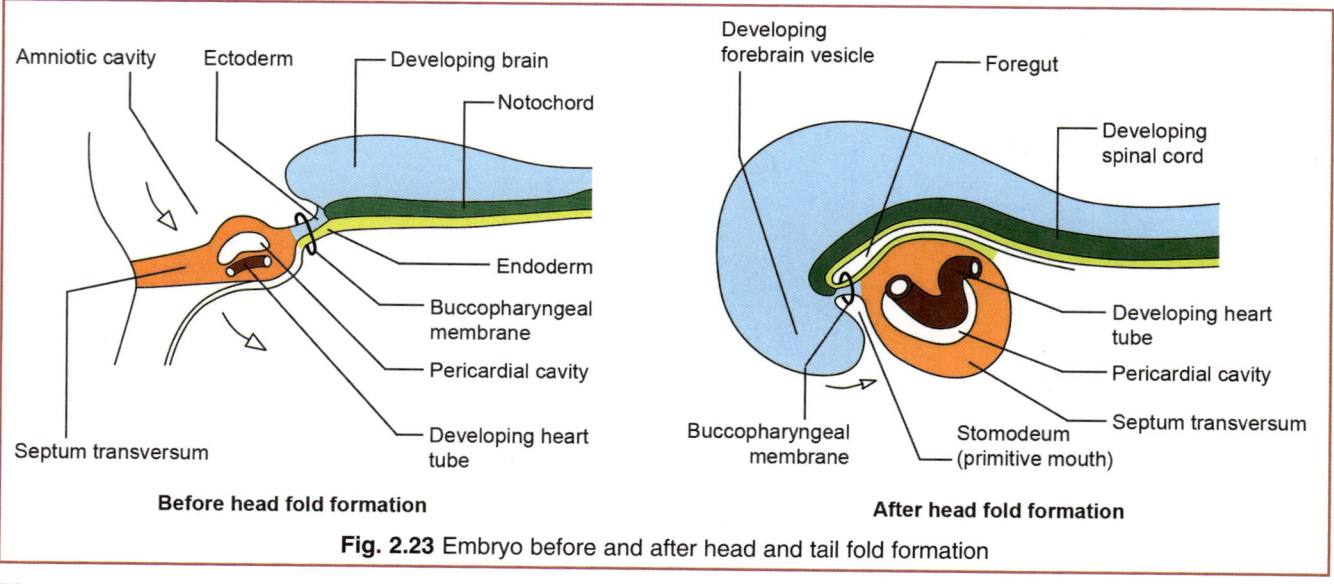

Fig. 2.23 Embryo before and after head and tail fold formation

With the formation of these folds the yolk sac becomes enclosed within the embryo and is called '**primitive gut**'. The portion of the yolk sac remaining outside the embryo is called umbilical vesicle.

The primitive gut is an endodermal tube externally surrounded by splanchnopleuric layer of the lateral plate mesoderm. The gut is now divisible into three parts namely— foregut, midgut and hindgut. Foregut occupies the head fold. The foregut continues caudally with mid gut, which further continues with hind gut in the tail fold. The gut gives rise to gastrointestinal tract and part of respiratory tract.

The foregut is related to notochord and hind brain posteriorly. The ventral portion of the foregut is now related to buccopharyngeal membrane, pericardial sac with

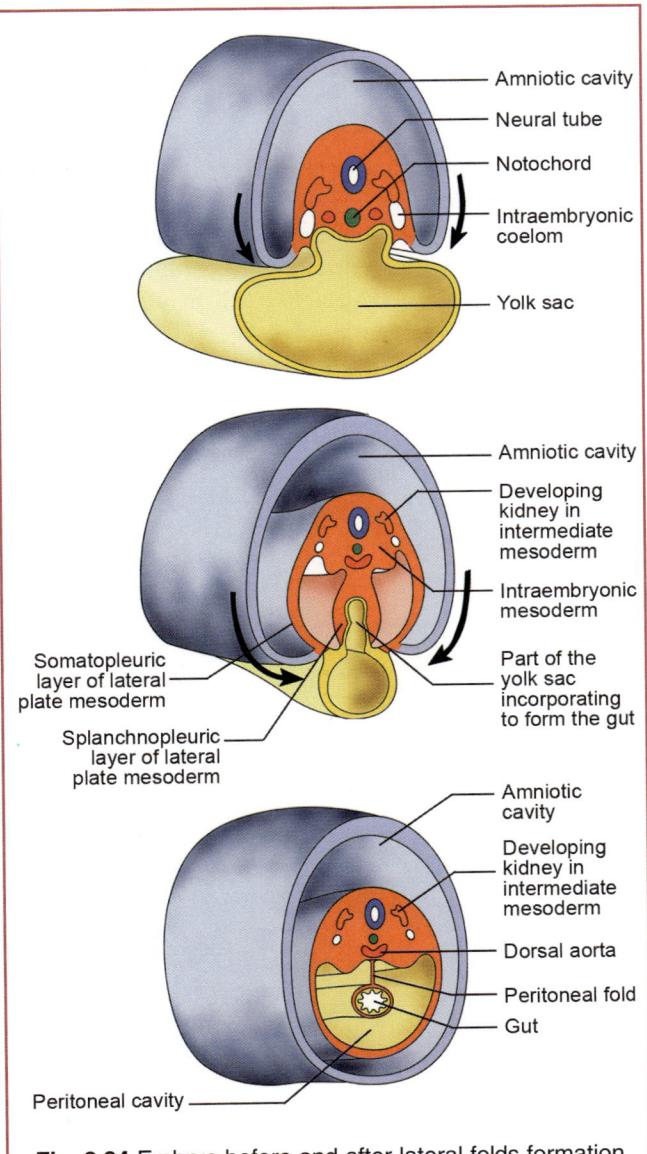

Fig. 2.24 Embryo before and after lateral folds formation

developing heart tube and septum transversum in cranio-caudal direction. The area in front of the buccopharyngeal membrane forms the stomodeum or primitive mouth. The stomodeum is bound above by forebrain vesicle and below by pericardial sac. Later pericardial sac is displaced more caudally to reach the thoracic region along with the septum transversum, which allows the formation of neck. The buccopharyngeal membrane ruptures during fourth week so that endodermal gut is continues cranially with stomodeum, which allows the amniotic fluid to enter the gut.

From the ventral wall of the hind gut, the allanto-enteric diverticulum (allantois) extends into the connecting stalk (umbilical cord). The distal part of the allantois persists as urachus and its proximal part is connected to apex of the developing bladder. Caudal to the allantois, the ventral wall of the hind gut presents 'cloacal membrane'. The surface depression in front of the membrane is called 'proctodeum' which forms the lower part of the anal canal.

With the formation of the right and left lateral folds, the yolk sac is incorporated inside the embryo as mid gut and the portion of the yolk sac outside the embryo forms umbilical vesicle (Fig. 2.24). The mid gut and umbilical vesicle are connected by 'vitello-intestinal duct' which traverses the connecting stalk. The vitello-intestinal duct disappears at birth but if persists, it presents as a diverticulum from the ileum as 'Meckel's diverticulum'.

FORMATION OF NEURAL TUBE (NEURULATION)

The notochord induces the formation of neural tube and in its absence the neural tube fails to develop (Figs 2.25 and 2.26).

- During third week of development the ectodermal cells overlying the notochordal process becomes thick to form the '**neural plate**'.

- The appearance of the neural plate extends from the primitive streak to the region of buccopharyngeal membrane.

- The lateral edges of the neural plate become more elevated to form '**neural folds**'.

- The depressed mid region between the neural folds form the '**neural groove**' (Fig. 2.25).

- Gradually the neural folds approach each other in the midline and fuses.

- With this fusion, the neural groove is transformed in to a neural tube. The fusion begins in the cervical region at

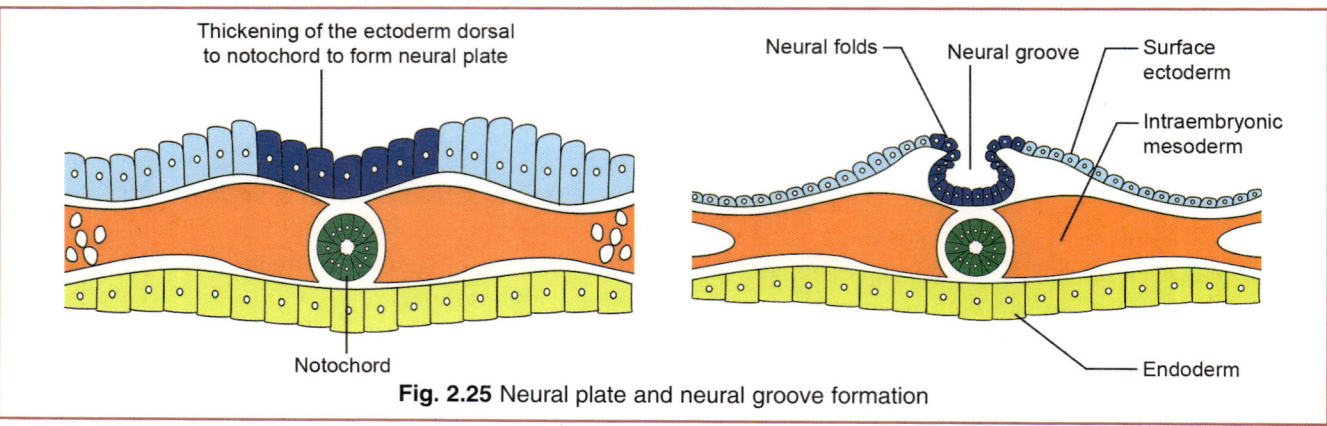

Fig. 2.25 Neural plate and neural groove formation

the level of fifth somite and then proceeds in both cranial and caudal direction.

- The cranial and caudal ends of the neural tube are called as cranial and caudal neuropores respectively which allows the amniotic fluid to pass through the neural tube.

- The cranial neuropore closes approximately on day 25 (18–20 somite stage), whereas the caudal neuropore closes on day 27 (25-somite stage).

- Thereafter the surface ectoderm of the two sides meet in the midline, thereafter the neural tube is detached from it.

- The conversion of neural plate into neural tube by a process of folding is called 'neurulation'.

The lower end of the neural tube forms the spinal cord while the broader cephalic end of the neural tube forms the brain (Fig. 2.26).

Neural tube defects (NCDs)

Most of the spinal cord defects result from abnormal closure of the neural folds, which are referred to as neural tube defects. These defects involve meninges, vertebrae/skull, muscles and skin.

Spina bifida: It is a general term for neural tube defects affecting the spinal region. It is characterized by splitting of the vertebral arches and may or may not involve underlying neural tube. Accordingly different types of spina bifida occurs

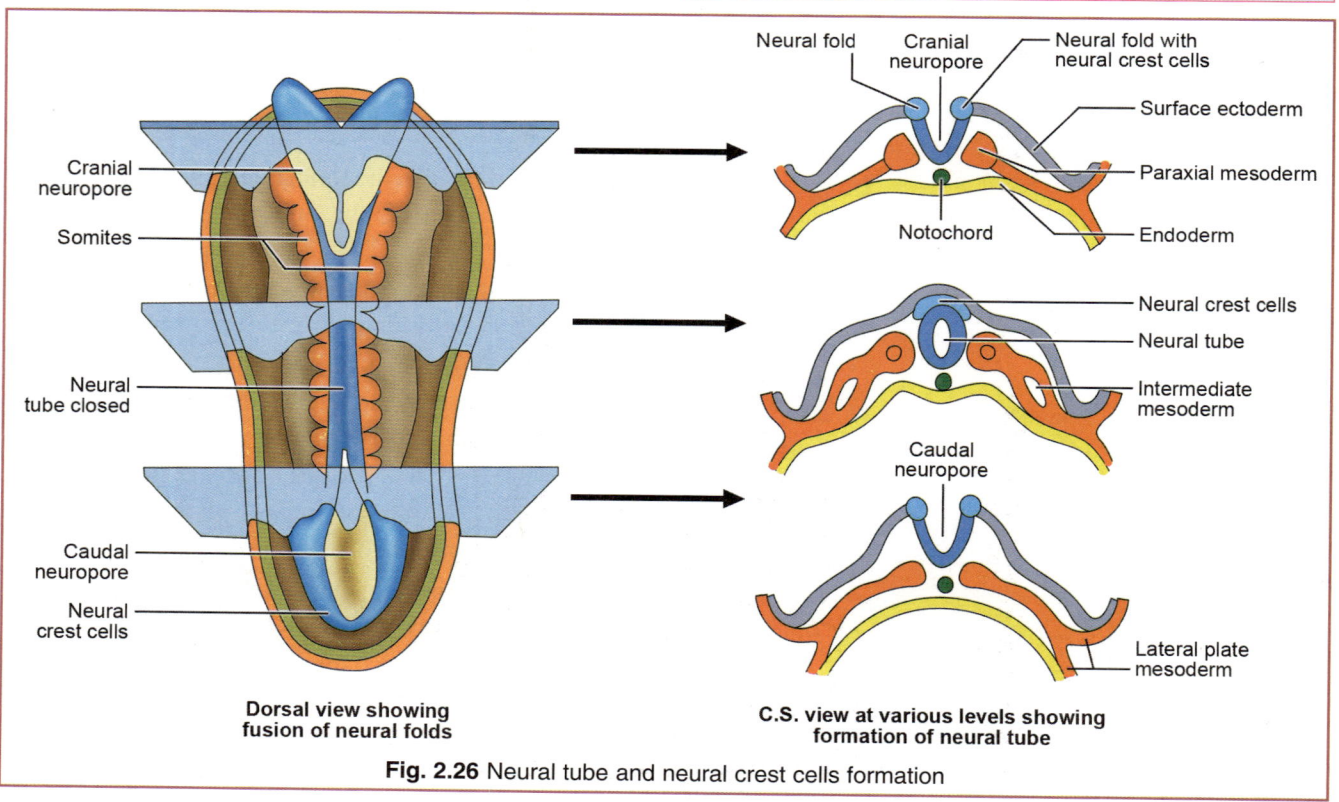

Dorsal view showing fusion of neural folds

C.S. view at various levels showing formation of neural tube

Fig. 2.26 Neural tube and neural crest cells formation

1. Spina bifida occulta: The sclerotome cells do not migrate over the neural tube, resulting in failure in the formation of neural arch of the vertebra. It often occurs at the level of L5 and S1 vertebra. It is covered by skin with patch of hair overlying the affected region.

2. Spina bifida cystica/aperta: In this condition the neural tissue and meninges protrude out through defective vertebral arch and is covered by skin. If CSF and meninges protrude as a cyst, then it is called meningocele. If the spinal cord also protrudes in to the cyst, then it is called meningomyelocele (Figs 2.27A to C).

Spina bifida can be diagnosed prenatally by ultrasound and by determination of α-fetoprotein levels in maternal serum and amniotic fluid. The defect in the closure of the vertebral arch can be visualized by 12 weeks. Valproic acids, hypervitaminosis A are known to cause neural tube defects supplementation with folic acid (400 μg) daily beginning from two months prior to conception and later throughout gestation is known to reduce the risks of neural tube defects.

Anencephaly: It occurs due to failure of cephalic part of the neural tube to close. In this condition the cranial vault is not formed, which exposes the malformed brain with mass of necrotic tissue (Fig. 2.28).

Craniorachischisis: Defect in closure of neural tube affecting caudal part of the spinal cord along with anencephaly.

Anencephaly interferes with swallowing reflex and can cause hydramnios.

Neural crest cells (Fig. 2.29)

These cells are derived from the two neural folds. The cells at the lateral border of the neural folds differentiate and dissociates from it during fusion of the neural folds. These cells now occupy the area between the surface ectoderm and the neural tube. These cells are called 'neural crest cells'. These cells undergo transformation from

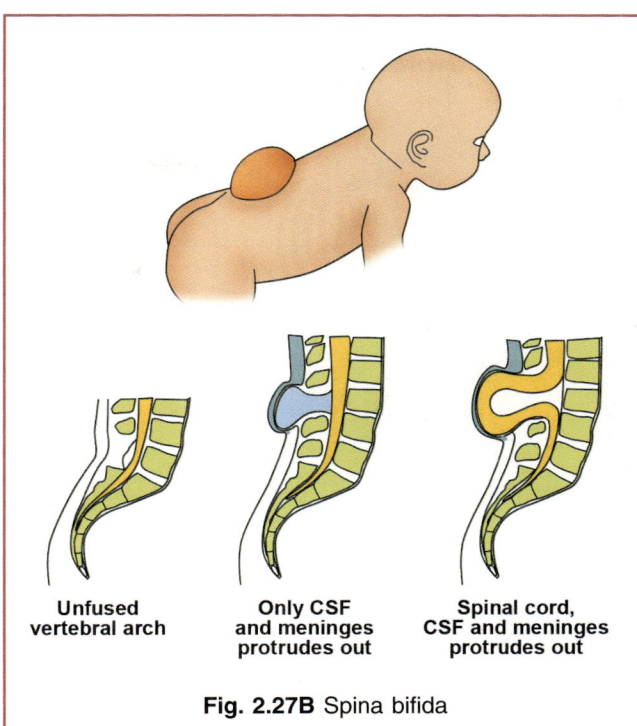

| Unfused vertebral arch | Only CSF and meninges protrudes out | Spinal cord, CSF and meninges protrudes out |

Fig. 2.27B Spina bifida

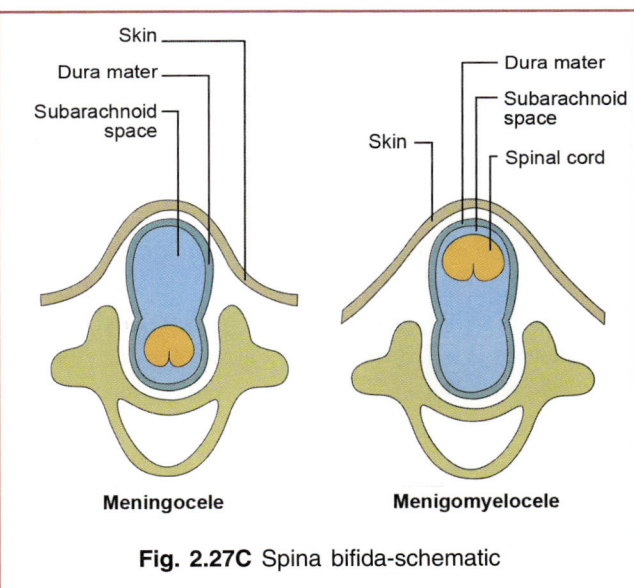

Skin
Dura mater
Subarachnoid space
Dura mater
Subarachnoid space
Skin
Spinal cord

Meningocele   Menigomyelocele

Fig. 2.27C Spina bifida-schematic

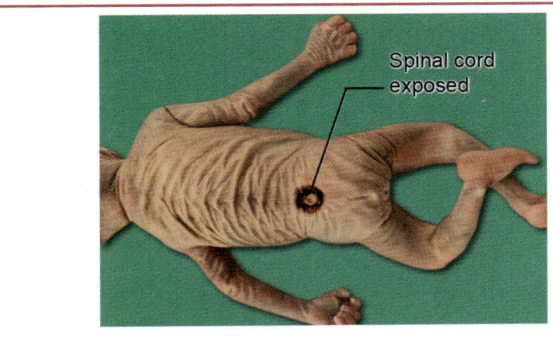

Spinal cord exposed

Fig. 2.27A Spina bifida

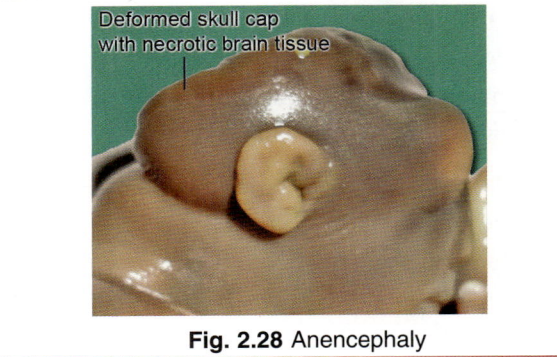

Deformed skull cap with necrotic brain tissue

Fig. 2.28 Anencephaly

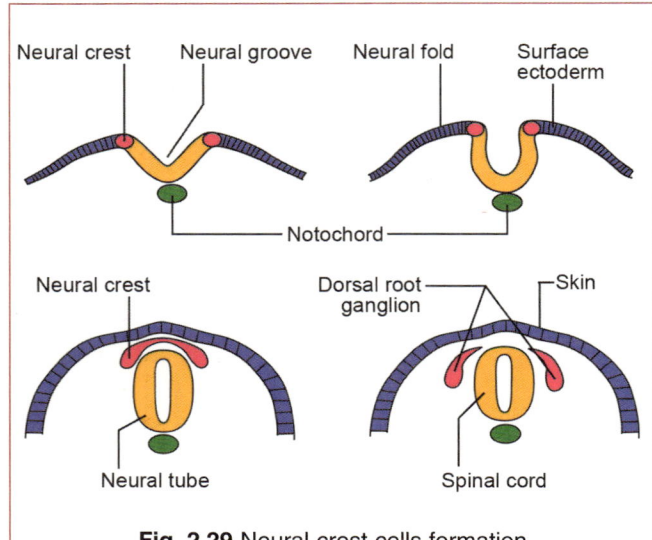

Fig. 2.29 Neural crest cells formation

Neural crest derivatives

- Migrates to craniofacial region to form its skeletal elements
- Neurons of the dorsal root ganglia
- Neurons of the ganglia of 5, 7, 8, 9 and 10 nerves
- Neurons of the sympathetic ganglia
- Schwann cells and Glial cells
- Ganglionic cells of the suprarenal medulla
- Chromaffin tissue
- Melanoblasts of the skin
- Piamater and Arachnoid mater
- C cells of the thyroid
- Conotruncal septum of the heart
- Odontoblasts
- Dermis of the head and neck
- Laryngeal cartilages are also known to be derived from neural crest cells
- Endocardial cushions of heart

its epithelial nature to mesenchymal tissue (Note that mesoderm refers to germ layer derived from epiblast while mesenchymal tissue refers to loosely organized embryonic tissue irrespective of its origin).

The neural crest cells migrate from this area to form many structures. Cells migrating in dorsal direction enter the surface ectoderm to form the melanocytes of the skin. Cells migrating in ventral direction forms sensory ganglia, sympathetic neurons, schwann cells and cells of the adrenal medulla. Cells migrating in cranial direction contribute to craniofacial skeleton.

At the time of closure of the neural tube, two bilateral ectodermal thickenings appear in the cephalic region of the embryo. The lens placodes appear more cranially, which invaginates during fifth week to form the lens. The otic placodes caudal to lens placodes also invaginates to form otic vesicles, which forms structures associated with hearing and maintenance of the equilibrium.

5th Week Development (Major events)

- Limb bud appears, differentiation of hand and feet
- Neural tube differentiation

6th Week Development (Major events)

- Facial region differentiation
- Chondrification starts in skeletal elements and ossification begins in mandible and clavicle.

7th and 8th week of development (Major events)

- Face appears in a human form
- Separation of digits
- Heart is completely developed
- Skeletal and smooth muscle differentiates

- Metanephric kidney starts functioning
- Testes or ovaries are developed

Upper limb buds grows during 5th week from the dorsolateral body wall. The lower limb buds appear at a somewhat later date from the dorsal body wall. The somatopleuric layer of the lateral plate extends within the limb buds as mesodermal core and later differentiates to form bones, joints and muscles of the limbs. The distal end of each limb bud forms an expanded and flattened plate, which later differentiates to digits.

Neuromuscular development is sufficient to allow fetal movement in the eighth week of life. Other features of week 8 include the first appearance of a thin skin, a head as large as the rest of the body, forward-looking eyes, appearance of digits on the hands and feet, appearance of testes and ovaries (but not distinguishable external genitalia), and a crown-rump length of approximately 30 mm. By the end of the eighth week, nearly all adult structures have at least begun to develop, and the fetus "looks like a baby".

Summary of the fate of the germ disc

ECTODERM

1. Entire CNS, PNS, including cranial, spinal and autonomic ganglia.

2. Epidermis of the skin including hair, nails, sebaceous and sweat glands.

3. Epithelial lining of cheek and gum, enamel of the teeth, roof of the mouth, nasal cavity, paranasal sinuses, salivary glands, lower part of the anal canal, terminal part of the urethra.

4. Pituitary gland and chromaffin organs

5. External acoustic meatus, outer lining of the tympanic membrane, internal ear.

6. Corneal epithelium, conjunctiva, lacrimal gland, nasolacrimal duct, lens and retina.

MESODERM

1. All connective tissue.

2. Teeth with the exception of enamel.

3. All muscles of the body except muscles of the iris and erector pilorum muscle of the skin.

4. Cardiovascular and lymphatic system.

5. Urogenital system except most of the bladder, prostate and urethra.

6. Supra renal cortex and gonads

7. Mesothelial cells of pericardial, pleural and peritoneal cavities

ENDODERM

1. Endodermal yolk sac is converted into gut, which is divisible into fore gut, mid gut and hind gut

2. Fore gut: Epithelial lining of the pharynx, esophagus, stomach, duodenum up to the opening of bile duct

3. Mucous membrane of the tongue

4. Epithelial lining of the respiratory system, auditory tube and tympanic cavity

5. Parenchyma of the tonsil, thyroid, parathyroid, thymus, liver and pancreas

6. Mid gut: Epithelial lining of the alimentary tract from duodenum (distal to opening of bile duct) to the junction of right 2/3rd and left 1/3rd of transverse colon.

7. Meckel's diverticulum if present

8. Hind gut: Epithelial lining of GI tract from left 1/3rd of the transverse colon to the anal canal (up to the pectinate line)

9. Most of the mucous membrane of the urinary bladder, urethra, parenchyma of the prostate, bulbo-urethral gland or greater vestibular gland.

10. Epithelial lining of the vagina.

PLACENTA

Placenta is a structure, which connects the fetus with the uterine wall of the mother. It is a structure, where maternal and foetal tissues come in direct contact without rejection. Structurally, it contains the bulk of the chorionic villi.

At full term the placenta is a 'disc' shaped structure 15 to 20 cm in diameter and 3 cm thickness in the central part. It weighs about 500 gms

The placenta presents foetal and maternal surfaces and peripheral margin

The foetal surface is smooth, covered by amnion and presents the attachment of the umbilical cord close to its centre. The maternal surface is rough and irregular. It shows 15–30 **cotyledons**, which are limited by fissures. The peripheral margin is continuous with the foetal membranes. At birth it is detached from the uterine wall and, is expelled approximately 15–30 minutes after birth of the child.

Structure of placenta

The placenta consists of chorionic plate on foetal side and basal plate on maternal side. These two plates are connected by stem villi, which present primary, secondary and tertiary chorionic villi. The space between the stem villi is called 'intervillous spaces, which are filled with maternal blood. A tertiary chorionic villus contains foetal blood vessels in the centre, surrounded successively by extra embryonic mesoderm, cytotrophoblast and syncytiotrophoblast.

The chorionic plate on foetal side is composed of (fetus to mother)

1. Extraembryonic mesoderm

2. Cytotrophoblast

3. Syncytiotrophoblast

The basal plate on maternal side is composed of (mother to fetus)

1. Decidua basalis

2. Outer layer of syncytiotrophoblast (which undergo fibrinoid degeneration)

3. Outer shell of trophoblast

4. Inner layer of syncytiotrophoblast

Formation of chorionic villi

While blastocyst is getting implanted in the uterine endometrium, the trophoblast cells are differentiated into inner cytotrophoblast and outer syncytiotrophoblast. The uterine endometrium is now called decidua which is now divided into basalis, capsularis and parietalis. The outer syncytiotrophoblast proliferate to form many layers with multiple nuclei and advances towards decidua basalis and capsularis. Meanwhile the inner cytotrophoblast forms extraembryonic mesoderm internally. The trophoblast and extraembryonic mesoderm layer together form 'chorion'.

1. A number of lacunar spaces appear within the syncytiotrophoblast. The adjacent lacunar spaces are separated by cords of syncytial tissue which are called trabeculae

2. The lacunae enlarge and uterine capillaries break into these lacunae. Therefore, lacunae are now filled with maternal blood

3. The trabeculae are converted into **primary chorionic villi** by entering of cytotrophoblast in the central axis in each trabeculae (Fig. 2.30).

4. The lacunar spaces are now called intervillous spaces.

5. From the tip of the primary chorionic villi, the cells of the cytotrophoblast spread outwards within the substance of the syncytiotrophoblast to form outer cyto-trophoblastic shell

6. The extraembryonic mesoderm now invade the central axis of the primary chorionic villi to form **secondary chorionic villi**

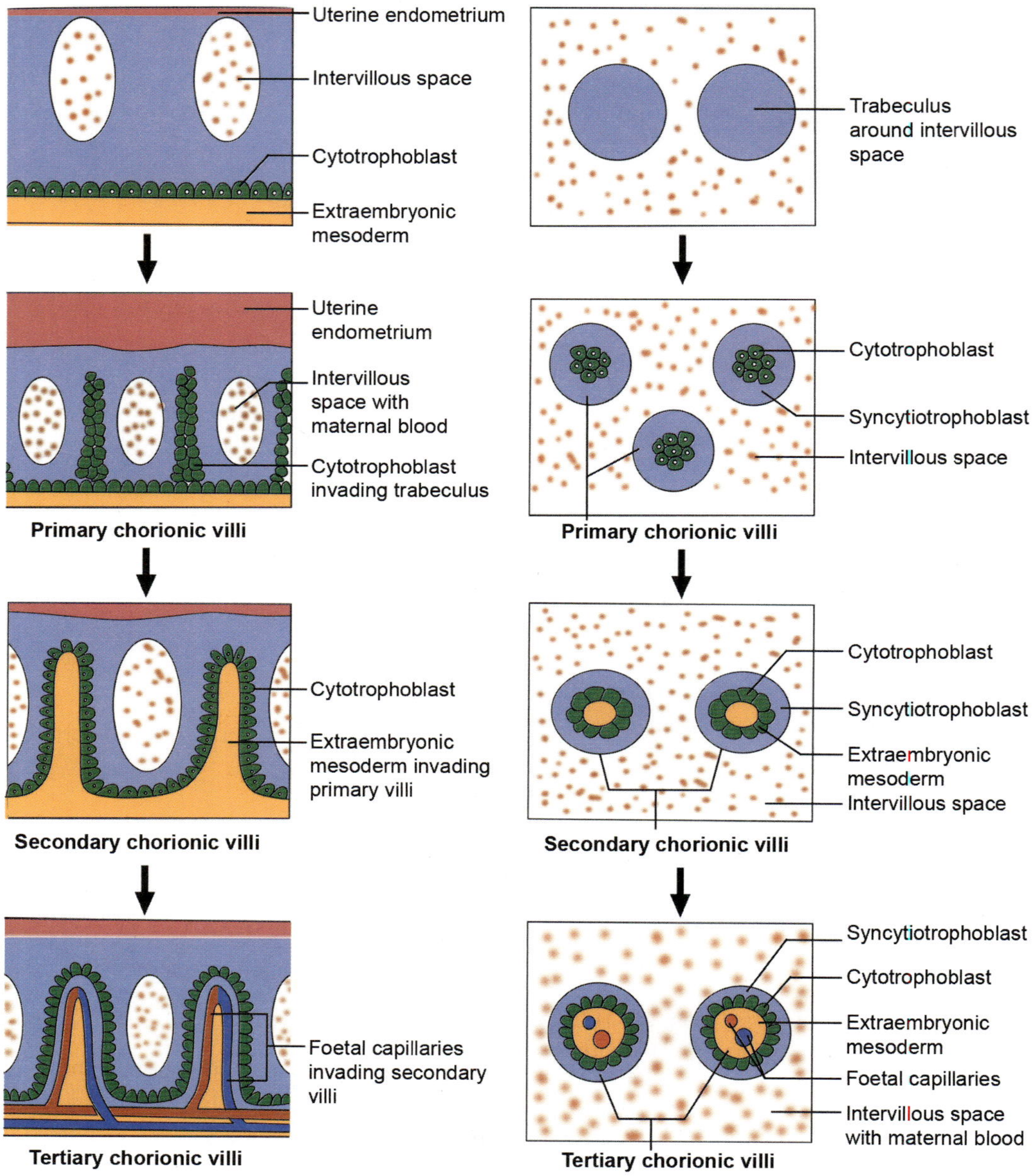

Fig. 2.30 Chorionic villi formation

7. Foetal blood vessels derived from the umbilical vessels appear within the extraembryonic mesoderm of the secondary villi, thus with the appearance of these vessels the secondary villi is converted into **tertiary chorionic villi.**

8. Later numerous branching villi project into the intervillous space

9. Chorionic villi attached to the deciduas basalis proliferate more rapidly and this part is called chorion frondosum. Rest of the chorionic villi disappears to form a smooth surface called chorion laeve (Fig. 2.31).

10. During third month of pregnancy the deciduas capsularis and parietalis are fused to obliterate chorion laeve.

Placental barriers

It consists of tissues, which intervene between foetal blood in the chorionic villi and maternal blood in the intervillous space. Through this barrier exchange of gases and metabolic products takes place between the foetus and the mother. The barrier consists of

1. Endothelium of the foetal blood vessels

2. Extra embryonic mesoderm

3. Cytotrophoblast and its basement membrane

4. Syncytiotrophoblast

In the later part of the pregnancy the barrier becomes thin by disappearance of cytotrophoblastic layer from most villi. However at the end of the pregnancy the amount of fibrous

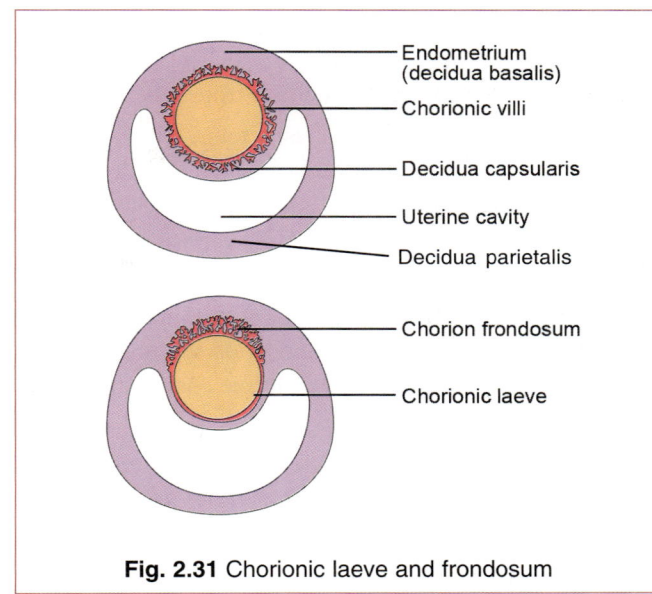

Fig. 2.31 Chorionic laeve and frondosum

tissue increases in the core of the villi and also thickening of the basement membrane of the foetal capillaries is observed. There is deposition of fibrinoid on the surface of the villi in the chorionic plate.

Functions of placenta (Fig. 2.32)

• Exchange of gaseous and metabolic products between the maternal and foetal blood

• Placenta prevents the entry of pathogenic organisms from mother to fetus. This is by Hofbauer cells of placental barrier which is phagocytic in function. However most

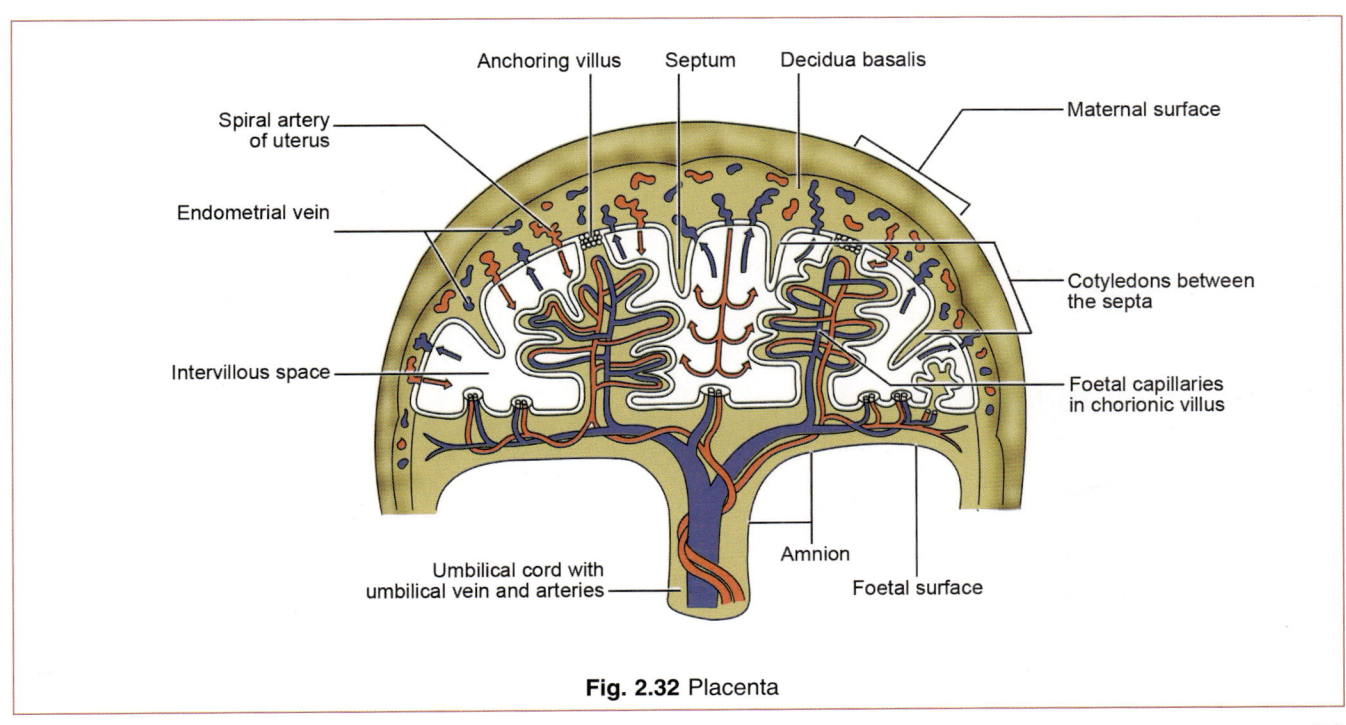

Fig. 2.32 Placenta

of the drugs consumed by the pregnant women pass through the placenta and cause embryotoxicity particularly when used in the first trimester

• Transfer of maternal antibodies to fetus, which provides immunity against infectious diseases like diphtheria, measles and small pox, but not against chicken pox

Secretion of hormones

1. **Progesterone:** It is responsible for decidual reaction in the endometrium to provide nutrition to the embryo. It maintains the integrity of the uterine endometrium.

2. **Oestrogen:** It causes enlargement of the uterus, breasts and relaxes the pelvic ligaments. The maternal blood oestrogen level rises towards the end of the pregnancy.

3. **Human Chorionic Gonadotropin (HCG):** It is synthesized by trophoblast cells and is excreted in the urine of the mother as early as 8 days of missed period. Detection of this hormone in the urine is an indicator of pregnancy. The level of HCG in the maternal blood decreases after the 16th week. Presence of high levels of HCG beyond 16th week of pregnancy may indicate molar pregnancy (hydatidiform mole).

   HCG maintains the growth of the corpus luteum up to 3rd month and also helps secretion of testosterone from the interstitial cells of testes in male foetus.

> **Placenta praevia:** Normally, the blastocyst implants along the anterior or posterior wall of the fundus or body of the uterus. Occasionally, the blastocyst implants close to the internal opening of the cervix. In such case the placenta bridges the internal opening of the cervix. The attachment of the placenta may extend partially or completely into the lower uterine segment (cervix of the uterus).
>
> This condition is called 'placenta praevia'. It causes difficulty during childbirth, and may cause even life-threatening bleeding.

Classification of placenta (Fig. 2.33)

1. According to the attachment of the umbilical cord

a. Velamentous placenta: It is a rare anomaly where umbilical cord is attached to the placental membrane instead of fetal surface

b. Placenta succenturiata: An accessory lobe of placenta may be connected to the main mass of placenta by foetal membrane

c. Battle-dore placenta: In this condition the umbilical cord is attached close to the margin of placenta

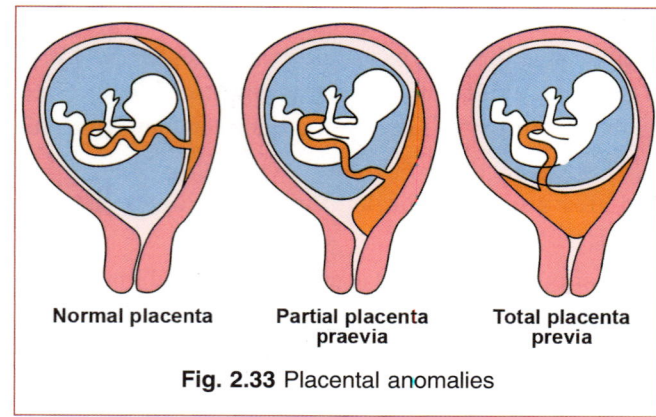

Fig. 2.33 Placental anomalies

2. According to the shape

a. Lobed placenta: Placenta may be present in the form of two or more lobes.

b. Placenta membranacea: It refers to thin placenta and is not present in the form of a disc. It presents chorionic villi all around the blastocyst.

3. According to the degree of penetration

a. Placenta accreta: Placenta is adherent to the deciduas basalis

b. Placenta increta: Placenta penetrates into the myometrium

c. Placenta percreta: Placenta penetrates the entire uterine wall.

Umbilical cord (Fig. 2.34)

It extends from the centre of the anterior abdominal wall of fetus to the placenta. At full term pregnancy, the length of the umbilical cord is about **50 cm.** It is tortuous presenting false knots. The cord contains two umbilical arteries, which carry deoxygenated blood towards the placenta and one umbilical vein, which carries oxygenated blood from the placenta to the embryo. These vessels are surrounded by a mucoid connective tissue called 'Wharton's jelly'. The umbilical cord is externally covered by **amnion**.

Umbilical cord develops from connecting stalk (unsplit extraembryonic mesoderm) which passes through the umbilical ring during fifth week of development. The connecting stalk contains allantois and umbilical vessels.

Along with the connecting stalk is yolk sac (vitelline duct) and a canal connecting intra- and extraembryonic coelomic cavities. With the enlargement of the amniotic cavity and obliteration of extraembryonic coelom, the connecting stalk becomes narrow to form the primitive umbilical cord which is now externally covered by amnion. The yolk sac gradually gets obliterated.

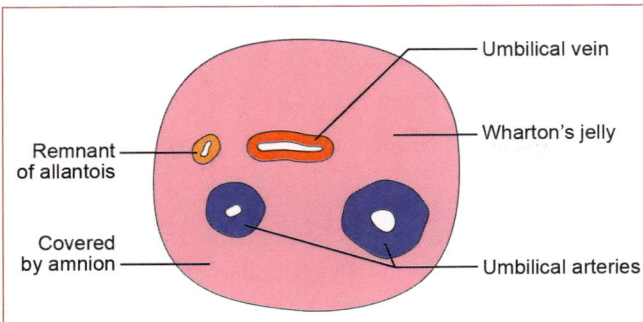

Fig. 2.34 Cross section through umbilical cord

The cord may be unusually long and may encircle the neck of the foetus producing strangulation, or may prolapse into the cervical canal. Too short a cord may create difficulty in parturition by pulling the placenta.

Contents of the umbilical cord:

1. Blood vessels: The cord contains two umbilical arteries, and one (left) umbilical vein. After birth the distal part of the artery is obliterated and proximal part remains as superior vesical artery. The left umbilical vein is fibrosed to form ligamentum teres (Fig. 2.35).

2. Vitello-intestinal duct: It communicates the mid gut with extraembryonic part of the yolk sac. In adult it may persists as Meckel's diverticulum

3. Extraembryonic mesoderm forms mucoid connective tissue called 'Wharton's jelly'

4. A small portion of the extraembryonic coelom

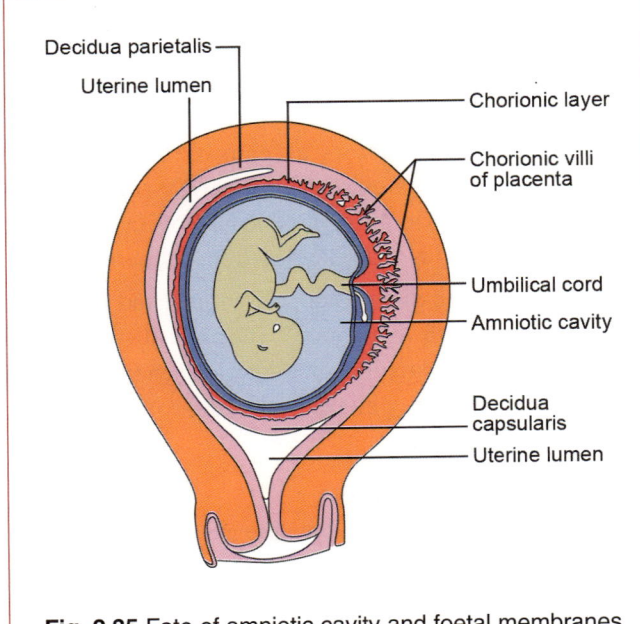

Fig. 2.35 Fate of amniotic cavity and foetal membranes

5. Distal part of the Allantoic diverticulum: In adults it forms urachus (from the apex of the bladder to umbilicus)

In 1 in 200 newborns, only one umbilical artery is present and these babies have approximately a 20% chance of having cardiac and other vascular defects

Amniotic fluid/Liquor amnii: It is a clear watery fluid which acts as a protective cushion for the embryo. It is produced partly by amniotic cells, but mainly from maternal blood. The embryo is suspended by the umbilical cord and literally swims in the fluid. The fluid maintains the uniform pressure for the symmetrical growth of the embryo. It cushions and protects the embryo. It allows the foetus to develop freely. The volume of the fluid is about 30 ml at 10 weeks of gestation and 450 ml at 20 weeks of gestation. At full term, the average volume of amniotic fluid is 1000 ml. The volume of amniotic fluid is replaced every three hours. The foetus starts swallowing the amniotic fluid from the beginning of fifth month and it is estimated that it drinks about 400 ml per day. Foetal urine is added to the amniotic fluid from fifth month onwards which is mostly watery.

Hydramnios (polyhydramnios): It is a term referred to increased volume of amniotic fluid (exceeds 2 liters). Maternal diabetes and congenital anomalies are the causes for hydramnios. When the foetus is unable to swallow the amniotic fluid due to oesophageal atresia or in neurogenic defect of the swallowing reflex in anencephaly or congenital pyloric stenosis, large amount of amniotic fluid is collected.

Oligamnios (oligohydramnios): It is a term referred to decreased volume of amniotic fluid. Oligamnios may be associated with the congenital agenesis of the metanephric kidney that results in the baby with hypoplastic lungs (underdeveloped lungs).

Parturition (Birth)

During the last 2 to 4 weeks of pregnancy the myometrium becomes thick in the upper region of the uterus and a softening and thinning of the lower segment and cervix. It signals for the labor. Labor is divided into 3 stages

1. Effacement: Uterine contraction forces the amniotic sac against the cervical canal (dilatation and thinning of the cervical canal) and rupture of amniotic sac (Fig. 2.36).

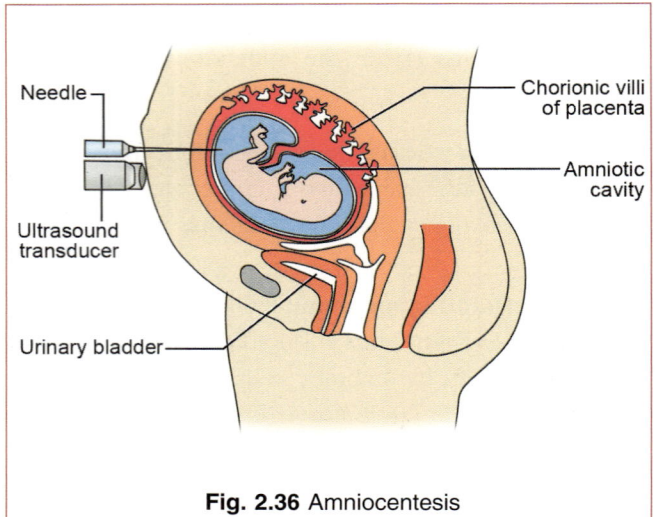

Fig. 2.36 Amniocentesis

2. Delivery of the fetus: Further uterine contraction and increased intra abdominal pressure

3. Delivery of the placenta and fetal membranes

To start with uterine contraction occurs at every 10 minutes interval, then during second stage of labor they may occur at every 1 minute and lasts for 30 to 90 seconds.

> Breech presentation: The baby enters the birth canal with the buttocks or feet first as opposed to the normal head first presentation. It is more common in those babies that are small for gestation and if the uterus is of abnormal shape.

Twinning

When mother gives birth to 2 young individuals in single pregnancy, it is referred as twinning. In twin-birth, boys are most common, next common are a boy and a girl and twin girls are least common.

Dizygotic twinning: Occasionally women's ovaries release two eggs at once that are fertilized by two different sperms. The result is non-identical or fraternal twins, who resemble one another no more closely than typical brothers and sisters. Fraternal twins are also called dizygotic twins.

The incidence of dizygotic twinning increases with the age of the mother.

Monozygotic twinning: In some pregnancies, the inner cell mass of a single blastocyst splits into two at the end of first week of development. This produces identical twins (monozygotic = from one zygote, single sperm/single ovum). They have identical genetic constitution, similarity in appearance, structure sex, fingerprints and in blood-groups. Transplantation of tissues/organs from one member of identical twins to the other member is accepted without rejection.

Types of Monozygotic twins:

- Monozygotic Bichorionic (25–30%)
- Monochorionic Biamniotic (70–75%)
- Monochorionic Monoamniotic (1–2%)

Conjoined twins (Siamese twins)

In this condition two separate organizing centers appearing simultaneously in the single germ disc (partial splitting of primitive streak and node) resulting in incomplete separation of two embryos. Such twins are equal in size. Most of the conjoined twins do not survive due to complication at parturition. Conjoined twins may be classified as follows (Fig. 2.38)

- Thoracophagus referring to fusion of the thoracic region
- Pyophagus refers to fusion of the sacral region
- Craniophagus refers to Siamese united by head

Superfetation

Under normal condition ovulation ceases during pregnancy. Aberrant ovulation when takes place during pregnancy, may lead to multiple births following fertilization at subsequent period. In superfetation, the embryos are of different ages.

TERATOLOGY AND PRENATAL DIAGNOSIS

Birth defects (congenital anomalies) refer to anatomical, behavioral, functional and metabolic disorders present at birth. Teratology refers to study of these birth defects. In majority (40 to 60%) of the birth defects the cause is unknown. The causes may be genetic, environmental or their combination.

A syndrome refers to a group of anomalies occurring together that has a common cause.

Chromosomal abnormalities

Some of the diseases observed in the humans have genetic and environmental factors as causative agents. The environmental factors can be physical (X-rays and UV rays), chemical (toxic affluents released by factories), or gaseous (harmful gases discharged from refineries).

Most of the genetic diseases appear at birth and are called congenital (or birth associated). Genetic disorders can be either due to structural or numerical changes in the chromosome(s) or gene(s) of autosomes or sex chromosomes.

1. Numerical abnormalities

Numerical abnormalities involve the gain or loss of one or more chromosomes known as aneuploidy or the addition of one or more complete haploid complements called euploid.

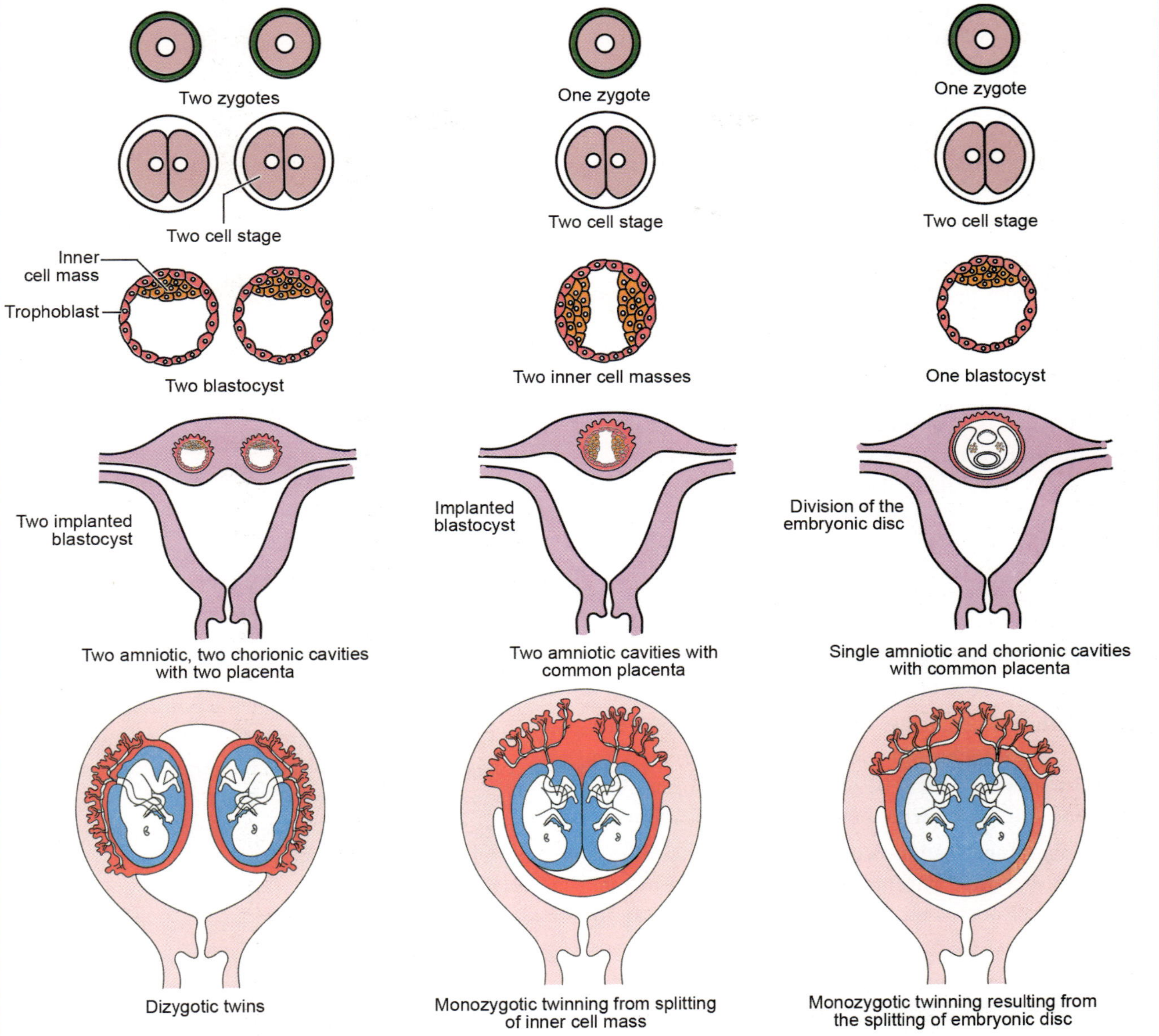

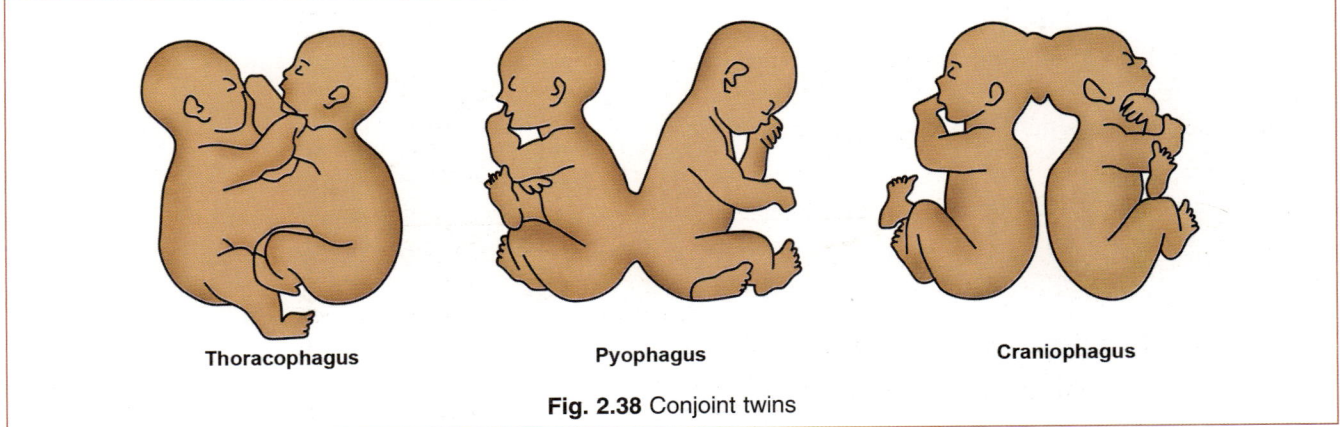

Two zygotes

Two cell stage

Inner cell mass

Trophoblast

Two blastocyst

Two implanted blastocyst

Two amniotic, two chorionic cavities with two placenta

Dizygotic twins

One zygote

Two cell stage

Two inner cell masses

Implanted blastocyst

Two amniotic cavities with common placenta

Monozygotic twinning from splitting of inner cell mass

One zygote

Two cell stage

One blastocyst

Division of the embryonic disc

Single amniotic and chorionic cavities with common placenta

Monozygotic twinning resulting from the splitting of embryonic disc

Fig. 2.37 Twinning

Thoracophagus   **Pyophagus**   **Craniophagus**

Fig. 2.38 Conjoint twins

SECTION 2

Ploidy: Cells containing multiples of 23 chromosomes are called ploidy. Some cancer cells contain triploid (69 chromosome) and tetraploidy (92 chromosome). Most ploidy conceptions are spontaneously aborted or have short-term survival.

Trisomy: The presence of an extra chromosome is called the trisomy 21, 13, 16, and 18, X etc. Down's syndrome (trisomy 21) is the most common trisomy in live borns.

Monosomy: The absence of a single chromosome is monosomy. Monosomy X (Turner syndrome) is the most common one.

Mosaicism: It is a postzygotic event and occurs after fertilization at an early cell division in the embryos. It results in an individual with two (rarely more) cell lines having different chromosomal constitutions. These numerical abnormalities are usually the result of non-dysjunction, which is the failure of a pair of chromosome to separate normally during either the first or the second meiotic division.

2. Structural abnormalities

Deletions: Deletion is caused due to a chromosome break and subsequently loss of genetic material.

Translocation: Interchange of genetic material between non-homologous chromosomes. The individual with balanced translocation can be phenotypically normal, but can produce offsprings with unbalanced translocation.

Robertsonian translocation occurs when the long arm of the two acrocentric chromosomes fuses to form one chromosome. Robertsonian translocation occurs only in chromosome 13, 14, 15, 21 and 22.

Inversions: Inversions are common structural anomalies and may be either pericentric (involving centromere) or paracentric (not involving centromere). Individuals with inversion are usually normal in phenotype but can produce offsprings with deletion or duplications.

Isochromosomes: This is caused due to an error in cell division when the chromosome divides along the axis perpendicular to its axis of division. The resultant chromosome will be either both 'p' or 'q' arm of the chromosome.

Genetic disorder involving autosomes

1. **Cri-du-chat syndrome:** The cause is partial deletion of short arm of chromosome number 5. It is characterized by cat-like cry of babies.

2. **Down's syndrome:** (Trisomy 21) 47, XY. In gametogenesis two 21 chromosomes are carried

due to non-disjunction. It is common in children born to elderly women. The syndrome is characterized by flattened occiput, short and flat-bridge nose, epicanthic folds, protruding tongue, simian crease (single line in palm), low IQ, short and stocky hands and feet.

Genetic disorder involving sex chromosomes

1. **Turner's syndrome:** The individual is female. It is due to the monosomy of the X chromosome (45, XO). It is characterized by growth retardation, webbed neck, short stature, cubitus valgus and impaired secondary sexual characteristics.

2. **Klinefelter's syndrome:** The individual is male. It is due to the presence of one extra X chromosome (47 XXY). It is characterized by gynecomastia, hypogonadism, and increased height.

Fragile X syndrome: It is a genetic condition involving changes in long arm of the X chromosome. It is the most common form of inherited intellectual disability (mental retardation) in boys. It is characterized by high forehead, large ears, long face and large testis. Fragile X syndrome is caused by a change in a gene called FMR1. A small part of the gene code is repeated on a fragile area of the X chromosome. The FMR1 gene makes a protein needed for brain to grow properly. Both boys and girls are affected. Since boys have only one X chromosome, a single fragile X is likely to affect them more severely. One can have fragile X syndrome even if one's parents do not have it.

Teratogens causing birth defects:

The teratogens associated with birth defects are listed below in the table.

In reviewing the history of teratogens two disasters need to be mentioned namely atomic bomb explosion in Japan and Thalidomide tragedy in Germany (1957)

The devastating effects of atomic bomb explosion over Hiroshima and Nagasaki during 1945 killed about 62,000 people and further its radiation effect killed many more. The pregnant women who survived after atomic bomb explosion had a higher percentage of abortions, death of children within first year of life and severe neurological defects in survived children.

Thalidomide tragedy: Thalidomide is an anti-nausea and sedative drug that was introduced in the late 1950s and was used in pregnant women for effects of morning sickness. It was sold from 1957 to 1962 and then withdrawn after being found to be a teratogen. More than 10,000 children in 46 countries were born with limb defects (phocomelia) as a consequence of thalidomide use.

Prenatal diagnosis

There are many prenatal diagnostic tools available to assess the growth and development of the foetus. This is helpful in early detection of birth defects.

1. **Ultrasonography:** It is a non invasive technique where sound waves are reflected from tissues to create images. It can be performed through abdominal wall or through vagina. This investigation reveals many parameters like

Teratogen	Birth defects
Maternal infections	
Rubella virus (German measles)	Cataracts, Heart defects (PDA), Glaucoma, Deafness, tooth abnormalities
Herpes simplex virus	Microcephaly, retinal dysplasia
Cytomegalovirus	Microcephaly, mental retardation, blindness, foetal death
Syphilis	Mental retardation, deafness
HIV	Microcephaly and growth retardation
Physical agents	
Radiation from X-ray	Microcephaly, skull defects, spina bifida, cleft palate, limb defects
Hyperthermia	Anencephaly, mental retardation, spina bifida, facial defects, limb and heart defects
Chemical agents	
Thalidomide	Limb defects, heart defects
Aminopterin	Anencephaly, hydrocephalus, cleft lip and palate
Anti-convulsant drugs (phenytoin, valproic acid)	Craniofacial defects, mental retardation, neural tube defects, heart defects, limb defects
Diazepam (valium)	Cleft lip
Warfarin	Chondrodysplasia and microcephaly
Alcohol	Holoprosencephaly-(explained separately)
Coccaine	Microcephaly, behavioral disorder, growth retardation, gastroschisis
Vitamin A	Craniofacial defects, eye defect, cleft palate
Organic mercury sprayed over food grains	Neurological defects
Lead	Neurological defects and growth retardation
Hormones	
Maternal diabetes	Heart and neural tube defects
Synthetic progesterones used in pregnancy to prevent abortion	Masculinising effect in female child, enlarged clitoris
Cortisone	Cleft palate
Maternal obesity	Heart defects, omphalocele

foetal age, growth, anomalies, amniotic fluid level, placental position and multiple gestations if present. Congenital anomalies like neural tube defects (spina bifida, anencephaly), abdominal wall defects (omphalocele and gastroschisis), heart defects, facial defects (cleft lip and palate) can be determined by ultrasonography.

Foetal age and growth is assessed by crown-rump length (CRL = sitting height) during 5th to 10th week of gestation or as the crown heel length (CHL = standing height/Vertex to heel), biparietal diameter (BPD) of the skull, femur length, and abdominal circumference. At the time of birth the weight of the normal foetus is about 3000 g to 3550 g, CR length is about 36 cm, and its CHL is about 50 cm.

The developing embryo can first be visualized at about 6 weeks gestation. Recognition of the major internal organs and extremities, abnormalities if any, can be best accomplished between 16 to 20 weeks of gestation. The limitation of this technique is that, subtle abnormalities may not be detected in early pregnancy, or may not be detected at all. A good example of this is Down's syndrome (trisomy 21) where the morphologic abnormalities are often not marked, but only subtle features such as nuchal thickening can be determined.

2. Maternal serum screening:

Serum α-fetoprotein (AFP): It is produced by fetal liver and its maternal serum level increases during second trimester and then begins to decline after 30 weeks of gestation. It is used for detection of neural tube defects, omphalocele, amniotic band syndrome, sacrococcygeal teratoma and intestinal atresia. Its level is decreased in Down's syndrome, trisomy 18, sex chromosomal abnormalities.

Human chorionic gonadotropin (HCG): The maternal blood HCG levels decreases after 16th week of development. But its level remains high in molar pregnancy.

3. Chorionic villus sampling (CVS) biopsy: It is a technique used to detect the genetic disorders much earlier than (carried out at 10–13 weeks after the last missed period) amniocentesis (16–20 weeks).

In **chorionic villus sampling biopsy**, a catheter is inserted through the cervix to the chorion and a sample of chorionic villi is obtained by suction or cutting. It has risk (0.2 to 0.3% fetal mortality, infection, amniotic fluid leak) and limitation (some but not all of the placental cells tested in the CVS will be abnormal). CVS cannot

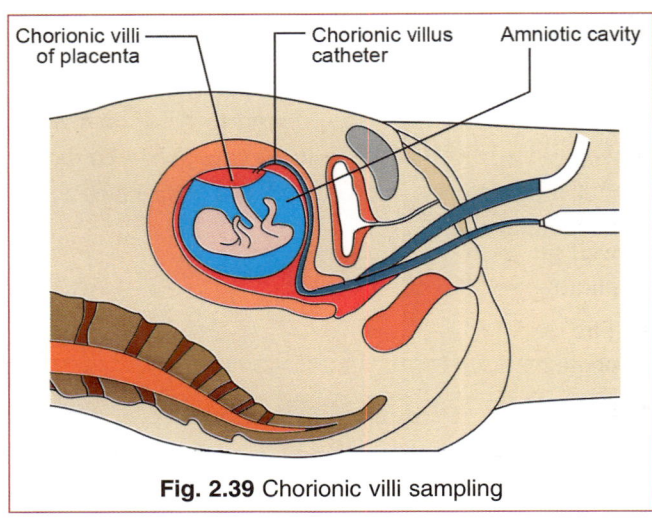
Fig. 2.39 Chorionic villi sampling

detect all birth defects. It is used for testing chromosomal abnormalities or any other specific genetic disorders only if there is family history or any other reason (Fig. 2.39).

1. **Amniocentesis:** The aspiration of amniotic fluid is known as amniocentesis. It is safely performed at 14th–16th weeks of pregnancy. This is done to investigate the nuclear sex of the fetus in some sex linked diseases. The enzyme estimation of the fluid and other chemical tests may be helpful to diagnose the gross fetal malformations.

2. **Cordocentesis (percutaneous umbilical blood sampling):** It is a diagnostic test that examines blood from the fetus to detect foetal abnormalities. It is an ultrasound guided procedure in which a thin needle is inserted through the abdomen and uterine walls to the umbilical cord. The needle is inserted into the umbilical cord to retrieve a small sample of foetal blood. The sample is sent to the laboratory for analysis. The procedure is similar to amniocentesis, but instead of amniotic fluid foetal blood is collected. Cordocentesis is usually done when diagnostic information cannot be obtained through amniocentesis, chorionic villus sampling, ultrasound or when the results of these tests are non conclusive. It is performed after 17 weeks of pregnancy. Cordocentesis detects chromosome abnormalities like Down's syndrome and blood disorders (i.e. foetal hemolytic disease).

3. **Karyotyping:** It is an orderly arrangement of chromosomes based on their overall size and position of centromere and banding pattern.
- Numerical abnormalities involving the gain or loss of one or more chromosomes can be detected by this technique.
- A small quantity of venous blood is collected and suspended in a suitable culture medium in which lymphocytes can multiply.

- The cell division is arrested at metaphase stage by adding colchicine or colcemid to the medium. The cells are then treated with hypotonic saline for proper spreading out of chromosomes.

- A suspension containing cells is spread out on a slide and stained with Giemsa in which the chromosomes are well spread out. A metaphase chromosomal plate is then photographed.

- The individual chromosomes are cut from the photographs and are arranged in a proper sequence.

- From this sequential arrangement of chromosomes (karyotype) any abnormalities in their number or form can be identified.

4. **Fluorescence *in situ* hybridization (FISH) technique:** This technique detects and locates the presence or absence of specific DNA sequence (gene) in a chromosome. It can also be used to detect and locate specific RNA target in cells.

5. **DNA recombinant technology:**
   Recombinant DNA technology is a technology that allows DNA to be produced via artificial means. This technology works by taking DNA from two different sources and combining it into a single molecule. That alone, however, will not do much. It only becomes useful when that artificially-created DNA is reproduced, in a process known as DNA cloning. There are two main types of cloning that recombinant DNA technology is used for: therapeutic cloning and reproductive cloning. Most people are familiar with reproductive cloning, which will produce an organism with the exact genetic information of one that already exists. Therapeutic cloning is explained below.

   Recombinant DNA is used to identify, map and sequence genes, and to determine their function

6. **Micro array**

   A DNA microarray (also commonly known as DNA chip or biochip) is a collection of microscopic DNA spots (proteins) attached to a solid surface, usually a silicon chip. Scientists use DNA microarrays to measure the expression levels of large number of genes simultaneously or to genotype multiple regions of a genome. Each DNA spot contains picomoles (10–12 moles) of a specific DNA sequence, known as probes (or reporters or oligos). These can be of short section of a gene or other DNA element that are used to hybridize a cDNA or cRNA (also called anti-sense RNA) sample (called *target*) under high-stringency conditions. DNA

Microarray technology helps researchers learn more about different diseases such as heart diseases, mental illness, infectious disease and especially the study of cancer.

Fetal therapy

1. **Foetal medical treatment:** Fetal treatment for infections, endocrine dysfunctions and other medical problems are provided through mother which cross the placental barrier to reach the fetus.

2. **Foetal surgery:** With advances in ultrasound and surgical procedures several types of surgeries may be performed, including placing shunts to remove fluid from organs or cavities. Surgeries are also performed after opening the uterus to repair diaphragmatic hernia and repairing spina bifida defects.

3. **Stem cell transplantation:** Foetus does not develop any immune-competence before 18 weeks gestation. It is possible to transplant tissue or cells without rejection.

4. **Gene therapy:** Gene therapy is the insertion of genes into an individual's cells and tissues to treat a disease, such as a hereditary disease in which a deleterious mutant allele is replaced with a functional one. The most common form of gene therapy involves using DNA that encodes a functional, therapeutic gene in order to replace a mutated gene. Although the technology is still in its infancy, it has been used with some success. Scientific breakthroughs continue to move gene therapy toward mainstream medicine.

Amniocentesis and stem cells:

Recent studies have discovered that amniotic fluid can be a rich source of multipotent mesenchymal, hematopoietic, neural, epithelial and endothelial stem cells.

Artificial heart valves, working tracheas, as well as muscle, fat, bone, heart, neural and liver cells have all been engineered through use of amniotic stem cells.

Therapeutic cloning (Somatic nuclear transfer):

It is fundamentally different from human reproductive cloning, that it produces stem cells, not babies (Fig. 2.40).

A nuclei taken from adult cells (e.g. skin) is introduced into enucleated oocytes. Oocytes are stimulated to differentiate into blastocysts and embryonic stem cells are harvested. Since the cells are derived from the host, they are genetically compatible. These stem cells would be used for replacement of an organ, piece of nerve tissue, or quantity of skin.

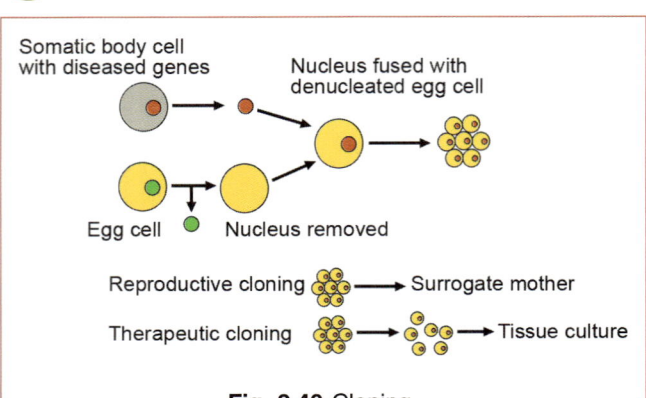

Somatic body cell
with diseased genes   Nucleus fused with
                             denucleated egg cell

Egg cell   Nucleus removed

Reproductive cloning ⟶ Surrogate mother

Therapeutic cloning ⟶ ⟶ Tissue culture

Fig. 2.40 Cloning

MCQs

1. An undescended testis of a prepubertal male is removed since it is at higher risk to develop testicular cancer. Histologic analysis reveals that cells of the germ line in this testis have advanced as far as which of the following stages of development?
   A. Primordial germ cell
   B. Spermatogonium
   C. Primary spermatocyte
   D. Secondary spermatocyte

2. A female patient with unexplained infertility is treated with menopausal gonadotropin and pure follicle stimulating hormone to induce follicular development. Several oocytes are aspirated from enlarged follicles and cultured in nutrient medium until they reach the normal second stage of meiotic arrest before they are fertilized. Fertilization is therefore carried out at which of the following stages of oocyte development?
   A. Prophase of the primary oocyte
   B. Metaphase of the primary oocyte
   C. Prophase of the secondary oocyte
   D. Metaphase of the secondary oocyte

3. Ultrasound examination of an anovulatory patient with polycystic ovary syndrome (PCOS) reveals that her ovaries contain multiple enlarged but immature follicles. The oocytes within these follicles have advanced to which of the following stages of meiosis?
   A. First meiotic prophase
   B. First meiotic metaphase
   C. Second meiotic prophase
   D. Second meiotic metaphase

4. A 23-year-old male with respiratory difficulties is diagnosed with a mediastinal germ cell tumor. The primordial germ cell that gave rise to this tumor inappropriately migrated to this site from which of the following tissues?
   A. Liver
   B. Yolk sac
   C. Testis
   D. Spleen

5. Gastrulation is the main event which takes during 3rd week of development. During this period which of the following structure induces the formation of intra-embryonic mesoderm?
   A. Notochord
   B. Prechordal plate
   C. Primitive streak
   D. Chorion

6. The sclerotome of the somite gives rise to
   A. Vertebral column
   B. Dermis of the skin
   C. Muscles of the body wall
   D. Epidermis of the skin

7. The sacrococcygeal teratoma is derived from the remnants of the
   A. Prechordal plate
   B. Notochord
   C. Trophoblast
   D. Primitive streak

8. The 3rd week of development is highly sensitive stage for teratogenic insults. Which of the following major event takes during this week?
   A. Completion of neural tube formation
   B. Fusion of heart tubes
   C. Rudimentary limb buds appears
   D. Formation of intraembryonic mesoderm

9. Which of the following structure induces the formation of neural tube?
   A. Primitive streak
   B. Prechordal plate
   C. Notochord
   D. Chorion

10. A foetus is suspected to have neural tube defect. Which of the following estimation from maternal serum would predict this anomaly?
    A. Progesterone
    B. α-fetoprotein
    C. Human Chorionic Gonadotropin (HCG)
    D. Estriol

11. Ultrasound of a fetus at the 6th month of development reveals a possible meningomyelocele in the lower lumbar region. History of the mother reveals that the anticonvulsant valproic acid was taken during the first trimester. This drug probably disrupted axial development through interference with the metabolism of which of the following factors?

    A. Progesterone
    B. Folic acid
    C. Human chorionic gonadotropin
    D. alpha-fetoprotein

12. The melanoblast of the skin is derived from

    A. Neural tube cells
    B. Surface ectoderm
    C. Neural crest cells
    D. Sclerotome

13. A 32-year-old lady gave birth to a siamese twins with fusion of the sacral region. It is referred as

    A. Craniophagus
    B. Thoracophagus
    C. Pygophagus
    D. Parasitic twins

14. Which of the following is not a feature of monozygotic twins?

    A. They have identical features
    B. They have identical genetic constitution
    C. They have identical sex
    D. The twins can be male and female

15. At full term, the placental barrier consists of
    A. Cytotrophoblast and Syncytiotrophoblast
    B. Syncytiotrophoblast only
    C. Mesoderm and Cytotrophoblast
    D. Mesoderm and Syncytiotrophoblast

16. A pregnant lady with the history of genetically abnormal child in the past was advised to undergo a procedure 'amniocentesis. This procedure is most safely performed after the
    A. 8th week of pregnancy
    B. 10th week of pregnancy
    C. 6th week of pregnancy
    D. 14th week of pregnancy

17. A female patient spontaneously aborts a hydatidiform mole (molar pregnancy). Which of the following hormone level remains elevated in maternal blood even after 16th week of development? (which would provide a basis to predict this anomaly)
    A. Progesterone
    B. Adrenocortical hormone
    C. Human chorionic gonadotropin (HCG)
    D. Follicle stimulating hormone

18. A 32-year-old pregnant lady diagnosed to have a condition 'Polyhydramnios'. Which of the following anomaly would be associated with this condition?
    A. Hydatidiform mole
    B. Hypoplasia of the lungs
    C. Oesophageal atresia
    D. Agenesis of the kidney

19. A pregnant woman is found to have her placenta attached to the lower uterine segment during ultrasound investigation. The Gynecologist is concerned about difficulty during child birth. This condition is called
    A. Placenta succenturiata
    B. Velamentous placenta
    C. Placenta accreta
    D. Placenta praevia

20. At the time of birth, the Crown-Rump (CR) length of the normal child is about
    A. 28–30 cm
    B. 31–33 cm
    C. 35–36 cm
    D. 38–41 cm

21. An infant is born with Meckel's diverticulum from the ileum. It is a remnant of
    A. Thyroglossal duct
    B. Vitello-intestinal duct from mid-gut
    C. Allantois
    D. Mesonephric duct

22. An infant born is known to have congenital cysts of the lung. The lungs are developed from
    A. Ectoderm
    B. Foregut
    C. Midgut
    D. Mesoderm of the 2nd pharyngeal arch

23. Which of the following muscle is developed from Ectoderm?
    A. Deltoid
    B. Musculature of the stomach
    C. Hamstring muscles
    D. Muscles of the iris
    E. Cardiac muscles

24. The following adult structures are derived from ectoderm lining the stomodeum *except*
    A. Anterior pituitary
    B. Epithelium of the paranasal air sinuses
    C. Salivary glands
    D. Thyroid gland

25. The remnant of the notochord in adult persists as
    A. Vertebral column
    B. Spinal cord
    C. Nucleus pulposus of the intervertebral disc
    D. Ligamentum flavum

26. The sclerotome of the somite give rise to
    A. Vertebral column
    B. Dermis of the skin
    C. Muscles of the body wall
    D. Epidermis of the skin

27. The heart develops in
    A. Splanchnopleuric layer of the lateral plate mesoderm in the midline cranial to prechordal plate before head fold formation
    B. Somatopleuric layer of the lateral plate mesoderm caudal to the prechordal plate before head fold formation
    C. Splanchnopleuric layer of the lateral plate mesoderm in the midline caudal to prechordal plate before head fold formation
    D. Somatopleuric layer of the lateral plate mesoderm cranial to the prechordal plate before head fold formation

28. An incomplete closure of the neural tube when it affects the spinal cord is called
    A. Myelocele
    B. Anencephalus
    C. Spina bifida occulta
    D. Meningocele
    E. Meningomyelocele

29. During routine ultrasound investigation of a pregnant lady, it was observed that the fetus had a serious neurological deficit in which the neural tube fails to close and also at the same region the vertebral arch failed to form. This condition is called
    A. Spina bifida occulta
    B. Spina bifida cystica
    C. Myelocele
    D. Anencephalus

30. The melanoblasts of the skin is derived from
    A. Neural tube cells
    B. Surface ectoderm
    C. Neural crest cells
    D. Sclerotome

31. The chorion frondosum is the bushy chorionic villi formed at
    A. Decidua capsularis
    B. Decidua basalis
    C. Decidua parietalis
    D. Abembryonic pole

32. Which of the following stage will the fertilized concept implant in the uterine endometrium?
    A. Zygote
    B. Morula
    C. Blastocyst
    D. Embryo

33. The umbilical cord is developed from
    A. Unsplit intraembryonic mesoderm
    B. Somatopleuric layer of extraembryonic mesoderm with trophoblast
    C. Splanchnopleuric layer of extraembryonic mesoderm
    D. Unsplit extraembryonic mesoderm

34. A pregnant lady is diagnosed to have a condition 'oligamnios'. Which of the following anomaly would be more commonly associated with this condition?
    A. Oesophageal atresia
    B. Anencephaly
    C. Agenesis of metanephric kidney
    D. Molar pregnancy

35. During full term pregnancy, the umbilical cord consists of all the structures *except*
    A. Remnant of Vitello-intestinal duct
    B. Remnant of the Allantoic diverticulum
    C. Right umbilical vein
    D. Two umbilical arteries

36. The normal site of fertilization is
    A. Uterus
    B. Ovary
    C. Pelvic cavity
    D. Ampulla of the uterine tube
    E. Isthmus of the uterine tube

37. The secretory/progestational phase of the uterine cycle is characterized by all the following features *except*
    A. Endometrium is divisible into compact, spongy and basal layers

B. Saw-toothed appearance of the uterine glands

C. Increased tortuosity of the spiral arteries

D. It is under the influence of both progesterone and oestrogen

E. It is under the influence of oestrogen alone

38. The oestrogen is secreted from
   A. Corpus luteum
   B. Cells of the tunica externa of the Graafian follicle
   C. Cells of the tunica interna of the Graafian follicle
   D. Corpus albicans

39. The normal chromosome number of a secondary oocyte is
   A. 22X
   B. 22Y
   C. 44XX
   D. 44XY

40. The acrosomal cap of the spermatozoa is derived from
   A. Nucleus of spermatid
   B. Mitochondria of the spermatids
   C. Proximal centriole of the spermatid
   D. Golgi apparatus of the spermatid

41. The average human gestational period after fertilization is
   A. 280 days
   B. 266 days
   C. 252 days
   D. 238 days

42. Crossing over (exchange of DNA) is an important event during meiosis cell division. In which of the following stage does it occur?
   A. Diakinesis
   B. Diplotene
   C. Pachytene
   D. Zygotene
   E. Leptotene

43. During a visit to a gynecologist, a patient reports she received Vitamin A treatment for her acne unknowingly during the first two months of an undetected pregnancy. Which organ systems in the developing fetus are most likely to be affected?
   A. The digestive system

B. The endocrine organs

C. The urinary and reproductive system

D. The skeletal and central nervous system

44. A 27-year-old pregnant woman is infected with the rubella virus. Her embryo or fetus is at the greatest risk from the development of a malformation if transplacental transmission occurs during which of the following time periods?
   A. Days 1–15
   B. Days 15–60
   C. The second trimester
   D. Third trimester

45. During embryological development, hemopoiesis occurs in different organs at different times. Which of the following are the correct organs, in the correct sequence, at which hemopoiesis occurs embryo-logically?
   A. Amnion, yolk sac, placenta, bone marrow
   B. Placenta, liver and spleen, yolk sac, bone marrow
   C. Yolk sac, bone marrow, liver and spleen
   D. Yolk sac, liver, spleen and lymphatic organs, bone marrow

46. A neonate is found to have a sacrococcygeal teratoma that contains several different tissue types resulting from a persistence of the primitive streak. The primitive streak normally gives rise to which of the following structures?
   A. Dorsal root ganglia
   B. Notochord
   C. Spinal cord
   D. Thyroid gland

47. A 27-year-old pregnant female presents to her obstetrician and reveals that twins run in her family. During ultrasound examination it has been confirmed that the embryo has split at the blastocyst stage. Splitting of the embryo at the blastocyst stage results in which of the following?
   A. Conjoined twins
   B. Dizygotic twins
   C. Fraternal twins
   D. Monozygotic twins

SECTION 2

Answers to MCQs

1. A
2. C
3. A
4. B
5. C
6. B
7. D
8. D
9. C
10. B
11. B
12. C
13. C
14. D
15. B
16. D
17. C
18. C
19. D
20. D
21. C
22. B
23. D

24. D
25. C
26. A
27. A
28. A
29. A
30. C
31. B
32. B
33. D
34. C
35. C
36. D
37. E
38. C
39. A
40. D
41. B
42. C
43. D
44. B
45. D
46. B
47. D

Write short notes on

General Anatomy

1. Epithelial tissue
2. Cell junctions
3. Collagen fibres
4. Fibroblast
5. Hyaline cartilage
6. Primary cartilaginous joint
7. Secondary cartilaginous joint
8. Fibrous joint
9. Cardiac muscle
10. Epiphysis
11. Blood supply to a long bone
12. Laws of ossification
13. Arterial anastomoses
14. Capillaries and sinusoids
15. Structure of a neuron
16. Glial cells
17. Lymph node
18. Periosteum
19. Dermatome
20. Structure of a typical synovial joint
21. Centre of ossification
22. Growing end of the long bone
23. Diaphysis

General Embryology

1. Spermatogenesis
2. Spermiogenesis
3. Structure of a matured spermatozoon
4. Oogenesis
5. Structure of a secondary oocyte
6. Graafian follicle

7. Corpus luteum
8. Fertlization
9. Implantation
10. Morula
11. Blastocyst
12. Trophoblast
13. Chorion
14. Amnion
15. Primitive streak
16. Yolk sac
17. Gastrulation
18. Intraembryonic mesoderm
19. Somite
20. Notochord
21. Umbilical cord
22. Derivatives of the germ layer
23. Neural tube and its defects
24. Neural crest cells
25. Septum transversum
26. Amniotic fluid
27. Prenatal diagnosis
28. Chromosomes
29. Karyotyping
30. Sex chromatin (Barr body)
31. Anomalies of the placenta
32. Teratogens
33. X Chromosome
34. Cri du chat syndrome
35. Klinefelter syndrome
36. Turner syndrome
37. Trisomy 21
38. Sex chromosomes

SECTION 2

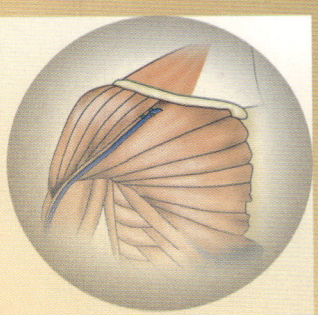

Upper Limb

Osteology of the Upper Limb

3

- Clavicle
- Scapula
- Humerus
- Radius
- Ulna
- Carpal bones, Metacarapals and Phalanges
- MCQs

Objectives
- To list the bones forming the skeleton of the upper limb
- To explain the major parts, articulations, attachment, blood supply and clinical relevance of each of them.

CLAVICLE (COLLAR BONE)

It is a prominent subcutaneous bone present on either side of the root of the neck connecting the trunk with the upper limb (Fig. 3.1).

- Medially it articulates with the manubrium sterni at the sternoclavicular joint.
- Laterally, it articulates with the acromial process of the scapula at the acromioclavicular joint.
- Its superior surface is subcutaneous. Its medial end is expanded and lateral end is flat (Figs 3.1 and 3.2).
- The medial 2/3 of the clavicle is convex forwards. It has following attachments

Anterior aspect—origin to pectoralis major muscle,

Posterior surface—origin of sternohyoid,

Superior surface—origin to sternomastoid

Inferior surface—costoclavicular ligament,

- The lateral 1/3rd of the clavicle is concave forwards. It has following attachments

Anterior border—origin to deltoid muscle

Posterior border—insertion of trapezius

Upper surface—subcutaneous

Lower surface—It has a conoid tubercle and trapezoid ridge, which provides attachments to coracoclavicular ligament (Fig. 3.2).

Peculiarities of clavicle

1. It is the only long bone placed horizontally in the body.
2. It is subcutaneous and can be easily palpated.
3. It is the first bone to ossify in the body.
4. It is the only long bone with two primary centres of ossification for shaft.
5. It is the only long bone to ossify in membrane.
6. It has no medullary cavity.

Ossification

It is the only long bone having 2 primary centre of ossification and they appear during 5th–6th week of intrauterine life (IUL) and fuse at 45th day of IUL. One

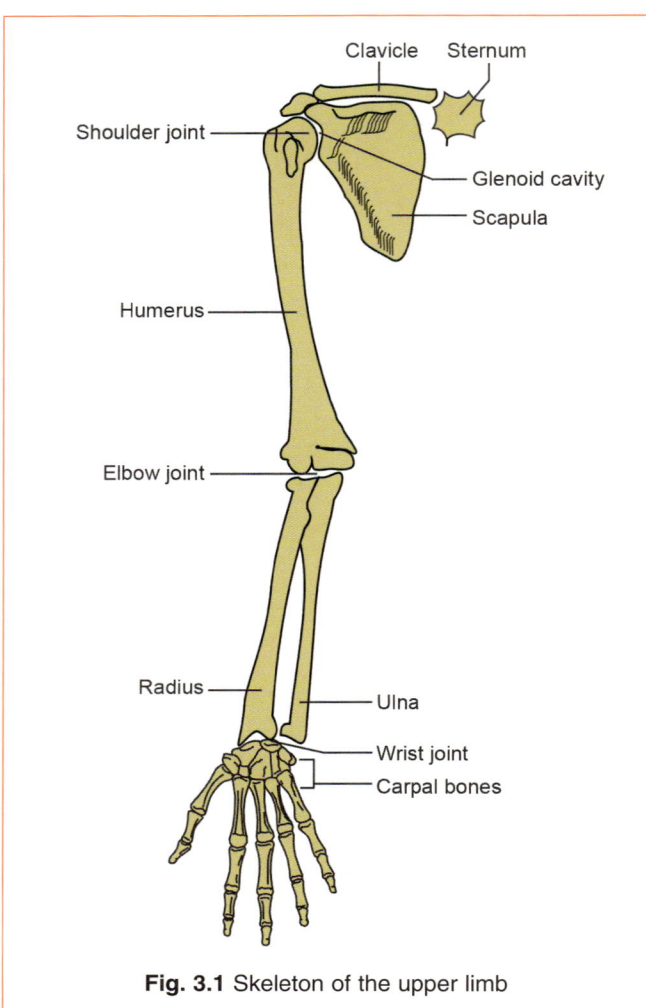

Fig. 3.1 Skeleton of the upper limb

SECTION 3

The junction of medial 2/3rd and lateral 1/3rd is the most common site of fracture in clavicle.

It usually occurs due to fall on the outstretched hand.

After fracture, the lateral segment displaces downwards due to the weight of the upper limb and it can also compress subclavian vessels. The medial segment is displaced upwards by the pull of the sternomastoid muscle.

Sometimes a vein connecting cephalic with external jugular vein may be torn during fracture of clavicle leading to severe bleeding.

Clavicle fracture is treated by immobilization with figure 8 bandage.

CASE-1

A 15-year-old boy while demonstrating his skills in bicycle, suddenly went off balance and fell onto the ground with all his body weight on his right outstretched hand. A distinctive cracking noise was heard, and he felt sudden pain in his right shoulder region. On examination, the smooth contour of his right clavicle was found to be absent. The shoulder and the lateral end of the clavicle were depressed and the medial part of the clavicle was elevated. The clavicle was fractured and the edges of the bony fragments could be palpated. From the knowledge of your anatomy answer the following questions.

1. Which part of the clavicle is most commonly fractured?

2. Why are the bony fragments displaced?

secondary centre appears for medial end at puberty and fuses with the shaft by 20 years.

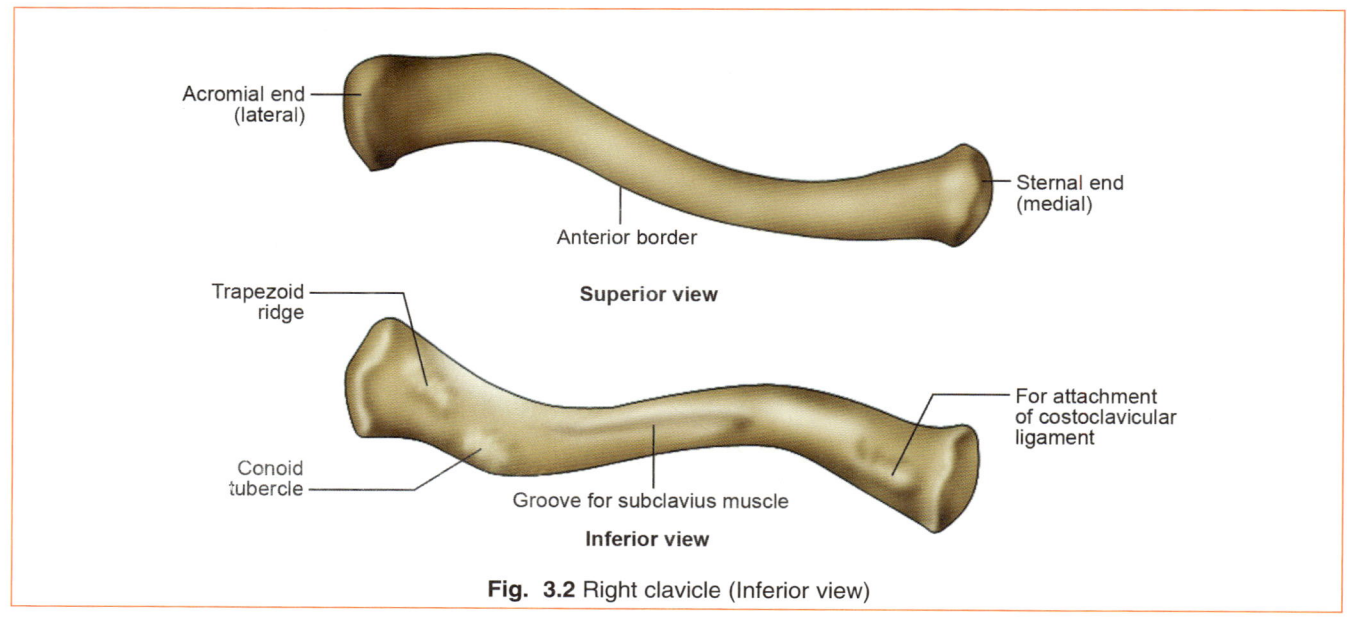

Fig. 3.2 Right clavicle (Inferior view)

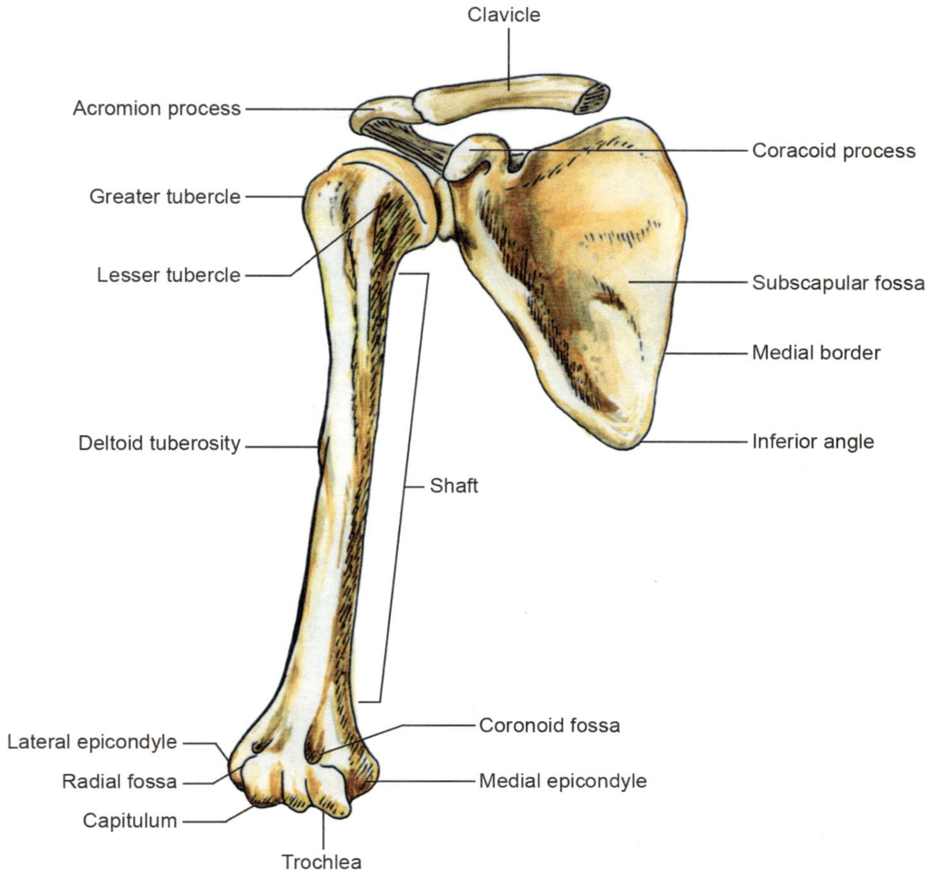

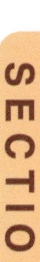

Clavicle

Acromion process

Greater tubercle

Lesser tubercle

Coracoid process

Subscapular fossa

Medial border

Inferior angle

Deltoid tuberosity

Shaft

Lateral epicondyle

Radial fossa

Capitulum

Coronoid fossa

Medial epicondyle

Trochlea

Fig. 3.3 Humerus and Scapula - Anterior View

3. Why do mechanical forces leads to clavicle fracture instead of dislocating the sternoclavicular and acromioclavicular joints?

4. What structures are likely to be damaged in a simple fracture of the clavicle?

SCAPULA (SHOULDER BLADE)

This bone is placed in the scapular region behind the upper 7 ribs. It gives attachments to many muscles (scapular muscles) that connect the upper limb with trunk (Fig. 3.3).

Scapula presents two surfaces and three borders.

a. Costal surface is also called 'subscapular fossa'. It provides attachment to the subscapularis muscle.

b. Dorsal surface is divided into an upper supraspinous and lower infraspinous fossa by spinous process. The two fossae are connected through spinoglenoid notch.

i. Superior border - It presents 'suprascapular notch' which is bridged by suprascapular ligament converting the

notch into a foramen. The suprascapular nerve passes beneath the ligament while the suprascapular artery passes above the ligament.

ii. Lateral border - It extends below the glenoid cavity and provides attachment to teres minor muscle in the upper 2/3rd and teres major muscle in the lower 1/3rd.

iii. Medial border - It faces the vertebral column and provides attachment to serratus anterior on costal surface and levator scapulae at the superior angle. The rhomboideus minor is attached on the medial border opposite the root of the spine and rhomboideus major attached on the medial border below the root of the spine.

Scapula also presents three processes (Figs 3.3 and 3.4).

1. Acromion process: It projects from the lateral end of the spine and overhangs the glenoid cavity. It is subcutaneous and is palpable. It articulates with the lateral end of the clavicle at the acromioclavicular joint. It's medial border provides insertion to trapezius muscle, lateral border

99

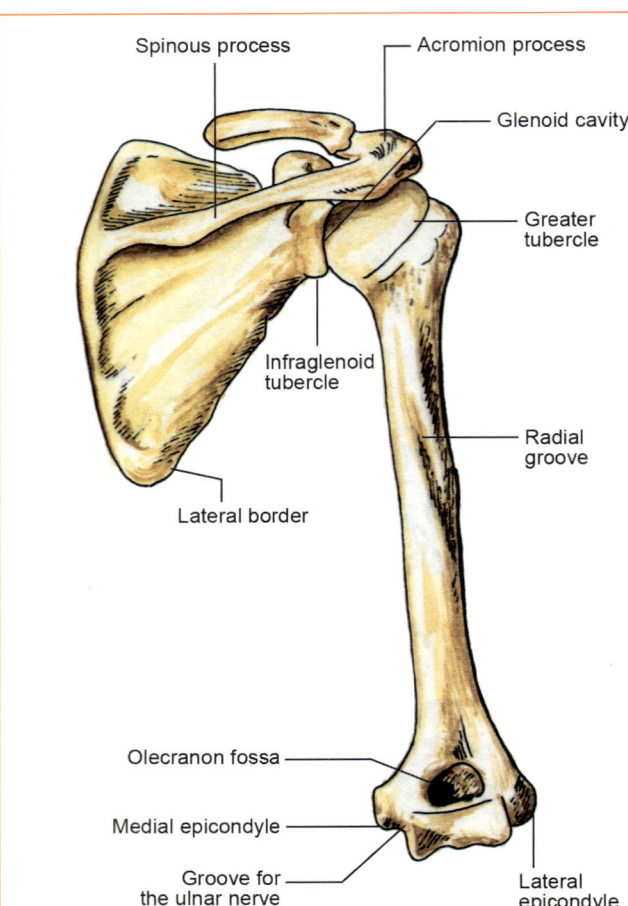

Fig. 3.4 Humerus and Scapula (Posterior View)

provides attachments to deltoid muscle. The coracoacromial ligament is attached to the medial side of its tip.

2. Coracoid process: It is a small forward projection from the scapula. It's tip provides origin to short head of biceps and corachobrachialis muscle. It's medial border and superior surface provides attachments to pectoralis minor muscle. The coracoacromial ligament is attached to its lateral border, coracoclavicular ligament on the superior surface and coracohumeral ligament at its root.

3. Spinous process: It can be felt in the living as a ridge on the back. It is present on the dorsal aspect of scapula, continues laterally as acromion process. The spine presents an upper lip and lower lips. The upper lip continues with the medial border of the acromion process. It provides insertion to trapezius muscle. The lower lip continues with the lateral border of the acromion process and provides origin to the deltoid muscle. The medial end of the spine corresponds to spine of the T3 vertebra.

Glenoid cavity: It projects on the lateral side. The glenoid cavity of the scapula articulates with the head of the humerus

(bone of the arm) to form the shoulder joint. The peripheral margin provides attachments to glenoidal labrum and fibrous capsule of the shoulder joint outside to it.

Supraglenoid tubercle: It provides attachment to long head of the biceps which is intracapsular.

Infraglenoid tubercle: It provides attachment to long head of the triceps which is extracapsular.

Ossification

One primary centre for the body appears during 8th week of IUL. There are 7 secondary centres – 1 each for medial border, inferior angle, coracoid process and lower part of the glenoid cavity and 2 for acromion process. The coracoid process fuses with the body during 15th year and rest of the secondary centres by 20th year.

> Paralysis of a muscle called serratus anterior causes winging of the scapula. The medial border of the scapula becomes prominent on the back and arm cannot be abducted.

HUMERUS

Humerus is the bone of the arm. It has an upper end, lower end and a shaft in-between (Figs 3.3 and 3.4).

Upper end

Head: It is rounded and covered by hyaline articular cartilage. It articulates with glenoid cavity of the scapula to form shoulder joint.

Greater tubercle: Greater tubercle is a long elevation behind the lesser tubercle. It has three impressions for the insertions of supraspinatus, infraspinatus and teres minor muscles (SIT).

Lesser tubercle: The lesser tubercle is the prominent, sharp projection on the anterior aspect of the upper end. It receives the insertion of subscapularis muscle.

Bicipital groove (intertubercular sulcus): It is an area between the greater and lesser tubercles. The floor of the sulcus provides insertion to latissimus dorsi, medial lip of the groove for teres major and lateral lip for pectoralis major muscle. The long head of the biceps with its synovial sheath traverses it.

a. **Surgical neck:** It is the junction between the upper end and shaft of the humerus. Axillary nerve and posterior circumflex humeral artery winds around it.

b. **Anatomical neck:** It is the constricted portion adjoining the head. It provides attachment to the capsule of the shoulder joint.

SECTION 3

c. **Morphological neck:** It is the line joining the epiphysis with diaphysis and connects the two tuberosities.

Shaft

- It is rounded in the upper part and triangular in the lower part and connects the upper and lower ends. It has following important features.
- It has anterior, medial and lateral borders, which are prominent in the lower part.
- The lateral border provides attachments to lateral intermuscular septum, and below it continues as lateral supracondylar ridge. The brachioradialis muscle takes origin from the upper 2/3rd of the ridge while extensor carpi radialis longus (ECRL) from the lower 1/3rd.
- The medial border provides insertion to coracobrachialis in the middle and medial intermscular septum in the lower part, which forms medial supracondylar ridge.
- The shaft presents anterolateral, anteromedial and posterior surfaces.
- The anterolateral surface presents a 'V' shaped deltoid tuberosity in the upper part for the insertion of deltoid muscle. Brachialis muscle takes origin from the lower part of the anterior surface.
- The posterior surface is obliquely traversed by radial groove.
- An oblique ridge above the radial groove provides origin to lateral head of the triceps while the posterior surface below the radial groove provides origin to medial head of the triceps.

Radial groove (spiral groove): The middle 1/3rd of the posterior surface is crossed by a groove called the radial groove. It is related to the radial nerve and the profunda brachii artery.

Lower end

Capitulum is a rounded projection on the lateral side and articulates with the head of the radius (elbow joint).

Trochlea is a pully shaped area present medially that articulates with the trochlear notch of ulna (elbow joint).

Medial epicondyle: A subcutaneous prominent bony projection on the medial side of the elbow. It is crossed posteriorly by the ulnar nerve and superior ulnar collateral artery. It gives origin to all the superficial flexor muscles of the forearm (common flexor origin). The ulnar collateral ligament is attached to its apex.

Lateral epicondyle: It is on the lateral side but smaller than the medial epicondyle. It provides origin to all the superficial extensor muscles of the forearm (common extensor origin). The radial collateral ligament is attached to its tip.

Coronoid fossa: Present just above the trochlea to accommodate the coronoid process of the ulna in a flexed elbow.

Radial fossa: Present above the capitulum, to accommodate the head of the radius in a flexed elbow.

Olecranon fossa: It is present posteriorly and accommodates the olecranon process of the ulna in an extended elbow.

Ossification

One primary centre appears during 8th week of IUL for shaft. There are 7 secondary centres-3 for upper end and 4 for lower end of the humerus. The secondary centre for head appears at 1st year and that for the greater tubercle at 3rd year and lesser tubercle at 5th year. All these fuses together to form one epiphysis at 7 years and fuses with the shaft at 20th year.

The secondary centre for capitulum and lateral flange of the trochlea appears at 2nd year, for medial epicondyle at 6th year, for medial part of the trochlea at 10th year and for the lateral epicondyle at 12th year. Two epiphyses are formed at lower end one for medial epicondyle and other for the rest. The rest fuses with the shaft at 16 while medial epicondyle fuses with the shaft at 18th year.

> Supracondylar fracture is common which can damage the median nerve and brachial artery (Volkman's ischemic contracture).
>
> Fracture of the mid shaft can damage the radial nerve, while fracture of medial epicondyle can damage the ulnar nerve. Fracture at the surgical neck can damage axillary nerve.

RADIUS

Radius is the lateral bone of the forearm. It has two ends (upper and lower) and a shaft (Figs 3.5 and 3.7).

Upper end

Head: It is a disc shaped structure separated from the shaft by neck. Its upper surface articulates with the capitulum of humerus (elbow joint). Medial margin of the head articulates with radial notch of the ulna to form the superior radioulnar joint. The lateral margin is surrounded by annular ligament.

Neck: It is the lower constricted part of the bone below the head.

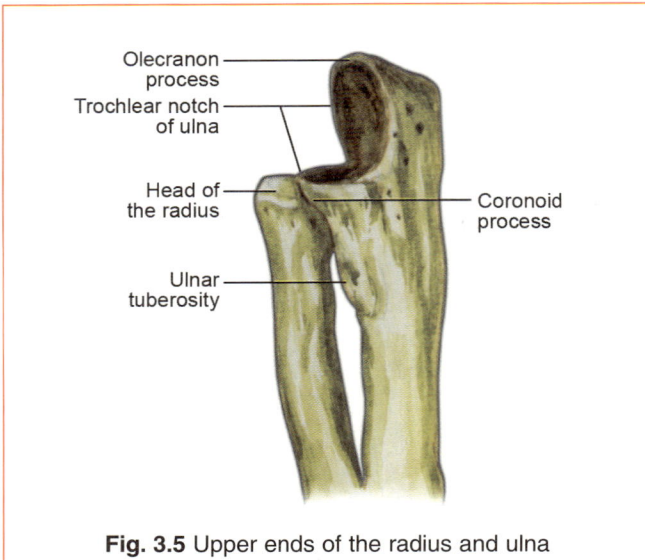

Fig. 3.5 Upper ends of the radius and ulna

Radial tuberosity: It is below the medial part of the neck and provides insertion to the biceps brachii muscle.

Shaft

• It is the elongated cylindrical part connecting the two ends. It presents three borders and three surfaces.

• The anterior border extends from radial tuberosity to the styloid process of the radius. Its upper part provides attachments to radial origin of flexor digitorum superficialis.

• The posterior border is well defined in the middle 1/3rd only.

• The interosseus (medial) border is sharp and provides attachment to interosseus membrane.

• The anterior surface provides attachments to flexor pollicis longus in the upper part and pronator quadratus in the lower part. A nutrient foramen is present in this surface.

• The posterior surface provides attachments to abductor pollicis longus in the upper part and extensor pollicis brevis in the lower part.

• The lateral surface provides attachments to supinator in the upper 1/3rd and pronator teres in the middle 1/3rd. The lateral surface continues downwards as styloid process.

Lower end

• The lower end presents 5 surfaces- anterior, posterior, medial, lateral and inferior.

• Inferior surface of the lower end articulates with scaphoid laterally and lunate medially (wrist joint).

• The posterior surface presents 4 grooves for extensor tendons and a dorsal tubercle.

  Lister's tubercle: The posterior aspect of the lower end presents a tubercle called dorsal tubercle (or Lister's tubercle).

• The groove lateral to the tubercle is traversed by extensor carpi radialis longus tendon and on the medial side by the tendon of extensor pollicis longus.

• Styloid process: It is a conical projection from the lower end at the lateral aspect. The brachioradialis muscle is attached to the lateral surface of the styloid process while its tip provides attachments to radial collateral ligament of the wrist joint.

• Medial part of the lower end presents **ulnar notch** articulates with the head of the ulna to form the inferior radioulnar joint. This part also gives attachment to the articular disc of the inferior radioulnar joint.

Ossification

One primary centre for the shaft appears during 8th week of IUL. There are 2 secondary centres one each for upper end and lower end. The secondary centre for upper end appears at 4 years and fuses with the shaft at 18 years. The secondary centre for lower end appears at 2 years and fuses with the shaft at 20 years.

> **Colle's fracture:** It is a fracture of the radius at about 2.5 cm proximal to its distal end. The distal segment (wrist and hand) is displaced posteriorly by the pull of brachioradialis muscle. It is often referred as 'dinner fork deformity' due to the shape of the resultant forearm. This fracture is most commonly caused by people

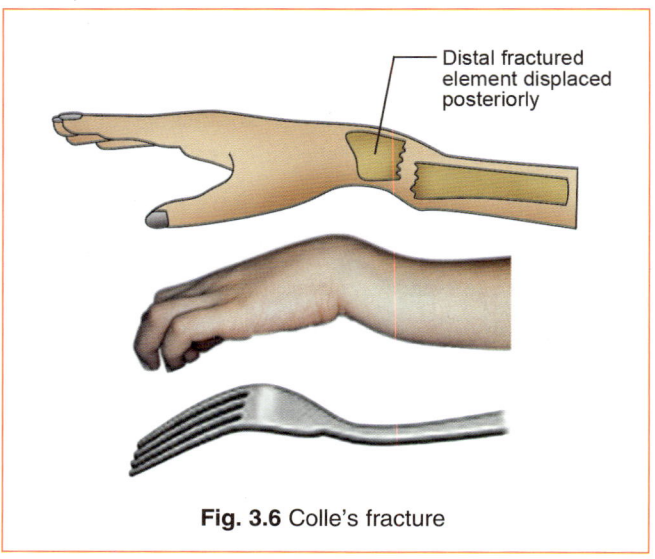

Fig. 3.6 Colle's fracture

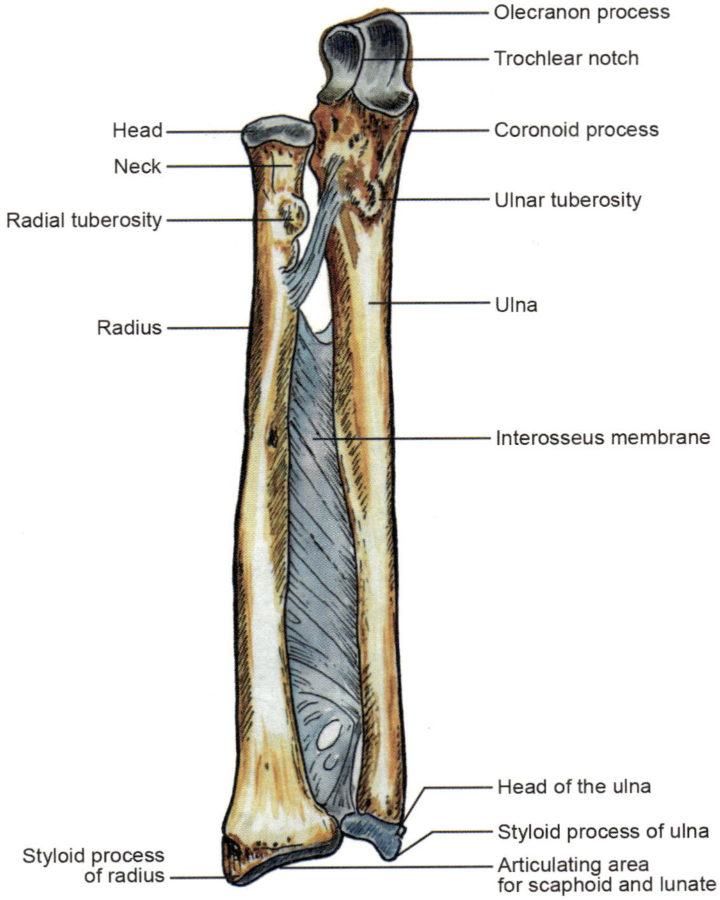

Olecranon process

Trochlear notch

Head

Coronoid process

Neck

Radial tuberosity

Ulnar tuberosity

Radius

Ulna

Interosseus membrane

Head of the ulna

Styloid process of ulna

Styloid process of radius

Articulating area for scaphoid and lunate

Fig. 3.7 Radius and Ulna (Anterior view)

falling onto a hard surface and tying to resist their fall with outstretched hand. It is a common fracture enountered by people with osteoporosis (Fig. 3.6).

Smith's fracture: It is a reverse of Colle's fracture which occurs due to fall with flexed wrist or a direct blow on dorsal aspect of the forearm. The fractured (distal) segment is displaced anteriorly.

The radius can be exposed in its whole length by an incision along the anterior border of the brachioradialis.

CASE-2

A 26-year-old woman fell while coming down the staircase and sustained a fracture of the lower end of the right radius. The orthopedic surgeon instructed the resident to make sure to immobilize the wrist joint in the position of function. What is "position of the function "means? What is its the clinical importance?

ULNA

It is the medial bone of the forearm. It has the following parts – upper end, shaft and lower end (Fig. 3.7).

Upper end

The important parts include:

- **Olecranon process:** It projects forwards from the upper part of the ulna. It bends forward, forming a beak like projection. It occupies the olecranon fossa of the humerus when the elbow is extended. **Triceps** muscle is inserted into its superior surface. Its medial surface provides attachments to flexor carpi ulnaris, flexor digitorum profundus and part of the ulnar collateral ligament of the elbow joint. Its lateral surface receives anconeus insertion.

- **Coronoid process:** It is a shelf-like projection from the upper end and anterior part of the shaft below the olecranon process. Its anterior aspect bears a rough impression, called the **ulnar tuberosity** which provides insertion to **brachialis** muscle. The medial margin of the anterior surface of the coronoid process provides attachments to ulnar collateral ligament, flexor digitorum superficialis and pronator teres. The lateral surface presents supinator crests which provides attachments to deep part of the supinator muscle.

- **Radial notch:** Lateral surface of the coronoid process presents a radial notch, to articulate with head of the radius to form the superior radioulnar joint. Its margins provide attachment to annular ligament.

- **Trochlear notch:** It is between the olecranon and coronoid process. It articulates with trochlea of the humerus.

Shaft

- It has three borders (lateral, anterior and posterior) and three surfaces (anterior, medial and posterior). The lateral (interosseus) border provides attachment to the interosseus membrane.

- The anterior border in its upper $3/4^{th}$ provides attachment to flexor digitorum profundus.

- The posterior border is subcutaneous and provides attachment to deep fascia. It provides attachments to flexor digitorum profundus, flexor carpi ulnaris and extensor carpi ulnaris muscle from above downwards.

- The anterior surface provides attachments to flexor digitorum profundus in the upper part and pronator quadrates in the lower part. This surface presents a nutrient foramen.

- The medial surface provides attachments to flexor digitorum profundus in its upper part. It is subcutaneous in the lower part.

- The posterior surface is between posterior and interosseus borders. It provides attachments to anconeus

in the upper part (above the oblique line), abductor pollicis longus, extensor pollicis longus and extensor indicis in the lower part (area lateral to the oblique line).

Lower end

Head: Its lateral part articulates with the ulnar notch of the radius (inferior radioulnar joint). Its inferior surface is separated from the carpal bones by an articular disc of the inferior radioulnar joint.

Styloid process: It projects from the posteromedial aspect of the lower end. It is palpable on posteromedial part of the wrist. It lies 1.25 cm above the level of the tip of the styloid process of the radius. Ulnar collateral ligament of the wrist is attached to its apex. The tendon of the extensor carpi ulnaris grooves the area between the head and the styloid process posteriorly.

Ossification

One primary centre appears for shaft during 8th week of IUL. There are 2 secondary centres one each for upper and lower ends. The secondary centre for upper end appears at 8 years and fuses with the shaft at 18 years. The secondary centre for lower end appears at 6 years and fuses with the shaft at 20 years.

> The tip of the olecranon process, medial and lateral epicondyles lie in same horizontal plane when the elbow is fully extended. These three bony points form an equilateral triangle when the elbow is flexed. This relationship is lost in dislocation of the elbow but maintained in supracondylar fracture of the humerus.
>
> Fracture of the shaft of the ulna alone is very rare. It often occurs with fracture of the radius. If one falls on the point of elbow, the olecranon may be fractured.

CARPAL BONES

The skeleton of the hand is made up of carpal, metacarpal and phalangeal bones (Figs 3.8 and 3.9).

Carpal bones are 8 in number, and are arranged in proximal and distal rows.

Proximal row consists of (from lateral to medial side)

- Scaphoid
- Lunate
- Triquetral
- Pisiform

Distal row consists of (from lateral to medial side)

- Trapezium
- Trapezoid

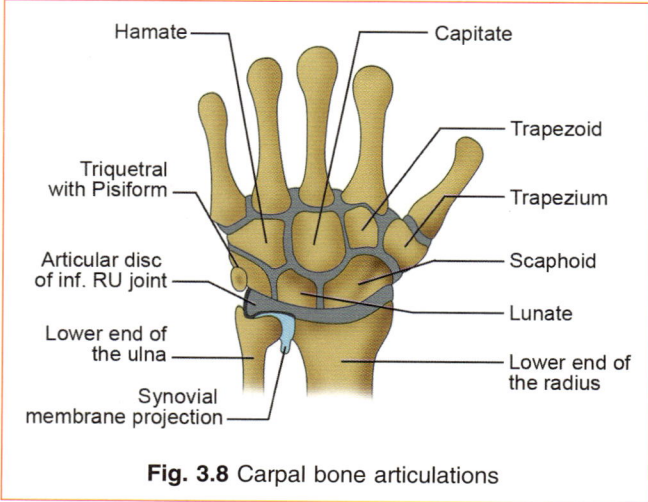

Fig. 3.8 Carpal bone articulations

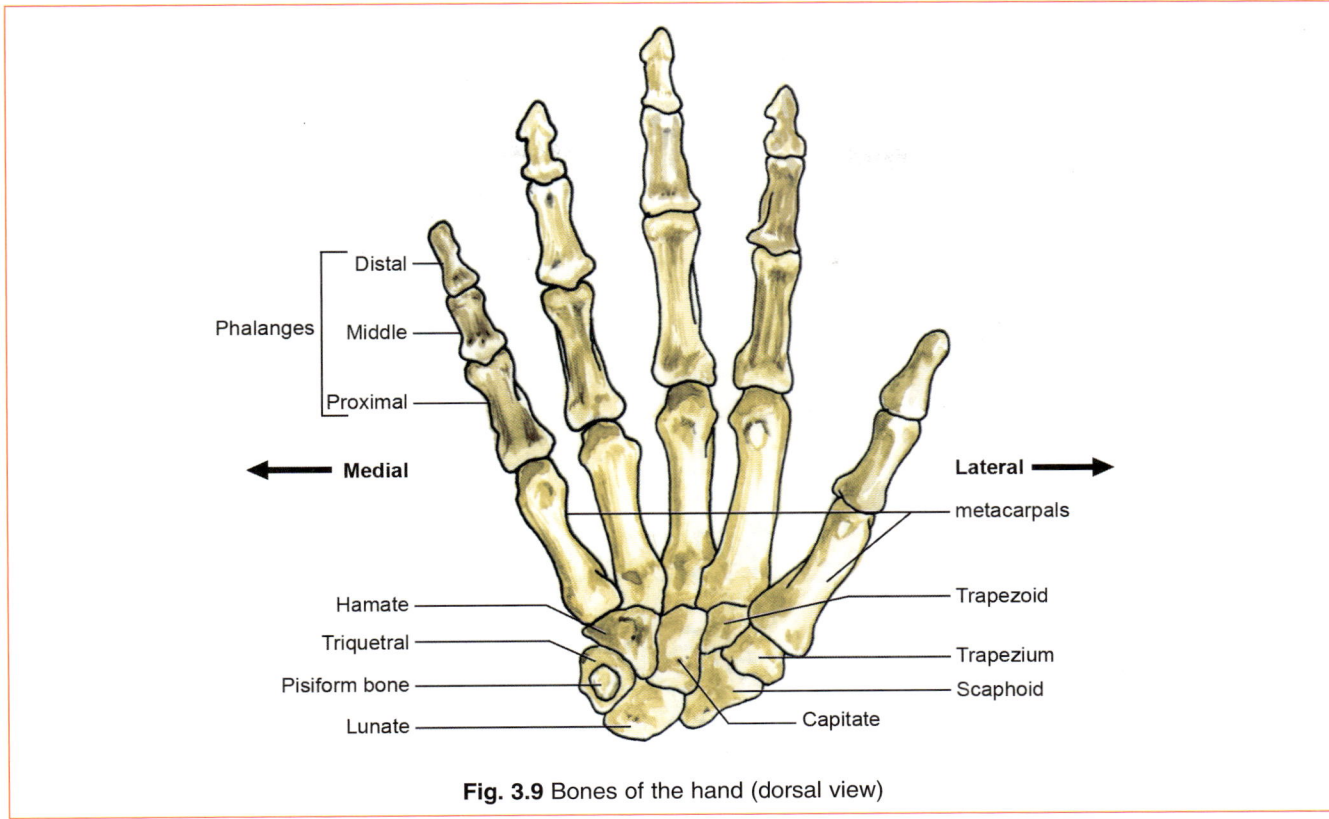

Fig. 3.9 Bones of the hand (dorsal view)

- Capitate
- Hamate

Scaphoid: It is boat shaped bone having proximal and distal segments with a constriction between them. Proximally it articulates with radius, medially with lunate and distally with trapezium, trapezoid and capitate. The tubercle of the scaphoid gives attachment to flexor retinaculum.

Lunate: It is half moon shaped. Proximally it articulates with radius, laterally with scaphoid, medially with triquetral and distally with capitate.

Triquetral: It is a pyramidal shaped bone with an oval facet for pisiform. Proximally it is related to the articular disc of the inferior radioulnar joint, on the palmar aspect it articulates with pisiform and distally with hamate.

Pisiform: It is 'pea' shaped bone. It is a sesamoid bone developed within the tendon of the flexor carpi ulnaris muscle. It provides attachments to flexor and extensor retinacula, pisohamate and pisometacarpal ligaments. Dorsally it articulates with triquetral.

Trapezium: It is a quadrilateral bone. It has a groove on its palmar aspect for the passage of the tendon of flexor carpi radialis, while its margin provides attachment to flexor retinaculum. Proximally it articulates with scaphoid,

medially with trapezoid and distally with base of the first metacarpal bone.

Trapezoid: It appears like a baby's foot. It articulates with scaphoid, trapezium, capitate and 2nd metacarpal bone.

Capitate: It is the largest carpal bone with a rounded head. Proximally it articulates with scaphoid and lunate, laterally with trapezoid, medially with hamate and distally with 3rd metacarpal bone.

Hamate: It is wedge shaped with a hook like process. The hook provides attachment to flexor retinaculum. The deep

Ossification of carpal bones	
Carpal bones	**Time of appearance**
• Capitate	3rd month
• Hamate	4th month
• Triquetral	3rd year
• Lunate	4th year
• Scaphoid and Trapezoid	5th year
• Trapezium	6th year
• Pisiform	12th year

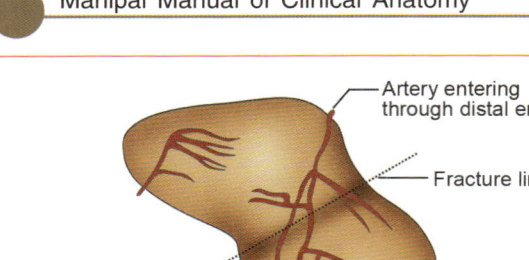
Fig. 3.10 Scaphoid-arterial supply

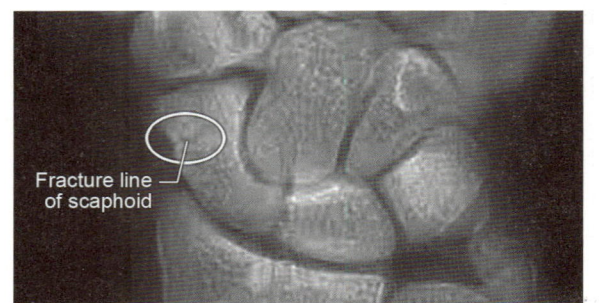
Fig. 3.11 Scaphoid non union-radiograph

branch of the ulnar nerve grooves it on the medial side. It articulates with triquetral, capitate, 4th and 5th metacarpal bones.

Ossification

Each carpal bone ossifies by single centre of ossification which appears after birth.

Remember capitate is the first to ossify, followed by hamate before 1st year. The triquetral is the 3rd carpal to ossify (its centre appear at 3rd year), followed by lunate (4th carpal to ossify and centre appear at 4th year). For scaphoid and trapezoid the centre appear at 5th year and for trapezium at 6 years.

Scaphoid fracture: Scaphoid is the most common carpal bone to be fractured due to fall on the outstretched hand. In scaphoid fracture there will be tenderness in the anatomical snuff box as well as over the volar aspect of the scaphoid. A fracture of scaphoid between its proximal and distal segments can lead to avascular necrosis of its proximal segment. This is because the artery supplying the scaphoid enters through distal segment and then proceeds to proximal segment (Figs 3.10 and 3.11)

Lunate dislocation: Though it is uncommon, its forward dislocation can cause carpal tunnel syndrome.

Triquetral fracture: It is characterized by pain and tenderness at the back of the wrist.

The ulnar nerve passes between the hook of the hamate and the pisiform bone in a fibro-osseous tunnel known as Guyon's canal. Ulnar nerve injury at Guyon's canal causes paraesthesia of the ulnar side of the hand and weakness of the intrinsic muscles of the hand.

CASE-3

A 22-year-old man fell of his bicycle on a outstretched left hand. He thought he had sprained his wrist, but when the pain in his wrist persisted, he sought medical advice. On physical examination of the back of the both hands, with the fingers and thumbs fully extended, a small amount of swelling was seen over the" anatomical snuff box" of his left hand. On deep palpation, a localized area of tenderness could be felt over the scaphoid bone. A diagnosis of a fracture of left scaphoid bone was made. For what anatomical reasons do fracture of this bone sometimes fail to unite.

Metacarpal bones

There are five metacarpal bones which are numbered from lateral to medial side. Each metacarpal bone has a head (placed distally), a shaft and a base (at the proximal end).

Ossification: One primary centre for shaft appears during 9th week of IUL, one secondary centre (at the base for 1st metacarpal and at the head for the remaining) appears during 2nd year. The fusion of epiphysis with diaphysis in 1st metacarpal bone occurs during 16 years and in the remaining metacarpals at 18 years.

Bennet's fracture: It is an oblique fracture involving the ulnar side of the base of the 1st metacarpal bone.

Phalanges

There are 14 phalanges in each hand, 3 for each finger and 2 for thumb. Each phalanx has a base, a shaft and a head.

Ossification: Each phalanx develops from one primary centre for shaft and one secondary centre (at 2nd year) for base. The primary centre for proximal phalanx appears at 10th week, for middle phalanx at 12th week and for distal phalanx at 8th week. The fusion between epiphysis and diaphysis occurs at the age of 16 years.

Mallet finger: It is a condition in which the distal phalanx undergoes extreme flexion due to detachment of extensor tendon on the distal phalanx. This is commonly seen in basket ball and cricket players.

S E C T I O N   3

Boxer's fracture: This occurs when an individual strike a blow with a closed fist. The most commonly injured sites for experienced boxers are the first and second metacarpals, whereas for unexperienced boxers the fifth metacarpal is the most common site of injury. The metacarpals have a good blood supply and thus heals rapidly.

CASE-4

A 54-year-old woman slipped on a shiny floor and sustained a fracture of the fifth right metacarpal bone. When a plaster cast is applied with the little finger flexed, in which direction should the little finger be pointing?

Solutions to the case studies

Case-1

1. Anatomically the weakest part of the clavicle is the junction of the medial 2/3 and lateral 1/3, and this is where a fracture usually occurs.

2. The lateral bony fragment is displaced downwards by the weight of the arm and pulled forward and medially by the pectoralis major muscle. The medial fragment is elevated by the sternocleidomastoid muscle.

3. Dislocation of the sternoclavicular joint is prevented by the ligaments of the joint, especially the very strong costoclavicular ligament. The very strong coraco-clavicular ligament prevents dislocation of the acromioclavicular joint. If the mechanical force is great

and if the clavicle is strong enough, the dislocation of medial or lateral end might occur.

4. The supraclavicular nerves, or a communicating vein between the cephalic and the internal jugular vein, may be damaged with a fractured clavicle.

Case-2

Its importance lies in the fact that should some part of the hand become stiff or fixed permanently by adhesions, the patient would have a hand positioned to give the maximum mechanical efficiency.

Case-3

The fracture line may deprive the proximal fragment of its arterial supply and result in ischemic necrosis of this fragment. Because of the articulation of the scaphoid with other bones, the fracture line may enter a joint and be bathed in synovial fluid. The presence of synovial fluid may inhibit union between the bony fragments. The scaphoid is a difficult bone to immobilize because of its position and small size.

Case-4

When flexed, all fingers (excluding the thumb) point toward the tubercle of the scaphoid in normalcy. When a finger is unstable following a fracture, it is attempting to align its long axis parallel to one of the borders of the hand, which is incorrect and will result in malfunction. Hence placing the finger in a normal position has to be done during immobilisation in a fracture (Fig. 3.12).

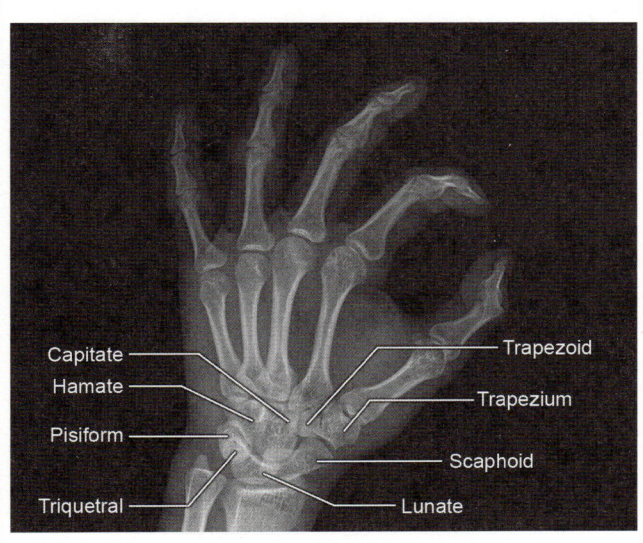

Fig. 3.12 Radiograph of the hand

MCQs

1. A 28-year-old volleyball player fell on her right outstretched arm during a game. She felt an immediate pain in her wrist, and the orthopedic surgeon at the emergency room described the deformity in her right wrist as similar to a "dinner fork." All wrist movements are painful. A plain radiograph revealed a transverse fracture of the distal end of the radius, where the fractured segment tilted backwards and upwards. The patient was diagnosed with typical Colle's fracture. Among the options given below, which bone/part of the bone is least likely to be fractured by a fall on an outstretched hand?

   A. Styloid process of the ulna

   B. Distal end of the radius

   C. Clavicle

   D. Distal phalanx of the thumb

2. Which of the following patients are MOST likely to suffer from differential radial and ulnar growth subsequent to this type of injury?

   A. A 10-year-old girl
   B. A 28-year-old woman
   C. A 42-year-old man
   D. A 60-year-old man

3. An unexperienced resident examines the x-ray of the forearm of a child after a fall. There appears to be a break through near, but not at the distal end of the ulna. Before diagnosing it as a fracture, the resident should also consider the possibility that this is actually _____

   A. Articular cartilage
   B. Epiphyseal plate
   C. Perichondrium
   D. Primary ossification center

4. A 32-year-old male was brought to the hospital with complaints of severe pain at right shoulder after falling from a tree. The X-ray reveals a fracture in the middle third of the right clavicle. The medial end of the fractured clavicle is displaced upward due to traction by the

   A. Serratus anterior muscle
   B. Rhomboideus muscles
   C. Pectoralis minor muscle
   D. Sternocleidomastoid muscle

5. A 36-year-old female presents to the emergency room after falling in the bathroom. She complains of wrist pain and numbness in her right palm. Based on her symptoms, you suspect that her lunate bone in the wrist has dislocated. Which of the following carpal bones articulates with lunate?

   A. Scaphoid, pisiform, hamate
   B. Scaphoid, triquetral and capitate
   C. Scaphoid and trapezoid
   D. Capitate and triquetral

6. An 18-year-old female visits the hospital with the complaints of "right hand clumsiness." Physical examination reveals decreased sensation over the fifth finger and a flattened hypothenar eminence. Assuming the involvement of ulnar nerve, where in following sites is this nerve likely to be injured?

   A. Carpal tunnel
   B. Surgical neck of the humerus
   C. Hook of the hamate
   D. Head of the radius

7. A 15-year-old boy is brought to the emergency department complaining of pain in his right hand following a fist fight. The physician tells the patient that he has broken his hand. Which of the following is a most likely site of fracture in this patient?

   A. Distal radius
   B. Hamate
   C. Metacarpals
   D. Scaphoid

8. While falling on an outstretched hand, the most common carpal bone that is likely to be fractured is

   A. Scaphoid
   B. Trapezoid
   C. Lunate
   D. Capitate

9. After falling on the ice, it was determined that a patient had a Colle's fracture. Care must be taken to relieve tension on the broken distal end of the radius. Which muscle would exert tension on radius in such cases?

   A. Extensor carpi ulnaris
   B. Brachioradialis
   C. Extensor carpi radialis longus
   D. Pronator quadratus

10. Which of the following injuries are least common to occur from a fall on an outstretched hand?

    A. Fracture of the clavicle
    B. Fracture of the distal radius (Colle's fracture)
    C. Dislocation of the lunate bone
    D. Fracture of the neck of the 1st, 2nd, or 5th metacarpal

Answers to MCQs	
1. D	
2. A	
3. B	
4. D	
5. B	
6. C	
7. C	
8. A	
9. B	
10. D	

Pectoral Region and Mammary Gland

- Pectoral region
- Mammary gland
- MCQs

Objectives
- To know the cutaneous innervation to the pectoral region
- To list the muscles of the pectoral region and to explain their attachments, nerve supply and actions.
- To explain the attachments and structures piercing the clavipectoral fascia
- To explain the structure, blood supply, lymphatic drainage and clinical anatomy of mammary gland

PECTORAL REGION

Pectoral region is the area in the upper part of the chest. The clavicle, different parts of the sternum, sternal angle and nipple can be seen or felt in this area.

Skin

The skin of the pectoral region is supplied by branches of (Fig. 4.1)

1. Supraclavicular nerves (C3,4): It divides into medial, intermediate and lateral branches. These branches supplies skin just inferior to the clavicle (Fig. 4.1).

2. Anterior and lateral cutaneous branches of second to sixth intercostal nerves (T2 to T6).

Note that the dermatomes of the pectoral region include C3, C4 and followed by T2. The C5 to T1 nerves forms the brachial plexus through which it supplies the upper limb.

Superficial fascia

It consists of fat and in females the breast (mammary gland) is located in the superficial fascia. It is explained separately.

A superficial muscle called 'platysma' is present in the upper part of the pectoral region.

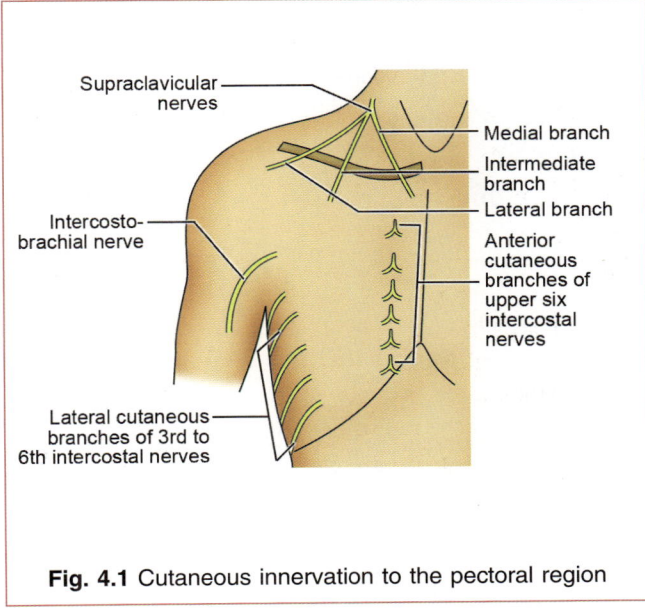

Fig. 4.1 Cutaneous innervation to the pectoral region

Supraclavicular nerves
Medial branch
Intermediate branch
Lateral branch
Anterior cutaneous branches of upper six intercostal nerves
Intercosto-brachial nerve
Lateral cutaneous branches of 3rd to 6th intercostal nerves

Deep fascia

The deep fascia of the pectoral region is called 'pectoral fascia'. It covers the pectoralis major muscle.

The muscles of the pectoral region connects the upper limb with trunk on its anterior aspect. These muscles mainly act on the shoulder joint. The name of the muscles, their attachment, actions and nerve supply is listed in Table 4.1.

Deltopectoral groove

It is an intermuscular groove between deltoid and pectoralis major muscle (Fig. 4.2). It is traversed by cephalic vein with delto-pectoral group of lymph nodes. These lymph nodes receive lymph from superficial tissue of the upper limb along the cephalic vein including the thumb. The groove also presents deltoid branch of the thoraco-acromial artery.

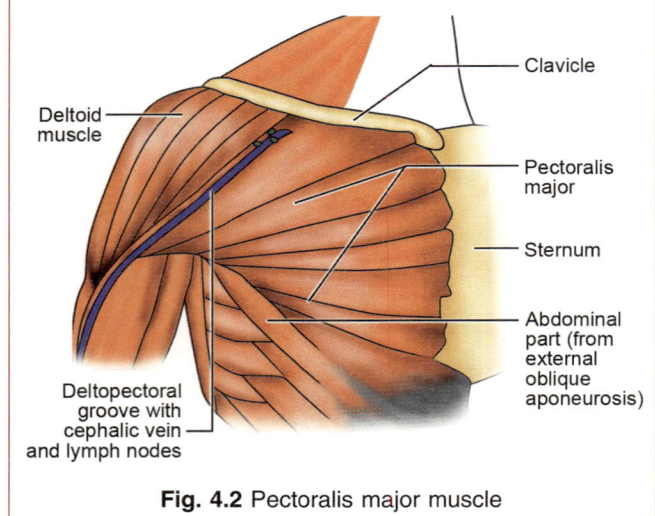

Fig. 4.2 Pectoralis major muscle

Paralysis of Serratus anterior muscle results in a condition called '**winging of the scapula**' (Fig. 4.5). The medial margin of the scapula becomes prominent on the dorsal side. In this case, a test is often done by asking the patient press forward against a wall with both hands simultaneously. The protraction of the scapula is produced by actions of both the serratus anterior and pectoralis minor muscle. In absence of action of serratus anterior, the rhomboideus muscle retract the scapula and makes medial border prominent.

Testing of Pectoralis major: By asking the patient to place hands on the hips and press firmly inwards and the examiner watches the prominence of anterior axillary fold (formed by pectoralis major muscle). It can also be tested by abducting the shoulder, followed by flexing (bringing the hand together).

Table 4.1 Muscles of the pectoral region

Name of the muscle and its origin	Insertion	Nerve supply	Actions
1. Pectoralis major • Anterior surface of the medial half of the clavicle • Lateral part of the anterior surface of the sternum • Second to sixth costal cartilages, aponeurosis of external oblique	Lateral lip of the bicipital groove of humerus (intertubercular sulcus)	Medial and lateral pectoral nerves	Medial rotation ⎤ Adduction ⎬ At shoulder joint Flexion ⎦
2. Pectoralis minor Third to fifth ribs	Medial margin and superior surface of the coracoid process of the scapula	Medial and lateral pectoral nerves	Along with serratus anterior protracts the scapula
3. Subclavius Junction of first rib and its costal cartilage	Undersurface of the middle third of the clavicle	Nerve to subclavius from upper trunk of brachial plexus	It steadies the clavicle during shoulder joint movement
4. Serratus anterior By 8 fleshy digitations from outer surfaces of upper 8 ribs	Medial border of the scapula on the costal surface	Nerve to serratus anterior (long thoracic nerve)	Protracts the scapula around the chest wall in pushing and punching movements

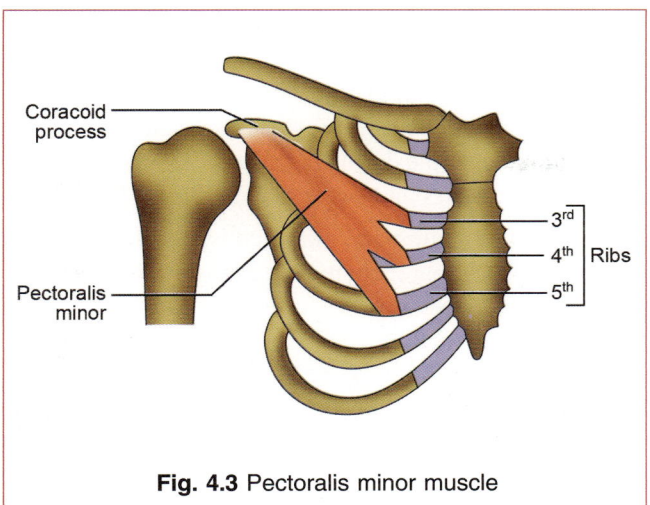

Fig. 4.3 Pectoralis minor muscle

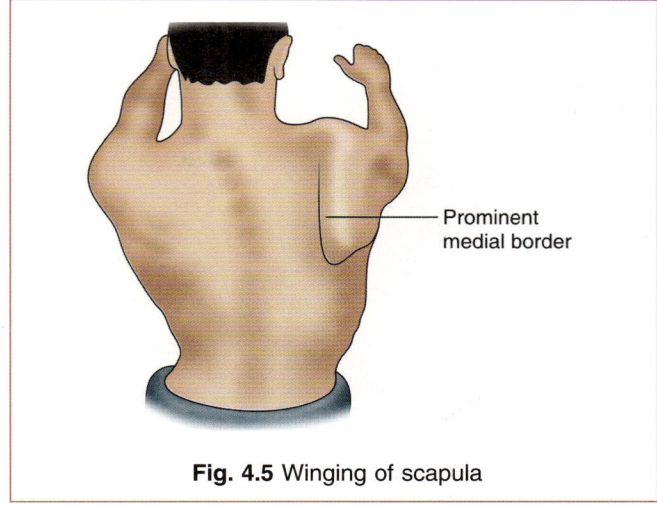

Fig. 4.5 Winging of scapula

Clavipectoral fascia

It is a well-defined fascia bridging the gap between the clavicle and the pectoralis minor muscle (Figs 4.3 and 4.6).

Attachments: Superiorly it arises by two slips from the undersurface of the clavicle where it encloses the subclavius muscle. Inferiorly first it splits to enclose the pectoralis minor muscle and at the lower border of this muscle the two layers reunites and extend downwards to the floor of the axilla (arm pit) as suspensory ligament of axilla. Medially it is attached to the first rib and laterally to coracoid process of the scapula. Sometimes this part of the fascia is thick and called 'costo-coracoid membrane'.

Structures piercing the clavipectoral fascia: The gap between the clavicle and the pectoralis minor muscle is pierced by

1. Cephalic vein: After piercing the fascia it ends in the axillary vein.

2. Lateral pectoral nerve

3. Thoraco-acromial artery and vein

4. Lymphatic vessels

MAMMARY GLAND (THE BREAST)

It is rudimentary in males and is well developed in females after puberty. It is an accessory organ of the female reproductive system and provides milk to the newborn.

Female mammary gland

Situation and extent: It is situated in the superficial fascia of the pectoral region. The base is connected to the chest wall and it extends vertically from second to sixth ribs. In the transverse plane it extends from lateral margin of the sternum to the mid-axillary line. The apex of the mammary gland presents nipple which lies at the level of fourth intercostal space.

Base: The major portion of the base rests on pectoralis major muscle, partly on serratus anterior and external oblique

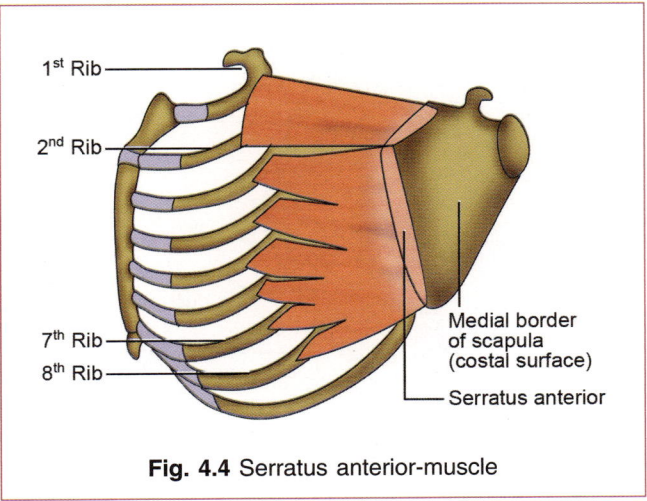

Fig. 4.4 Serratus anterior-muscle

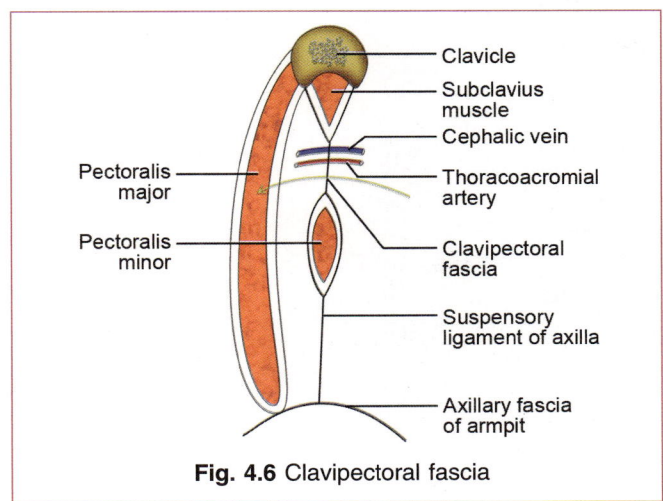

Fig. 4.6 Clavipectoral fascia

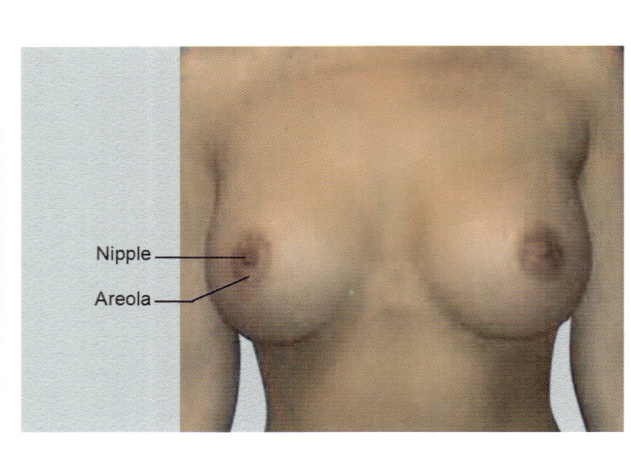

Fig. 4.7 Female breast

abdominis muscles (Fig. 4.4). The base is separated from it by a 'retromammary space', which is filled with loose connective tissue. This space provides some degree of mobility to the mammary gland.

A small portion of the mammary gland in the upper lateral part extends into the axilla. This part is called '**axillary tail**' (of Spence). This part of the mammary gland is closely related to anterior axillary lymph nodes. A carcinoma affecting this part of the mammary gland can be mistaken for enlarged anterior axillary lymph nodes.

Nipple

It is a conical projection in the skin covering the mammary gland. It has many sensory receptors. The lactiferous ducts draining the milk from the alveoli (about 15–20) pierce the nipple to open at its summit (Fig. 4.7).

A pigmented circular area surrounding the nipple is called **areola**. It has plenty of modified sebaceous glands and they enlarge during pregnancy and lactation. The oily secretion from these glands provides lubricant and prevents cracking of the nipple during lactation. The areola also has involuntary muscles and sweat glands (Fig. 4.7).

Structure: The mammary gland consists of mainly fat (adipose tissue), parenchyma (secretory units/glandular tissue) and blood vessels.

Glandular tissue

The gland consists of 15–20 lobes. Each lobe consists of many alveoli. The alveoli are lined by columnar epithelium during lactation. The alveoli are drained by lactiferous ducts. Each lactiferous duct receives many small ducts on their way to the nipple. The lactiferous ducts converge towards the nipple, where it presents a dilatation to form lactiferous sinus deep to the areola (Fig. 4.9). The secretion is controlled by the hormone prolactin secreted by the anterior lobe of the pituitary gland.

Suspensory ligaments (ligaments of Cooper): Some fibrous tissue extends from the skin to underlying pectoral fascia forming suspensory ligaments (Fig. 4.8).

In case of carcinoma of the mammary gland, these suspensory ligaments may be involved. It results in dimpling or puckering of the skin due to its attachment to the skin. It also results in fixation of the gland reducing the mobility.

Arterial supply

Mammary gland is supplied by branches of the following arteries (Fig. 4.10).

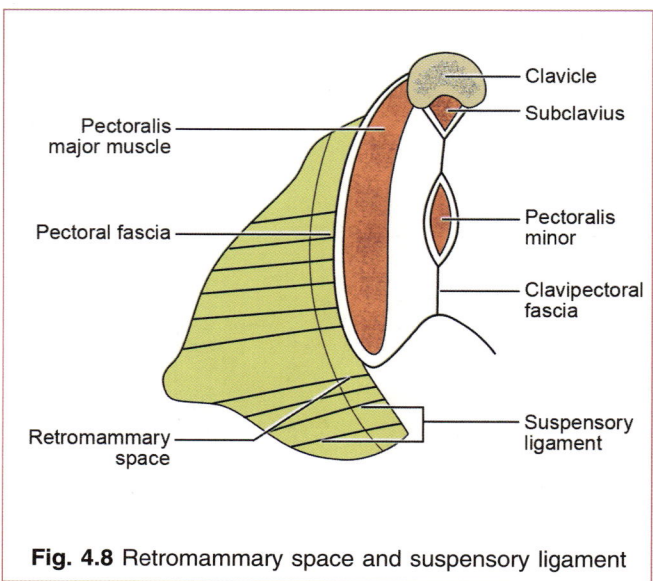

Fig. 4.8 Retromammary space and suspensory ligament

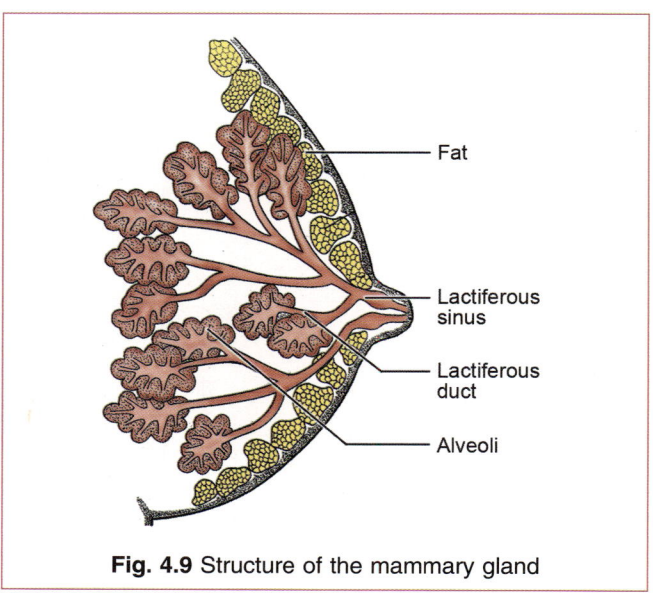

Fig. 4.9 Structure of the mammary gland

a. Branches from lateral thoracic artery.

b. Perforating branches from internal thoracic artery in the medial part.

c. Branches from the posterior intercostal arteries.

d. Branches from acromiothoracic and superior thoracic artery.

Venous drainage

The venous blood drains into axillary, internal thoracic and posterior intercostal veins.

> The posterior intercostal veins communicate with internal vertebral venous plexus. Hence a carcinoma of the mammary gland can spread into vertebral column and skull through these venous communications.

Lymphatic drainage

The lymphatic vessels and lymph nodes of mammary gland is clinically very important as lymph vessels form the major route for spread of carcinoma. It can be studied under superficial and deep lymphatic vessels.

Superficial lymphatic vessels: They drain the skin of the mammary gland except nipple and areola.

1. From the upper part of the gland the vessels drain into supra clavicular and deltopectoral group of lymph nodes

2. From the medial part drains into internal mammary (parasternal) nodes. Some of these vessels crosses the midline to reach the internal mammary nodes of the opposite side

3. The remaining major part drains into anterior axillary lymph nodes.

4. Few lymphatics from the lower part reach the abdominal cavity through rectus sheath where they communicate with subperiotoneal plexus (Fig. 4.12).

> • The lymphatic communication with subperitoneal plexus provides a route for carcinoma to spread into abdominal lymph nodes (for example hepatic nodes). It is possible that few cancerous cells drop into the peritoneal cavity and spread into abdominal or pelvic organs especially the ovary. This transcoelomic spread is referred as Krukenberg's tumors.
>
> • The blockage of superficial lymphatic vessels in case of carcinoma results in edema of the overlying skin. The edema does not occur at the points where the ducts of the sweat gland open on the skin. This gives resembles of an orange peel (peau d'orange appearance) to the mammary gland.

Deep lymphatic vessels: It drains the parenchyma of the mammary gland and also nipple and areola. The lymphatic vessels in the form of plexus deep to the areola are referred as sub-areolar plexus of Sappey. These plexus communicate with lymph vessels draining the parenchyma.

• Lymph vessels from the parenchyma mainly drain into anterior axillary lymph nodes. Few lymphatic vessels drain into inter pectoral group (located between pectoralis major and minor), posterior and lateral axillary group of lymph nodes (Fig. 4.10).

• From these nodes, lymph drain into central axillary group and then into apical axillary group of nodes. The apical group also receives few direct lymph vessels from the

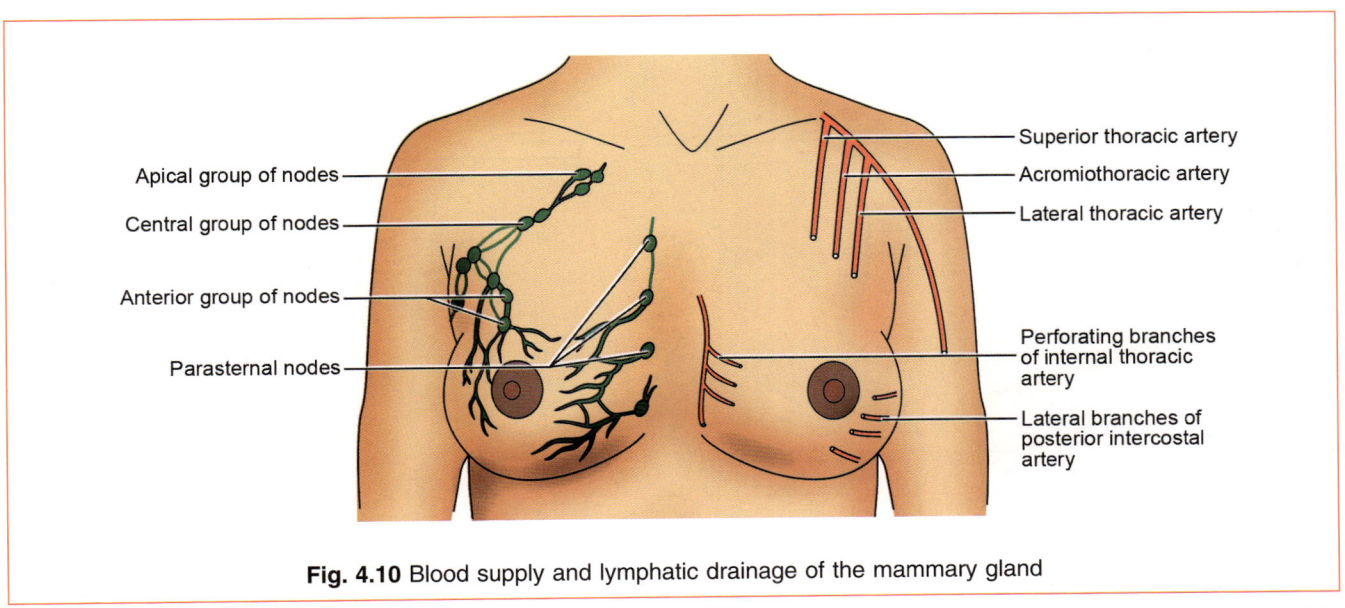

Fig. 4.10 Blood supply and lymphatic drainage of the mammary gland

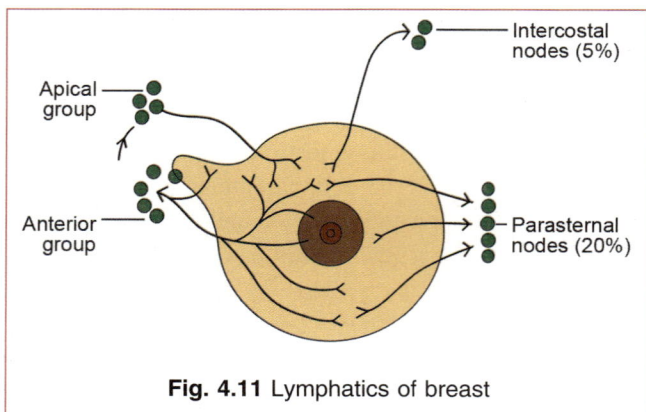

Fig. 4.11 Lymphatics of breast

upper part of the gland. Finally lymph vessels form subclavian trunk in the neck which joins thoracic duct on the left side and right lymphatic duct on the right side (Fig. 4.12).

• Lymph vessels emerging from the deep surface of the gland drains into intercostal nodes located at the posterior end of the intercostal spaces.

• Lymph from the medial side drains into parasternal (internal mammary) group of nodes (Fig. 4.11).

Lymph from the breast mainly drains into axillary (about 75%) and internal mammary group (about 20%) of lymph nodes and posterior intercostal nodes (5%).

Breast is the frequent site of carcinoma, which is manifested as painless hard lump in the initial stage. Through lymphatic communications cancer may spread from one breast to the other or into the peritoneal cavity.

In case of carcinoma of the mammary gland the anterior axillary group is first to be involved.

The sentinel lymph node is the hypothetical first lymph node or group of nodes draining a cancer. In case of diagnosed cancerous condition it is postulated that the sentinel lymph node/s is/are the target organs primarily reached by metastasizing cancer cells from the tumor In case of carcinoma of the mammary gland, the anterior axillary group nodes are considered as sentinel node.

For confirmation of diagnosis, biopsies of the axillary lymph nodes are necessary. The anterior, posterior and lateral group of axillary nodes are considered as level-I nodes, which are located inferior to the pectoralis minor muscle. The central and interpectoral groups of nodes are considered as level-II nodes. The apical axillary nodes belong to level-III nodes. In carcinoma of the breast the level-I is first to be involved, followed by level-II and level-III.

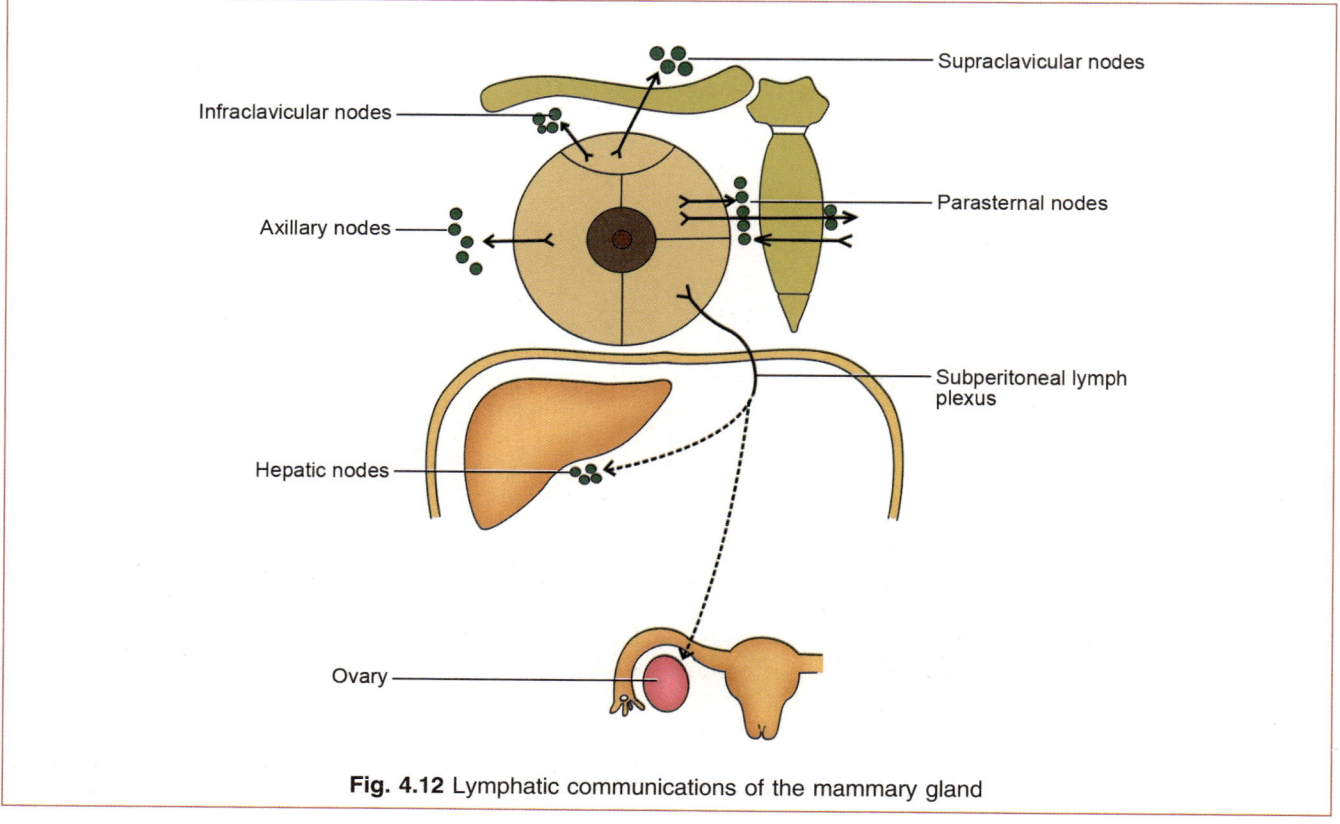

Fig. 4.12 Lymphatic communications of the mammary gland

The surgical removal of the mammary gland is called 'mastectomy', which is done in case of carcinoma of the breast along with the removal of axillary lymph nodes (level-I and II, which is often involved). During removal of axillary lymph nodes, the nerve to serratus anterior, the nerve to latissimus dorsi and intercostobrachial nerves are likely to be injured. Involvement of nerve to serratus anterior can cause difficulty in overhead abduction at the shoulder joint and results in winging of the scapula. Involvement of intercostobrachial nerve may lead to loss of cutaneous sensation in the arm pit and upper medial part of the arm.

Mammography is an X-ray of the mammary gland to detect the malignancy.

Though the mammary gland is rudimentary in males, abnormal enlargement of male mammary gland is referred as Gynecomastia. It is a feature of Klinefelter's syndrome (XXY).

Accessory nipples may be found anywhere along the milk line which extends from axilla to the inguinal region.

CASE-1

A 54-year-old woman, concerned about a mass that she detected during a breast self examination, visited the hospital. The physician also detected the mass in the left breast and ordered a mammogram. The results of these studies revealed a solid mass. A core biopsy of the mass was obtained and sent to the pathologist. The pathologist's reported as carcinoma. She underwent mastectomy and thereafter she recovered well. After couple of weeks she experienced weakness in her left shoulder and had difficulty in raising her left arm above her head. During her next visit to the hospital, the physician noticed that her left scapula was protruded posteriorly to a greater extent than on her right side. With relation to this case answer the following.

1. Name the lymph nodes receiving lymph from different parts of the breast and locate each group.

2. What is a sentinel node biopsy? (warning node)

3. What could be the cause of difficulty in raising the arm above the head in this patient?

Solution to the case history

Case-1

1. Refer text

2. The sentinel node is hypothetical first lymph node or group of nodes draining a cancer. In case of carcinoma

of the mammary gland the axillary group is considered as sentinel nodes. For confirmation of diagnosis these groups of lymph nodes are primarily considered for biopsy.

3. The difficulty in raising the arm above the head (overhead abduction at shoulder) is due to the paralysis of the serratus anterior muscle. The nerve to serratus anterior was injured during removal of axillary lymph nodes.

MCQs

1. A 24-year-old man is brought to the emergency department with a stab injury to his right upper limb. The knife has penetrated an area in front of the shoulder in a groove between deltoid and pectoralis major muscle. Which of the following structures could be the source for massive bleeding in this patient?

   A. Basilic vein
   B. Cephalic vein
   C. Axillary vein
   D. Subclavian vein

2. A 38-year-old woman notices a rock-hard lump in one breast. She is diagnosed with breast cancer, and undergoes a mastectomy. During the procedure, the surgeon notes that the breast tumor has spread to involve the muscle which is present immediately deep to the breast. Which of the following muscles is affected?

   A. Platysma
   B. Internal oblique abdominis
   C. Pectoralis minor
   D. Pectoralis major

3. While observing a mastectomy on a 56-year-old female patient, you are asked by the surgeon to identify an artery that supplies medial side of the mammary gland which he was tying off. Your correct answer has to be

   A. Posterior intercostal
   B. Lateral thoracic
   C. Internal thoracic
   D. Acromiothoracic

4. A woman with breast cancer subsequently develops metastasis in her vertebral column. The direct route for spread of the tumour to the vertebral column was via

   A. Lymphatic vessels draining into the axilla
   B. Veins draining into the posterior intercostal veins
   C. Veins draining into the axillary vein
   D Lymphatics communicating with subperitoneal plexus

115

5. The prognosis in breast cancer is poor as more of proximal lymph nodes are found to have cancerous cells in them. Which of the following axillary nodes if affected, would indicate the worst prognosis?

   A. Apical
   B. Central
   C. Lateral
   D. Anterior

6. A 53-year-old female diagnosed with carcinoma of the right breast. Having known the lymphatic drainage of the breast where would you consider the metastasis to occur first?

   A. Hepatic lymph nodes
   B. Axillary lymph nodes
   C. Parasternal lymph nodes
   D. Supraclavicular lymph nodes

7. In the process of doing an axillary lymph node dissection in a 48 year-old patient, the surgeon cleans the space between the pectoralis major and minor muscles in an attempt to remove all the lateral pectoral lymph nodes. Upon recovery it was noted that the patient's lower part of pectoralis major was paralyzed. The nerve that was most likely to be injured was

   A. Long thoracic
   B. Lateral pectoral
   C. Medial pectoral
   D. Intercostobrachial

8. A 17-year-old male, thrown from a motorcycle moving at high speed was admitted to the hospital. He was found to have a paralysis of right pectoralis major muscle. Which set of movements at the shoulder joint would be found greatly weakened?

   A. Adduction and medial rotation
   B. Abduction and flexion
   C. Abduction and extension
   D. Adduction and lateral rotation

9. A 48-year-old woman is diagnosed with a malignant tumour in the upper lateral quadrant of the right breast. Tumour metastasis is possible through lymphatics. Which of the following options best describes the sequence in which the lymph nodes would be affected by metastasis?

   A. Anterior to central to apical axillary nodes
   B. Posterior to parasternal to anterior axillary nodes
   C. Lateral to apical to central
   D. Posterior to supraclavicular to parasternal

10. A 58-year-old woman with a history of breast cancer underwent mastectomy with radical axillary node dissection. A neck exploration was performed for an enlarged cervical node as secondary concern about metastasis. Several weeks later she presents with a swollen right arm and swollen fingers along with right facial edema. Which of the following is the most likely cause of these findings?

   A. Disruption of the right lymphatic duct
   B. Disruption of the thoracic duct
   C. Thrombosis of the axillary vein
   D. Thrombosis of the cephalic vein

11. A 43-year-old woman notices a rock-hard lump in one breast. She is diagnosed with breast cancer, and undergoes a mastectomy. During the procedure, the surgeon notes that the breast tumour has spread involving the muscle layer immediately deep to the breast, hence this muscle was removed. Which of the following functions were most likely to be compromised?

   A. Adduction and lateral rotation
   B. Adduction and medial rotation
   C. Abduction and medial rotation
   D. Abduction and lateral rotation

Answers to MCQs

1. B
2. D
3. C
4. B
5. A
6. B
7. C
8. A
9. A
10. A
11. B

- Axilla
- Brachial plexus
- Axillary artery
- Axillary lymph nodes
- MCQs

Objectives

- To explain the boundaries and contents of the axilla.
- With the help of a schematic diagram explain the formation of brachial plexus and its branches and explain the injuries affecting different parts of the brachial plexus.
- To explain the course, parts, branches and distribution of axillary artery.
- Classify the axillary group of lymph nodes, give their location, areas of drainage and clinical anatomy.

SECTION 3

AXILLA (ARMPIT)

It is a space situated between the upper part of the arm and the chest wall. It is pyramidal in shape with its apex directed towards the root of the neck and a base directed below. It has anterior, posterior, medial and lateral walls.

Apex: The apex is blunt and is called **cervico-axillary canal**. This canal is bounded in front by clavicle, posteriorly by upper border of the scapula and medially by first rib. The brachial plexus and axillary artery enter the axilla through this canal. The axillary veins and lymphatics enter the neck through this canal.

Base: It is formed by skin, superficial fascia, deep fascia (axillary fascia) and suspensory ligament of the axilla. The base is bounded in front by anterior axillary fold, which is formed by the fibres of the pectoralis major muscle and posteriorly by posterior axillary fold. It is formed by the fibres of latissimus dorsi and teres major muscles (Fig. 5.1). The boundaries of the axilla are (Fig. 5.2):

Anterior wall: Pectoralis major, pectoralis minor and subclavius muscles.

Posterior wall: Subscapularis, latissimus dorsi and teres major.

Medial wall: Upper four intercostal spaces (upper thoracic wall) with upper part of the serratus anterior muscle.

Lateral wall: Shaft of the humerus with coracobrachialis and short head of the biceps brachii muscle.

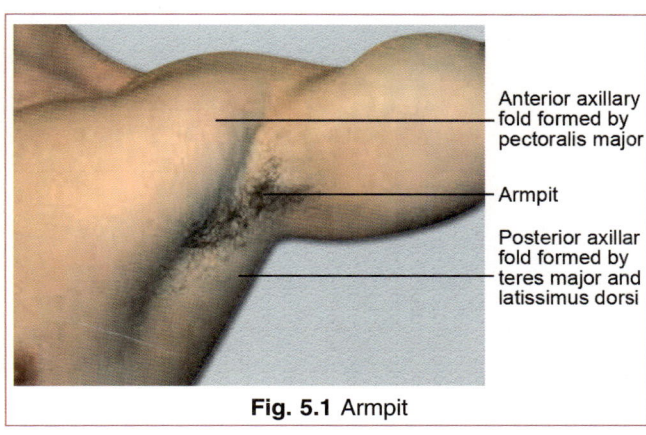

Anterior axillary fold formed by pectoralis major

Armpit

Posterior axillar fold formed by teres major and latissimus dorsi

Fig. 5.1 Armpit

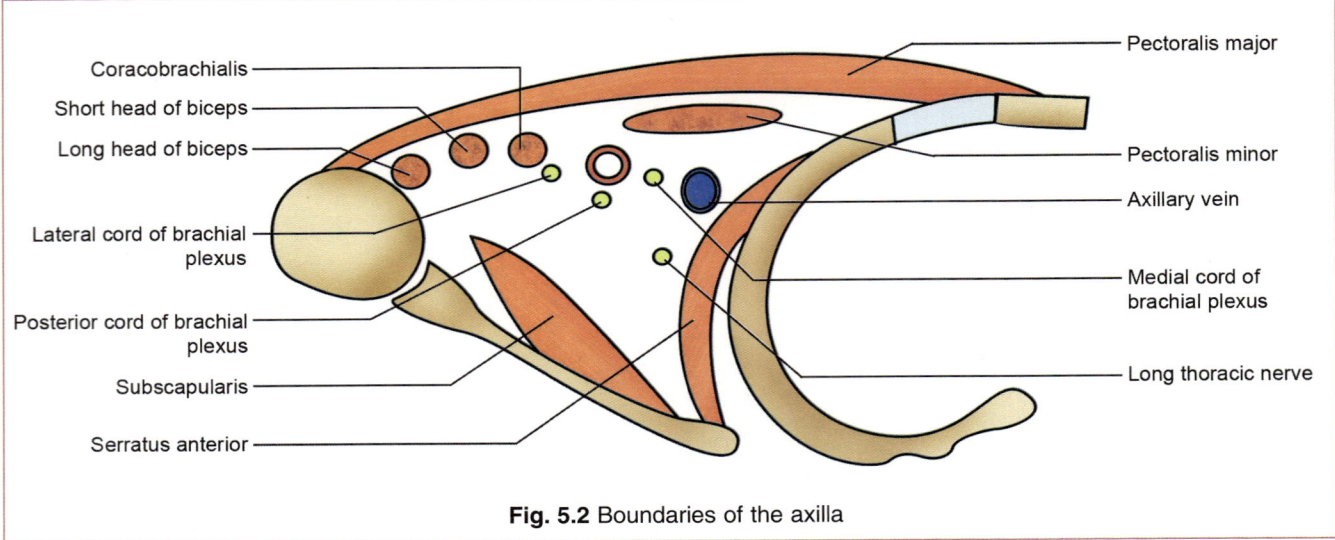

Fig. 5.2 Boundaries of the axilla

Contents

1. Axillary artery and vein (Fig. 5.3)
2. Infraclavicular part of the brachial plexus
3. Intercostobrachial nerve
4. Axillary lymph nodes
5. Axillary pad of fat.

- Axilla has abundant axillary hairs. Infections of the hair follicles and sebaceous glands give rise to boils (Fig. 5.4).
- Examinations of axillary lymph nodes are important in clinical practice.
- An abscess originating from the cervical vertebrae can track down to the axilla along the neurovascular bundle.

- While draining the abscess from the axilla incision is placed midway between anterior and posterior margin closer to the chest wall to avoid injury to the neurovascular structures.

BRACHIAL PLEXUS

It is a plexus of nerves that supplies the upper limb.

Formation

It is formed by ventral rami of lower four cervical and first thoracic nerves (C5, 6, 7, 8 and T1).

Pre-fixed condition: Contribution from C4 nerve constitutes 'pre-fixed condition' of the brachial plexus with reduced T1 contribution.

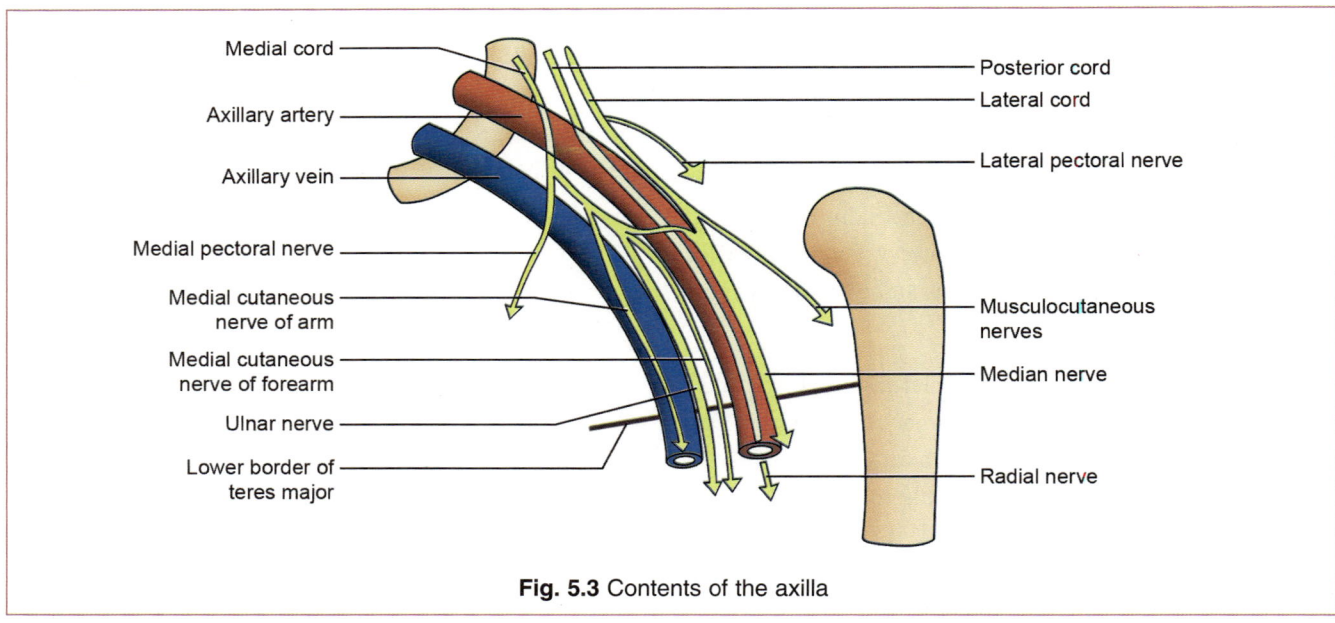

Fig. 5.3 Contents of the axilla

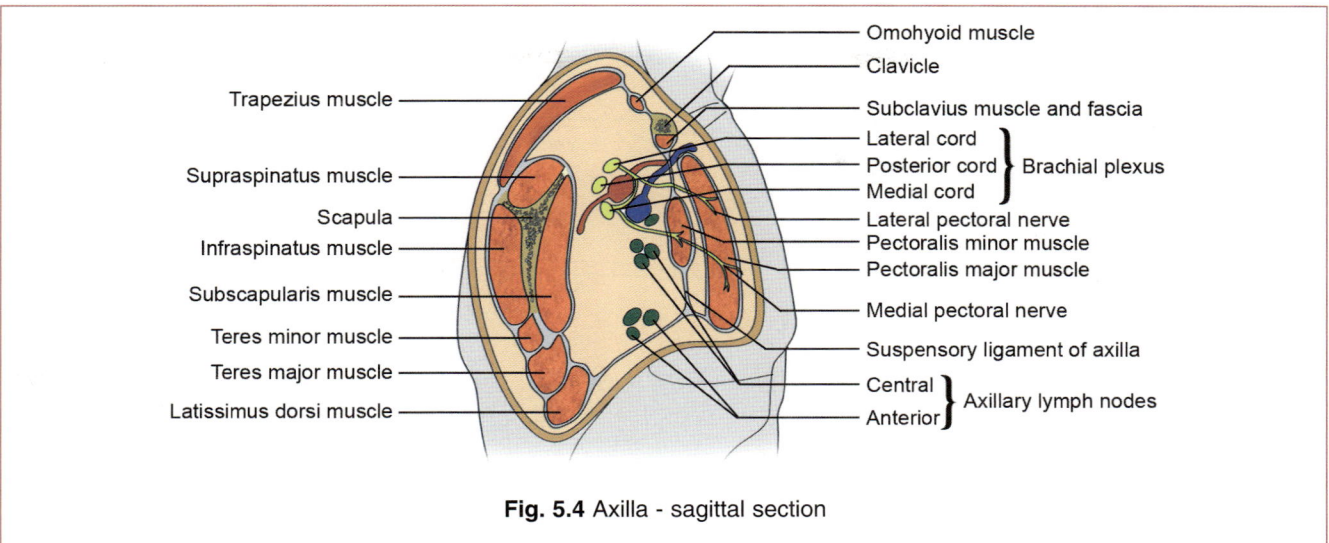

Fig. 5.4 Axilla - sagittal section

Post-fixed condition: Contribution from T2 nerve constitutes post-fixed condition of the brachial plexus with reduced C5 contribution.

Parts

The proximal part of the brachial plexus occupies the posterior triangle of the neck. This part is called '**supra-clavicular part**'. The distal part of the plexus occupy the axilla (armpit) and it is called '**infra clavicular part**'. For convenience both parts are discussed together. The brachial plexus consists of roots, trunks, divisions and cords. The roots, trunks and divisions are present in the posterior triangle of the neck as supraclavicular part. These nerve emerge between Scalenus anterior and medius muscles (Figs 5.5 and 5.6).

Roots

- The ventral rami of C5 and C6 joins to form '**upper trunk' (superior trunk).**

- The ventral ramus of C7 continue as '**middle trunk'.**

- The ventral rami of C8 and T1 joins to form '**lower trunk' (inferior trunk).**

The upper and middle trunk lies above the level of the subclavian artery, while the lower trunk is present on the upper surface of the first rib along with the subclavian artery. Each trunk divides into ventral and dorsal divisions behind the clavicle. The cords are formed at the cervico-axillary canal as follows.

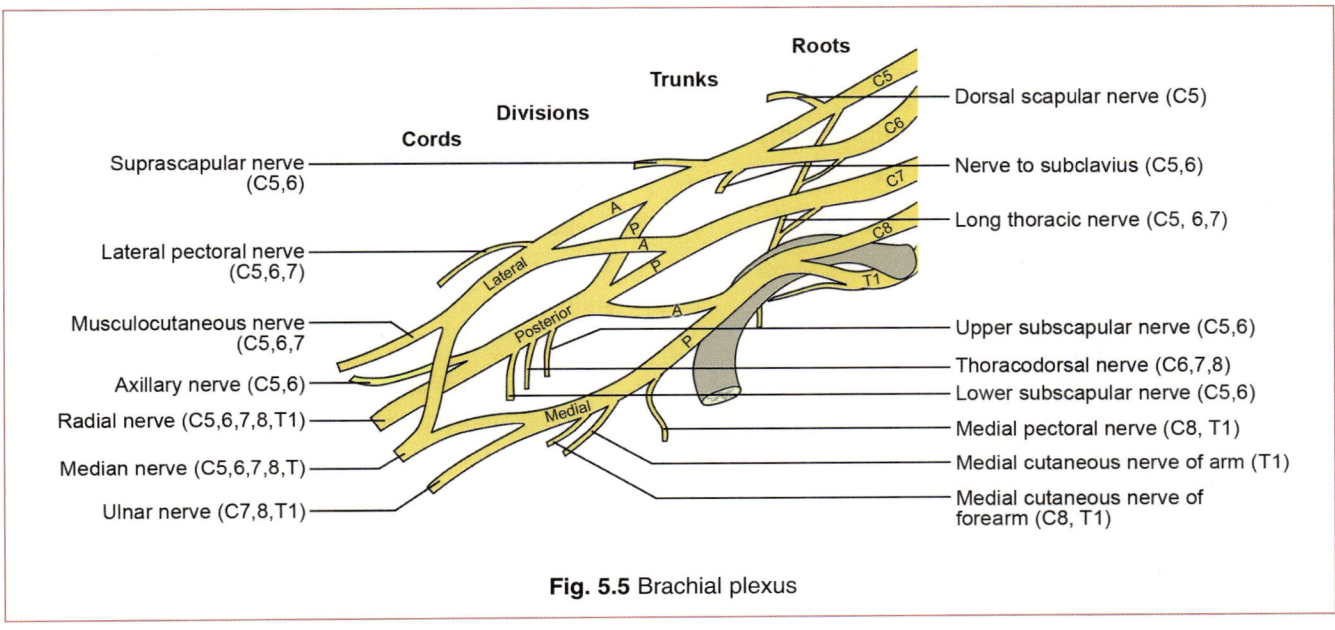

Fig. 5.5 Brachial plexus

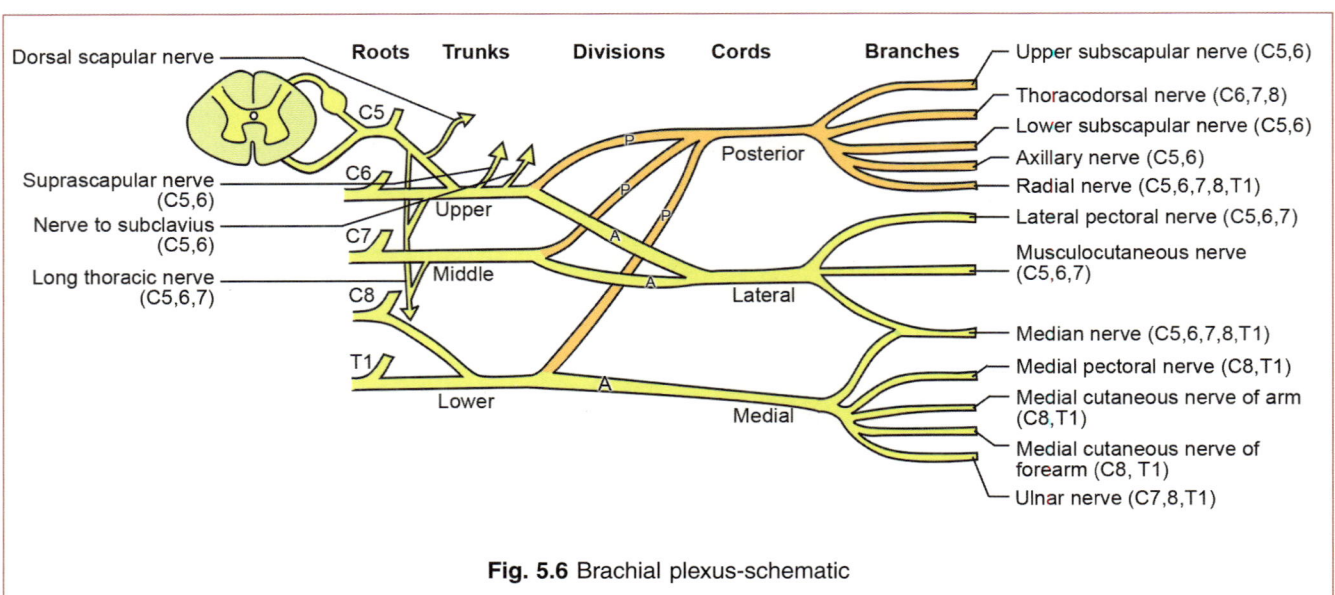

Fig. 5.6 Brachial plexus-schematic

Cords

- The ventral divisions of upper and middle trunks join to form 'lateral cord'
- The ventral division of lower trunk continues as 'medial cord'
- The dorsal divisions of all the trunks (upper, middle and lower) join to form 'posterior cord'.

The cords are named according to their relation to the second part of the axillary artery. The lateral cord is lateral, medial cord is medial and the posterior cord is posterior. However their relations to first part of the axillary artery is different, where medial cord is posterior, lateral and posterior cords are lateral in position.

The lateral cord will have C5, 6 and 7 fibres. The medial cord will have C8 and T1 fibres. The posterior cord has fibres from all the roots of the brachial plexus with reduced T1 fibres. The ulnar nerve contains fibres from C7,8 and T1. The C7 fibre is provided by either lateral cord or by median nerve to supply flexor carpi ulnaris muscle.

Branches

The branches arise from root level, from the upper trunk and from the cords.

Branches from the roots:

1. **Nerve to serratus anterior** (long thoracic nerve) C5, 6, 7: It is also called nerve of Bell. It descends in the medial wall of the axilla to supply serratus anterior muscle.

2. **Nerve to rhomboideus** (dorsal scapular nerve) C5: This nerve does not enter the axilla. It arises in the neck region and courses backwards to supply rhomboideus major, rhomboideus minor and levattor scapulae muscles.

Branches from the upper trunk (Erb's point):

1. Supra scapular nerve (C5, 6)

2. Nerve to subclavius (C5, 6)

Both these branches does not enter the axilla. The suprascapular nerve proceeds backwards and supplies supraspinatus and infraspinatus muscles.

Branches from the lateral cord:

1. **Lateral pectoral nerve (C5, 6, 7):** It pierces the clavipectoral fascia and enters the substance of pectoralis major. It gives a branch to pectoralis minor.

2. **Musculocutaneous nerve (C5, 6, 7):** It is the continuation of the lateral cord. It pierces the coracobrachialis muscle and supplies muscles in front of the arm and skin of the lateral side of the forearm as lateral cutaneous nerve of the forearm.

3. **Lateral root of the median nerve (C5, 6, 7):** It joins with the medial root arising from the medial cord in front of the axillary artery to form the median nerve.

Branches from the medial cord:

1. **Medial root of the median nerve (C8, T1):** It joins with the lateral root arising from the lateral cord to form median nerve.

2. **Medial pectoral nerve (C8, T1):** It pierces the pectoralis minor muscle and supplies pectoralis minor and major.

3. **Medial cutaneous nerve of the arm (C8, T1):** It supplies the skin of the medial side of the arm.

4. **Medial cutaneous nerve of the forearm (C8, T1):** It supplies skin of the medial side of the forearm.

5. **Ulnar nerve (C7, 8, T1):** It mainly supplies intrinsic muscles of the hand.

Branches from the posterior cord

1. **Upper subscapular nerve (C5, 6):** It supplies the subscapularis muscle.

2. **Lower subscapular nerve (C5, 6):** It supplies subscapularis and teres major muscles.

3. **Nerve to latissimus dorsi** (C6, 7, 8): It is also called **thoracodorsal nerve.** It supplies latissimus dorsi muscle. The terminal part of the nerve is accompanied by continuation of subscapular artery, which is then referred as thoracodorsal artery.

4. **Axillary nerve** (C5, 6): It is also called circumflex nerve. It leaves the axilla by passing posteriorly through a muscular interval called 'quadrangular space' along with posterior circumflex humeral artery. It winds around the surgical neck of the humerus, supplies deltoid and teres minor muscles and also skin over the deltoid.

5. **Radial nerve** (C5, 6, 7, 8, T1): It is the nerve of the posterior compartment. It leaves the axilla by passing through a muscular interval called 'lower triangular space'. It supplies extensor muscles of the arm and forearm.

Brachial plexus injury

Brachial plexus may be injured during labour (forceps delivery), automobile injury, stab injury, compression by enlarged lymph nodes or aneurysm of the axillary artery.

Erb's paralysis

The upper trunk of the brachial plexus where six nerves (C5 and 6 roots, nerve to subclavius and suprascapular nerve, anterior and posterior divisions of upper trunk) meet is called Erb's point. An injury to the Erb's point results in paralysis of muscles of the upper limb supplied by C5 and 6 fibres (Fig. 5.7).

Causes of injury:

Birth injury (excessive stretching of upper trunk)

Fall on the shoulder

During anesthesia (Brachial plexus block)

Clinical features:

- The arm hangs by the side of the body and medially rotated. The arm cannot be abducted and laterally rotated.
- The elbow is extended and flexion is not possible.

- The forearm is pronated and supination is not possible.
- The wrist and fingers are flexed.

  This position of the upper limb is referred to as policeman's tip or waiter's tip hand (Fig. 5.7).

Muscles involved:

- Deltoid (hence abduction at shoulder is not possible)
- Biceps, Brachialis and Brachioradialis (Hence flexion at elbow is not possible)
- Supinator (hence supination of forearm is not possible)
- Supraspinatus (hence initiation of abduction is not possible)
- Teres minor (hence lateral rotation is not possible)
- Infraspinatus (hence lateral rotation is not possible)

Klumpke's paralysis

It occurs due to injury to the lower trunk of the brachial plexus (C8, T1).

Causes of injury (Fig. 5.8):

- Undue abduction of arm (as in clutching something with hands while falling from a height.
- Birth injury
- Presence of cervical rib

Clinical features:

This results in paralysis of intrinsic muscles of hand and long flexors of the hand. The hand muscles are

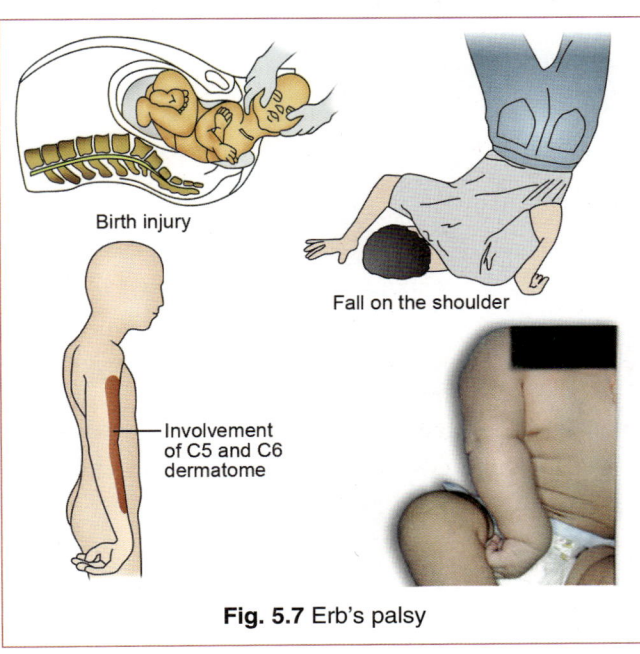

Fig. 5.7 Erb's palsy

Birth injury

Fall on the shoulder

Involvement of C5 and C6 dermatome

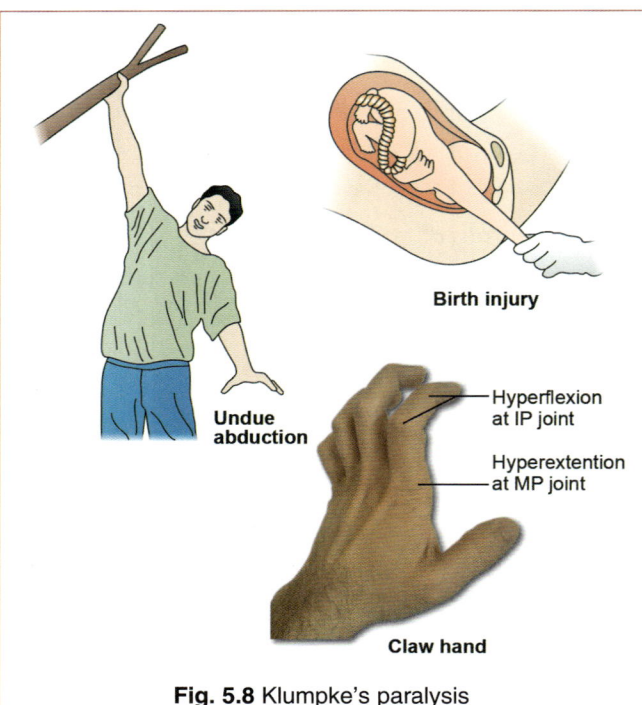

Birth injury

Undue abduction

Hyperflexion at IP joint

Hyperextention at MP joint

Claw hand

Fig. 5.8 Klumpke's paralysis

palmar and dorsal interossei and lumbricals. They are innervated mainly by ulnar nerve and also by median nerve with **C8** and **T1** fibres. These muscles are responsible for flexion at the metacarpophalangeal joint and extension at the inter phalangeal joint. Hence medial four fingers are hyperextended at metacarpo-phalangeal joint and hyper flexed at inter phalangeal joint. This condition is called '**claw hand**'. The wrist joint is hyper extended due to paralysis of wrist flexors. There will be wasting of thenar and hypothenar muscles. There is pain and numbness along the medial side of the arm, forearm and medial one and half finger.

Involvement of ventral ramus of T1 or its white ramus communicantes causes '**Horner's syndrome**'. This is because the sympathetic innervation to the head area (sweat glands of the face, dilator pupillae muscle of the eye and superior tarsal muscle of the upper eyelid) is conveyed through ventral ramus of first thoracic nerve.

Injury to the long thoracic nerve: It results in paralysis of Serratus anterior muscle, which is manifested by backward projection of scapula (**winging of scapula**). This nerve may be injured while removing the lymph nodes of the axilla as well.

Sympathetic fibres to the upper limb

The sympathetic fibres for the erector pilae muscle of the dermis (pilomotor), smooth muscles of the blood vessels (vasomotor) and sweat glands (sudomotor) are conveyed through the branches of the brachial plexus. The nerve roots (C5 to T1) contributing to the formation of brachial plexus receive post ganglionic grey rami communicantes from middle and inferior cervical sympathetic ganglia. These ganglia receive preganglionic sympathetic fibres from white ramus communicantes, which join the first thoracic ganglion and convey through ventral ramus of T1 nerves. (Remember sympathetic is thoracolumbar outflow).

Cervical rib syndrome/Scalenus anterior syndrome/thoracic outlet syndrome:

Presence of cervical rib or a congenitally hypertrophied scalenus anterior muscle would affect upper limb as it involves subclavian vessels and brachial plexus. The clinical manifestation and structures involved are listed below.

- Subclavian artery-pallor (pale) and coldness of the upper limb, feeble radial pulse.
- Subclavian vein-distension of the superficial veins, edema and pain in the upper limb
- Lower trunk of the brachial plexus-numbness, tingling and pain along the medial border of the hand and little finger, wasting of small muscles of the hand
- Treatment - Removal of cervical rib or scalenotomy

CASE-1

A baby was delivered with a breech presentation. During the second stage of labour, the right arm was carried up above the head, severely stretching the lower part of the brachial plexus. Assuming that six months later you were asked to examine the child.

a. Describe exactly the position assumed by the fingers of the right hand and name the muscles that would show evidence of wasting.

b. It is assumed that 1st thoracic root of the brachial plexus had been severely damaged. Do you expect any sensory loss to occur in this case?

CASE-2

Following a prolonged and difficult labour at 42 weeks of gestation, a newborn baby is noted to have an adducted and medially rotated shoulder with an extended elbow and pronated forearm. The X-ray films of the arm and forearm do not reveal any evidence of fracture or dislocation. This case was diagnosed as Erb's paralysis.

a. Draw a neat labelled diagram showing the formation and branches of brachial plexus.

b. What is Erb's point?

c. How do you correlate the position of the arm, elbow and forearm in this patient with respect to Erb's paralysis?

CASE-3

Following a left radical mastectomy, a 53-year-old woman found that she was unable to raise her left arm above the head to comb the hair. During the physical examination, she was asked to face a wall and push hard against it with both outstretched hands. It was noted that the inferior angle and medial border of the left scapula projected markedly posteriorly during this maneuver.

1. Which nerve had been cut during the mastectomy operation?

2. Explain in anatomical terms the inability of the patient to raise her left arm above her hand

3. Why does she demonstrate ''winging'' of her left scapula?

AXILLARY ARTERY

It is the continuation of the subclavian artery and is present in the axilla (Figs 5.9 and 5.10).

It extends from the outer border of the first rib to the lower border of the teres major muscle and it is divided into three parts by pectoralis minor muscle.

Branches

It gives the following branches. (The first part gives one branch, second part two branches and the third part three branches.)

From the first part:

1. **Superior thoracic artery:** It enters the thoracic wall and supplies upper 2 intercostal spaces.

From the second part:

2. **Thoraco-acromial artery (acromiothoracic artery):** It pierces the clavipectoral fascia beneath the clavicular fibres of the pectoralis major muscle. It soon divides into clavicular, deltoid, pectoral and acromial branches.

3. **Lateral thoracic artery:** It enters the thoracic wall along the lower border of the pectoralis minor muscle. It is related to anterior group of axillary lymph nodes. In females it one of the major artery supplying the mammary gland.

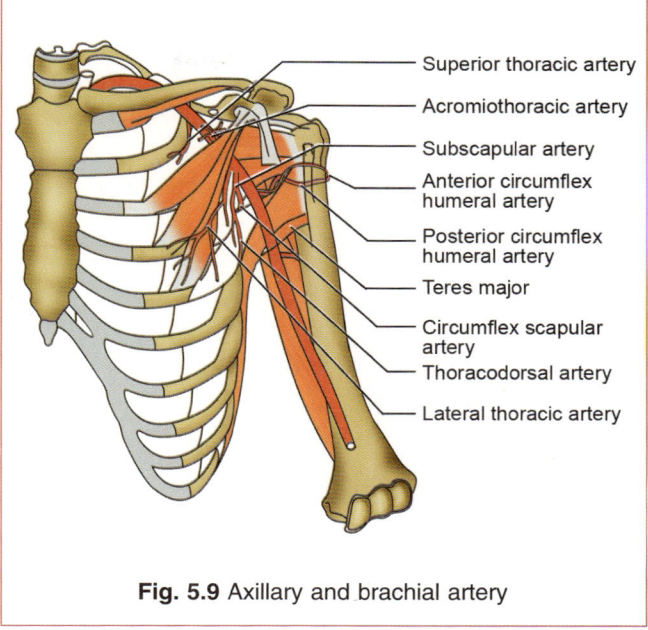

Fig. 5.9 Axillary and brachial artery

From the third part:

4. **Subscapular artery:** It is the largest branch from the axillary artery. It passes downwards along the posterior wall of the axilla on the subscapularis muscle. It gives circumflex scapular branch, which winds around the lateral border of the scapula through a triangular space to reach the back of the scapula where it anastomoses with supra scapular artery. The terminal part of the subscapular artery accompanies thoracodorsal nerve and is then called as 'thoracodorsal artery'.

5. **Anterior circumflex humeral artery:** It passes in front of the surgical neck of the humerus to anastomose with posterior circumflex humeral artery. It mainly supplies shoulder joint and humerus.

6. **Posterior circumflex humeral artery:** It is larger than anterior circumflex humeral artery, passes posteriorly

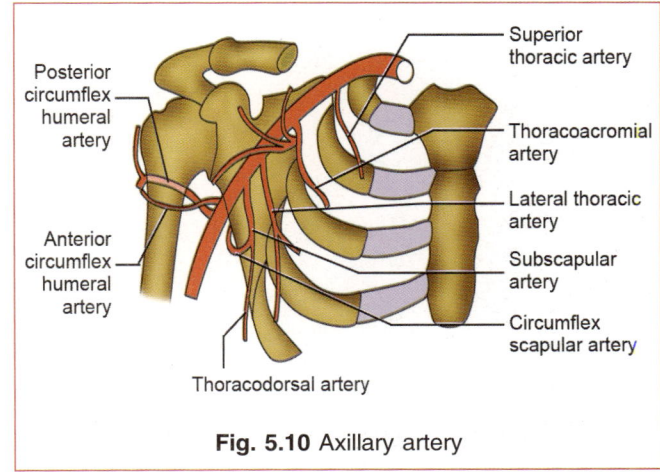

Fig. 5.10 Axillary artery

through quadrangular space along with the axillary nerve. It anastomose with anterior circumflex humeral artery at the surgical neck of the humerus. It supplies deltoid muscle and shoulder joint. It gives a descending branch which anastomoses with a branch from profunda brachii artery (first branch from brachial artery).

Major relations

First part:

Anteriorly: Pectoralis major, clavipectoral fascia, a communicating branch between medial and lateral pectoral nerves.

Posteriorly: Medial cord of the brachial plexus, first two digitations of serratus anterior muscle and long thoracic nerve.

Laterally: Lateral and posterior cord of the brachial plexus.

Medially: Axillary vein.

Second part:

Anteriorly: Pectoralis major and minor muscles.

Posteriorly: Posterior cord of the brachial plexus and subscapularis muscle.

Medially: Medial cord of the brachial plexus.

Laterally: Lateral cord of the brachial plexus.

Third part:

Anteriorly: Pectoralis major muscle and crossed in front by medial root of the median nerve

Posteriorly: Axillary and radial nerves, Subscapularis and teres major muscles

Medially: Medial cutaneous nerves of the arm and forearm, ulnar nerve and axillary vein.

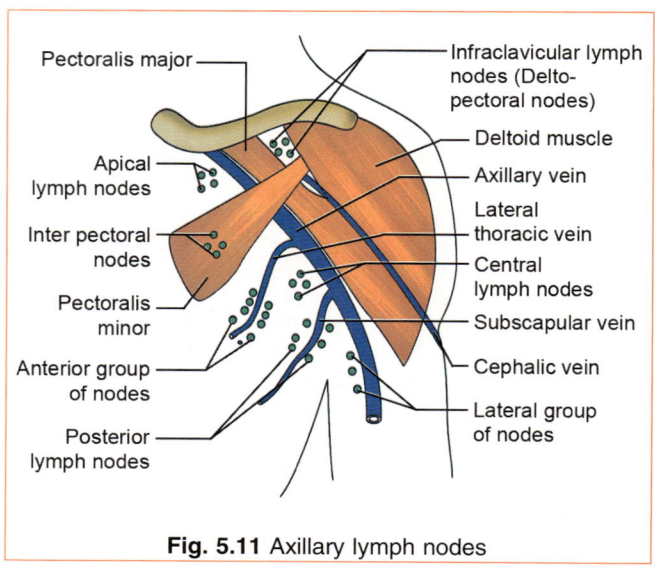

Pectoralis major
Apical lymph nodes
Inter pectoral nodes
Pectoralis minor
Anterior group of nodes
Posterior lymph nodes
Infraclavicular lymph nodes (Delto-pectoral nodes)
Deltoid muscle
Axillary vein
Lateral thoracic vein
Central lymph nodes
Subscapular vein
Cephalic vein
Lateral group of nodes

Fig. 5.11 Axillary lymph nodes

Laterally: Musculocutaneous nerve and coracobrachialis muscle

Surface markings

Axillary artery is marked on the body by abducting the arm to 90° and palm facing up. The first point is at the midpoint of the clavicle. The second part is at the junction of anterior 2/3rd and posterior 1/3rd of the line joining the anterior and posterior axillary folds. A line connecting these two points corresponds to axillary artery.

> Aneurysm of the axillary artery can compress the brachial plexus.

Axillary vein

It is formed by the continuation of basilic vein at the level of the lower border of the teres major muscle. At this point the two veins accompanying the brachial artery (venae comitantes) also join with basilic vein. Axillary vein continues as subclavian vein at the level of outer border of the first rib. It is medial to the axillary artery throughout its course.

> Axillary vein thrombosis occurs in people who work with hyper abducted arm for long period (for example painting the ceiling).
>
> Axillary vein is closely related to axillary group of lymph nodes, hence during removal of these nodes the vein may be injured.

AXILLARY LYMPH NODES

Axillary lymph nodes are anatomically classified into 5 groups, namely-anterior, posterior, lateral, central and apical (Figs 5.11 and 5.12).

Anterior group (Pectoral group): They are located along the course of lateral thoracic vessels in relation to the lower border of the pectoralis minor muscle. It receives lymph from mammary gland and also from superficial tissue of the front of the chest and anterior abdominal wall up to the level of umbilicus. The efferent vessels from these nodes drains into central group.

Posterior group (Subscapular group): They are located along the subscapular vessels. They receive lymph from mammary gland, posterior chest wall up to the level of iliac crest. The efferent vessels from these nodes drains into central group.

Lateral group (Brachial group): These groups of nodes are located along the axillary vein. They receive lymph from the entire upper limb except the area drained by cephalic vein, which drains into deltopectoral group of lymph nodes.

Central group: They are located in the fatty tissue of the axilla along the axillary vein. These nodes receive afferents from anterior, posterior and lateral groups and sends efferents to apical group. The intercostobrachial nerve passes through these nodes. Hence enlargement of these nodes may cause pain in the skin of the base of the arm pit and upper medial side of the arm. The nerve may be damaged during removal of these nodes.

Apical group: They are located near the apex of the axilla along the axillary vein close to the first rib and upper margin of the pectoralis minor muscle. They receive lymph from central group, deltopectoral group (infraclavicular group) and inter pectoral group. It also receives lymph from upper part of the mammary gland directly. The apical nodes are the terminal nodes of the upper limb. The efferent vessels arising from them forms subclavian trunk. The subclavian trunk joins with jugular trunk (bringing lymph from head and neck area) and opens into thoracic duct on the left side and right lymphatic duct on the right side.

Clinical classification

Clinically the axillary lymph nodes are classified into three levels by pectoralis minor muscle.

Level-I nodes: They are located inferior to the pectoralis minor muscle. It includes anterior, posterior and lateral group of axillary lymph nodes.

Level-II nodes: They are located in front and posterior to the pectoralis minor muscle. It includes central and interpectoral group of nodes.

Level-III nodes: They are located superior to the pectoralis minor muscle. It include apical group.

> Carcinoma of the breast spreads mainly by lymphatics and involve axillary group of nodes. It may cause painless enlargement of nodes in the axilla.
>
> **Examination of the axillary lymph nodes:** The patient's arm is held in a slightly abducted position to relax the floor and walls of the axilla. The physician uses his/her right hand for examining the left axilla and vice versa. The floor of the axilla is firmly pushed standing in front of the patient for palpating the anterior, lateral, central and apical nodes while for palpating posterior group the physician stands behind the patient.

Solutions to the case studies:

Case-1

a) An injury to the lower trunk of the brachial plexus results in claw hand. The medial four fingers are hyper extended at metacarpophalangeal joints and hyper flexed at inter phalangeal joints. There will be wasting of thenar and hypothenar muscles.

b) Yes. There is pain, numbness or loss of sensation along the medial side of the arm and forearm (T1 dermatome area).

Case-2

a) Refer text

b) Erb's point is located on the upper trunk of brachial plexus formed by meeting of six nerves C5 and C6, anterior and posterior divisions, nerve to subclavius and suprascapular nerve.

c) Refer text

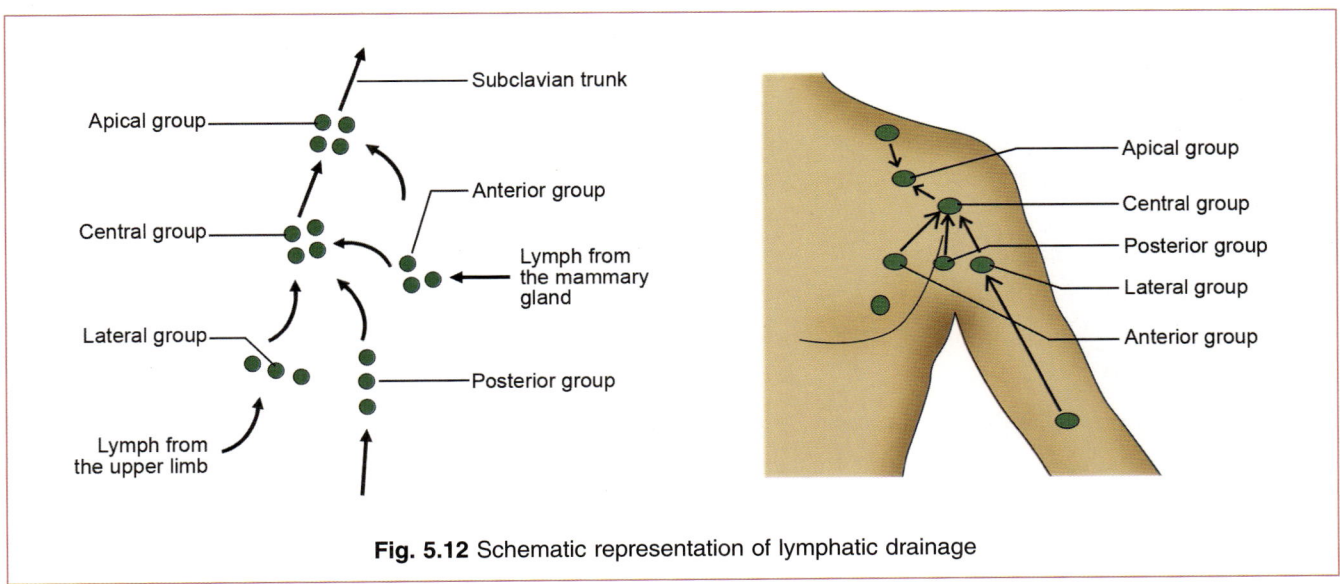

Fig. 5.12 Schematic representation of lymphatic drainage

Case-3

a) When removing the fat and lymph nodes from the axilla, the surgeon endeavours to preserve the long thoracic nerve. Sometimes it is cut by accident or has to be sacrificed because of its involvement in cancerous metastatic deposits.

b) In this case, the nerve removed was long thoracic nerve which resulted in paralysis of serratus anterior muscle. To raise the arm above the head (overhead abduction at shoulder) requires serratus anterior and trapezius muscles. The paralysis of serratus anterior explains why the patient experienced difficulty in combing her hair.

c) Another important function of the serratus anterior is to keep the scapula applied to the chest wall. Paralysis of this muscle resulted in "winging" scapula.

MCQs

1. A 54-year-old electrician reports pain in his left upper limb, tingling and numbness in 4th and 5th digits of his left hand. There is mild swelling of the left hand. He reports that pain and numbness is more when he is doing electrical work with his arms overhead. The X-ray reveals the presence of a cervical rib. Which of the following structures is most likely to be compressed be a cervical rib?

   A. Subclavian artery
   B. Brachial artery
   C. Brachiocephalic artery
   D. Axillary artery

2. A person sustains a left brachial plexus injury in an auto accident. After initial recovery the following is observed: a) the diaphragm functions normally, b) there is no winging of the scapula, c) abduction cannot be initiated, but if the arm is helped through the first 45 degrees of abduction, the patient can fully abduct the arm. From these findings and your knowledge of the formation of the brachial plexus where would you expect the injury to have occurred?

   A. Suprascapular nerve
   B. Axillary nerve
   C. Roots of plexus
   D. Superior trunk

3. The cords of the brachial plexus is present

   A. At or below the clavicle, closely related to the axillary artery.
   B. At or below the clavicle, closely related to the axillary vein.

C. Above the clavicle, medial to the scalenus anterior muscle.
D. Above the clavicle, behind the scalenus anterior muscle.

4. A patient underwent mastectomy with the subsequent removal of axillary lymph nodes that was lying inferior to the pectoralis minor muscle . Which of the following axillary lymph nodes are left behind without resection?

   A. Anterior
   B. Apical
   C. Lateral
   D. Posterior

5. You are attending an axillary lymph node dissection in a patient with a melanoma in the upper limb. The surgeon says, "We are going to sample the level II lymph nodes posterior to the pectoralis minor muscle." Having excelled in anatomy, you realize that she is referring to the anatomical nodes known as

   A. Apical axillary nodes
   B. Central axillary nodes
   C. Lateral axillary nodes
   D. Subscapular axillary nodes

6. In the axilla the pectoralis minor is a landmark, being closely related to all of the following structures except:

   A. Cords of the brachial plexus
   B. Cephalic vein
   C. Lateral thoracic artery
   D. Medial pectoral nerve

7. In a patient with Erb-Duchenne's palsy, a nerve arising from the upper trunk of the brachial plexus is lesioned. Due to this the patient is not able to initiate the abduction at his shoulder joint. The nerve involved is

   A. Dorsal scapular
   B. Long thoracic
   C. Suprascapular
   D. Lateral pectoral

8. Which of the following is not a direct branch of the axillary artery?

   A. Thoracodorsal
   B. Posterior circumflex humeral
   C. Thoracoacromial
   D. Subscapular

9. In a case of Erb's palsy where C5 and C6 roots of the brachial plexus are avulsed (torn out) ,which muscle is paralyzed?

   A. Latissimus dorsi

B. Pectoralis minor

C. Supraspinatus

D. Triceps brachii

10. A 38-year-old woman comes to the clinic complaining of pain radiating down the medial aspect of the left forearm and into the medial aspect of the left hand. She states that her left hand is weaker than her right hand. You note that her thenar and hypothenar eminences are smaller in the left hand compared with the right. Compression of what neural structure might account for the patient's symptoms?

A. Upper trunk of the brachial plexus

B. Median nerve

C. Ulnar nerve

D. Lower trunk of the brachial plexus

11. The middle trunk of the brachial plexus is lesioned. Axons in all of the following nerves will be affected *except* the

A. Median nerve

B. Axillary nerve

C. Musculocutaneous nerve

D. Radial nerve

12. The medial cord contains fibers derived from which of the following divisions of the brachial plexus?

A. Anterior divisions of middle and lower trunks

B. Anterior division of lower trunk only

C. Posterior division of lower trunk only

D. Anterior divisions of upper and middle trunks

13. A 28-year-old man fell from a tree while trimming limbs. As he fell, he grabbed a limb with his right hand, jerking his arm upward, but could not hold on. Which of the following conditions is most likely to be diagnosed in this patient?

A. Erb's palsy

B. Horner syndrome

C. Klumpke's paralysis

D. Wrist drop

14. A 21-year-old male is involved in street fight and sustains a knife wound to the neck. After the bleeding is controlled in the emergency department an ultrasound is obtained to rule out injury to the axillary artery. On neurologic examination, there is evidence of an injury to the posterior cord of the brachial plexus. Which of the following muscles would most likely be paralyzed?

A. Deltoid

B. Supraspinatus

C. Teres major

D. Subclavius

15. While riding his bicycle, a 16-year-old boy falls, striking the ground with his head and right shoulder. He is brought to the emergency department. On physical examination the physician notes that the boy holds his right upper limb at rest with the palm facing posteriorly. He is unable to abduct his arm at his shoulder and has diminished sensation over the lateral side of his arm. Which of the following neural structures was most likely injured?

A. Suprascapular nerve

B. Upper trunk of the brachial plexus

C. Musculocutaneous nerve

D. Axillary nerve

16. Following a difficult breech delivery in which the baby is delivered with an arm in the extended position, the neonate is noted to have unilateral loss of function of the intrinsic hand muscles. The baby is treated with physical therapy for this condition, the intrinsic muscle functions has not returned even after 3 years of age and examination now shows numbness along the inner aspect of the hand. Which of the following is the most likely diagnosis?

A. Radial nerve lesion

B. Erb's palsy

C. Median nerve lesion

D. Klumpke's paralysis

17. A 28-year-old man was admitted in the hospital with complaints of weakness in his left arm. On examination he has weak radial and ulnar pulses. The ultrasound reveals an aneurysm of the axillary artery in the axilla. This aneurysm is most likely to compress which of the following structures?

A. Suprascapular nerve

B. Long thoracic nerve

C. Lower trunk of the brachial plexus

D. Medial cord of the brachial plexus

Answers to MCQs

1. A		9. C	
2. D		10. D	
3. A		11. B	
4. B		12. B	
5. B		13. C	
6. B		14. A	
7. C		15. B	
8. A		16. D	
		17. D	

SECTION 3

Shoulder Region and Shoulder Joint

- Muscles of the upper back
- Muscles of the scapular region
- Maxillary nerve
- Shoulder joint
- Shoulder girdle
- MCQs

Objectives

- To explain the attachments, nerve supply, actions of muscles of the upper back and scapular region.
- To list the boundaries and structures passing through quadrangular and triangular spaces.
- To explain the anastomosis around the scapula and its functional significance.
- To explain the origin, course and distribution of axillary nerve and its clinical relevance.
- To explain the bones articulating, ligaments stabilizing, relations, movements occurring and muscles producing them in the shoulder joint.

MUSCLES OF THE UPPER BACK

The muscles on the back of the thorax are connected to upper limb. They are arranged in superficial and deep layers. The superficial layer includes trapezius and latissimus dorsi and the deep layer includes levator scapulae, rhomboideus major and minor muscles. The attachments, nerve supply and actions of these muscles are summarized in Table 6.1.

Axillary arch: Sometimes a muscular slip known as axillary arch extends from the lower border of the latissimus dorsi and crosses in front of the axillary vessels to join with the pectoralis major or sometimes with coracobrachialis.

After reflecting the skin and fascia of the upper back two triangular intervals are observed. They are

1. Triangle of auscultation

It has following boundaries
Inferiorly-upper horizontal border of latissimus dorsi

Medially-lateral border of the trapezius
Laterally-medial border of the scapula

Floor: 6th and 7th ribs with the intercostal space between them (sixth intercostal space). Sounds of the swallowed liquid in the lower end oesophagus is heard with the help of a stethoscope placed in this space.

2. Lumbar triangle (Petit's triangle)

It has following boundaries.
Base-iliac crest
Anteriorly-posterior border of the external oblique muscle
Posteriorly-lateral margin of the latissimus dorsi
Floor-internal oblique muscle

It is a weak area and a potential site for lumbar hernia ,that may occur through this interval.

> Testing the latissimus dorsi muscle function: The muscle can be felt in the posterior axillary fold when the patient adducts the abducted arm against resistance.

Table 6.1 Muscles of the back

Name of the muscle and its origin	Insertion	Nerve supply	Actions
1. Trapezius (Fig. 6.1) • Medial part of the superior nuchal line of the occipital bone • Ligamentum nuchae (fibrous structure connecting cervical spines) • Spinous processes and supraspinous ligaments of all 12 thoracic vertebrae	• Upper fibres inserted to posterior border of the lateral one third of the clavicle • Middle fibres to medial border of the acromion and upper lip of the crest of the spine of scapula • Lower fibres to the triangular area at the medial end of the spine of the scapula	Spinal part of the accessory nerve and ventral rami of C3 and C4 nerves are proprioceptive	• Upper fibres elevate the scapula • Middle fibres retract the scapula • Upper and lower fibres acting together with serratus anterior rotates the scapula for overhead abduction at shoulder joint.
2. Latissimus dorsi (Fig. 6.1) • Lower 6 thoracic spines and their supraspinous ligaments • Spines of all the lumbar and sacral vertebrae through the posterior layer of thoracolumbar fascia • Outer lip of the iliac crest • Lower 4 ribs • Inferior angle of the scapula	The muscle forms a tendon and is inserted to the floor of the bicipital groove.	Nerve to latissimus dorsi from posterior cord of the brachial plexus	Extension Medial rotation Adduction Helps in climbing (lifting the trunk) } At shoulder joint
3. Rhomboideus minor • Lower part of the ligamentum nuchae • Spinous processes of C7 and T1 vertebrae	Medial border of the scapula on the dorsal aspect	Nerve to rhomboideus (C5)	Retract the scapula
4. Rhomboideus major Spinous process of T2 to T5 vertebrae and their supraspinous ligaments	Medial border of the scapula on the dorsal aspect (from spine to inferior angle)	Nerve to rhomboideus (C5)	Retract the scapula

Dorsal scapular nerve (Nerve to Rhomboideus)

It is a nerve arising from ventral ramus of C5 in the posterior triangle of the neck. It appears in this triangle by piercing the Scalenus anterior muscle. It descends in front of the levator scapulae muscle along with the deep branch of the transverse cervical artery or dorsal scapular artery. It leaves the neck in relation to the anterior surface of the levator scapulae. In the back, the nerve and the artery descends deep to the levator scapulae (anterior surface of the muscle) and then deep to the rhomboideus muscles. It supplies rhomboideus major and minor and also levator scapulae.

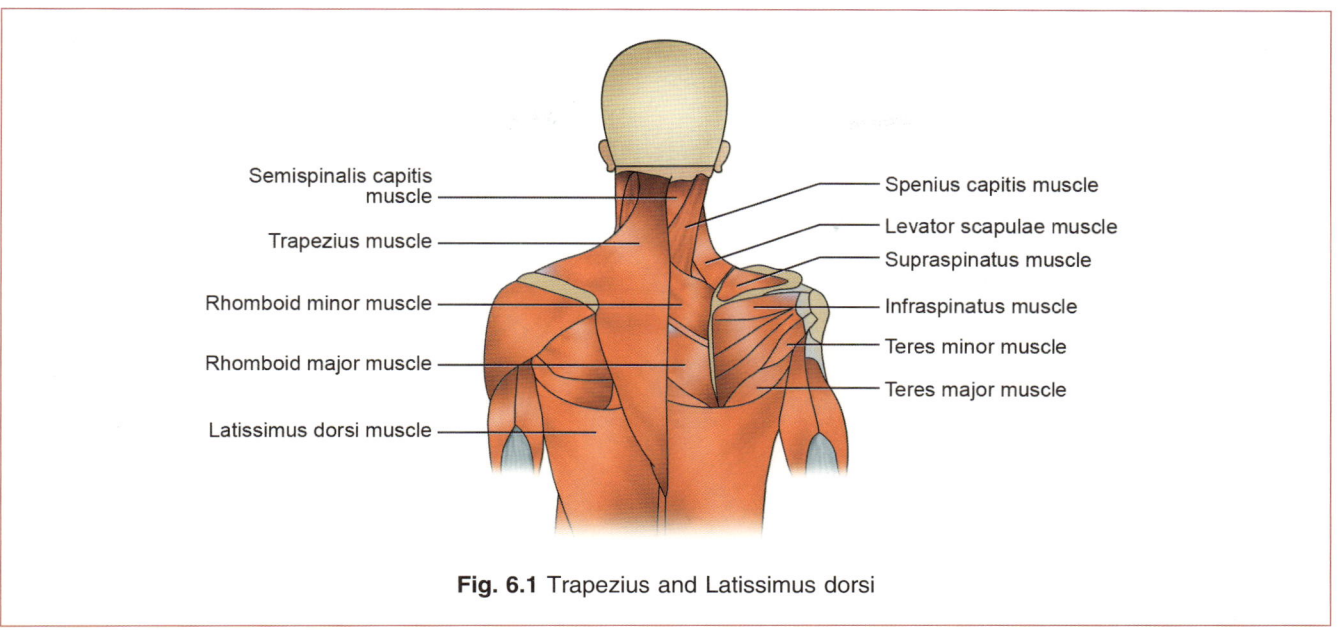

Fig. 6.1 Trapezius and Latissimus dorsi

Spinal part of the accessory nerve:

Though this nerve is identified in this region supplying trapezius muscle, it is discussed in detail in Chapter 70.

MUSCLES OF THE SCAPULAR REGION

These muscles act on shoulder joint. Their name, attachments, nerve supply and actions are listed in Table 6.2. The deltoid muscle is explained in next page.

Table 6.2 Muscles of the scapular region

Name of the muscle and its origin (Fig. 6.2)	Insertion	Nerve supply	Actions
1. **Supraspinatus** Medial 2/3rd of supraspinous fossa of scapula	Tendon passes beneath the coraco acromial arch and inserted into upper impression of greater tubercle of humerus	Suprascapular nerve (C 5, 6)	Initiates the abduction at shoulder joint (first 15°)
2. **Infraspinatus** Medial 2/3rd of the infraspinous fossa of scapula	Middle impression of the greater tubercle of the humerus	Suprascapular nerve (C5, 6)	Lateral rotation at shoulder joint
3. **Teres minor** Upper 2/3rd of the lateral border of the scapula	Lowest impression of the greater tubercle of humerus	Axillary nerve (C5, 6)	Lateral rotation at the shoulder joint
4. **Teres major** Lower 1/3rd of the lateral border of the scapula	Medial lip of the bicipital groove of humerus	Lower subscapular nerve (C5, 6)	Medial rotation and adduction at shoulder joint
5. **Subscapularis** Medial 2/3rd of the subscapular fossa of the scapula	Lesser tubercle of the humerus	Upper and lower subscapular nerves (C5, 6)	Medial rotation and adduction at shoulder joint

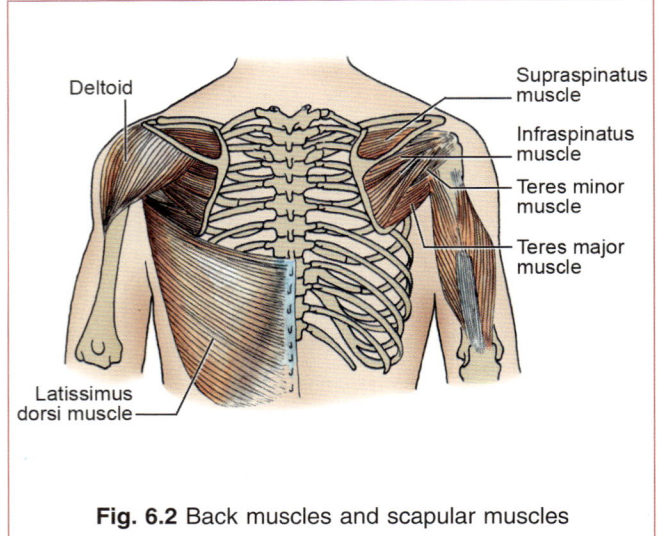

Fig. 6.2 Back muscles and scapular muscles

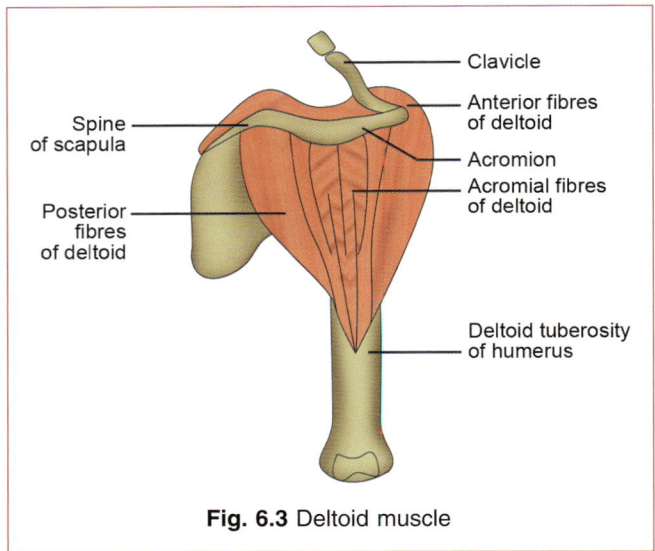

Fig. 6.3 Deltoid muscle

Deltoid

Deltoid is a powerful muscle that surrounds the shoulder region. It is one of the sites for giving intramuscular injections (Fig. 6.3).

Origin

The anterior fibres arise from anterior border of the lateral 1/3rd of the clavicle.

The middle fibres are multipennate and arise from lateral margin of the acromion process.

The posterior fibres arise from lower lip of the crest of the spine of the scapula.

Insertion: A 'V' shaped deltoid tuberosity of the humerus.

Nerve supply: Axillary nerve (C5, 6)

Actions

1. Anterior fibres cause flexion and medial rotation at shoulder joint.
2. Posterior fibres cause extension and lateral rotation of the shoulder joint.
3. Middle fibres abduct the arm at shoulder joint from 15° to 90°.

A multipennate arrangement allows the muscle to accommodate lot of fibres in a smaller volume and the force of contraction of the muscle is directly proportional to the number of muscle fibres. Functionally the middle fibres are important as abduction is against the gravity. The lateral border of the acromion process sends four fibrous septa downwards. From the deltoid tuberosity three fibrous septa ascend upwards between the four septa arising from the acromion process. The muscle fibres traverses between the septa.

Testing the deltoid muscle function: The person is asked hold the arm in abducted position against the resistance.

Structures under cover of Deltoid

Bones: Coracoid process, Greater and lesser tubercle of the humerus with inter tubercular sulcus, surgical neck of the humerus.

Muscles: Muscles attached to the coracoid process (pectoralis minor, coracobrachialis, short head of the biceps), muscles attached to the greater and lesser tubercles (supraspinatus, infraspinatus, teres minor and subscapularis).

Nerves and vessels: Anterior and posterior circumflex humeral vessels and axillary nerve.

Bursa: Subacromial bursa.

> **Intramuscular injections:** Deltoid muscle is often a site for intramuscular injection. The needle is inserted at 90° angle on the lateral multipennate portion of the deltoid, below the acromion process.

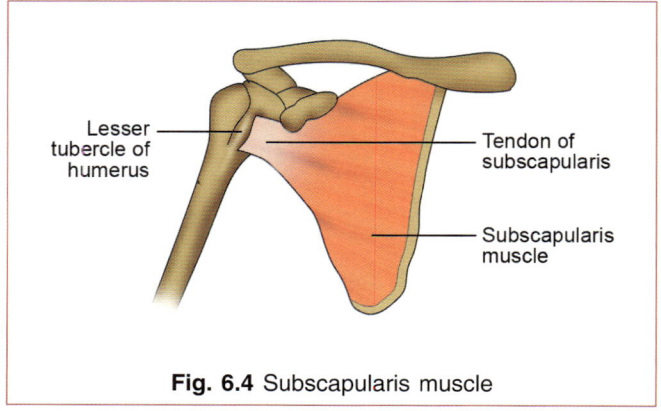

Fig. 6.4 Subscapularis muscle

Intermuscular spaces: The arrangement of the scapular muscles leaves three intermuscular spaces for the passage of the neurovascular structures. These spaces can be better defined or seen from behind (Fig. 6.4).

Quadrangular space (Fig. 6.5)

It has following boundaries

Above (from before backwards): Subscapularis, capsule of the shoulder joint and teres minor

Below: Teres major

Medially: Long head of the triceps

Laterally: Surgical neck of the humerus

Structures passing through it:

1. Axillary nerve
2. Posterior circumflex humeral vessels

Upper triangular space

It has following boundaries

Above: Teres minor

Below: Teres major

Laterally: Long head of the triceps

Structure passing through it: Circumflex scapular artery winds around the lateral margin of the scapula and passes through this space. It may pass through the substance of the teres minor muscle also.

Lower triangular space (Fig. 6.5)

It has following boundaries

Above: Teres major

Medially: Long head of the triceps

Laterally: Shaft of the humerus

Structure passing through it:

1. Radial nerve
2. Profunda brachii vessels.

Axillary nerve (Circumflex nerve- C5, 6)

- It arises from the posterior cord of the brachial plexus.
- First it present posterior to the third part of the axillary artery along with the radial nerve, resting on subscapularis muscle
- It passes through the quadrangular space below the shoulder joint along with the posterior circumflex humeral artery.
- The main trunk gives branches to the shoulder joint and then divides into anterior and posterior divisions.

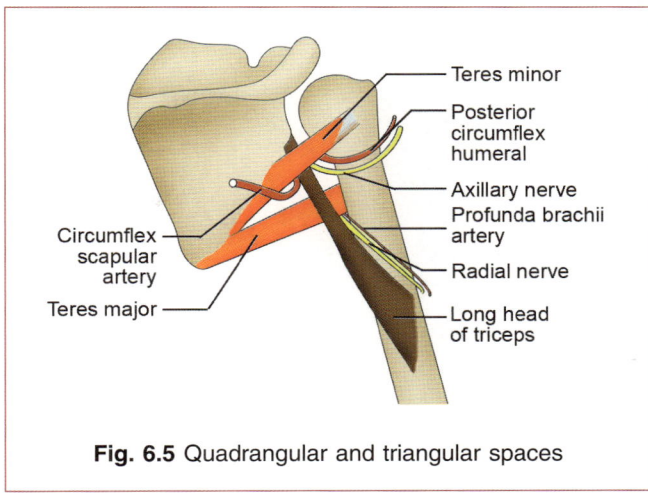

Fig. 6.5 Quadrangular and triangular spaces

- The anterior division along with the posterior circumflex humeral artery **winds around the surgical neck of the humerus.** The anterior division supplies deltoid and couple of branches supplies skin over the deltoid.
- The posterior division supplies teres minor muscle and posterior part of the deltoid. The branch to teres minor presents a pseudoganglion (connective tissue thickening around the nerve). After supplying these muscles the posterior division continues as upper lateral cutaneous nerve of the arm.

Fracture of the surgical neck of the humerus can cause injury to the axillary nerve, which results in loss of power of abduction at shoulder joint. There is also a sensory loss on the skin over the deltoid muscle.

In case of fracture of surgical neck or downward dislocation of the shoulder the axillary nerve function is tested by gently pricking on the skin over the deltoid.

Anastomosis around the scapula

This arterial anastomosis connects the first part of the subclavian artery with the third part of the axillary artery. The arteries taking part are (Fig. 6.6)

1. **Suprascapular artery:** It is a branch from the thyrocervical trunk of the first part of the subclavian artery. It enters the back of the scapula above the transverse scapular ligament to the supraspinous fossa. It enters the infraspinous fossa through spinoglenoid notch. Branches arising from it anastomose with branches of circumflex scapular and deep branch of the transverse cervical artery.

2. **Circumflex scapular artery:** It is a branch from the subscapular artery, passes through the upper triangular space to wind around the lateral border of the scapula.

133

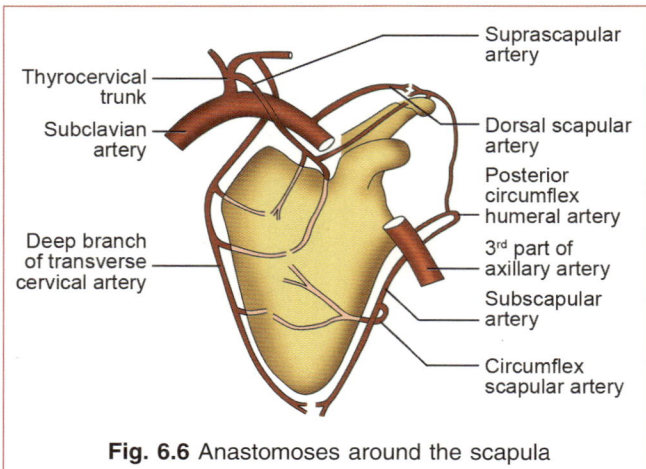

Fig. 6.6 Anastomoses around the scapula

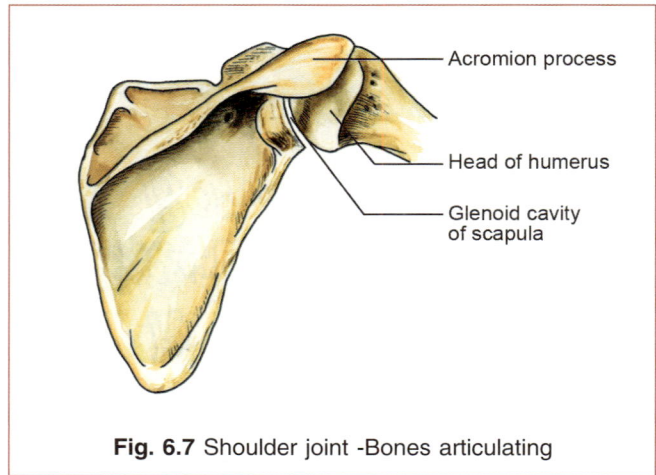

Fig. 6.7 Shoulder joint -Bones articulating

Its branches anastomose with branches of suprascapular and deep branch of the transverse cervical artery.

3. **Deep branch of the transverse cervical artery:** It arises as a branch from the thyrocervical trunk of the first part of the subclavian artery. It divides into superficial and deep branches. The deep branch accompanies the dorsal scapular nerve passes deep to the levator scapulae and rhomboideus muscles. Sometimes this artery is replaced by a dorsal scapular artery having similar course, but arises from third part of the subclavian artery.

Significance: These anastomoses connect the first part of the subclavian artery with the third part of the axillary artery. In case of obstruction in distal part of the subclavian artery or proximal part of the axillary artery these anastomotic vessels enlarge considerable to provide collateral circulation. This may give rise to a clinical sign called 'pulsating scapula'.

SHOULDER JOINT

Type: It is a ball and socket variety of synovial joint.

Bones articulating: The head of the humerus covered by articular hyaline cartilage with glenoid cavity of the scapula, which is also covered by hyaline cartilage (Fig. 6.7).

Structures stabilizing

1. **Capsular ligament (fibrous capsule):** It is made up of collagen and elastic fibres. Medially, it is attached to the peripheral margin of the glenoid cavity outside the glenoidal labrum. The attachment encloses the origin of long head of biceps brachii. Laterally, it is attached to the anatomical neck of the humerus but extending a

little below on the inferomedial aspect up to the surgical neck (Fig. 6.8).

Synovial membrane lines the inner aspect of capsule and also invests the tendon of the long head of biceps brachii muscle.

1. **Glenohumeral ligaments:** These are thickened part of the anterior aspect of the fibrous capsule and better defined from the inner aspect

a. *Superior glenohumeral ligament:* It extends from the base of the coracoid process to the upper part of the anatomical neck at the level of the upper edge of the lesser tubercle.

b. *Middle glenohumeral ligament:* It extends from the anterior margin of the glenoid cavity to the level of lower part of the lesser tubercle of the humerus. The subscapular bursa communicates with the joint cavity between the superior and middle bands.

c. *Inferior glenohumeral ligament:* It extends from the lower part of the anterior and posterior margin of the glenoid cavity to the lower part of the anatomical neck.

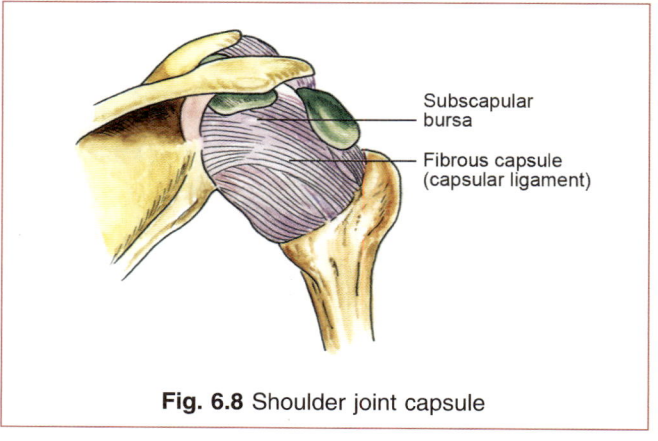

Fig. 6.8 Shoulder joint capsule

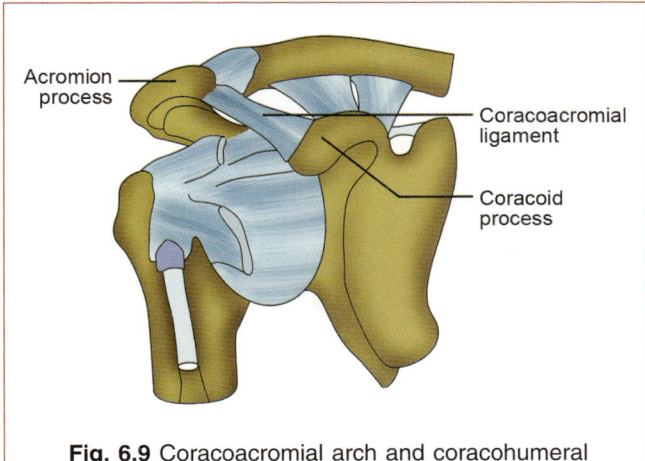

Fig. 6.9 Coracoacromial arch and coracohumeral ligament

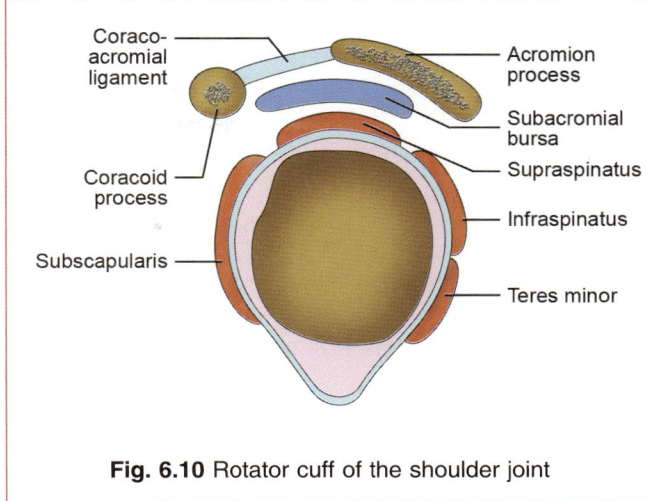

Fig. 6.10 Rotator cuff of the shoulder joint

In traumatic anterior dislocation, the inferior glenohumeral ligament is stretched or it's attachment to glenoid labrum is torn. This is known as Bankart lesion, which predisposes recurrent dislocation of the joint

3. **Glenoidal labrum:** It is a fibro-cartilaginous rim attached to the periphery of the glenoid cavity. It deepens the glenoidal cavity. On cross section it is triangular in shape with its base attached to the peripheral margin of the glenoid cavity.

4. **Coracohumeral ligament:** It extends from the root and lateral border of the coracoid process of scapula to anatomical neck of the humerus. Morphologically it is considered as divorced part of the insertion of the pectoralis minor muscle. The ligament resists the lateral rotation and adduction (Fig. 6.9).

5. **Musculo-tendinous rotator cuff:** The tendons of the muscles around the shoulder joint on their way to insertion blend with the fibrous capsule. It keeps the head of humerus in contact with glenoidal cavity. The tendons are:

    Subscapularis – in front

    Supraspinatus – above

    Infraspinatus – behind

    Teres minor   – behind

The lower part of the capsule however is least supported and is separated from the long head of the triceps by axillary nerve. Lower part of the capsule is stretched in abduction and is more prone for dislocation of the humeral head.

Rotator cuff disorders

The 2 main disorders of the rotator cuff are impingement and tendinopathy.

• The muscle most commonly involved is supra-spinatus

• Swelling of supraspinatus muscle, excessive fluid in subacromial bursa or subacromial bony spurs may produce significant impingement when arm is abducted

• The blood supply to supraspinatus tendon is poor, repeated trauma leads to degenerative changes with calcification of tendon, producing extreme pain (painful arc syndrome).

• Frozen shoulder: Tendinitis of the entire rotator cuff (Fig. 6.10).

6. **Coracoacromial arch:** It is formed by three structures-coracoid process, acromion process and coraco-acromial ligament. It acts as a secondary synovial socket for the head of the humerus. It prevents the upward displacement of the head of the humerus. Between the supra-spinatus tendon and coraco-acromial arch is the **subacromial bursa.** This accommodates the greater tubercle of the humerus during overhead abduction (Fig. 6.9).

Inflammation of subacromial bursa causes pain when pressure is applied just below the acromion. However, the pain at the same point is not felt after abduction of arm. This is known as Dawbarn's sign.

7. **Transverse humeral ligament:** It connects the medial and lateral lips of the upper part of the intertubercular sulcus. Its function is to keep the tendon of long head of the biceps in position.

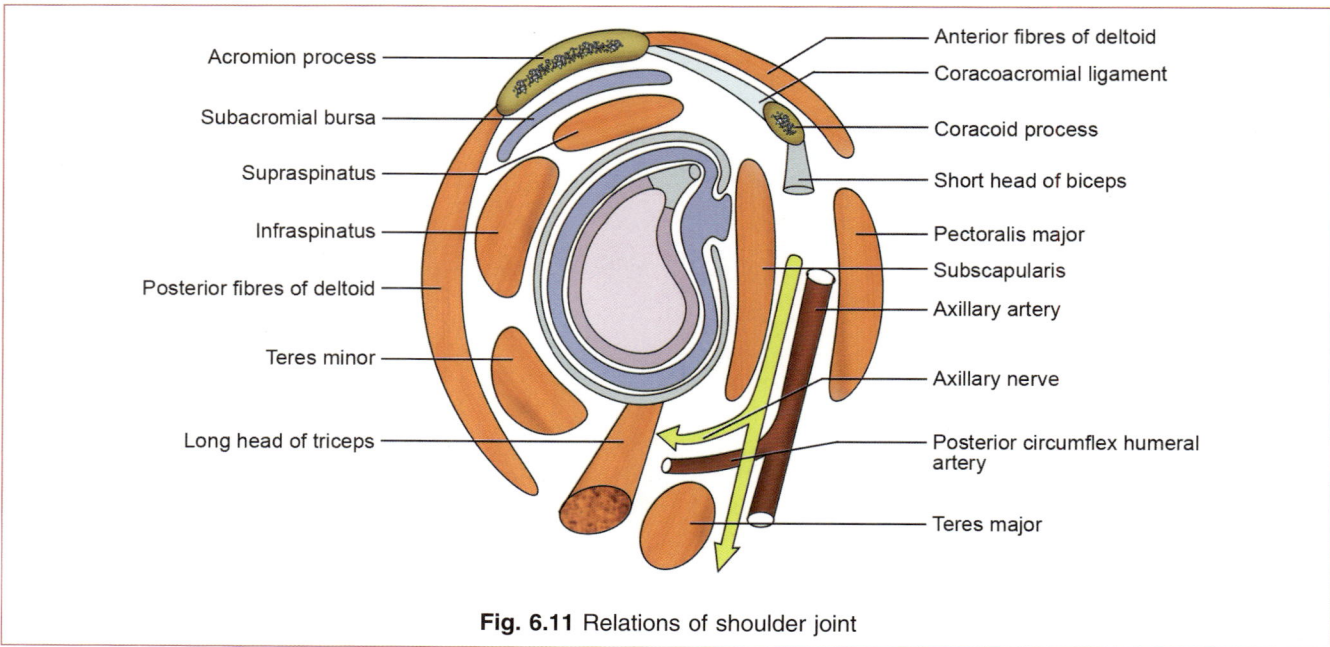

Fig. 6.11 Relations of shoulder joint

Arterial supply

Shoulder joint is supplied by anterior and posterior circumflex humeral arteries.

Nerve supply

Shoulder joint is supplied by axillary nerve, suprascapular nerve and lateral pectoral nerve.

Relations of the shoulder joint

Above: Tendon of supraspinatus, subacromial bursa, coracoacromial arch and deltoid muscle one above the other (Figs 6.11 and 6.13).

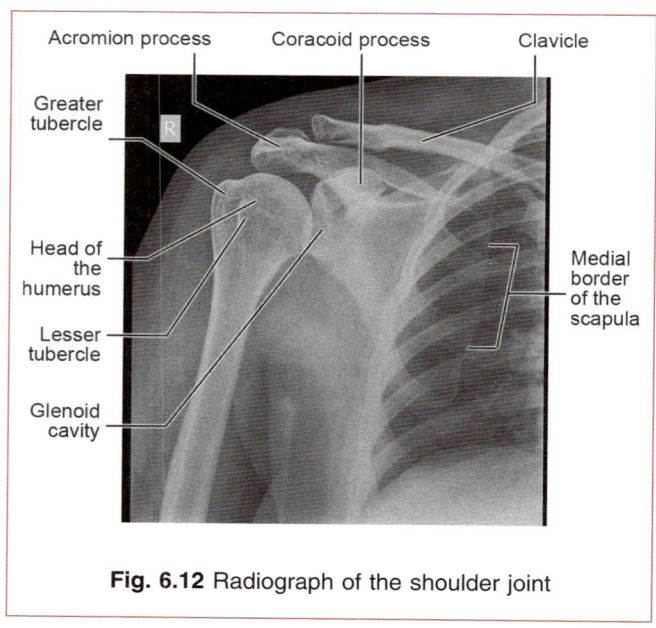

Fig. 6.12 Radiograph of the shoulder joint

Below: Long head of the triceps separated by quadrangular space with axillary nerve and posterior circumflex humeral artery.

Anteriorly: Insertion of subscapularis, coracoid process with muscles attached to it.

Posteriorly: Insertion of infraspinatus, teres minor and deltoid muscle.

Movements and muscles producing them

Shoulder joint is a multiaxial ball and socket variety of synovial joint. The humeral movements are analysed with reference to the direction of the glenoid cavity of the scapula (Fig. 6.12).

- Flexion and extension takes place at an angle which passes perpendicular to the centre of the glenoid cavity.

- Adduction and abduction movements take place at an angle which passes parallel to the direction of the glenoid cavity. Therefore abduction carries the arm lateral and forwards, while adduction medial and backwards.

- Circumduction is a succession of above mentioned four movements in an order.

The movements and the muscles producing them are listed in the table (next page).

Overhead abduction at the shoulder joint

1. Initiation of the abduction (may be up to 15°) is by the action of supraspinatus muscle.

2. Abduction between 15 to 90–120° is by the middle (acromial) fibres of the deltoid muscle. During this

S E C T I O N   3

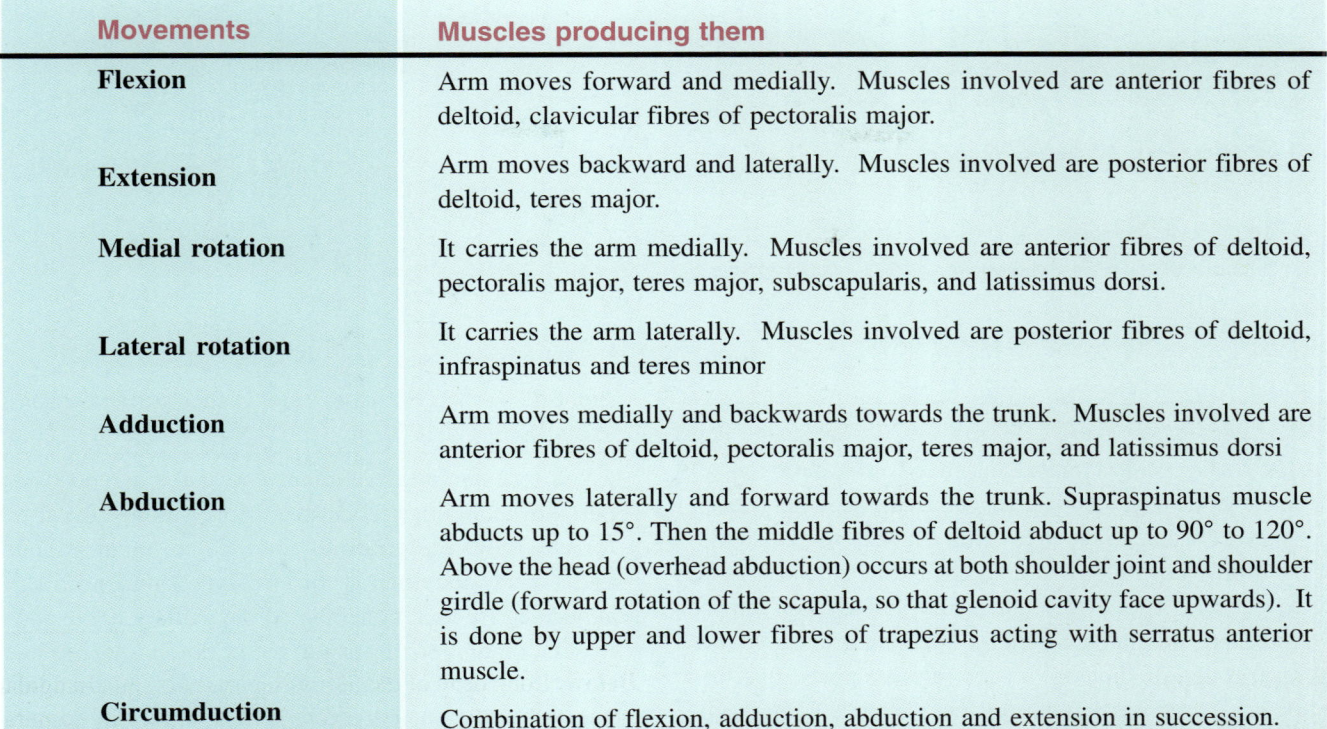

Movements	Muscles producing them
Flexion	Arm moves forward and medially. Muscles involved are anterior fibres of deltoid, clavicular fibres of pectoralis major.
Extension	Arm moves backward and laterally. Muscles involved are posterior fibres of deltoid, teres major.
Medial rotation	It carries the arm medially. Muscles involved are anterior fibres of deltoid, pectoralis major, teres major, subscapularis, and latissimus dorsi.
Lateral rotation	It carries the arm laterally. Muscles involved are posterior fibres of deltoid, infraspinatus and teres minor
Adduction	Arm moves medially and backwards towards the trunk. Muscles involved are anterior fibres of deltoid, pectoralis major, teres major, and latissimus dorsi
Abduction	Arm moves laterally and forward towards the trunk. Supraspinatus muscle abducts up to 15°. Then the middle fibres of deltoid abduct up to 90° to 120°. Above the head (overhead abduction) occurs at both shoulder joint and shoulder girdle (forward rotation of the scapula, so that glenoid cavity face upwards). It is done by upper and lower fibres of trapezius acting with serratus anterior muscle.
Circumduction	Combination of flexion, adduction, abduction and extension in succession.

movement, subscapularis, infraspinatus and teres minor acts as 'synergists', which pushes the humeral head downwards and medially to keep it in the socket.

3. Overhead abduction up to 180° occurs by humeral head movement at shoulder joint (120°) and also scapular forward rotation at the shoulder girdle (60°).

4. In every 15° elevation, shoulder joint contributes 10° and shoulder girdle 5° (2:1 ratio).

5. Humerus movement at the shoulder joint involves lateral rotation of the humerus by infraspinatus and teres minor.

6. The scapular forward rotation involves both acromioclavicular joint (20°) and sternoclavicular joint (40°).

7. Initial elevation of the acromial end of the clavicle (upper fibres of trapezius and levator scapulae) is followed by downward swing of the sternal end of the clavicle (upper and lower fibres of the trapezius with serratus anterior)

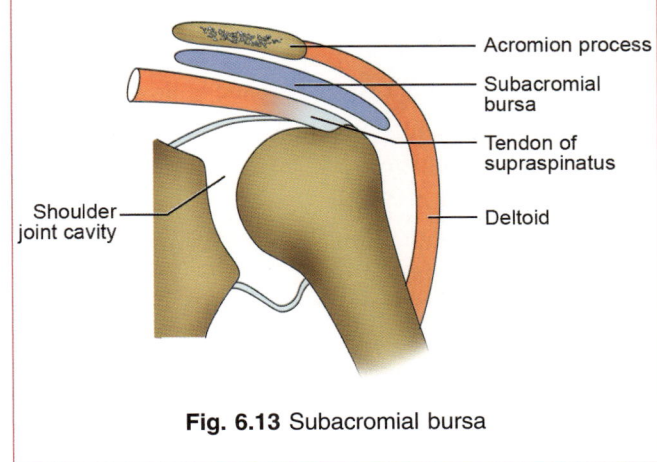

Fig. 6.13 Subacromial bursa

Dislocation of the shoulder (Fig. 6.14): The anterior dislocation can be sub-coracoid, sub-glenoid or sub-clavicular. The downward dislocation is more common in abducted position of arm. It can injure the axillary nerve, which is closely related to the lower part of the joint capsule.

To reduce the dislocation, the elbow must be flexed under traction, humerus laterally rotated first, adducted and then rotated medially. An X-ray is taken to ensure proper reduction, and axillary nerve function is assessed by asking the patient to abduct the shoulder while supporting the arm.

Frozen shoulder: In this condition, shoulder movements are restricted due to tendinitis of the rotator cuff.

Aspiration of the fluid from the joint cavity is done by introducing the needle through the deltopectoral groove.

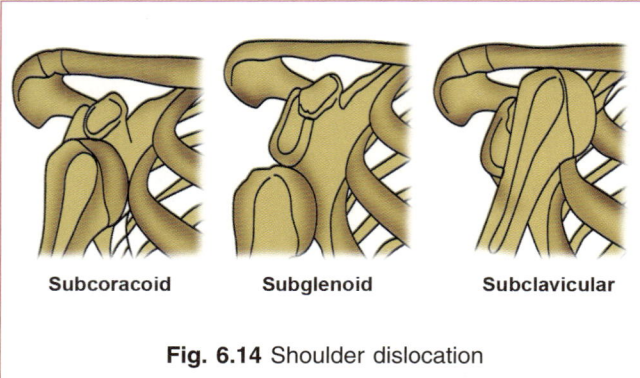

Subcoracoid   Subglenoid   Subclavicular

Fig. 6.14 Shoulder dislocation

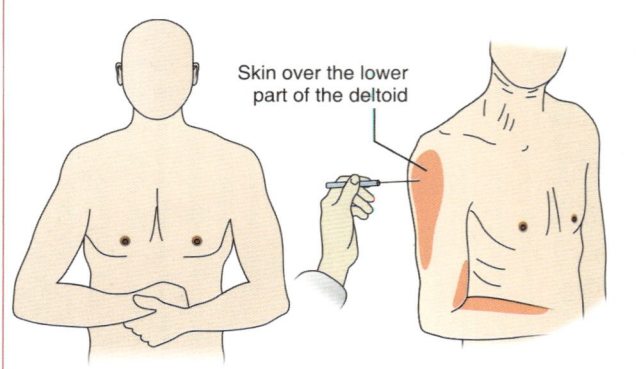

Skin over the lower
part of the deltoid

Fig. 6.16 Testing the nerve injury in shoulder dislocation

CASE -1

The goalkeeper in a football match fell on his outstretched left arm. He felt an immediate pain in the shoulder region and was unable to move his arm. On examination in the hospital his arm appeared abducted and the deltoid muscle looked flat. The injured upper limb looked "too long", and there was intense pain on attempting to move the arm. A plain radiograph of the region showed that the humeral head was lying below the glenoidal labrum and that there was no fracture of the humerus. The diagnosis was an anterior dislocation of the shoulder, and the orthopedic surgeon recom-mended Kocher's maneuver for management (Fig. 6.16).

1. Why did the deltoid appear flat and hollow?

2. What neurovascular structures are liable for injury in such a condition. How do you rule out the involvement of nerve?

3. What is the anatomical principle in reducing a dislocated shoulder?

CASE-2

A 47-year-old woman was brought to the hospital after her right shoulder dislocation. A resident student was

asked to examine the patient and make a report on possible nerve injuries. He carefully examined the arm for neurological defects of the median, ulnar, radial and musculocutaneous nerves, but found nothing abnormal. He then remembered the axillary nerve and its relation to the inferior surface of the shoulder joint. He also remembered that this nerve supplies deltoid muscle, which abducts the shoulder joint. He asked the patient to abduct the dislocated shoulder; she could not, of course because of the severe pain. The resident student reported to the physician that he was unable to test the axillary nerve for a neurological deficit. What test will you carry out, using your knowledge of anatomy?

CASE-3

A 45-year-old man fell off from a truck when he was unloading and struck the ground on his left arm and side. On getting up, he experienced severe pain and limitation of movement of his left shoulder. On examination, the normal rounded contour of the left shoulder was seen to be lost, the long axis of the left arm passed upward and medially, and some kind of fullness was noted below the lateral part of the clavicle. Very little passive movement of the left shoulder was permitted by the patient. The skin sensation was normal over the lower part of the left deltoid muscle. Using your knowledge of anatomy, explain what was wrong with the patient. Why had the shoulder lost its normal contour? Why was the region below the lateral end of the clavicle appeared full?

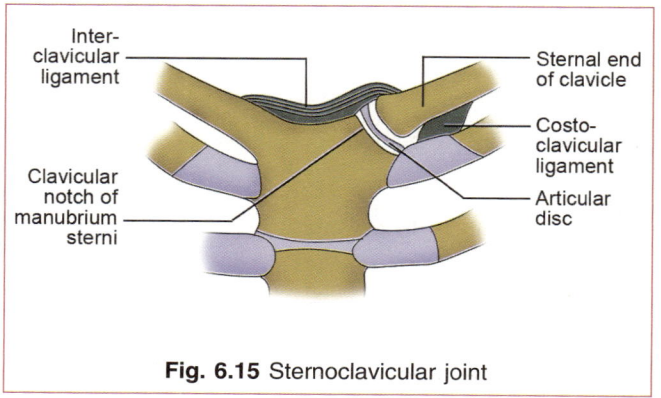

Inter-
clavicular
ligament

Sternal end
of clavicle

Costo-
clavicular
ligament

Clavicular
notch of
manubrium
sterni

Articular
disc

Fig. 6.15 Sternoclavicular joint

SHOULDER GIRDLE

Shoulder or pectoral girdle connects the bones of the upper limb with the axial skeleton. It consists of two joints:

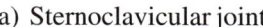

a) Sternoclavicular joint

b) Acromioclavicular joint

Sternoclavicular joint

Type: It is a saddle variety of synovial joint.

Bones articulating: Sternal end of the clavicle articulates with clavicular notch of sternum and also first costal cartilage (Fig. 6.15).

An articular disc made up of fibrocartilage intervenes between the articulating surfaces of the bones in the joint

The joint is stabilized by capsular ligament, interclavicular ligament and costoclavicular ligament.

Costoclavicular ligament: It extends from the inferior surface of the medial (sternal) end of the clavicle to the junction of 1st rib and its costal cartilage.

Interclavicular ligament: It stretches between the non-articular part of the right and left clavicle at their medial end, occupying the suprasternal notch.

Acromioclavicular joint

Type: It is a plane synovial joint.

Bones articulating: Lateral end of the clavicle with medial margin of acromion process of scapula.

The joint is stabilized by fibrous capsular ligament and coracoclavicular ligament.

Coracoclavicular ligament: It forms the strong bond of union between the scapula and the clavicle. It consists of conoid and trapezoid parts. The conoid part stretches between conoid tubercle on the undersurface of the clavicle to the root of the coracoid process.

The trapezoid part stretches between trapezoid ridge on the under surface of the clavicle to the upper surface of the coracoid process.

The weight of the upper limb is transmitted through costoclavicular ligament.

The acromioclavicular joint is prone for dislocation or shoulder separation, in which the coracoclavicular ligament is likely to be torn.

Movements of the shoulder girdle

Elevation of scapula: The lateral end of the clavicle is elevated while the medial end moves downward.

Muscles involved – Upper fibres of trapezius and levator scapulae.

Depression of scapula: The medial end of the clavicle is rotated upward by the weight of the upper limb and also by lower fibres of serratus anterior muscle.

Forward movement of the scapula (pushing and punching movements): The lateral end of the clavicle advances forward and medial end swings backward. This action is brought by serratus anterior and pectoralis minor muscle.

Retraction of the scapula: The medial end of the clavicle swings forward and the lateral end swings backwards. This action is brought by middle fibres of trapezius and rhomboideus muscles.

Forward rotation of the scapula: This movement occurs during abduction of the arm above the level of shoulder. The glenoid cavity is directed almost vertically upward and greater tuberosity of the humerus is accommodated in subacromial bursa. This action is produced by upper and lower fibres of trapezius with serratus anterior.

CASE-4

A 14-year-old boy fell on his left shoulder while bicycling down a steep incline. He immediately complained of severe pain in the area of his collar bone. All movements of his left arm were painful. He tried to avoid painful motion by holding his left arm close to his body and by supporting the left elbow with his right hand. The boy was brought to the hospital and the X-ray confirmed the diagnosis of fractured clavicle. The fracture was present at the junction of the medial $2/3^{rd}$ and lateral $1/3^{rd}$. Upon passing the fingers along the borders of the clavicle the examiner could make out the projecting ends of the fragments. These are felt as overriding, with the sternal fragment being angulated upward and the medial end of the lateral fragment pointing backward and medially. Passive movement of the left shoulder was quite painful.

1. How is the clavicle fracture reduced?

2. Clavicle fracture is one of the most common fractures in the body. How do explain this?

3. How do you explain the direction of displacement of fractured segments anatomically?

4. Which large muscle connecting the thorax with the arm would adduct(pull the arm towards the thorax), and causing a decrease in the distance between acromion and midline and therefore leading to overriding of the fragments?

5. Since medial rotators of the arm are stronger than the lateral, and the bracing action of the clavicle is

nullified by the fracture and thus the arm is also medially rotated. What are the muscles responsible for this action?

6. Which part of the brachial plexus may be involved in fractures of the clavicle?

CASE-5

A 44-year-old man visited his physician complaining of pain since three week in his right shoulder. On examination, the patient could actively abduct his right shoulder for about 40 degrees after which he experienced severe pain that prevented further movement. If the arm was then raised passively above 90 degrees, then he could hold it actively in that position without pain. If the patient attempted to lower the arm, he again experienced severe pain in the mid range of abduction. Using your knowledge explain the condition in anatomical terms.

Solution to the case study

Case-1

1. Because of the downward dislocation of the humeral head.

2. Axillary nerve and posterior circumflex humeral artery. Axillary nerve function is assessed by looking for intact cutaneous sensation over the deltoid muscle.

3. The elbow is flexed under traction, humerus laterally rotated first, adducted and then rotated medially. An X-ray (check X-ray) is taken to ensure proper reduction.

Case-2

The axillary nerve gives motor fibres to the deltoid and teres minor muscles. If the shoulder joint is dislocated, it is impossible to test for activity of these muscles. The axillary nerve, however, also supplies the skin covering the lower half of the deltoid muscle, and it is a simple task to ask the patient if she can feel a pinprick or light touch with a piece of cotton over this area. Damage to the axillary nerve produces paresthesia or anesthesia of the skin overlying the lower half of the deltoid muscle.

Case-3

The patient had a subcoracoid dislocation of the left shoulder joint. The head of the humerus was dislocated downwards through the weakest part of the capsule of the joint. It was then displaced medially in front of the scapula and behind the subscapularis muscle. The greater tubercle of the humerus no longer held the deltoid muscle laterally, thus the normal contour of the shoulder was therefore lost.

The head of the humerus that had come below the coracoid process of the scapula was responsible for the fullness below the lateral end of the clavicle.

Case-4

1. The fracture is reduced by pulling the shoulder upwards and backwards for proper alignment of the fragments and is retained by application of Figure '8' bandage.

2. Clavicle is the only bone connecting the shoulder girdle to the trunk. It maintains the shoulder and arm at the proper distance from the chest. If unbroken, the clavicle maintains a constant distance between the acromion and the middle of the body so that a decrease in this distance, as compared with the normal side, is a rough indication of the amount of overriding of the fragments.

3. The clavicular head of the sternocleidomastoid muscle is responsible for the upward tilt of the medial fragment. On the other hand, the deltoid arises from lateral third of the clavicle and combined with the weight of the arm is responsible for this downward displacement. These factors cause the left arm to hang lower than right.

4. The pectoralis major, supported by the latissimus dorsi and smaller muscles is responsible for this displacement.

5. The pectoralis major, the subscapularis, the teres major and the latissimus dorsi are the medial rotators of the arm that explains why the medial end of the lateral fragment points posteriorly.

6. The lower trunk of the brachial plexus (C8, T1) may be injured in clavicle fractures.

Case-5

This patient had supraspinatus tendinitis. During the mid range of abduction, the tendon of the supraspinatus impinges against the outer border of the acromion. Normally, the large subacromial bursa intervenes and ensures that the movement is relatively free of friction and is painless. In this condition, the bursa has degenerated and the supraspinatus tendon exhibits a localized area of collagen degeneration.

MCQs

1. An elderly patient complains of shoulder pain and has difficulty in abducting his arm. Arthroscopy is done in which a dye is injected into the shoulder joint and an X-ray is taken. The radiologist notes that the dye has leaked from the shoulder joint into the subacromial bursa. Which tendon might have ruptured for this to occur?

A. Deltoid

B. Infraspinatus

C. Teres minor

D. Supraspinatus

2. The rotator cuff is composed of all of the following muscles except:

A. Infraspinatus

B. Subscapularis

C. Supraspinatus

D. Teres major

3. During a strenuous game of tennis ,a 50 year old woman complained of severe shoulder pain that forced her to quit the game. During physical examination it was found that she could not initiate abduction of her arm, but if her arm was elevated to 45 degrees from the vertical (at her side) position, she had no trouble fully abducting it. Which muscle is paralysed for this condition to occur?

A. Deltoid

B. Infraspinatus

C. Supraspinatus

D. Teres major

4. Which of the following dislocations is seen commonly in the shoulder joint ?

A. Anterior

B. Inferior

C. Posterior

D. Superolateral

5. In a fracture of the surgical neck of the humerus, which artery may be injured?

A. Subscapular artery

B. Posterior circumflex humeral artery

C. Profunda brachii artery

D. Circumflex scapular artery

6. It was determined that a football player tore his coracoclavicular ligament. This is an example of a:

A. Pulled elbow

B. Rotator cuff tear

C. Separated shoulder

D. Dislocated shoulder

7. A football player suffered a severe shoulder separation. Although this is a dislocation of the acromioclavicular joint, several associated structures could also be torn including the one that gives the joint its greatest strength and stability, namely:

A. Acromioclavicular ligament

B. Coracoacromial ligament

C. Coracoclavicular ligament

D. Supraspinatus tendon

8. You are in the emergency room when a KMC student is brought in with a shoulder injury sustained while playing football. In comparing the symmetry of his two shoulders, you notice a marked elevation of the distal end of his clavicle with respect to the acromion on the injured side. The X-ray reveals a grade III shoulder separation. For this to have occurred, which ligament might have torn?

A. Coracoacromial

B. Coracoclavicular

C. Costoclavicular

D. Superior glenohumeral

9. A man riding a motorcycle hit a wet spot in the road, lost control, and was thrown from his bike. He landed on the right side of his head and the tip of his shoulder, bending his head sharply to the left and stretching the right side of his neck. Subsequent neurological examination revealed that the roots of the 5th and 6th cervical nerves had been torn away from the spinal cord. Following the above injury, which of the movements of the arm at the shoulder would you expect to be totally lost?

A. Adduction

B. Abduction

C. Flexion

D. Extension

10. In a fracture of the surgical neck of the humerus, which nerve may be injured?

A. Subscapular

B. Circumflex

C. Median nerve

D. Thoracodorsal

11. Which muscle is the strongest medial rotator of the arm?

A. Coracobrachialis

B. Infraspinatus

C. Subscapularis

D. Supraspinatus

12. An elderly man complained of pain in his shoulder when he brought his forearm and hand behind his back while dressing. It was determined that the pain was caused by stretching of the lateral rotators of his arm during this movement. Which muscle was most likely to be involved?

A. Infraspinatus

B. Latissimus dorsi

SECTION 3

C. Subscapularis

D. Supraspinatus

13. In old age, the supraspinatus tendon is sometimes ruptured where it blends with the capsule of the shoulder joint. Following this kind of injury one might expect

A. Difficulty in adducting the arm

B. Difficulty in flexing the arm

C. Difficulty in abducting the arm

D. Difficulty in extending the arm

14. While performing an arthrogram to study an apparent rotator cuff injury, it was noted that the contrast material had spread from the shoulder joint onto the anterior lateral surface of the scapula near the joint. When asked, the postgraduate student responded that this was due to an anterior tear in the cuff. Having just studied the shoulder joint you respond that the contrast is in a normal extension of the joint cavity called the:

A. Subacromial bursa

B. Subscapular bursa

C. Bicipital bursa

D. Olecranon bursa

15. A football player suffers downward dislocation of the shoulder. The cutaneous sensation over the deltoid muscle is impaired. These findings suggest damage to which of the following nerves?

A. Axillary

B. Median

C. Musculocutaneous

D. Radial

16. Your patient has been thrown from a motorcycle and suffers trauma to the upper limb. In the hospital, the left arm of the patient hangs at his side with loss of abduction and weakness of flexion and lateral rotation at the glenohumeral joint. What else might you expect to observe in the patient?

A. Atrophy of the hypothenar eminence

B. Weakness in the ability to protract the scapula

C. Weakness in supination

D. Inability to abduct and adduct the fingers

17. Your patient suffers from a progressive compression of the axillary artery posterior to the pectoralis minor.

Collateral circulation develops bypassing the blockage. With which artery does the suprascapular artery anastomose to establish a collateral circulation?

A. Dorsal scapular artery

B. Thoracoacromial artery

C. Subscapular artery

D. Radial artery

18. A 53-year-old male visits the hospital with complaints of a dull ache in his shoulder that interferes with his sleep. Local tenderness is present just below the acromion. Active abduction of the right arm into an overhead position is accompanied by severe pain. A tendon of which of the following muscles is most likely inflamed in this patient?

A. Biceps brachii

B. Supraspinatus

C. Levator scapulae

D. Pectoralis minor

Answers to MCQs

1. D

2. D

3. C

4. B

5. B

6. C

7. C

8. B

9. B

10. B

11. C

12. A

13. C

14. B

15. A

16. C

17. C

18. B

Dermatomes, Superficial Veins and Lymphatics of the Upper Limb

7

- Dermatomes of the upper limb
- Superficial veins of the upper limb
- Lymphatics of the upper limb
- MCQs

Objectives
- To know the dermatomes of the upper limb and their clinical relevance.
- To know the superficial veins and lymphatics of the upper limb and their clinical relevance.

DERMATOMES OF THE UPPER LIMB

A dermatome is an area of the skin supplied by a single spinal segment. The dermatome representation differs in trunk and limbs. In trunk there they are arranged successively one below another and each dermatome is extending from anterior to posterior midline. There is a considerable overlapping of adjacent dermatomes so that injury to a single spinal nerve results in very little sensory loss in the corresponding dermatome.

In case of upper limb nerve supply is through brachial plexus and not directly by spinal nerves, hence there is greater overlapping of adjacent dermatomes.

Apart from the branches of the brachial plexus (C5 to T1), the skin of the upper limb also receives intercostobrachial nerve (T2) and branches of supraclavicular nerve (C3, C4). Hence dermatomes of the upper limb include C5 to T1 and also C4 and T2.

Dermatomes of the upper limb and its developmental basis

- The first two dermatomes of the brachial plexus – C5 and C6 are arranged in preaxial border (C5 being proximal and C6 up to the base of the thumb).

- The last two dermatomes of the brachial plexus – C8 and T1 are arranged in postaxial border (T1 being proximal and C8 up to the base of the little finger).

- The C7 part of the dermatome is present only in the hand and it includes middle three fingers.

- The C4 dermatomes (branches of supraclavicular nerves) overlies the shoulder and T2 dermatome is present at the base of the axilla (intercostobrachial nerve-lateral cutaneous branch of the second intercostal nerve)

The picture of the dermatome differs in ventral and dorsal aspects (Figs 7.1 and 7.2). The line of separation between preaxial and postaxial borders are represented by an axial line.

143

The area of C5 dermatome includes lower lateral part of the shoulder, lateral part of the arm and upper lateral part of the forearm. These areas are supplied by axillary nerve, lower lateral cutaneous nerves of the arm (radial nerve) and musculocutaneous nerve (C5, 6,7).

The area of C6 dermatome includes a strip of area lateral to the axial line, medial to C5 dermatome, lower lateral aspect of the forearm and the thumb (radial nerve).

The area of C7 dermatome includes ventral and dorsal aspects of the middle three fingers. On the dorsal aspect the area extends more proximally (mainly by branches of median and radial nerves).

The area of C8 dermatome includes a small strip of area along the medial border of the lower part of the forearm including ventral and dorsal aspect of the little finger.

The area of T1 dermatome in the upper limb includes medial part of the lower arm and upper part of the forearm.

The area of T2 dermatome is the skin of the floor of the axilla through intercostobrachial nerve.

> Knowledge of the cutaneous distribution of the spinal nerve is important. A lesion affecting the spinal nerve or the spinal segment results in sensory loss in the area of distribution of that nerve. Though there is overlapping of dermatome, but while examining the sensory loss in

> a patient provides information about the probable nerve or spinal segment involved. Similarly in confirmed nerve lesion (by MRI in case of disc prolapse) you can look for the area is involved in sensory loss.
>
> In case of upper limb, T1 and T2 dermatomes (medial side of the arm and armpit) is important as pain fibres from heart in case of angina will also reach spinal cord through dorsal root ganglia of T1 and T2. This explains referred pain in the medial side of the arm in angina pectoris.

Cutaneous nerves of the upper limb

1. **Supraclavicular nerve (C3, 4):** The skin in front of the clavicle up to the second rib (pectoral region) and also skin over the shoulder is supplied by supraclavicular nerve.

2. **Intercostobrachial nerve (T2):** It is the lateral cutaneous branch of the second intercostal nerve supplying skin of the floor of the axilla.

3. **Upper lateral cutaneous nerve of the arm (C5, 6):** It is a branch from the axillary nerve supplies skin over the deltoid muscle

4. **Lower lateral cutaneous nerve of the arm (C5, 6):** It is a branch from the radial nerve given in the spiral

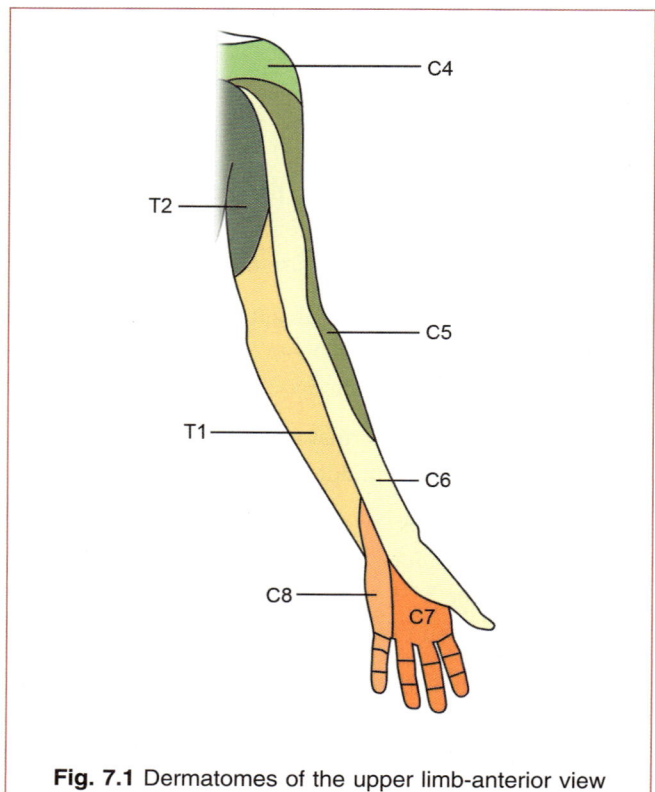

Fig. 7.1 Dermatomes of the upper limb-anterior view

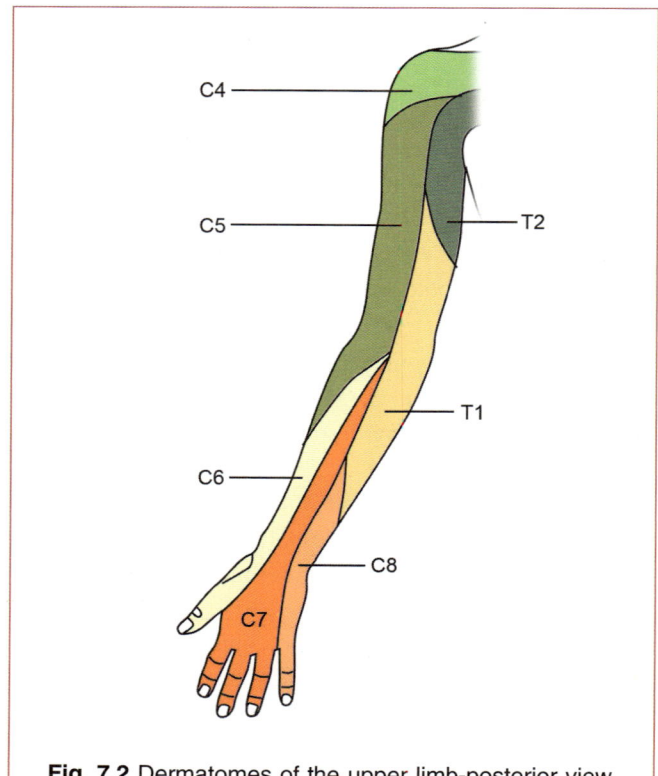

Fig. 7.2 Dermatomes of the upper limb-posterior view

SECTION 3

groove, supplies the skin of the lower lateral aspect of the arm.

5. **Posterior cutaneous nerve of the arm (C5):** It is a branch from the radial nerve in the axilla. It supplies the skin of the back of the arm up to the level of olecranon process.

6. **Medial cutaneous nerve of the arm (T1):** It is a branch from the medial cord of the brachial plexus, supplies skin of the medial side of the lower arm.

7. **Posterior cutaneous nerve of the forearm (C6,7, 8):** It is a branch from the radial nerve in the spiral groove. It supplies the skin of the back of the forearm.

8. **Lateral cutaneous nerves of the forearm (C5, 6):** It is the continuation of the musculocutaneous nerve. It supplies the skin of the anterolateral and posterolateral surfaces of the forearm.

9. **Medial cutaneous nerve of forearm (C8, T1):** It is a branch from the medial cord of the brachial plexus. It supplies the skin of the anteromedial and posteromedial surfaces of the forearm.

10. **Superficial terminal branch of the radial nerve (C6,7, 8):** It supplies the lateral $2/3^{rd}$ of the dorsum of the hand and skin of the lateral two and a half finger on the dorsal side.

11. **Palmar cutaneous branch of the median nerve (C6, 7, 8):** It supplies the skin of the lateral aspect of the palm.

12. **Palmar digital branches of median nerve (C6, 7, 8):** It supplies the skin of the palmar aspect of the lateral three and a half finger. These branches crosses the palmar side to dorsal side and supplies the nail bed and the skin up to the level of the middle phalynx.

13. **Palmar cutaneous branch ulnar nerve (C8, T1):** It supplies the skin of the medial part of the palm

14. **Dorsal cutaneous branch of the ulnar nerve (C8, T1):** It supplies the skin of the medial part of the dorsum of the hand and also dorsal aspect of the medial one and a half fingers.

15. **Palmar digital branch of the ulnar nerve (C8, T1):** It supplies the skin of the palmar aspect of the medial one and half finger.

SUPERFICIAL VEINS OF THE UPPER LIMB

Dorsal venous arch

It is an irregular network of veins located in the superficial fascia on the dorsum of the hand. It receives three dorsal metacarpal veins from the adjacent sides of the four fingers. On the lateral side the network receives veins from the radial side of the index finger and two veins from the thumb. On the medial side it receives a vein from the medial side of the little finger.

Cephalic vein

Formation: It is formed by the union of lateral end of the dorsal venous arch with a vein arising from the thumb at the lateral aspect of the dorsum of the hand (Figs 7.3 and 7.4).

Course and relations: It ascends superficial to the anatomical snuff box where it is related to the superficial terminal branch of the radial nerve. Then it ascends along the posterolateral side of the forearm, where it is related to lateral cutaneous nerve of the forearm. It ascends on the lateral side of the arm. Then it courses along the delto-pectoral groove where it is related to delto-pectoral lymph nodes. Just below the clavicle the vein takes a sharp turn to pierce the clavipectoral fascia and enters the axilla to terminate in the axillary vein. The cephalic vein is superficial throughout its major part of the course.

Median cubital vein

It is a large tributary of the cephalic vein arises from the cephalic vein in the forearm. It crosses superficially in the roof of the cubital fossa in front of the elbow. It rests on the bicipital aponeurosis, which separates the median cubital vein from the underlying brachial artery. The median cubital vein joins the basilic vein on the medial side of the arm just proximal to the elbow. Perforating veins arising from the median cubital vein pierces the bicipital aponeurosis to join the deeper veins. The median cubital vein relieves the load of cephalic vein by transferring blood into the basilic vein (Fig. 7.4).

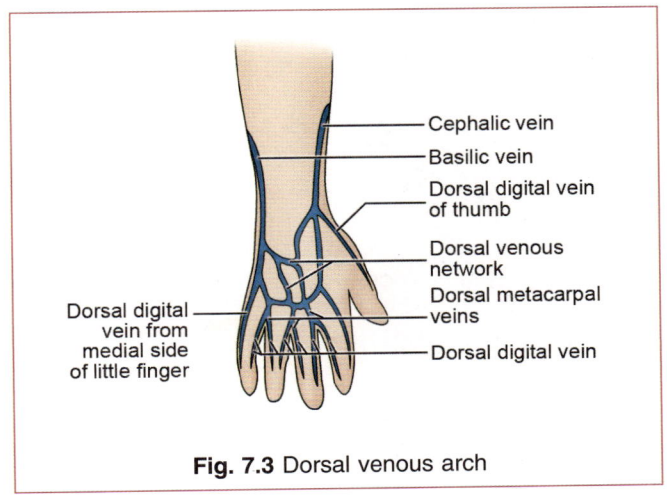

Cephalic vein
Basilic vein
Dorsal digital vein of thumb
Dorsal venous network
Dorsal metacarpal veins
Dorsal digital vein
Dorsal digital vein from medial side of little finger

Fig. 7.3 Dorsal venous arch

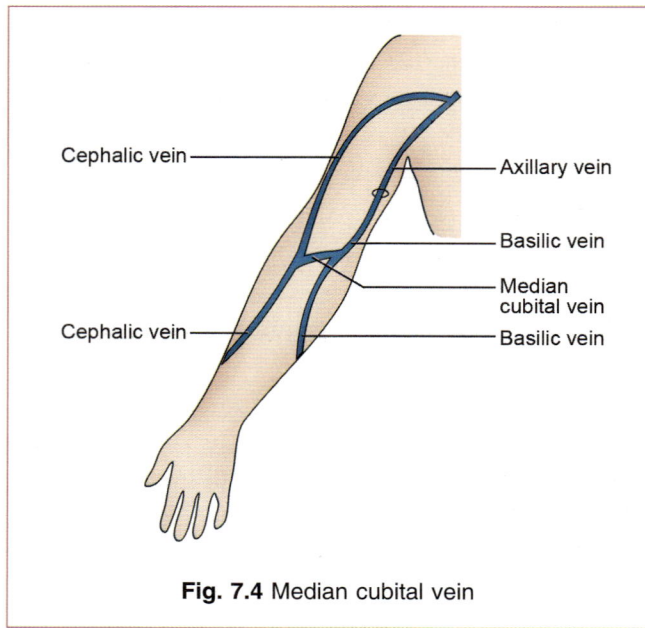

Fig. 7.4 Median cubital vein

The clinical relevance of the median cubital vein is discussed in Chapter 8—Arm and cubital fossa (Fig. 7.4).

Basilic vein

It is formed from the medial end of the dorsal venous arch. It ascends on the medial side of the posterior surface of the forearm. Just below the elbow it ascends on the anterior surface of the forearm and crosses the medial part of the front of the elbow. Here it is closely related to the medial cutaneous nerve of the forearm. It receives median vein just proximal to the elbow. The basilic vein pierces the deep fascia at the mid-arm level to become deep. In its further course it is placed medial to the brachial artery. At the lower

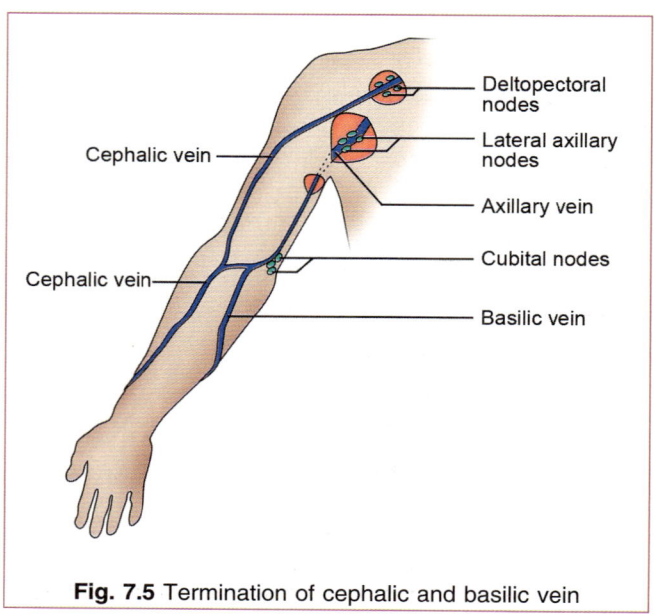

Fig. 7.5 Termination of cephalic and basilic vein

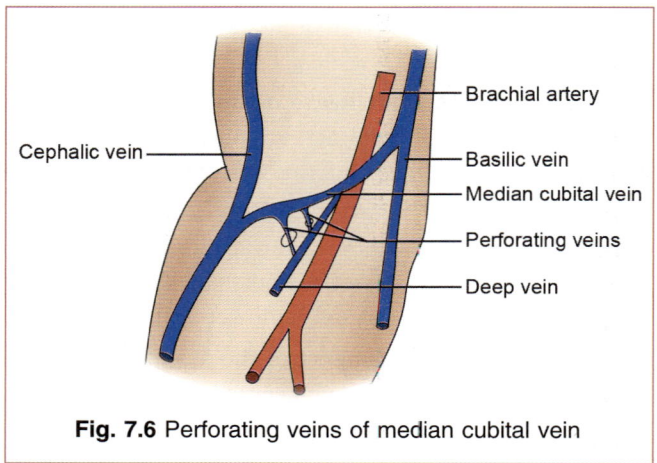

Fig. 7.6 Perforating veins of median cubital vein

margin of the teres major muscle it joins with two veins accompanying the brachial artery to form the axillary vein. It is also described that 'basilic vein continues to form axillary vein at the lower margin of the teres major muscle (Fig. 7.5).

Median vein of the forearm

This vein (s) present in front of the forearm. It ascends in front of forearm to open into the median cubital or basilic vein (Fig. 7.6).

LYMPHATIC DRAINAGE OF THE UPPER LIMB AND LYMPH NODES OF THE UPPER LIMB

The lymph vessels of the upper limb can be divided into superficial and deep set.

The superficial vessels drains skin and superficial fascia.

a. Lymph from the superficial tissue of the thumb, lateral side of the forearm, and arm form plexus along the cephalic vein and drains into deltopectoral group of lymph nodes (infraclavicular nodes).

b. Lymph from superficial tissue of the medial side of the forearm follows the basilic vein and drain into superficial cubital nodes.

The deep lymph vessels draining deeper tissue, forms plexus along the main blood vessels and drain into lateral group of axillary lymph nodes. From the lateral group it drains into central and then into apical group of axillary lymph nodes.

MCQs

1. A 17-year-old boy receives a superficial cut on the thumb side of his forearm. The superficial vein most likely affected is the:

A. Basilic
B. Cephalic
C. Median vein of the forearm
D. Median cubital

2. 18-year-old boy received a superficial cut on the ulnar side of his forearm. The superficial vein most likely to be affected is the:

A. Basilic
B. Cephalic
C. Median antebrachial
D. Median cubital

3. Following an insertion of IV cannula in the median cubital vein, the patient suddenly lost sensation on the radial side of the forearm. Which nerve was accidentally injured in the process?

A. Lateral cutaneous nerve of the forearm
B. Medial cutaneous nerve of the forearm
C. Musculocutaneous nerve
D. Posterior cutaneous nerve of the forearm

4. A 48-year-old man presents with severe neck pain and weakness in his left upper limb. He did not get relief from over-the-counter medications. He denies any history of trauma. On examination the patient is thin and walks with his neck tilted to the left side. The patient has limited neck flexion and extension secondary to pain. The patient has a normal motor and sensory functions of all extremities, with the exception of the left upper extremity. His radial side of left forearm and thumb are numb to the touch (decreased sensation to light touch). The patient has a decreased brachioradialis reflex and slight weakness of his wrist extensors. Plain radiographs appears normal. Which of the following is most likely to be the diagnosis?

A. Compression of his left C6 nerve root
B. Compression of his left thoracic first nerve root
C. Compression of his right Tl nerve root
D. A tumour in his lumbar spine

5. A surgeon while suturing the hand of a patient did not gave anesthetics since the area between his thumb and

index finger on the dorsal side was already numb. Which nerve must have been injured (most likely by the fracture of his wrist) for this area to be numb?

A. Lateral cutaneous nerve of the forearm
B. Medial cutaneous nerve of the forearm
C. Median nerve
D. Superficial terminal branch of the radial nerve

6. Because of scarring of a patient's median cubital vein, the nurse chooses to insert an infusion needle into her basilic vein on the medial side of the front of the elbow. Despite the certainty that the needle does not pass through the deep (investing) fascia, there is still a chance that it might nick or impale which of the following structures?

A. Brachial artery
B. Lateral cutaneous nerve of the forearm
C. Medial cutaneous nerve of the forearm
D. Median nerve

7. A patient with a herniated intervertebral disc injury has lost sensation at the base of his right thumb and along the lateral side of his forearm. The strength of shoulder abduction and elbow flexion is diminished. The fingers and thumb move normally. The intervertebral disc herniation is most likely at which of the following levels

A. C3/C4
B. C5/C6
C. C6/C7
D. C7/Tl

Answers to MCQs

1. B
2. A
3. A
4. A
5. D
6. B
7. B

SECTION 3

Arm and Cubital Fossa

8

- Front of the arm
- Cubital fossa
- Back of the arm
- MCQs

Objectives
- To list the muscles of the anterior and posterior compartments of the arm, their insertion, nerve supply and actions
- To explain the origin, course, distribution of musculocutaneous nerve.
- To explain list the boundaries, contents and clinical relevance of cubital fossa.
- To explain the anastomoses around the elbow and its functional significance

The arm is divided into anterior and posterior compartments by the deep fascia. The medial and lateral intermuscular septa are the extension of the deep fascia, attached to the medial and lateral supracondylar ridges of humerus. They are better defined in the lower part of the arm, hence the division of the arm into anterior and posterior compartment is just arbitrary in the upper part.

The anterior compartment is considered as flexor compartment because two of its muscle are responsible for flexing the elbow joint.

The posterior compartment is considered as extensor compartment because the triceps muscle in this compartment is responsible for extension at the elbow joint. The structures present in each compartment are explained below.

The medial intermuscular septum is pierced by ulnar nerve, superior ulnar collateral vessels. The lateral intermuscular compartment is pierced by radial nerve with radial collateral vessels.

FRONT OF THE ARM (FLEXOR COMPARTMENT)

The anterior compartment presents three muscles namely - coracobrachialis, biceps brachii and brachialis. All these muscles are supplied by musculocutaneous nerve. The lower part of the arm also presents origins of brachioradialis and extensor carpi radialis longus muscles. Apart from these muscles it also contains the median nerve and the brachial artery.

1. Biceps brachii

Origin: It has two heads of origin. The short head arises from the tip of the coracoid process along with coracobrachialis. The long head arises from the supraglenoid tubercle of the scapula within the shoulder joint cavity.

The tendon of the long head traverses the shoulder joint cavity and emerges through a gap in the attachment of the capsule between greater and lesser tubercles. At this area the tendon is superficially crossed by transverse humeral ligament which holds the tendon in its position during the

149

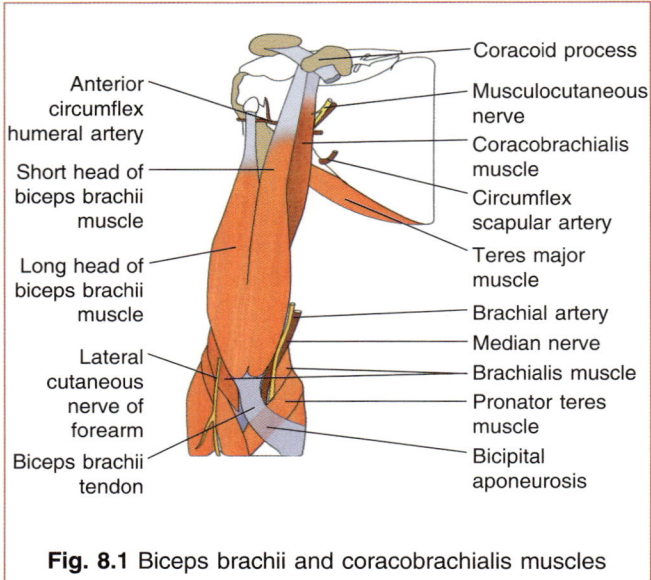

Fig. 8.1 Biceps brachii and coracobrachialis muscles

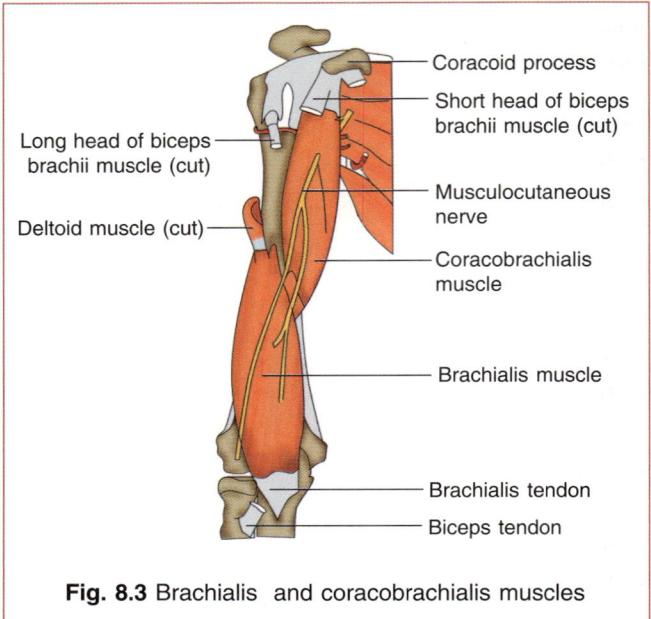

Fig. 8.3 Brachialis and coracobrachialis muscles

movement of shoulder joint. The long head is enclosed in a synovial sheath which prevents the friction during the movements of the joint. The long head descends in the bicipital groove (Figs 8.1 and 8.2).

Insertion: The two heads join in the front of the arm. It is inserted by a tendon to the tuberosity of the radius. The tendon gives an expansion called 'bicipital aponeurosis' from its medial margin, which joins the deep fascia of the forearm. The aponeurosis separates the median cubital vein from the brachial artery and is pierced by the perforating veins.

Nerve supply: Musculocutaneous nerve

Actions: It supinates the forearm at the radioulnar joint and flexes the elbow joint. It is also a weak flexor of the shoulder joint. The long head stabilizes the head of the humerus during shoulder movements.

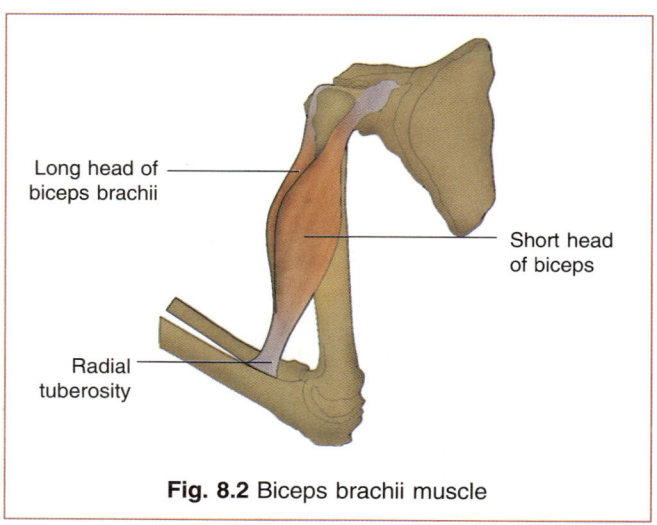

Fig. 8.2 Biceps brachii muscle

2. Coracobrachialis

Origin: It takes origin from the tip of the coracoid process of the scapula along with the short head of the biceps brachii muscle. The upper part of the muscle is pierced by the musculocutaneous nerve (Fig. 8.3).

Insertion: It is inserted into the middle of medial surface of the humerus.

Nerve supply: It is supplied by musculocutaneous nerve.

Action: It is a weak flexor of the arm at the shoulder joint.

3. Brachialis

Origin: It arises from the lower part of the shaft of the humerus. It descends in front of the elbow joint forming the floor of the cubital fossa.

Insertion: It is inserted into the ulnar tuberosity.

Nerve supply: It has two nerves supplying it, the musculocutaneous and the radial nerve.

Action: It is the chief flexor of the elbow joint.

Median nerve of the arm

The median nerve is formed by the union of two roots (medial root from the medial cord and the lateral root from the lateral cord). It descends in the anterior compartment of the arm and enters the cubital fossa. In the upper part of the arm it is related lateral to the brachial artery. At the level of the insertion of the coracobrachialis it crosses in front of the artery from lateral to medial side. In the lower part of the arm the median nerve is related medial to the brachial artery. In the arm it gives vascular branches to the brachial artery. The first muscular branch (to pronator teres

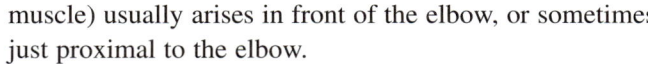

muscle) usually arises in front of the elbow, or sometimes just proximal to the elbow.

Musculocutaneous nerve (C5, 6, 7)

- It has both muscular and cutaneous distribution.
- It arises from the lateral cord of the brachial plexus
- It pierces the coracobrachialis muscle on its way to the front of the arm.
- In the arm it descends posterior to the biceps brachii and anterior to the brachialis muscle.
- It emerges from the interval between the above said muscles on the lateral side and becomes superficial.
- Further continuation of the nerve is called lateral cutaneous nerve of the forearm, which descends in the lateral part of the roof of the cubital fossa.
- It supplies three muscles in the front of the arm - coracobrachialis, biceps brachii and brachialis.
- The lateral cutaneous nerve of the forearm supplies the skin in front and back of the forearm along the lateral side (Fig. 8.4)

An injury to the musculocutaneous nerve can cause loss of cutaneous sensation on the lateral side of the forearm and also weakens the flexion movement at the elbow joint.

Brachial artery

- Brachial artery is the continuation of the axillary artery, and is present in the arm.
- It extends from the lower border of the teres major muscle up to the neck of the radius in the cubital fossa where it divides into radial and ulnar arteries.

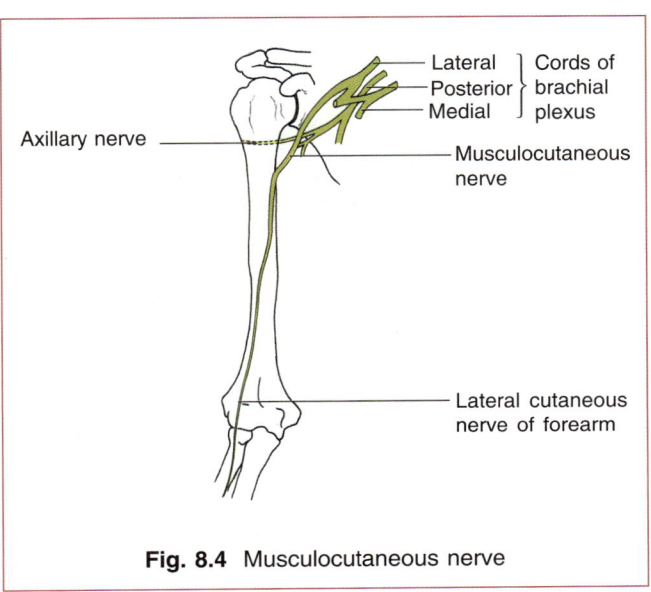

Fig. 8.4 Musculocutaneous nerve

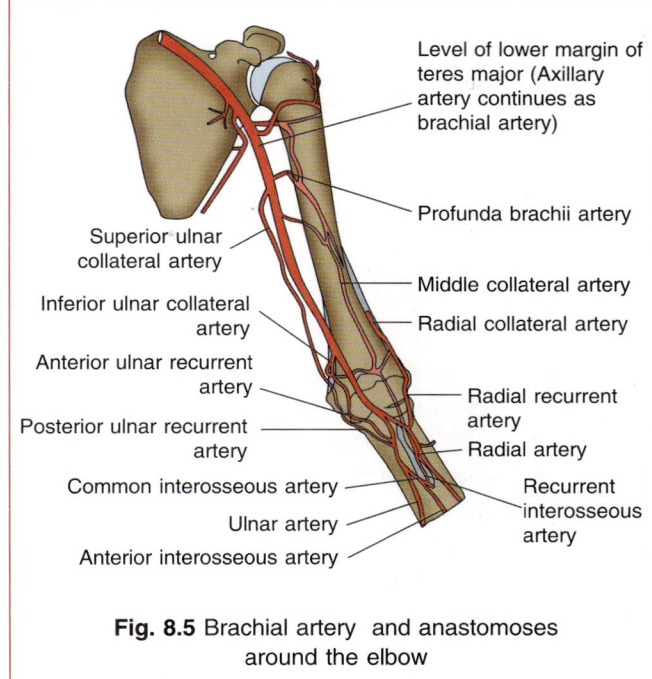

Fig. 8.5 Brachial artery and anastomoses around the elbow

- The brachial artery is related to median nerve on its medial side in the upper part of the arm, lateral to the nerve in the lower part.
- The artery successively rests on long head of the biceps brachii, medial head of the triceps, coracobrachialis and brachialis muscles.
- It is accompanied by a pair of veins (vena comitantes)
- In the cubital fossa the artery lies lateral to the median nerve and medial to the tendon of the biceps brachii. It is separated from superficially placed median cubital vein by bicipital aponeurosis.

Branches: The brachial artery gives many named and unnamed branches (Fig. 8.5). The important branches include

1. **Profunda brachii artery**, which accompanies the radial nerve and enters the spiral groove through lower triangular space. It gives muscular branches to triceps muscle, nutrient branch to the humerus, an ascending 'deltoid' branch which anastomoses with a descending branch of the posterior circumflex humeral artery.

   The two terminal branches are radial collateral (anterior descending) and middle collateral (posterior descending). The radial collateral accompanies the radial nerve pierces the lateral intermuscular septum to descend in front of the lateral epicondyle. The middle collateral descends posterior to the lateral epicondyle. These branches take part in anastomoses around the elbow joint.

2. Superior ulnar collateral artery: It accompanies the ulnar nerve, pierces the medial intermuscular septum and descends posterior to the medial epicondyle.

3. Inferior ulnar collateral artery: It descends in front of the medial epicondyle

4. Muscular branches

Arterial pulsations are felt or auscultated in front of the elbow just medial to the tendon of the biceps while recording the blood pressure.

Compression of the brachial artery is possible with tight plaster cast or tourniquet to the arm. Injury to the artery is also possible in supracondylar fracture of the humerus, where the proximal fractured segment of the bone is displaced anteriorly and can compressing or injuring the brachial artery. Compression of the brachial artery reduces the blood flow to the forearm and the hand. It is clinically manifested by 5 Ps (**p**allor, **p**ain, **p**uffiness, **p**ulselessness and eventually **p**aralysis of muscle). Impaired blood supply to the muscle for a prolonged period leads to necrosis and fibrosis of the muscle, which leads to **Volkmann's ischemic contracture,** in which there is flexion contracture of the metacarpophalangeal and interphalangeal joints (Fig. 8.6).

CASE-1

A 53-year-old male was admitted in the hospital for generalized arteriosclerosis, aortic valve defects and cardiac failure. During his stay in the hospital, he suddenly complains of sharp pain and paresis of the right forearm of about one hour's duration. On examination, the forearm is cold and pale, with the hand and fingers drawn up in a contracted position. There is loss of movement and sensation below the elbow. Radial and ulnar arterial pulsations are absent. This case was diagnosed as occlusion of the brachial artery

by a blood clot. An individual suffering from aortic valve disease is known to develop an arterial embolism.

1. Give the course of the blood clot from the left ventricle to the right brachial artery

2. Where do you feel for the pulsation of the radial and ulnar arteries?

3. What is the cause for paresis and the loss of sensation?

4. How does the collateral circulation take place if the block in the brachial artery is above the origin of the profunda brachii artery?

CASE-2

A 9-year-old boy fell off a swing and sustained a supracondylar fracture of his left humerus. Following the reduction of the fracture, a plaster cast was carefully applied, and the child was sent home. Few hours later, the child complained of pain in the forearm, which persisted. Four hours later, the parents decided to return to the hospital, since the child's left hand looked dusky white, and the pain in forearm was still present. On examination, it was found the cutaneous sensation of the hand was completely lost. The colour of the skin was bluish white. The lower part of the plaster cast was removed but pulse of the radial and the ulnar arteries could not be palpated. Every possible effort was made to restore the circulation of the forearm. What deformity would you expect this child to have one year later? Explain the deformity on anatomical grounds.

CUBITAL FOSSA

This is a triangular space situated in front of the elbow (homologous with the popliteal fossa present on the back of the knee).

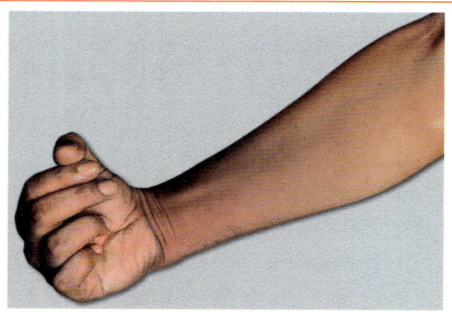

Fig. 8.6 Volkmann's ischemic contracture

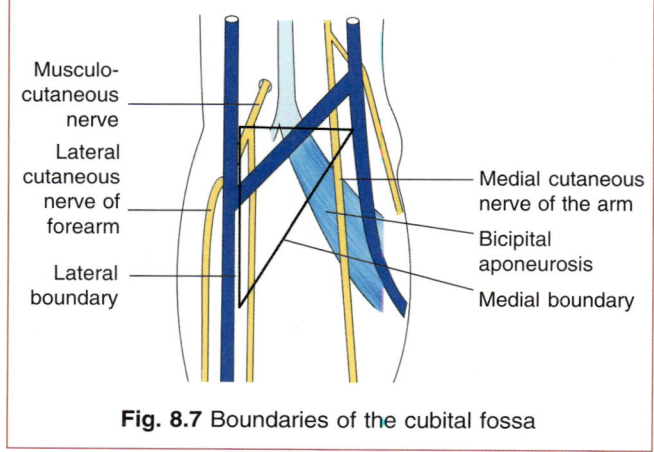

Musculo-cutaneous nerve

Lateral cutaneous nerve of forearm

Lateral boundary

Medial cutaneous nerve of the arm

Bicipital aponeurosis

Medial boundary

Fig. 8.7 Boundaries of the cubital fossa

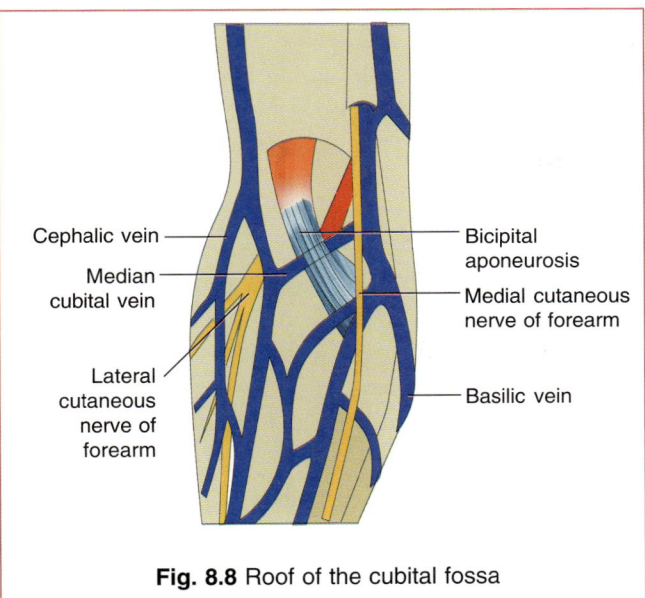

Fig. 8.8 Roof of the cubital fossa

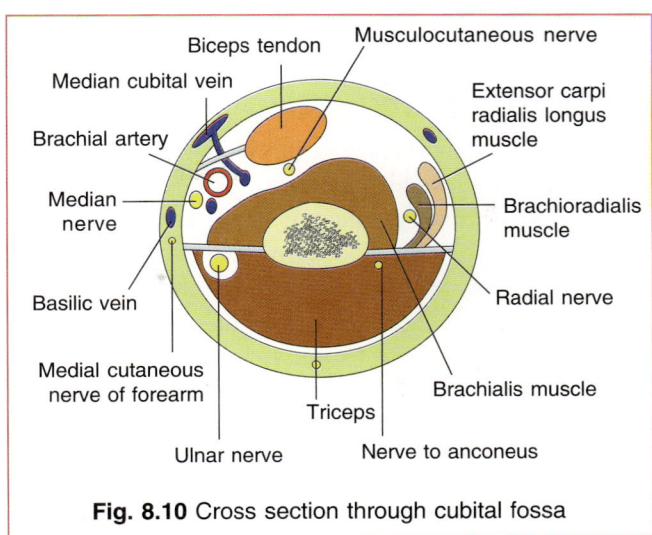

Fig. 8.10 Cross section through cubital fossa

Boundaries

Base: An imaginary line connecting the two epicondyles of the humerus (Fig. 8.7).

Medially: Lateral border of the pronator teres muscle.

Laterally: Medial border of the brachioradialis muscle.

Apex: Meeting point of the medial and lateral borders.

Roof: It consists of skin, superficial fascia and the deep fascia. The roof has a superficial vein called the median cubital vein, which courses obliquely. The roof also presents cephalic vein and lateral cutaneous nerve of the forearm on the lateral side, basilica vein and medial cutaneous nerve of the forearm on the medial side. The deep fascia presents

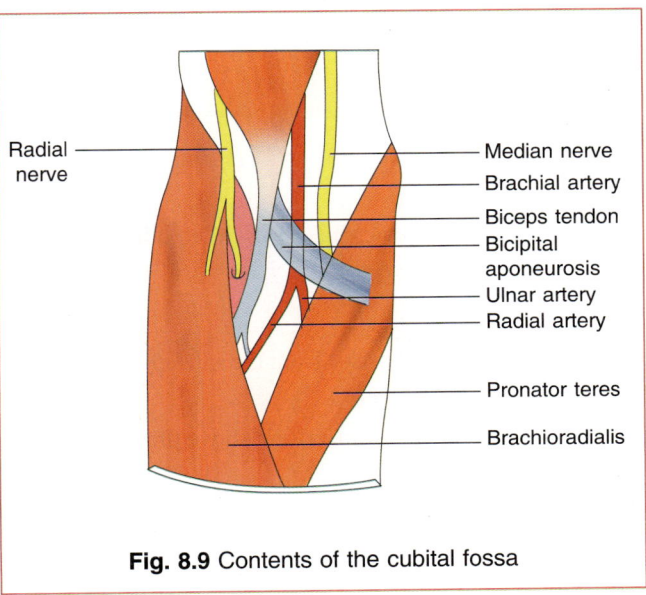

Fig. 8.9 Contents of the cubital fossa

bicipital aponeurosis which also contributes to the roof (Fig. 8.8).

Floor: The floor is formed by brachialis muscle in the upper part and supinator muscle in the lower part.

Contents (Fig. 8.9)

The contents of the fossa from medial to lateral side are

1. **Median nerve:** Further down it leaves the fossa by passing between the two heads of the pronator teres muscle.

2. **Brachial artery:** It terminates in the fossa at the level of the neck of the radius by dividing into ulnar and radial arteries. In the fossa the ulnar artery gives anterior and posterior ulnar recurrent branches, common interosseus artery. The radial artery in the fossa gives radial recurrent branch (Fig. 8.10). The blood pressure is recorded by auscultating the brachial artery in front of the elbow. The pulsation of the artery can be felt medial to the biceps brachii tendon.

3. **Tendon of the biceps brachii muscle** (which is inserted into the radial tuberosity).

4. **Radial nerve** appears on the lateral side between brachialis and brachioradialis muscles. It terminates by dividing into a superficial branch and deep branch. The deep branch pierces the supinator muscle and in its further course it is called as posterior interosseus nerve.

Median cubital vein

It is a large communicating vein between cephalic and the basilic vein. It begins from the cephalic vein below the elbow and ends in the basilic vein (Fig. 8.8). It receives tributaries from the front of the forearm and is connected to the deep veins by perforating veins, which perforates the bicipital aponeurosis. Since it is fixed to deep veins through the perforating veins, it is the vein of choice for intravenous injections and for cardiac catheterization.

> There is a possibility of injuring brachial artery and median nerve during intravenous injection or procedures through median cubital vein. Variations in the median cubital vein is also possible. Injury to the brachial artery results in spurting of blood from the injured vessel.

CASE-3

A 45-year-old male patient got admitted to the hospital for cardiac medication. For the first few days of treatment the intravenous route was chosen in order to accelerate the medication effect. The first three injections into the median cubital vein were painless and well tolerated ,on fourth injection the patient complained immediately of burning pain at the site of injections in the lateral part of the cubital fossa. The pain increased during the day and radiated over the anterior aspect of the forearm. In the evening, the patient complained of numbness and prickling over the dorsal aspect of the forearm. Intravenous medication was continued in the other arm. Under prescribed treatment the patient improved gradually and was discharged from the hospital. However, the numbness over the lateral part of the forearm persisted. Palpation of the cubital fossa showed an abnormally hard area at the previous site of painful injection. There is no muscular atrophy and movements of the forearm and hand is normal. However there is complete loss of all modalities of sensation over most of the area supplied by the lateral cutaneous nerve of the forearm (Fig. 8.10).

1. What is the rationale behind choosing an intravenous route ?

2. Which is the favorite site for a venipuncture and why is this location chosen?

3. Which two superficial veins are connected by the median cubital vein ?

4. How do you increase the state of distention of the superficial veins for the purpose of venipuncture ?

5. What is the effect of the latter procedure and what is the complication if the tourniquet is applied too tightly?

6. In case of leakage of the injected drug from the vein after withdrawal of the needle or through faulty extravenous injection of part of the drug, two nerves may readily be damaged. Identify them.

7. What is the origin of these two cutaneous nerves and what cutaneous areas do they supply?

8. Which nerve was involved in this case?

9. Another complication during a venipuncture is an accidental intra-arterial injection. Which artery may be involved and what separates this artery from the median cubital vein?

Anastomosis around the elbow

This anastomosis is important in providing collateral circulation in case of compression of the brachial artery. It connects the axillary artery with radial and ulnar arteries. The anastomosis can be studied by knowing the specific branches taking part in front and behind the epicondyles of the humerus.

1. Anterior to the medial epicondyle: Superiorly the inferior ulnar collateral artery (from the brachial artery) and inferiorly the anteriror ulnar recurrent branch from the ulnar artery anastomose with each other.

2. Posterior to the medial epicondyle: Superiorly the superior ulnar collateral artery (from the brachial artery) accompanying ulnar nerve and inferiorly the posterior ulnar recurrent branch from the ulnar artery anastomose with each other.

3. Anterior to the lateral epicondyle: Superiorly the radial collateral (anterior descending) branch from the profunda brachii artery that accompanies the radial nerve and inferiorly the radial recurrent branch from the radial artery anastomose with each other.

4. Posterior to the lateral epicondyle: Superiorly the middle collateral (posterior descending) branch from the profunda brachii artery and inferiorly the interosseus recurrent branch from the posterior interosseus artery (a branch from the common interosseus artery) anastomose with each other.

BACK OF THE ARM

Muscles of the back of the arm (Posterior or extensor compartment)

Only one muscle occupies this area, called **triceps brachii.** It has three heads of origin.

Triceps brachii

Origin: The long head arises from the infraglenoid tubercle of the scapula (Fig. 8.11).

The lateral head arises from a ridge above the radial groove of the humerus.

The medial head arises from the posterior surface of the humerus below the radial groove. The long and lateral head converge together and descends superficial to the medial

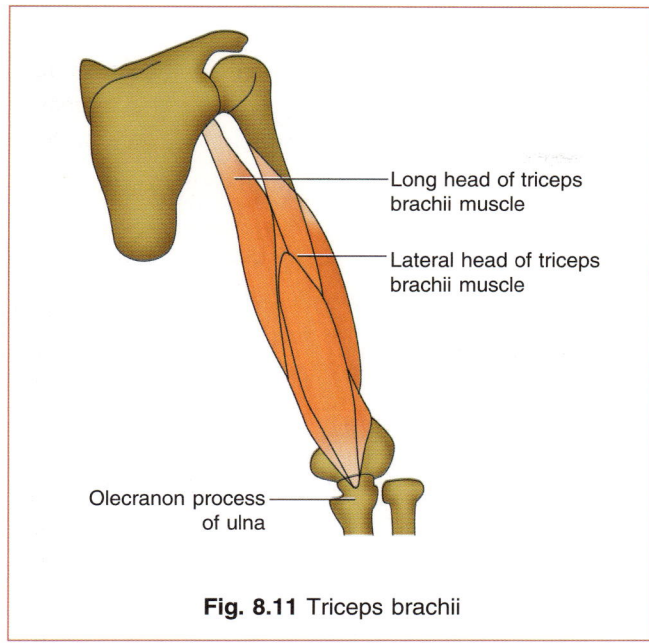

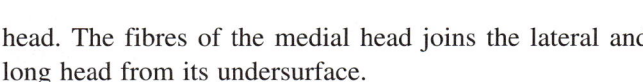

Fig. 8.11 Triceps brachii

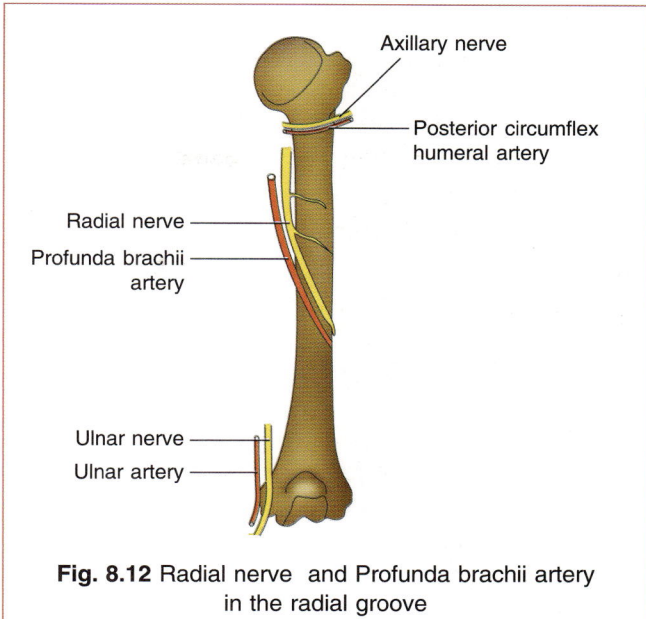

Fig. 8.12 Radial nerve and Profunda brachii artery in the radial groove

head. The fibres of the medial head joins the lateral and long head from its undersurface.

Insertion: To the olecrenon process of the ulna. A few fibres from the tendon is attached to the capsule of the elbow joint, which is referred as 'articularis cubiti' or 'subanconeus'. It prevents the nipping of the capsule during extension of the elbow.

Nerve supply: It is supplied by radial nerve. In the axilla it gives branches to long and medial head of the triceps. In the spiral groove it gives branches to lateral and medial heads.

Action: It is a chief extensor of the elbow joint.

Radial nerve in the spiral groove

- The radial nerve enters the spiral groove through lower triangular space along with the profunda brachii artery

- In the spiral groove the nerve and the artery descends between lateral and medial head of the triceps muscle and is in close contact with the periosteum of the humerus.

- At about 5 cm below the deltoid tuberosity the nerve pierces the lateral intermuscular septum along with the radial collateral artery to enter the anterior compartment. At the same level on the medial side the ulnar nerve pierces the medial intermuscular septum and enters the posterior compartment.

- The radial nerve appears in front of the elbow between the brachialis medially and brachioradialis laterally.

- In front of the elbow it ends by dividing into superficial and deep terminal branches.

Branches:

Before entering the spiral groove (in the axilla)

1. Muscular branches to long and medial head of the triceps brachii. The branch to the medial head is sometimes referred as ulnar collateral nerve because it descends parallel to the ulnar nerve.

2. Posterior cutaneous nerve of the arm, which supplies the skin of the back of the arm.

In the spiral groove

1. Muscular branches to lateral and medial head of the triceps brachii. The branch to the medial head passes through the substance of the muscle and also supplies anconeus.

2. The cutaneous branches includes

a) Lower lateral cutaneous nerve of the arm: It supplies skin of the upper lateral aspect of the arm.

b) Posterior cutaneous nerve of the forearm: It supplies the skin of the posterior aspect of the forearm.

In front of the elbow

1. Muscular branches to brachialis, brachioradialis and extensor carpi radialis longus muscles.

2. Articular branches to the elbow joint.

3. Terminal branches- Superficial and deep.

a. **Superficial terminal branch:** It is purely a cutaneous branch. It descends deep to the brachioradialis along the lateral side of the forearm. It becomes superficial after emerging from the lateral border of the brachioradialis muscle in the middle of the forearm. In its further course it is related to cephalic vein. It crosses superficial to the anatomical snuff box to reach the dorsum of the hand. It supplies the skin of the lateral part of the dorsum of the hand and dorsal aspect of the lateral three and a half fingers.

b. **Deep terminal branch:** It pierces the supinator muscle and enters the posterior compartment. The nerve is called as posterior interosseous nerve. It is purely a motor nerve supplying all the extensor muscles of the forearm whose main action is extension at the wrist joint.

Radial nerve is injured in fracture affecting the shaft of the humerus (in the spiral groove). The nerve may be also injured by prolonged hanging of the arm in an arm chair during sleeping by a drunken person, which may compress the radial nerve (**Saturday night palsy**). The nerve can also be compressed in the armpit by using crutch (**Crutch paralysis**). The signs and symptoms vary depending upon the extent of lesion.

An injury in the spiral groove may not affect much on extension of the elbow, because the long and medial head receives branches from the radial nerve even before entering the spiral groove. Injury to the radial nerve in the spiral groove has both motor and sensory effects. The motor effect is manifested by '**wrist drop**' as extensor muscles of the forearm are paralyzed. It also includes finger drops and thumb drops. The sensory loss is the lower lateral aspect of the arm, back of the forearm and the lateral part of the dorsum of the hand including dorsal aspect of the lateral three and a half fingers.

CASE-4

A 12-year-old boy fell from a tree and fractured the left humerus about midway between the two ends of the bone. The left hand immediately assumed a flexed position and, regardless of effort, the boy could not extend the hand at the wrist or any of the fingers including the thumb. In addition, flexion and supination of the left forearm were weakened but not abolished. Abduction of the thumb was greatly weakened. Further examination observed that the boy had lost cutaneous sensation over part of posterior aspect of the arm, entire posterior forearm and dorsum of the left hand from thumb to middle finger. The boy was scheduled for neurosurgery, followed by orthopaedic manipulation of the broken bone. The arm was put in cast, which

was removed 8 weeks later. A year after the accident the boy had regained complete control of the left upper limb and reported no sensory loss.

1. Which structure other than the humerus was damaged and what is this clinical condition called?
2. Discuss the of involvement of musculocutaneous nerve in this case with respect to motor and sensory deficit as observed by the neurologist.
3. Does any other structure accompany the damaged structure in its course around the humerus?

Solutions to the case studies

Case-1

1. The clot travelled from the left ventricle to the ascending aorta, then to the arch of aorta, brachiocephalic trunk, right subclavian artery and right axillary artery.

2. Remember that the pulse is best felt in areas where the artery is superficial and resting on a firm structure such as a bone or a ligament or a tendon. The ulnar artery lies superficial to flexor retinaculum on the radial side of the pisiform bone. The pulse of the radial artery is felt on the lateral side of the wrist a little more proximally, lateral to the tendon of the flexor carpi radialis in front of the lower end of the radius.

3. The nerves and muscles can function only in the presence of sufficient blood supply, which was interrupted in this case by the arterial embolus (clot).

4. This is a most unfavorable site and the circulation relies on the anastomosis between the descending branch of the posterior circumflex humeral artery and an ascending branch of the profunda brachii artery.

Case-2

At the time of the fracture of the humerus or following the application of the plaster cast, there was compression of the brachial artery in the region of the cubital fossa. This was followed by Volkmann's contracture.

Case-3

1. The intravenous route is chosen when rapid action of the drug is required.
2. The median cubital vein is most frequently utilized for venipuncture (taking of a blood sample), venesection (blood letting), intravenous injections and blood transfusions because the vein is superficially located and therefore easily seen and felt. It is mechanically fixed by perforating veins which connects the deeper veins with median cubital vein after perforating the bicipital aponeurosis.

3. The median cubital vein connects cephalic vein with basilic vein and crosses the roof of the cubital fossa.

4. The following procedure are customarily employed – a) Keeping the arm in a dependent position for some time which slows the venous return. b) Compressing the veins by a tourniquet 1.5 to 2 inches proximal to the site of puncture. c) Applying heat by means of hot water bag, moist towels or by immersing the hand and forearm into a basin of hot water. d) Alternating opening and closing of the hand.

5. Muscular activity will increase the amount of arterial blood flow to the distal portion of the upper limb. It is also possible that the opening and closing of the hand will enhance the blood flow from the deep to superficial veins by means of the perforating veins. On the other hand, applying tight tourniquets may obstruct the arterial flow to the forearm.

6. They are the lateral cutaneous nerve of the forearm, which is related to cephalic vein and medial cutaneous nerve of the forearm which is related to basilic vein.

7. The lateral cutaneous nerve of the forearm is the continuation of musculocutaneous nerve, which supplies skin in front and back on the lateral side of the forearm. The medial cutaneous nerve of the forearm is a branch from the medial cord of the brachial plexus, which supplies skin in front and back on the medial side of the forearm.

8. In the present case the injection injured anterior branch of the lateral cutaneous nerve of the forearm.

9. The artery involved is the brachial artery. It is separated from median cubital vein by bicipital aponeurosis . The aspirated blood would be bright red and not dark red, but this criterion could be nullified if the needle at first entered the vein and only in the course of the injection pierced the venous wall and slipped into the artery.

Case-4

1. The fracture of the humerus severed the radial nerve, which comes in contact with the bone in the spiral groove. The resultant clinical condition is known as wrist drop due to paralysis of all of the extensors of the wrist.

2. With paralysis of extensors of the wrist, the wrist and the fingers go into an exaggerated flexed position due to the unopposed action of flexors. Extension of the forearm was weakened, but not lost, because the branches of the radial nerve to the long head and medial head normally emerge from above the site of lesion. The brachioradialis muscle is actually a flexor of the forearm,

and its loss explains somewhat reduced strength of flexion, such reduction is barely noticeable. The loss of cutaneous sensation at the back of the arm, forearm and lateral part of the dorsum of the hand were due to the involvement of the cutaneous branches of the radial nerve

3. Profunda brachii artery

MCQs

1. A man suffers a penetrating wound through the anterior axillary fold, resulting in damage to one of the main terminal branches of the brachial plexus, effect is a significant weakening of flexion of the elbow. The other effect to be expected is

   A. Weakening of flexion at the shoulder
   B. Loss of cutaneous sensation on the anterolateral surface of the forearm
   C. Loss of cutaneous sensation on the tips of several fingers
   D. Only weakening of flexion at the shoulder

2. A 35-year-old construction worker arrives in the emergency room after an accident. The tendon of the biceps brachii at the elbow has been severed by a laceration that extends 2 cm medially from the tendon. Which of the following structures is likely to have been injured by medial extension or the laceration?

   A. Brachial artery
   B. Musculocutaneous nerve
   C. Ulnar nerve
   D. Radial nerve

3. In street fight while escaping a stab, a 34-year-old man injures his anterior surface of the middle of the right arm. The stab severs all the tissues till the bone. When examined in the emergency room it is noted that the patient can weakly flex his elbow and the lateral side of his forearm is numb. In addition to the muscles, which nerve is injured?

   A. Median
   B. Ulnar
   C. Radial
   D. Musculocutaneous

4. While riding a bike, a person fell against a tree and fractured the shaft of the humerus at mid length. Which nerve may be injured that lie in proximity to the injury?

   A. Ulnar
   B. Radial
   C. Axillary
   D. Median

SECTION 3

5. In a fracture of the mid shaft of the humerus, which artery is most likely to be injured?

   A. Profunda brachii
   B. Subscapular
   C. Posterior circumflex humeral
   D. Radial recurrent

6. As an inexperienced phlebotomist (blood drawer) attempts to insert the needle to draw blood from the median cubital vein, the patient suddenly screams and complains of pain and burning in the middle and thumb side of his palm. The nerve accidentally impaled by the needle was the

   A. Medial cutaneous nerve of the forearm
   B. Lateral cutaneous nerve of the forearm
   C. Ulnar
   D. Median

7. Supination of the hand and forearm would be diminished by loss of radial nerve function. But one of the following powerful supinator would remain intact and unaffected, namely:

   A. Supinator
   B. Brachialis
   C. Brachioradialis
   D. Biceps brachii

8. If the musculocutaneous nerve is severed at its origin from the brachial plexus, flexion at the elbow is greatly weakened but not abolished. What muscle remains operative and can contribute to flexion?

   A. Triceps brachii
   B. Brachialis
   C. Coracobrachialis
   D. Long head of biceps brachii

9. An elderly patient faints on her outstretched arm. She complains of pain at her elbow. Physical examination reveals a palpable defect at the location of her biceps tendon. The elbow flexion causes pain, but she is still able to actively flex her elbow. Radiographs do not show evidence of a fracture or dislocation. She is diagnosed with a biceps tendon rupture. Which of the following muscles allow the patient to continue flexing her elbow?

   A. Brachialis and brachioradialis
   B. Flexor carpi ulnaris and flexor carpi radialis
   C. Flexor digitorum superficialis and flexor digitorum profundus
   D. Pronator teres and supinator

10. During insertion of an IV cannula in the median cubital vein, the patient suddenly lost feeling on the radial side of the forearm. Which nerve was injured?

   A. Lateral cutaneous nerve of the forearm
   B. Medial cutaneous nerve of the forearm
   C. Posterior cutaneous nerve of the forearm
   D. Superficial terminal branch radial nerve

Answers to MCQs

1.B
2.A
3.D
4.B
5.A
6.D
7.D
8.B
9.A
10.A

Forearm, Elbow Joint, Radioulnar Joints and Wrist Joint

- Anterior compartment of the forearm
- Posterior compartment of the forearm
- Elbow joint
- Radioulnar joints
- Wrist joint
- MCQs

Objectives

- To list the muscles of the anterior and posterior compartments of the forearm, their insertion, nerve supply and actions
- To explain the attachment of extensor retinaculum of the wrist and to identify the structures passing deep to it
- To know the course, branches of radial and ulnar arteries in the forearm
- To explain the bones articulating, ligaments stabilizing, movements occurring and muscles producing them in the elbow, radio-ulnar, wrist and first carpo-metacarpal joints

ANTERIOR COMPARTMENT OF THE FOREARM

The two bones of the forearm, radius and ulna with interosseus membrane between them divides the forearm into anterior and posterior compartments. The anterior compartment consists of muscles, vessels and nerves.

Muscles: The muscles of the anterior compartment are described in superficial and deep groups. The primary action of these muscles is flexion at the wrist joint with few exceptions. The superficial group has a common origin from the medial epicondyle of the humerus which is referred as 'common flexor origin'. Majority of these muscles enter the palm after traversing deep to the flexor retinaculum of the hand. All the muscles in the anterior compartment are supplied by median nerve or its branch, anterior interosseus nerve except for flexor carpi ulnaris and medial half of the flexor digitorum profundus. The attachments, specific nerve supply and actions are explained in Tables 9.1 and 9.2.

Vessels: The radial and ulnar arteries on their way to the hand traverse the anterior compartment with number of branches.

Nerves: The median and the ulnar nerve traverse the anterior compartment.

Muscles of the front of the forearm

It consists of superficial and deep groups. These muscles mainly cause flexion at the elbow and wrist joints. Hence, this compartment is called the flexor compartment (Figs 9.1 and 9.2).

Superficial muscles

These superficial muscles have a common origin from the medial epicondyle of the humerus (common flexor origin).

1. Pronator teres
2. Flexor carpi radialis
3. Palmaris longus
4. Flexor carpi ulnaris
5. Flexor digitorum superficialis (sublimis)

Muscle	Origin	Insertion	Nerve supply	Actions
Table 9.1 Superficial flexor muscles of the forearm				
Pronator teres	Medial epicondyle of humerus	Middle of lateral aspect of shaft of radius	Median nerve	Pronation of forearm
Flexor carpi radialis	Medial epicondyle of humerus	Bases of second and third metacarpals	Median nerve	Flexes and abducts the hand at the wrist
Palmaris longus	Medial epicondyle of humerus	Flexor retinaculum and palmar aponeurosis	Median nerve	Flexes wrist joint
Flexor digitorum superficialis • **Humero ulnar head** • **Radial head**	Medial epicondyle of humerus; medial border of coronoid process of ulna Anterior oblique line of shaft of radius	Divided into 4 tendons. Each tendon splits into two, gets inserted to the sides of middle phalanx of 2nd to 5th digits	Median nerve	Flexes the middle phalanx and assists in flexing of proximal phalanx and the wrist joint
Flexor carpi ulnaris • **Humeral head** • **Ulnar head**	Medial epicondyle of humerus Medial aspect of olecranon process and posterior border of ulna	Pisiform bone; further tendon extends and gets inserted to the hook of the hamate and base of fifth metacarpal bone	Ulnar nerve	Flexes and adducts hand at the wrist joint

SECTION 3

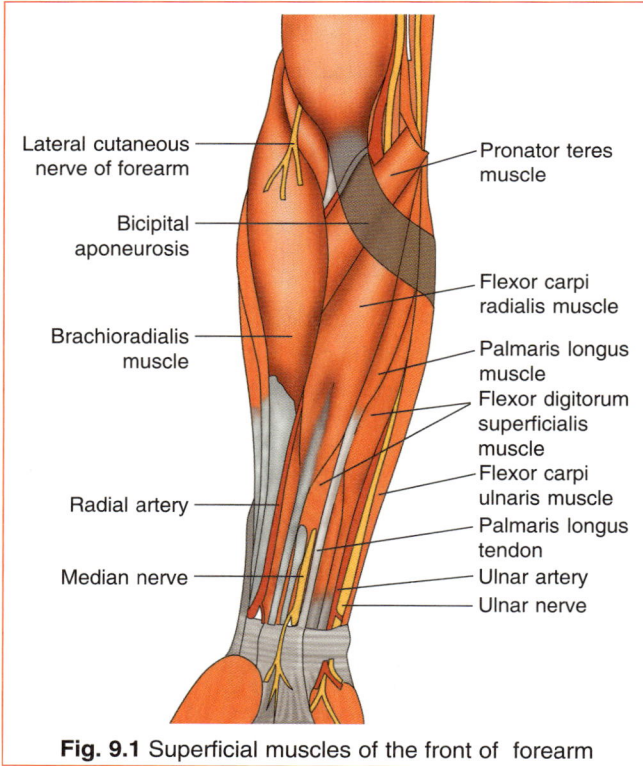

Fig. 9.1 Superficial muscles of the front of forearm

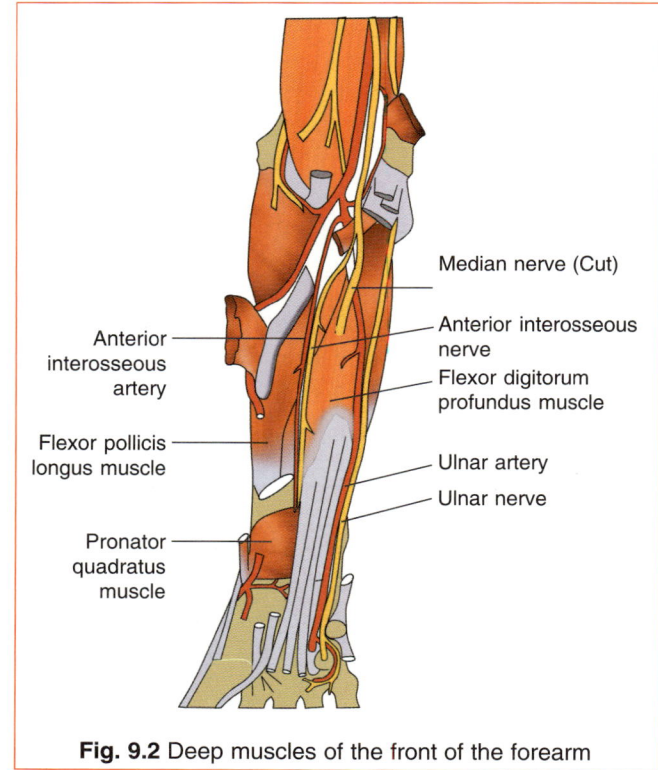

Fig. 9.2 Deep muscles of the front of the forearm

All these muscles are supplied by **median nerve** except flexor carpi ulnaris ,which is supplied by **ulnar nerve**.

Deep muscles

1. Flexor digitorum profundus

2. Flexor pollicis longus

3. Pronator quadratus

The long tendons of these muscles (Flexor digitorum superficialis, flexor digitorum profundus and flexor pollicis longus) while passing through the hand (over the carpal bones) are held in position by a fibrous band called **flexor retinaculum**.

Testing of flexor digitorum superficialis: This muscle is required for flexing the middle phalanx of the medial four fingers. The person is asked to flex the middle phalanx of the finger (to be examined), but other fingers needs to be held in extended position to eliminate the action of flexor digitorum profundus.

Testing of flexor digitorum profundus: This muscle is required to flex the distal phalanx. The person is asked to flex the finger (to be examined) with resistance applied to remaining fingers not flex at both proximal and distal inter phalangeal joints.

Radial artery

- It is one of the terminal branches of the brachial artery given at the neck of the radius in the cubital fossa.

- It descends superficially in the forearm along the lateral border. It leaves the forearm by turning posteriorly to enter the anatomical snuffbox.

- The artery is superficial in the distal part of the forearm, covered by skin and fascia. In the proximal part of the forearm it is covered superficially by brachioradialis muscle.

- While descending in the forearm, the radial artery is related to many structures from above downwards. These posterior relations of the radial artery in the forearm is

Table 9.2 Deep muscles of the front of the forearm

Muscle	Origin	Insertion	Nerve supply	Actions
Flexor digitorum profundus	Upper ¾ of anterior and medial surface of shaft of ulna. Upper ¾ of posterior border and medial surface of olecranon and coronoid processes of ulna. Adjoining anterior surface of interosseous membrane.	Forms 4 tendons for medial 4 digits. Passes deep to flexor retinaculum to enter the palm. Perforates the tendon of flexor digitorum superficialis at the level of proximal phalanx. Inserted to palmar surface of base of distal phalanx	Medial half by ulnar nerve. Lateral half by anterior interosseous nerve.	Flexes the distal phalanx combined with the action of flexor digitorum superficialis. Flexes other joints of digits, fingers and wrist. Acts better when wrist is extended
Flexor pollicis longus	Upper ¾ of anterior surface of shaft of radius ;adjoining anterior surface of interosseous membrane	Passes deep to the flexor retinaculum to enter the palm Inserted into palmar surface of distal phalanx of the thumb	Anterior interosseous nerve	Flexes the distal phalanx of thumb Flexes the proximal joints that is crossed by the tendon
Pronator quadratus	Oblique ridge on the lower ¼ of anterior surface of shaft of ulna and adjoining medial area	Superficial fibres- lower ¼ of anterior surface and anterior border of radius Deep fibres- triangular area above ulnar notch	Anterior interosseous nerve	Superficial fibres- pronates the forearm Deep fibres- fixes the lower ends of radius and ulna

SECTION 3

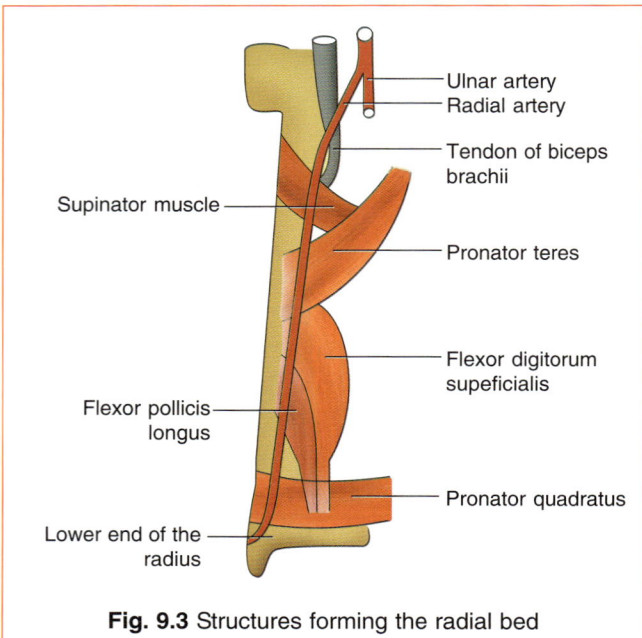

Fig. 9.3 Structures forming the radial bed

SECTION 3

referred as 'radial bed'. The following structures form the radial bed (Fig. 9.3)

1. Tendon of biceps brachii
2. Supinator
3. Pronator teres
4. Flexor digitorum superficialis
5. Flexor pollicis longus
6. Pronator quadratus
7. Lower end of the radius

• The terminal part of the radial artery appears in the hand where it forms deep palmar arch.

• The radial artery gives following branches in the forearm.

a. Radial recurrent: This branch arises in the cubital fossa and take part in anastomoses with radial collateral artery

b. Muscular branches to muscles of the front of the forearm

c. Palmar carpal branch: It arises at the level of the distal border of the pronator quadratus muscle and enters the palm. It anastomose with palmar carpal branch of the ulnar artery and recurrent branch from the deep palmar arch

d. Dorsal carpal branch (posterior radial carpal branch) for the formation of dorsal carpal arch with similar branch from the ulnar artery.

e. Superficial palmar branch: It enters the palm through the thenar muscle and joins the superficial palmar branch of the ulnar artery to complete the superficial palmar branch.

Radial pulse is felt against the anterior surface of the lower end of the radius, lateral to the tendon of flexor carpi radialis muscle. For the blood gas analysis, the radial artery is punctured, this being most superficial artery compared to the remaining arteries.

CASE-1

Palpation of the radial arterial pulse at the wrist can provide the experienced physician a considerable insight into the state of the patient's circulatory system. The degree of hardness of the arterial wall can be appreciated by the examining finger, the pulse rate, quality and rhythm can be determined. The amount of pressure required to occlude the vessel can be used to assess the blood pressure. What are the relations of the radial artery at the site where the pulse is taken?

Ulnar artery

• It is the larger terminal branch of brachial artery arises in the cubital fossa at the level of neck of the radius.

• It leaves the cubital fossa by descending deep to the deep head of the pronator teres muscle which separates the artery from the median nerve.

• In the forearm the ulnar artery passes deep to the superficial flexors of the forearm in the proximal part. In the distal part it is under the cover of flexor carpi ulnaris muscle. Further down it becomes superficial covered by skin and fascia (Fig. 9.4).

• It enters the palm, superficial to the flexor retinaculum lateral to the ulnar nerve. In the palm, the ulnar artery divides into superficial and deep branches.

• The superficial branch continues to form **superficial palmar arch**, which is joined on the lateral side by branches of the radial artery.

• The deep branch of ulnar artery joins the terminal part of the radial artery to form the **deep palmar arch**.

• Hence the two terminal branches of brachial artery anastomose with each other and help in collateral circulation in case of thrombosis of any one of the arteries.

• The ulnar artery gives following branches

a. In the cubital fossa it gives anterior and posterior ulnar recurrent branches which take part in anastomoses around the elbow joint.

b. Common interosseous artery: It arises from the lateral side of ulnar artery in the cubital fossa. At the upper border of the interosseus membrane it divides into anterior and posterior interosseous arteries.

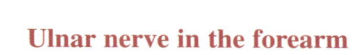

Anterior interosseus artery: It descends on the anterior surface of the interosseous membrane along with the anterior interosseous nerve. At the proximal border of the pronator quadrates muscle it pierces the interosseous membrane to enter the posterior compartment. It enters the dorsum of the hand deep to the extensor retinaculum of the hand. The anterior interosseous artery gives nutrient branches to radius and ulna and a median artery that accompanies the median nerve.

c. Muscular branches to the muscles of the front of the forearm.

d. Palmar and dorsal carpal branches

e. The superficial and deep terminal branches

Median nerve in the forearm

• It leaves the cubital fossa by passing between the two heads of the pronator teres muscle.

• In the forearm it descends deep to the flexor digitorum superficialis and superficial to flexor digitorum profundus muscles.

• In the distal part of the forearm the nerve becomes superficial to the tendons of flexor digitorum superficialis and posterior to the palmaris longus tendon. It enters the palm by passing deep to the flexor retinaculum.

Branches:

In the cubital fossa it gives muscular branches to pronator teres, palmaris longus, flexor carpi radialis and flexor digitorum superficialis.

Articular branches to elbow and radioulnar joints.

In the forearm

1. Anterior interosseus nerve:

It arises from the median nerve just distal to the cubital fossa. It descends in front of the interosseus membrane along with the anterior interosseus artery. The nerve passes posterior to the pronator quadratus to end in front of the wrist.

It supplies the lateral half of the flexor digitorum profundus (which gives origin to the tendons for index and middle fingers), flexor pollicis longus and pronator quadratus. It also supplies the distal radioulnar joint, wrist joint and intercarpal joints.

2. Muscular branch to the flexor digitorum superficialis which gives origin to the tendon of index finger.

3. Palmar cutaneous nerve: It descends superficial to the flexor retinaculum and supplies the skin of the palm over the thenar eminence.

Ulnar nerve in the forearm

• The ulnar nerve passes behind the medial epicondyle.

• It passes between the two heads of the flexor carpi ulnaris in close relation to the ulnar collateral ligaments.

• The nerve descends in the medial side of the forearm superficial to the flexor digitorum profundus and deep to the flexor carpi ulnaris.

• In the lower part of the forearm, the nerve becomes superficial covered by skin and fascia.

• It enters the palm superficial to the flexor retinaculum along with the ulnar artery lateral to the pisiform bone. Some fibres of flexor retinaculum passes superficial to the nerve and the artery to form 'Guyon's canal.

Branches:

In the forearm the ulnar nerve gives

a. Articular branches to the elbow joint

b. Muscular branches to the flexor carpi ulnaris and medial half of the flexor digitorum profundus, that sends tendons to ring and little fingers.

c. Palmar cutaneous branch arises near the wrist, which passes superficial to the flexor retinaculum, supplying the skin over the hypothenar eminence of the palm.

d. Dorsal cutaneous branch supplies the skin of the medial part of the dorsum of the hand.

POSTERIOR COMPARTMENT OF THE FOREARM

The posterior compartment consists of 12 extensor muscles which are arranged in superficial and deep groups. Apart from these muscles, the posterior interosseus nerve and artery and in the distal part of the forearm, the anterior interosseus artery is present.

Muscles of the back of the forearm

This compartment (extensor) consists of superficial and deep groups. These muscles mainly causes extension at the wrist joint and are supplied by **radial nerve** (OR its branch called posterior interosseus nerve). Paralysis of these muscles causes 'wrist drop'.

Before passing into the dorsum of the hand, the tendons of these muscles are held in their proper position by a fibrous band called **extensor retinaculum** opposite to the wrist.

Superficial muscles

1. Anconeus—Extends the elbow joint

2. Brachioradialis—Flexes the elbow joint in midprone position.

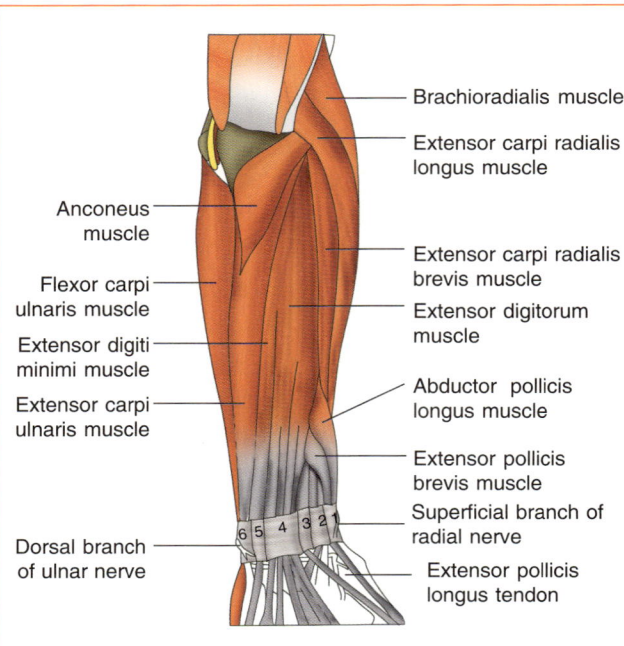

Anconeus muscle

Flexor carpi ulnaris muscle

Extensor digiti minimi muscle

Extensor carpi ulnaris muscle

Dorsal branch of ulnar nerve

Brachioradialis muscle

Extensor carpi radialis longus muscle

Extensor carpi radialis brevis muscle

Extensor digitorum muscle

Abductor pollicis longus muscle

Extensor pollicis brevis muscle

Superficial branch of radial nerve

Extensor pollicis longus tendon

Fig. 9.4 Superficial extensors of the forearm

3. Extensor carpi radialis longus—Extends and abducts the wrist.

4. Extensor carpi radialis brevis—Extends and abducts the wrist.

5. Extensor digitorum—It divides into four tendons for medial four fingers.

6. Extensor digiti minimi—Extends the little finger.

7. Extensor carpi ulnaris—Extends and adducts the wrist joint.

Deep muscles (Figs 9.5 and 9.6)

1. Supinator

2. Abductor pollicis longus—Abducts the thumb.

3. Extensor pollicis brevis—Extends the thumb.

4. Extensor pollicis longus—Extends the thumb.

5. Extensor indicis—Extends the index finger.

The attachments, actions and nerve supply of these muscles are explained in the Table 9.3

Table 9.3 Superficial muscles of the back of forearm				
Muscle	*Origin*	*Insertion*	*Nerve supply*	*Actions*
Anconeus	Lateral epicondyle of humerus	Lateral surface of olecranon process of ulna	Radial nerve	Extends the elbow joint
Brachioradialis	Upper 2/3rd of lateral supracondylar ridge of humerus	Base of styloid process of radius	Radial nerve	Flexes the forearm at elbow joint in mid prone position
Extensor carpi radialis longus	Lower 1/3rd of supracondylar ridge of humerus	Posterior surface of base of 2nd metacarpal	Radial nerve	Extends and abducts hand at wrist joint
Extensor carpi radialis brevis	Lateral epicondyle of humerus	Posterior surface of base of 3rd metacarpal	Radial nerve (deep branch)	Extends and abducts hand at wrist joint
Extensor digitorum	Lateral epicondyle of humerus	Bases of middle phalanx of 2nd–5th digits	Radial nerve (deep branch)	Extends the digits of hand
Extensor digiti minimi	Lateral epicondyle of humerus	Dorsal digital expansion of little finger	Radial nerve (deep branch)	Extensor of meta-carpophalangeal joint of little finger
Extensor carpi ulnaris	Lateral epicondyle of humerus	Bases of 5th metacarpal	Radial nerve (deep branch)	Extends and adducts the hand at wrist joint

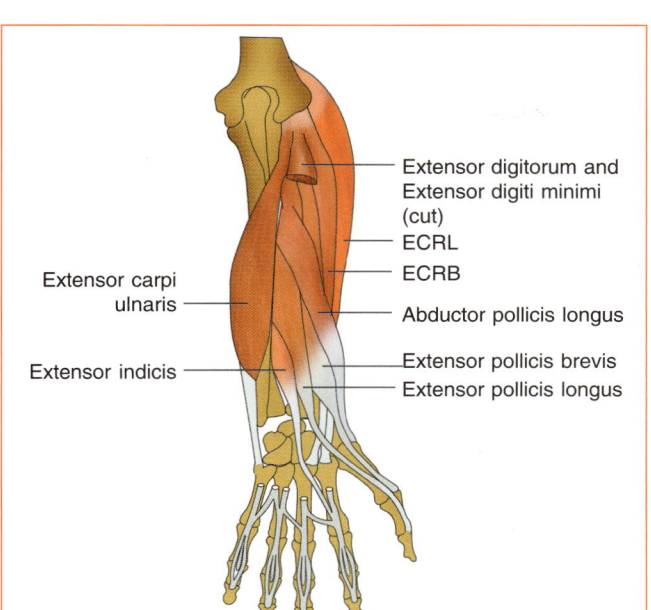

Fig. 9.5 Deep extensors of the forearm

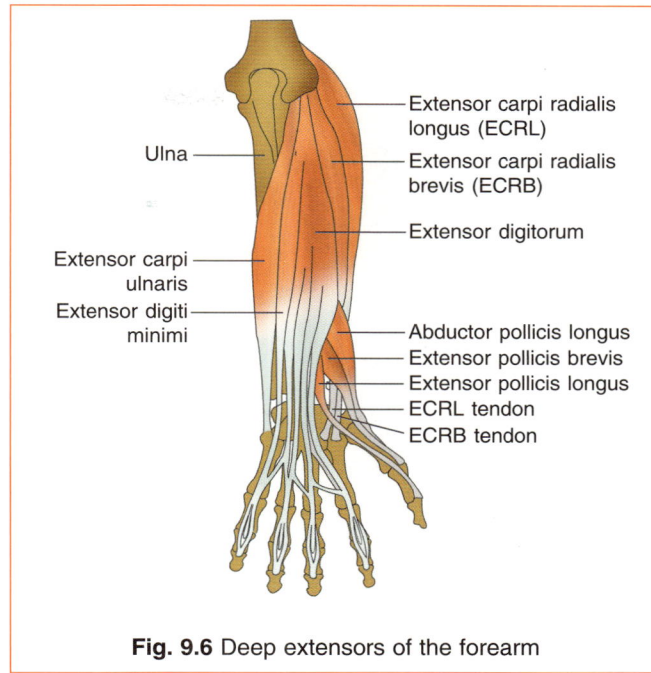

Fig. 9.6 Deep extensors of the forearm

Extensor retinaculum of the wrist

It is formed by the modification of the deep fascia present at the back of the wrist. Functionally it holds the long extensor tendons in their respective position during the movements at the wrist joint (Fig. 9.7).

Attachments: Medially it is attached to the pisiform and triquetral bones. Laterally to the anterior border of the lower end of the radius.

Table 9.4 Deep muscles of back of forearm

Muscle	Origin	Insertion	Nerve supply	Actions
Supinator	Lateral epicondyle of humerus, Annular ligament of superior radioulnar joint, Supinator crest of ulna and a depression behind it	Neck and complete shaft of upper 1/3rd of radius	Radial nerve (deep branch)	Supination of forearm in extended elbow
Abductor pollicis longus	Posterior surface of shaft of radius and ulna	Base of first metacarpal on the dorsal surface	Radial nerve (deep branch)	Abducts and extends thumb
Extensor pollicis brevis	Posterior surface of shaft of radius	Base of proximal phalanx of thumb	Radial nerve (deep branch)	Extends metacarpophalangeal joint of thumb
Extensor pollicis longus	Posterior surface of shaft of ulna	Base of distal phalanx of thumb	Radial nerve (deep branch)	Extends distal phalanx of thumb
Extensor indicis	Posterior surface of shaft of ulna	Dorsal digital expansion of index finger	Radial nerve (deep branch)	Extends the metacarpophalangeal joint of index finger

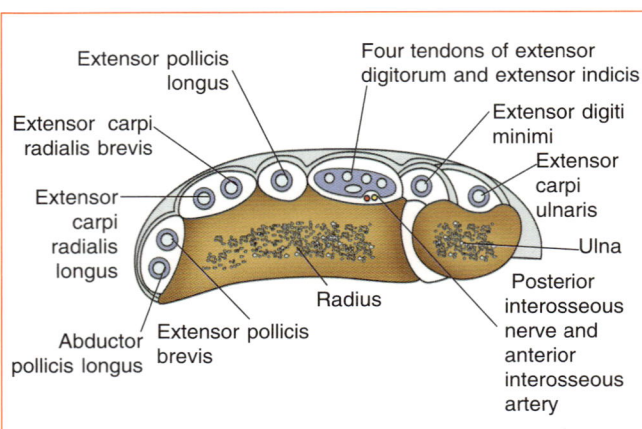

Fig. 9.7 Extensor retinaculum of the wrist

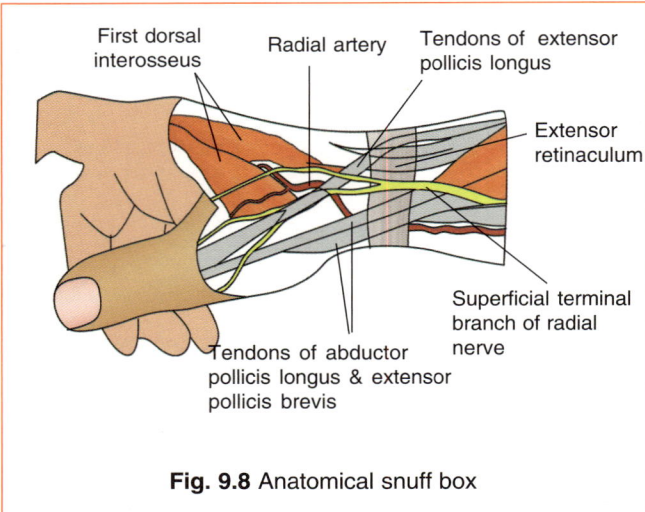

Fig. 9.8 Anatomical snuff box

Relations: It is crossed superficially by superficial terminal branch of the radial nerve, cephalic vein and cutaneous branch of the ulnar nerve.

From the under surface of the retinaculum septa passes deep and is attached to the dorsal surface of the distal end of the radius forming 6 osseofascial compartments. Each compartment is traversed by extensor tendons with their synovial sheaths. The compartment and their contents from lateral to medial side are

1. Abductor pollicis longus

   Extensor pollicis brevis

2. Extensor carpi radialis longus (ECRL)

   Extensor carpi radialis brevis (ECRB)

3. Extensor pollicis longus

4. Extensor digitorum (4 tendons)

   Extensor indicis

   Posterior interosseous nerve

   Anterior interosseous artery

5. Extensor digiti minimi (between radius and ulna)

6. Extensor carpi ulnaris

Anatomical snuff box

It is a hollow space present at the lateral side of the back of the wrist. It becomes visible with extended digits and the thumb (Fig. 9.8).

Boundaries

Anteriorly (laterally): Tendons of abductor pollicis longus and extensor pollicis brevis

Posteriorly (medially): Tendon of extensor pollicis longus

Roof: Superficial terminal branch of the radial nerve and the cephalic vein.

Floor: The trapezium, **scaphoid** and styloid process of the radius.

1. The anatomical snuff box is traversed by the radial artery. Pulsation of the artery can be felt in the floor.

2. Among the carpal bones, the scaphoid is more vulnerable to fracture. If the fracture is suspected there will be tenderness in the anatomical snuff box.

Dorsal digital expansion (Fig. 9.9)

The extensor tendons expands to form dorsal digital expansion. It is triangular in shape present dorsal to the metacarpophalangeal joint and the proximal phalanx. The tendon of the extensor digitorum occupies the central part of the expansion. The posterolateral corners of the expansion

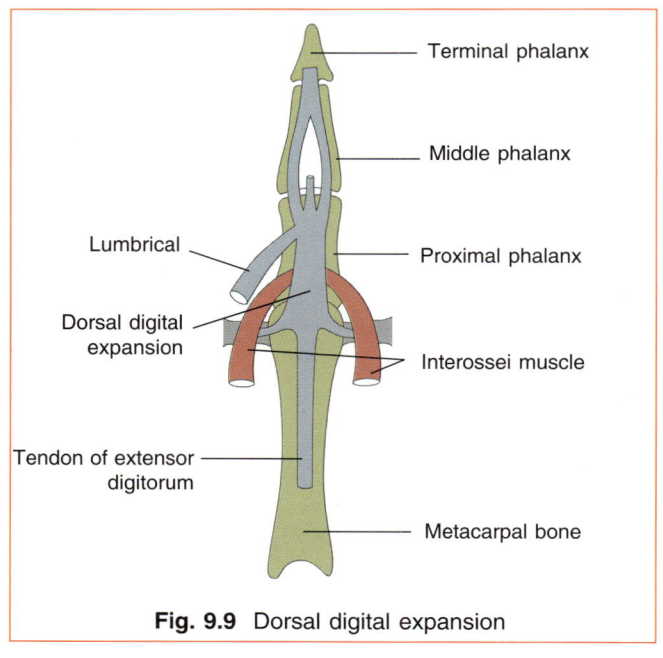

Fig. 9.9 Dorsal digital expansion

receives insertion of interossei and lumbricals. Distally each expansion divides into a central and 2 collateral slips. The central slip is attached to dorsum of the base of the middle phalanx, while collateral slips to base of the distal phalanx. Through these attachments, the lumbricals and interossei bring extension at the interphalangeal joints.

Muscles inserted into each expansions:

1. Index finger: First lumbrical, first dorsal interosseus and second palmar interosseus.
2. Middle finger: Second and third dorsal interossei and second lumbricals,
3. Ring finger: Fourth dorsal interosseus, third lumbrical and third palmar interosseus
4. Little finger: Fourth palmar interosseus, fourth lumbrical.

Posterior interosseous nerve

- It is the deep terminal branch of the radial nerve. It pierces the supinator muscle and appears in the posterior compartment of the forearm as posterior interosseous nerve.
- It is closely related to lateral aspect of the neck of the radius.
- The nerve descends between the superficial and deep extensor muscles of the forearm.
- In it's course downwards, it directly rests on the interosseous membrane.
- It is accompanied by posterior interosseus artery in the proximal part but in the distal part it is accompanied by anterior interosseous artery.
- It passes deep to the extensor retinaculum occupying the fourth compartment and ends in a pseudoganglion (accumulation of connective tissue around the terminal part of the nerve)

Branches:

1. Before piercing the supinator it gives branches to the supinator and extensor carpi radialis brevis.
2. Muscular branches to extensor digitorum, extensor digiti minimi and extensor carpi ulnaris, extensor pollicis longus, extensor indicis, abductor pollicis longus and extensor pollicis brevis

> The posterior interosseous nerve is vulnerable to injury in dislocation of the head of the radius.

ELBOW JOINT

Type

It is a hinge variety of synovial joint. It is also a compound joint since three bones are taking part in the joint formation.

Bones articulating

The lower end of the humerus presents trochlea and capitulum. The trochlea of the humerus articulates with trochlear notch of ulna and capitulum with upper surface of the head of the radius (Fig. 9.10). The elbow joint and the superior radioulnar joints have a common capsule.

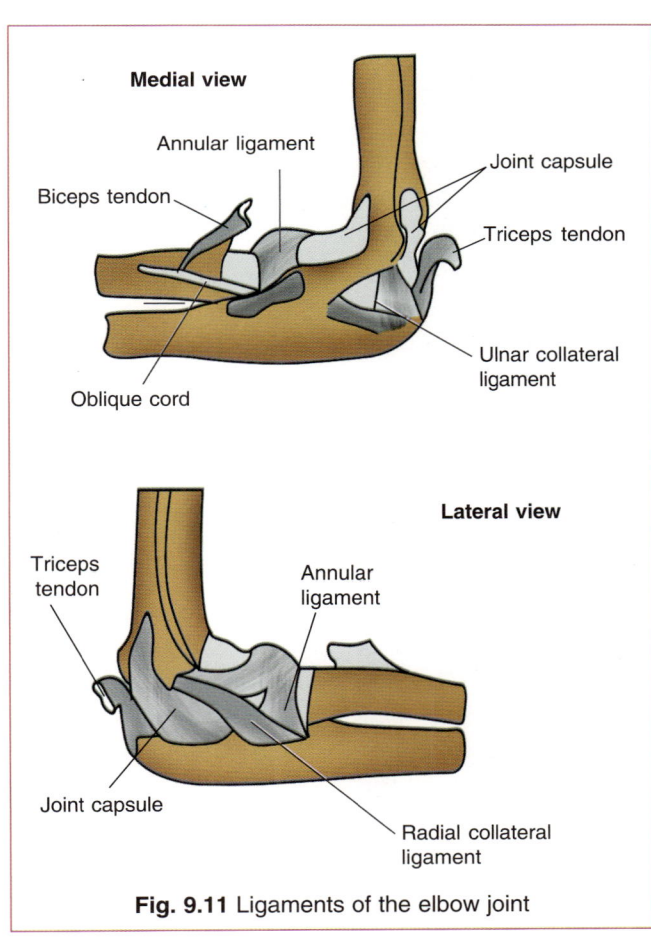

Fig. 9.11 Ligaments of the elbow joint

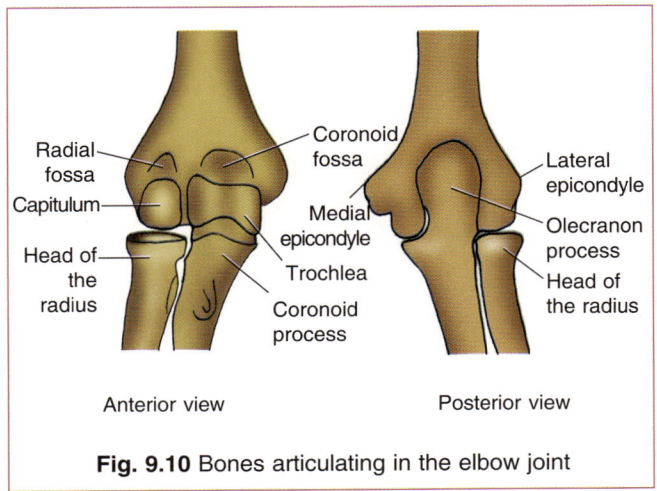

Fig. 9.10 Bones articulating in the elbow joint

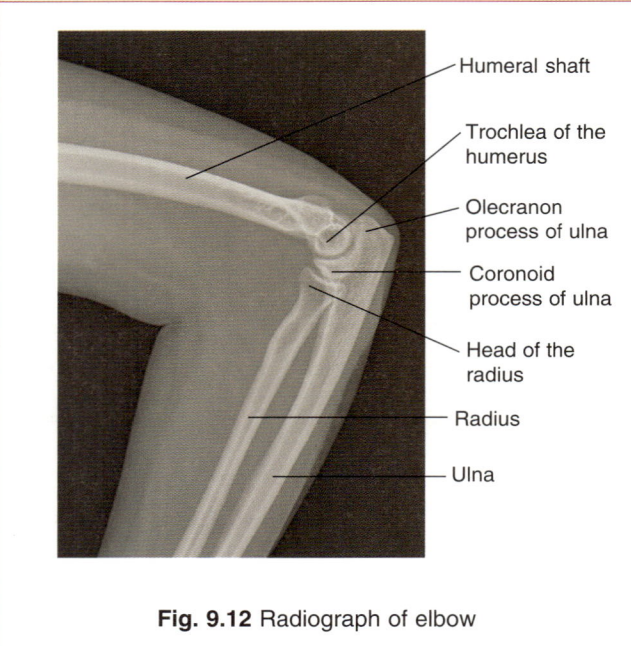

Fig. 9.12 Radiograph of elbow

Labels (top to bottom):
- Humeral shaft
- Trochlea of the humerus
- Olecranon process of ulna
- Coronoid process of ulna
- Head of the radius
- Radius
- Ulna

Structures stabilizing the joint

1. **Capsular ligament (fibrous capsule):** It is attached to the lower end of the humerus in such a way that it encloses coronoid, radial fossae in front and olecranon fossa behind. However, the two epicondyles of the humerus are outside the attachment of fibrous capsule. Below it is attached to the margins of trochlear notch of ulna medially. Laterally, it blends with annular ligament of the superior radio ulnar joint (Fig. 9.11). The fibrous capsule is lined by synovial membrane.

Inside the joint cavity there are three fat filled fossae. On the anterior aspect the coronoid fossa is present above the trochlea and radial fossa above the capitulum. On the posterior aspect there is an olecranon fossa. During flexion of the elbow joint, the coronoid and radial fossae are occupied by coronoid process of ulna and head of the radius respectively. During extension the olecranon fossa is occupied by olecranon process of the ulna.

2. **Ulnar collateral (Medial ligament):** It is thickening of fibrous capsule on the medial side. It is triangular in shape with its apex attached to the medial epicondyle of the humerus. It has an anterior band that is attached to the medial margin of the trochlear notch of the ulna and the posterior band attached to the medial border of the olecranon process. The lower ends of these two bands are connected by an oblique band (Fig. 9.11). The ulnar nerve is related to medial surface of the ligament. The ligament also provides attachment to few fibres of flexor carpi ulnaris muscle.

3. **Radial collateral (Lateral) ligament:** It is the lateral thickening of the fibrous capsule. Above it is attached to the lateral, epicondyle of the humerus and below it blends with annular ligament. The ligament provides origin to some fibres of the supinator muscle.

Relations

Anteriorly: It is related to brachialis muscle, biceps tendon, median nerve, brachial artery.

Posteriorly: Insertion of triceps brachii with olecranon bursa

Medially: Ulnar nerve and common flexor origin.

Laterally: Common extensor origin.

Arterial supply

Elbow joint is supplied by arterial anastomoses around the elbow. The anastomoses is formed by branches of brachial, ulnar, radial and profunda brachii arteries (Fig. 9.12).

Nerve supply

The elbow joint is supplied by branches of musculo-cutaneous, radial and ulnar nerves.

Movements and muscles producing them

Flexion: Brachialis, biceps brachii, brachioradialis and superficial flexors of forearm.

Extension: Triceps and anconeus.

Examination of three important bony land marks around the elbow is a common practice to differentiate posterior dislocation of the elbow joint and supracondylar fracture of humerus. The 3 bony points are medial and lateral epicondyles on each side and olecranon process posteriorly. In extended elbow these three points lie in a straight horizontal line. When the elbow is flexed they form an equilateral triangle. In posterior dislocation this triangle is distorted with backward movement of the olecranon process. But in humeral head fracture the normal bony relation is retained since olecranon moves along with the lower end of the humerus.

The aspiration of the fluid from the joint is performed usually around the olecranon process.

Tennis elbow: It occurs due to the inflammation of the radial collateral ligament and periosteum around the lateral epicondyle. Inflammation or tearing of muscles attached to the lateral epicondyle especially extensor carpi radialis brevis results in pain around the lateral epicondyle. The common cause for this injury is abrupt pronation with fully extended elbow

(Fig. 9.13). It is characterized by severe pain and tenderness in the area of lateral epicondyle.

Golfer's elbow: It is a condition with inflammation at the medial epicondyle. It may be due to inflammation of the ulnar collateral ligament or involvement of muscles attached to the medial epicondyle.

CASE-2

A 19-year old tennis player developed pain and tenderness in the upper lateral aspect of the right forearm following a tennis match. The area surrounding and just distal to the lateral epicondyle of the humerus was most sensitive to pressure. Also, the pain was intensified during backhand shots but was minimal in the forehand stroke. His trainer instructed the player to use a tight elastic band around the upper forearm during play. This helped somewhat initially, but the pain continued and became chronic and severe. The local orthopedic surgeon, who examined the arm and ordered a radiograph of the area involved. The radiograph did not show any bone or joint injury or pathology. The player was instructed to give up tennis until the condition cleared up and he was able to return to active competition after 6 weeks.

1. What are the scientific and layman terms for this condition?

2. What specific action of this portion of the upper limb is responsible for this type of injury?

3. Are there any other activities that would similarly affect this or the medial epicondylar area of the upper limb?

4. Briefly review the position and actions of the muscles of the forearm that are significant in the producing these symptoms.

Carrying angle: It is the angle of deviation of forearm from the axis of the arm when forearm is extended and supinated. The angle ranges from 10–15°. The carrying angle permits the arm to be swung without contacting the hips. The angle is slightly more in females. The angle is due to more downward projection of trochlea of humerus when compared to capitulum.

In **cubitus valgus**, the forearm is deviated more laterally than the normal with increase in the carrying angle. A childhood injury to the lateral epicondyle could cause cubitus valgus, which may gradually stretch the ulnar nerve behind the medial epicondyle (tardy ulnar palsy).

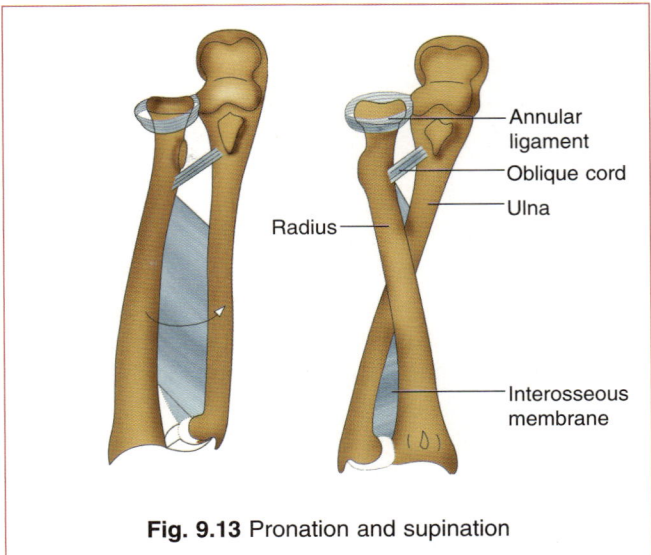

Fig. 9.13 Pronation and supination

In **cubitus varus**, the forearm is deviated medially and the carrying angle is reduced.

Carrying angle may also be defined as an angle between the arm and forearm and is measured from lateral side, which ranges from 160–170°.

CASE-3

A 32-year-old man visits hospital with complaints of intermittent pain and numbness over the anterior and posterior aspect of the ring and little fingers of the right hand. The patient had also noticed a weakness of his fingers of the right hand, especially when performing

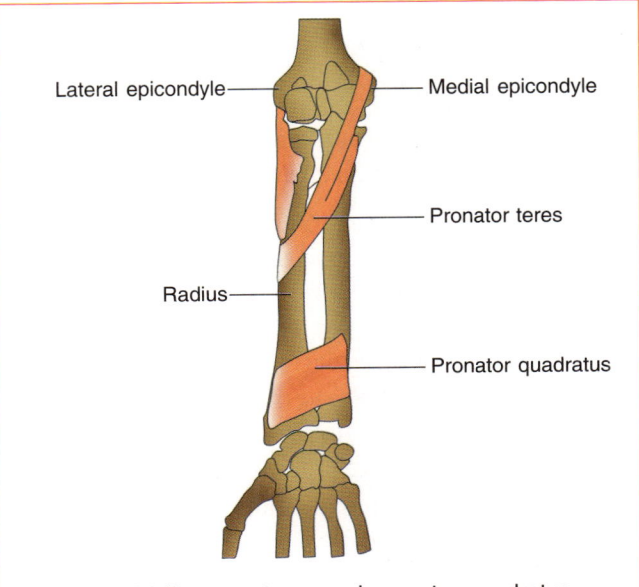

Fig. 9.14 Pronator teres and pronator quadratus

SECTION 3

the upstroke in writing. While taking case history, it was found that at the age of 11 he had a fracture of the lower end of the right humerus in an automobile accident. On examination, his carrying angle on the right side was noted to be greater than the left (cubital valgus), and there was some flattening (wasting) along the medial border of the right forearm. There was also a flattening of hypothenar eminence. On the dorsum of the hand there was evidence of ''hollowing-out'' between the metacarpal bones. The patient could draw his thumb across the palm (opposition), but if asked to pinch a piece of paper between his thumb and index finger, the terminal phalanx of the thumb had to be flexed to grip a piece of paper. Using your anatomical knowledge, explain this patient's disability, remembering that in his young age suffered from a supracondylar fracture of the humerus.

1. Why was the medial border of the forearm flattened?

2. Why was the hypothenar eminence flattened?

3. Why was there ''hollowing-out'' on the dorsum of the hand?

4. Why the patient could not adduct his thumb or his index finger?

RADIOULNAR JOINTS

The two bones of the forearm are connected at their proximal and distal ends by synovial joints. They are called superior and inferior radioulnar joints respectively. However, the shafts of radius and ulna are connected by a fibrous interosseous membrane (fibrous joint).

Superior radioulnar joint

Type: It is a pivot variety of synovial joint.

Bones taking part: The head of the radius articulates with radial notch of ulna and annular ligament.

Annular ligament: It keeps the radial head in position and is attached to the anterior and posterior margins of radial notch of ulna. The annular ligament is continuous above with fibrous capsule of the elbow joint. The ligament enables the head of the radius to rotate during pronation and supination. The annular ligament is internally lined by synovial membrane which continues with synovial membrane of the elbow joint.

The annular ligament in the adult is 'cup' shaped and is firmly attached to the neck of the radius which prevents downward displacement of the radial head. In children the annular ligament is tubular and the size of the head is

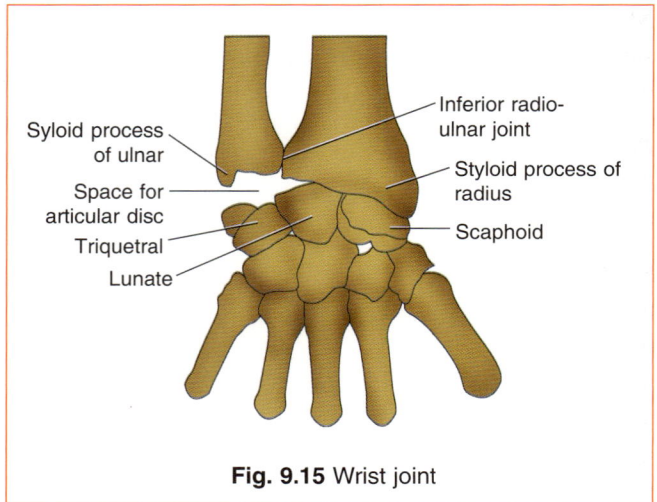

Fig. 9.15 Wrist joint

Labels: Syloid process of ulnar; Space for articular disc; Triquetral; Lunate; Inferior radio-ulnar joint; Styloid process of radius; Scaphoid

smaller. This factor is responsible for downward displacement of radial head in children and is referred as ''**pulled elbow**''.

Quadrate ligament: It extends between the neck of the radius and the lower margin of the radial notch of the ulna.

Inferior radioulnar joint

Type: It is a pivot variety of synovial joint.

Bones taking part: The head of the ulna articulates with ulnar notch of the radius.

The two articulating parts are enclosed in a fibrous capsule which is attached to the articular margin. The capsule is lined internally by a synovial membrane. The synovial membrane projects in front of interosseous membrane behind the pronator quadratus muscle as a narrow recess. The two articulating bones are also connected below by an articular disc (Fig. 9.14).

Articular disc: It is a white fibro cartilagenous structure and is triangular in shape. It separates the head of the ulna from the wrist joint (It is between the head of ulna and triquetral bone) (Fig. 9.15).

Middle radioulnar joint

It is formed by the interosseous membrane which extends between the interosseus borders of the radius to ulna. Proximally the membrane begins about 2 to 3 cm below the radial tuberosity and distally up to the inferior radioulnar joint. The interosseous membrane transmits weight from radius to ulna. The membrane is taut at midprone position. It also provides attachments to many muscles.

Oblique cord: It extends from the lateral aspect of the ulnar tuberosity to the lower end of the radial tuberosity.

Movements: The radioulnar joint permits pronation and supination movements. During these movements the head of the radius and ulna rotate in their bony sockets.

Pronation: The palmar aspect of the hand is turning to face downwards. Pronation is brought by pronator teres and pronator quadratus

Supination: The palmar aspect of the hand turns to face upward (screwing movement). Supination is brought by biceps brachii and supinator muscle.

The axis of movement at the radioulnar joint is not fixed. The vertical axis of movement of the radius passes through head of the radius to ulnar attachment of the articular disc below. The axis moves laterally during pronation and medially during supination, since lower end of the ulna is not fixed.

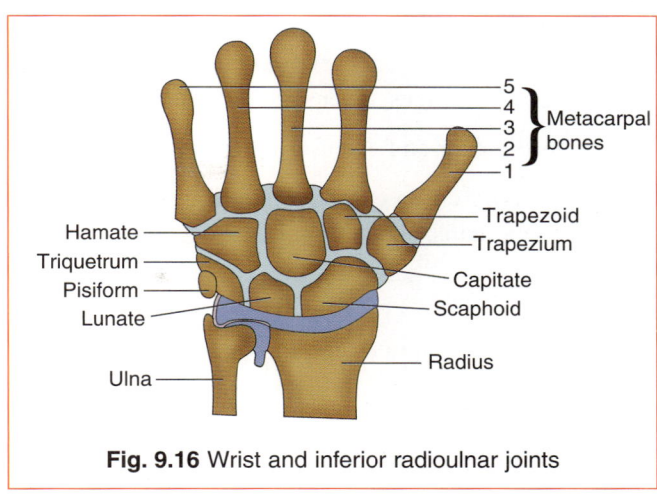

Fig. 9.16 Wrist and inferior radioulnar joints

WRIST JOINT (RADIO CARPAL JOINT)

Type: It is an ellipsoid variety of synovial joint.

Bones taking part:
* From above: The inferior surface of the lower end of the radius and the articular disc of the inferior radioulnar joint.
* From below: Scaphoid, lunate and triquetral bones (from lateral to medial side) below.

The joint is stabilized by a capsular ligament which is thickening on either side forming medial and lateral collateral ligaments (Fig. 9.16).

Fibrous capsule: It is attached to the articular margins of proximal and distal articular areas including the articular disc. Internally it is lined by synovial membrane.

The radial collateral ligament extends from the styloid process of the radius to the scaphoid and the trapezium.

The ulnar collateral ligament extends from the styloid process of the ulna to the triquetral and pisiform bone.

Relations:

Anteriorly: Tendons of flexor digitorum profundus and superficialis, flexor pollicis longus, flexor carpi radialis and ulnaris, median and ulnar nerves.

Posteriorly: Tendons of extensor digitorum, extensor indicis, extensor digiti minimi, extensor carpi radialis longus and brevis, extensor carpi ulnaris, posterior interosseous nerve and anterior interosseous artery.

Arterial supply: Palmar and dorsal carpal arches.

Nerve supply: Anterior and posterior interosseous nerves.

Movements and muscles producing them

Flexion: Flexor carpi radialis and ulnaris Flexor digitorum superficialis and profundus and palmaris longus

---

CASE-4

While playing in the ground, a father picked up his four-year-old daughter by his hand and started swinging her around in a circle. At first the girl giggled, but all of a sudden, she cried out in pain. When her father put her down, he noticed that she was holding her elbow. Her arm was partially flexed and pronated, and she was unable to supinate her hand without considerable pain. She was taken into the hospital. When the physician palpated her elbow, she found that the joint was tender, especially on the lateral side, but all of the bony landmarks were in their normal locations. The physician suspected that the head of the radius has slipped out of the annular ligament. Radiographs proved inconclusive. Fairly certain of the diagnosis, however, the physician attempted to reposition the head of the radius by supinating the forearm fully and then flexing the elbow. The head of the radius slipped back into position.

1. What is the annular ligament and where is it located?

2. What are the bony landmarks that are readily palpable at the elbow?

3. Why this kind of dislocation of the head of the radius common in pre-school children?

4. What other types of elbow dislocations are common and how do they present?

5. Why might the radiographs have been unhelpful in this situation?

Extension: Extensor carpi radialis longus and brevis, extensor carpi ulnaris, extensor digitorum, extensor indicis extensor pollicis longus, extensor digiti minimi

Adduction: Flexor and extensor carpi ulnaris.

Abduction: Extensor carpi radialis longus and brevis flexor carpi radialis, abductor pollicis longus.

CASE-5

A 27-year-old man met with a motor cycle accident. While falling from the motor cycle he stretched out his right hand injuring his wrist. He went to a clinic nearby. The physician advised him for X-ray of the wrist. The injured was reluctant for X-ray as he could move his wrist freely and requested for some pain-killer. After the medication the patient went home with relief of pain. However, he began to experience more pain and a loss of movement in the injured wrist. He visited the hospital and the X-ray was taken. The X-ray confirmed a fracture of the scaphoid bone in the wrist joint.

1. Where do you palpate the scaphoid bone in examining the wrist injuries?

2. What are the boundaries of this space?

3. What is the complication anticipated in a scaphoid fracture?

Solutions to the case studies:

Case-1

The radial artery lies in front of the distal part of the shaft of the radius; it is directly in contact with the front of the bone. On its lateral side lies the terminal part of the tendon of the brachioradialis and on the medial side is the tendon of the flexor carpi radialis muscle. The artery is covered anteriorly by skin and fascia.

Case-2

1. The scientific term for this condition is lateral epicondylitis and the layman term is 'tennis elbow'

2. The usual cause for this condition is repeated extension of the wrist against some force as might occur during the backhand stroke in tennis. This is the result of the fact that majority of the extensors of the wrist and fingers originate from lateral epicondyle. Contraction of these muscles against an oppositely directed force may cause a strain on the tendon of the muscle fibres in the area

around the lateral epicondyle, resulting in the pain and tenderness observed in this patient. The pain could be due to the result of tension on the periosteum of the lateral epicondyle, or a tear in the muscle attached to lateral epicondyle or a tear in the radial collateral ligament of the elbow.

3. Activities such as throwing a baseball can create strain on the medial epicondylar areas especially in young children in whom secondary ossification centres for these areas have not yet fused to the main body of the humerus. Also the golfers are very likely to get medial epicondylitis due to excessive strain over medial epicondyle.

4. Refer text.

Case-3

The patient's old supracondylar fracture of the right humerus had increased the carrying angle on the right side to such an extent that the ulnar nerve posterior to medial epicondyle would move like a string around a pulley when the elbow joint was flexed and extended. Repeated friction caused interstitial neuritis of the ulnar nerve and consequent interference with the motor and sensory functions of the nerve. The upstroke of writing is produced by flexion of the metacarpophalangeal joint and extension of the interphalangeal joints; both movements are normally carried out by the lumbricals and the interossei, which are supplied by the ulnar nerve.

1. Medial border of the forearm was flattened due to the involvement of the flexor carpi ulnaris and medial part of the flexor digitorum profundus.

2. Hypothenar muscles are supplied by ulnar nerve.

3. Hollowing out of the dorsum of the hand is due to the paralysis of dorsal and palmar interossei muscles which are supplied by ulnar nerve.

4. Adduction of the thumb required adductor pollicis and 1st palmar interossei, both are supplied by ulnar nerve.

Case-4

1. The annular ligament is a circular ligament which encloses the head of the radius, holding it firmly in place without directly attaching to the radius. This allows relatively free rotatory movement of the radius at its proximal articulation with the capitulum of the humerus. The annular ligament is attached to the anterior and posterior margins of the radial notch on the ulna.

2. The olecranon process of the ulna, lateral and medial epicondyles of the humerus, and the head of the radius are readily palpable at the elbow. The three-dimensional relationships of these landmarks are important in diagnosing injuries to the elbow joint.

3. This sort of elbow dislocation (pulled elbow, or subluxation of the head of the radius) is common in pre-school children, whose radial heads are small relative to the size of the annular ligament.

4. Other common injuries to the elbow include:

a) Posterior dislocation of the elbow: These are common in children and generally result from falling on an outstretched hand with the elbow flexed. These are easily recognized by unusual protrusion of the olecranon posteriorly along with displacement of the distal end of the humerus anteriorly, disrupting normal articulation with the forearm at the radial head and trochlear notch.

b) Avulsion of the medial epicondyle: Also common in children, this injury results from a fall that causes severe abduction of an extended elbow. The ulnar collateral ligament, which is stronger than the fusion of the diaphysis and epiphysis of the humerus at the medial epicondyle pulls the medial epicondyle away from the humerus. This epiphyseal plate does not usually fuse until 20 years of age.

c) Separation of the proximal radial epiphysis: This injury again happens only in children and is a displacement of the radial head following a fall that places a compression and abduction force on the elbow. This epiphysis usually fuses around 14–17 years of age. In adults, fractures of the elbow tend to occur more frequently than dislocations.

5. The radiographs probably were not helpful because this injury is not likely to tear the joint capsule and as a result, the head of the radius may not be obviously displaced on films. Furthermore, obtaining them was likely difficult in itself because of the age of the patient and the severity of pain caused by manipulation of the elbow.

Case-5

1. In the anatomical snuff box

2. Refer text

3. Refer Chapter 3 (osteology)

MCQs

1. A worker doing repetitive lifting develops an inflammation in the tendon of origin of the extensor carpi radialis brevis muscle, commonly called "tennis elbow". The focal point of pain would most likely be near which palpable bony landmark?

   A. Coronoid process of ulna
   B. Lateral epicondyle of humerus
   C. Lateral supracondylar ridge of humerus
   D. Medial epicondyle of humerus

2. In an attempt to commit suicide by slashing the ventral side of the wrist, the two tendons of the flexor digitorum superficialis located most superficially were completely severed. What movement would be affected?

   A. Flexion of the distal interphalangeal joints of middle and ring fingers
   B. Flexion of the proximal interphalangeal joints of middle and ring fingers
   C. Flexion of the proximal interphalangeal joint of index and little finger
   D. Flexion of the thumb

3. Which muscle is innervated by branches of both the median and ulnar nerves?

   A. Flexor digitorum superficialis
   B. Flexor carpi ulnaris
   C. Flexor digitorum profundus
   D. Flexor pollicis longus

4. While playing basketball, a player jams her middle finger against the ball. She experiences severe pain and she can no longer extend the distal phalanx of that finger. The injury has avulsed (torn away from the bone) which structure from her distal phalanx to produce this condition?

   A. Extensor digitorum
   B. Extensor carpi radialis brevis tendon
   C. Extensor carpi radialis longus tendon
   D. Extensor digiti minimi tendon

5. Development of "tennis elbow" (lateral epicondylitis) may involve inflammation of

   A. Ulnar collateral ligament
   B. Annular ligament
   C. Coracoacromial ligament
   D. Radial collateral ligament

6. The pulse of the radial artery at the wrist is felt immediately lateral to which tendon?

   A. Abductor pollicis longus

SECTION 3

B. Extensor pollicis longus

C. Flexor carpi radialis

D. Flexor digitorum profundus

7. A two-year-old child's hand was forcibly pulled by her mother. The child screams and holds her elbow. The mother notices that the forearm was pronated and she tries to supinate the forearm, which aggravated the pain. Which joint was dislocated?

A. Elbow

B. Superior radioulnar

C. Wrist

D. Inferior radioulnar

8. What sesamoid bone develops in the tendon of flexor carpi ulnaris?

A. Capitate

B. Lunate

C. Pisiform

D. Scaphoid

9. In order to check the pulse of a child whose forearm is in a cast, the pediatrician presses her finger into the depth of the "anatomical snuffbox". What tendon bounds this space posteriorly?

A. Brachioradialis

B. Extensor carpi radialis brevis

C. Extensor carpi radialis longus

D. Extensor pollicis longus

Answers to MCQs

1. B

2. B

3. C

4. A

5. D

6. C

7. B

8. C

9. D

SECTION 3

Hand and Nerves of the Upper Limb

10

- Skin of the palm
- Flexor retinaculum of the hand
- Palmar aponeurosis
- Fibrous flexor sheaths
- Intrinsic muscles of the hand
- Arterial arches
- Nerves of the hand
- Fascial spaces of the hand
- Digital pulp spaces
- Dorsum of the hand
- Major nerves of the upper limb
- MCQs

Objectives
- To know the cutaneous innervation of the hand
- To explain the attachments, structures passing superficial and deep to the flexor retinaculum of the hand
- To explain the attachment and significance of palmar aponeurosis
- To list the muscles of thenar and hypothenar, lumbricals and interossei muscles, their insertion, nerve supply and actions
- To explain the formation, branches and functional relevance of palmar arches
- To explain the course, distribution and clinical relevance of median and ulnar nerves in hand
- To explain the boundaries and clinical relevance of spaces of the hand
- To explain the origin, course, major relations, branches, distribution and clinical relevance of median, ulnar and radial nerves

SKIN OF THE PALM

The skin of the palm is very thick with plenty of sweat glands, but sebaceous glands are absent. The skin is firmly attached to the underlying palmar aponeurosis. The skin of the palm presents several skin lines or creases. They include

Flexure lines: These are transverse markings overlying the joints; where the skin is tightly adherent to the deep fascia.

Papillary ridges: They are better defined in the flexor surface of the distal phalanges of the fingers. These papillary ridges vary from person to person and differ from finger to finger in same person. The ducts of the sweat glands open along the ridges. Papillary ridges are explained in 3 types-whorl, loop and arch. Pattern of finger print is constant in an individual.

Langer's line or cleavage lines: These are the lines produced by the direction in which the collagen fibres are arranged in the dermis. In the palm it is known to be present in longitudinal direction. An incision parallel to the direction of Langer's line will disturb minimum collagen fibres.

Nerve supply to the skin of the palm (Cutaneous innervation)

1. Skin over the thenar eminence is supplied by palmar cutaneous branch of the median nerve arising in the forearm.
2. Skin of the palmar surface of the lateral 3½ fingers including the skin of the dorsal aspect of the terminal phalanges of the corresponding fingers are supplied by digital branches of the median nerve arising in the hand.
3. Skin over the hypothenar eminence is supplied by palmar cutaneous branch of the ulnar nerve arising in the forearm.
4. Skin of the palmar surface of the medial 1½ fingers are supplied by superficial terminal branch of the ulnar nerve in the hand (Figs 10.1 and 10.2).

The dermatomes of the palm includes C6, C7 and C8. The middle three is by C7, thumb by C6 and little finger by C8.

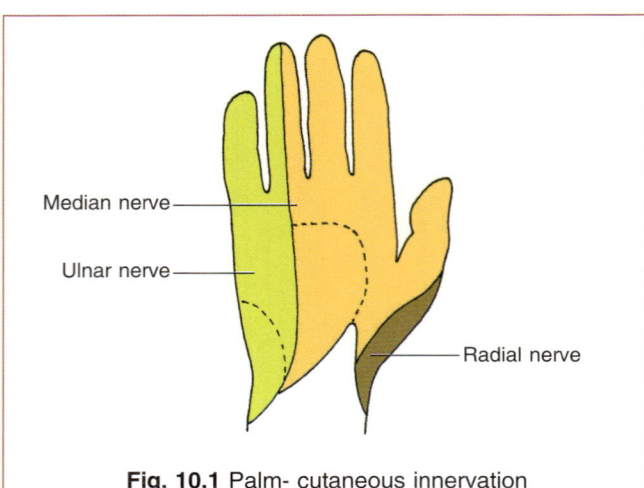

Fig. 10.1 Palm- cutaneous innervation

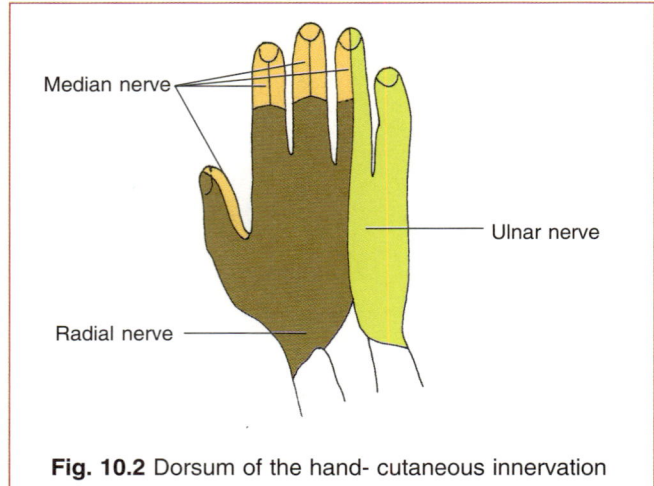

Fig. 10.2 Dorsum of the hand- cutaneous innervation

Superficial fascia

The superficial fascia is made up of fat which connects the skin with palmar aponeurosis. The Palmaris brevis is a subcutaneous muscle present on the medial side.

Deep fascia

The deep fascia of the hand is modified in different ways.

1. It forms flexor retinaculum opposite to the carpal bones.
2. It forms palmar aponeurosis in the central part of the palm.
3. It forms the fibrous flexor sheaths in the palmar aspect of the fingers for the passage of flexor tendons.

FLEXOR RETINACULUM OF THE HAND

It is a modified deep fascia with thick transversely running glistening fibres present opposite to the level of carpal bones. Functionally it holds the long flexor tendons in their position during movements of the wrist joint.

Attachments

Medially it is attached to the pisiform bone and the hook of the hamate. However a superficial slip is attached to the pisiform bone making a tunnel (Guyon's canal) for the passage of ulnar vessels and nerves (Fig. 10.3).

Laterally it is attached to the tubercle of scaphoid and the crest of the trapezium. A deep slip on the lateral side is attached to medial lip of the groove of trapezium forms a tunnel for the passage of flexor carpi radialis tendon.

Structures passing superficial to it

1. Ulnar nerve and vessels
2. Palmaris longus tendon
3. Palmar cutaneous branch of the ulnar nerve

4. Palmar cutaneous branch of the median nerve
5. Superficial palmar branch of the radial artery

Structures passing deep to the flexor retinaculum

1. Median nerve
2. Tendons of flexor digitorum superficialis
3. Tendons of flexor digitorum profundus
4. Tendon of flexor pollicis longus

The tendons of superficialis and profundus are enclosed in a common synovial sheath called ulnar bursa, while tendon of flexor pollicis longus has a separate synovial sheath called radial bursa.

Carpal tunnel: It is an osseo-fibrous tunnel between superficially placed flexor retinaculum and palmar surface of the carpal bone on the deeper side. All the structures passing deep to the flexor retinaculum are the contents of the carpal tunnel. Among them median nerve is clinically

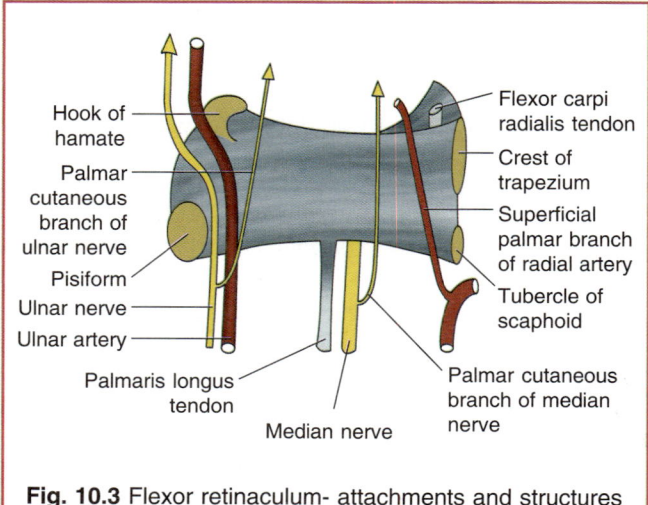

Fig. 10.3 Flexor retinaculum- attachments and structures superficial to it

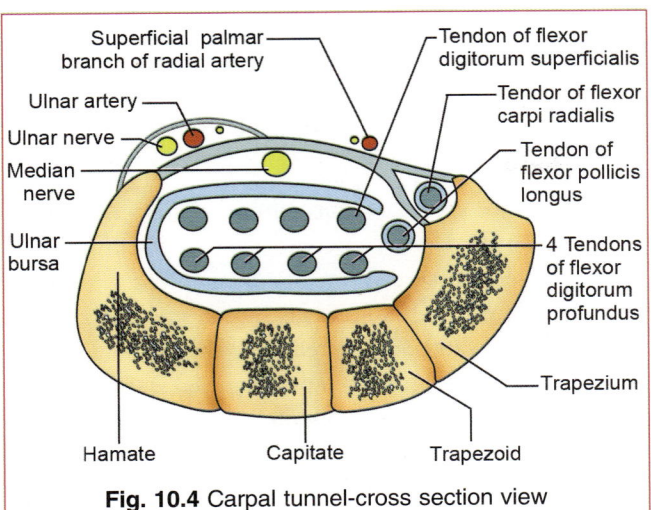

Fig. 10.4 Carpal tunnel-cross section view

significant because in case of inflammation of these tendons in the carpal tunnel the nerve is likely to be compressed. This is referred as 'carpal tunnel syndrome' which will be discussed after explanation of median nerve in the hand (Fig. 10.4).

PALMAR APONEUROSIS

- It is the modification of the deep fascia in the palm, better defined in the central portion of the palm. On medial and lateral side it covers the hypothenar and thenar muscles where it is thin.

- Palmar aponeurosis is triangular in shape with its apex directed proximally and the base distally.

- Proximally it continues with the tendon of the Palmaris longus muscle

- Distally it divides into four digital slips for the medial four fingers. Each slip divides into superficial and deep

slip. The superficial slip blends with the dermis of the skin. The deep slip blends with deep transverse ligament of the palm, metacarpophalangeal joint and base of the proximal phalanges (Fig. 10.5).

- The intervals between the slips are traversed by digital vessels, nerves and tendons of the lumbricals.

- From the medial and the lateral margins of the palmar aponeurosis the medial and lateral palmar septa extends dorsally. The medial septum is attached to the shaft of the 5th metacarpal bone, while lateral septum to shaft of the 1st metacarpal bone. These septa forms the boundary of the fascial spaces of the hand.

- The palmar aponeurosis protects the underlying superficial palmar arterial arch.

- It also provides a firm attachment to the overlying skin to improve the grip.

Dupuytren's contracture

Inflammation of the palmar aponeurosis may result in contracture and thickening of the aponeurosis. It usually affects the medial part of the aponeurosis where it undergoes shortening. This causes flexion deformity of the little and ring fingers. The flexion contracture affects proximal and middle interphalangeal joints but not the distal interphalangeal joint. It is repaired by surgically cutting the affected part of the aponeurosis (Fig. 10.6).

CASE-1

A 60-year-old man consulted his physician because he had noticed a thickening of the skin at the base of his left ring finger during the past three months. He described it as "There appears to be a band of tissue that is pulling my ring finger towards the palm. On examination of the palm of both hands, a localized thickening of the palmar aponeurosis could be felt at the base of the left ring and little fingers. The metacarpophalangeal joint of the ring finger could not

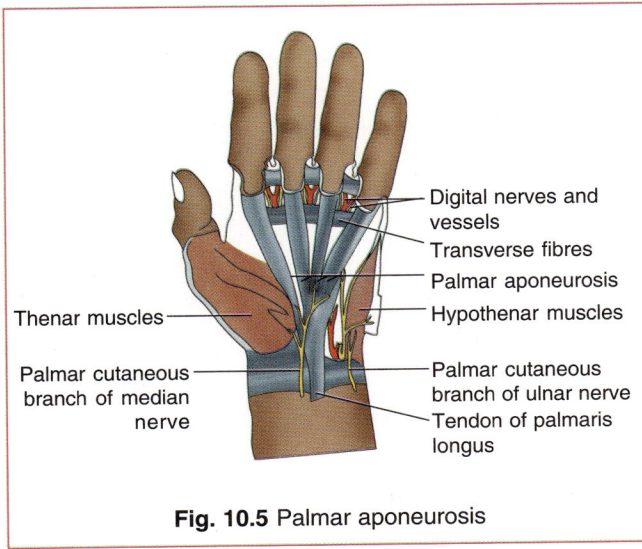

Fig. 10.5 Palmar aponeurosis

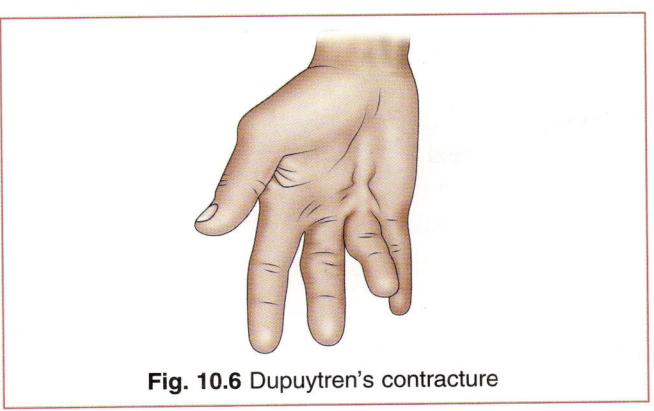

Fig. 10.6 Dupuytren's contracture

SECTION 3

be fully extended, either actively or passively. What was wrong anatomically with the left ring finger?

FIBROUS FLEXOR SHEATHS OF THE FINGERS

- The deep fascia is modified in the form of strong unyielding fibrous sheath on the palmar aspect of the all the fingers.

- It extends from the level of heads of the metacarpal bone to the base of the distal phalanx.

- The fibrous sheath of the thumb contains only tendon of flexor pollicis longus with radial bursa.

- In the medial four fingers, each fibrous sheath contains tendons of flexor digitorum superficialis and profundus.

- The fibrous sheath is thick opposite to the phalanges, but thin opposite to the joints to allow the free movements.

- To prevent the friction within the fibrous sheath the tendons are enclosed by **digital synovial sheath** in ring, middle and index finger. The sheath is closed at both ends. Proximally these synovial sheaths extend up to the level of metacarpal heads.

- But in the thumb the digital synovial sheath continues proximally with radial bursa, while digital synovial sheath of the little finger is continues proximally with the ulnar bursa.

- The under surface of the tendons are connected with the shafts of the phalanges by 2 types of vinculae, which are synovial folds. The vincula brevia are triangular folds which are 2 in number. One connects the superficial tendon to the proximal phalanx and the other connects

the profundus tendon with middle phalanx. The vincula longa are filliform folds connecting superficial and profundus tendons into the proximal phalanx. The vinculae provide passage for the blood vessels to reach the tendon.

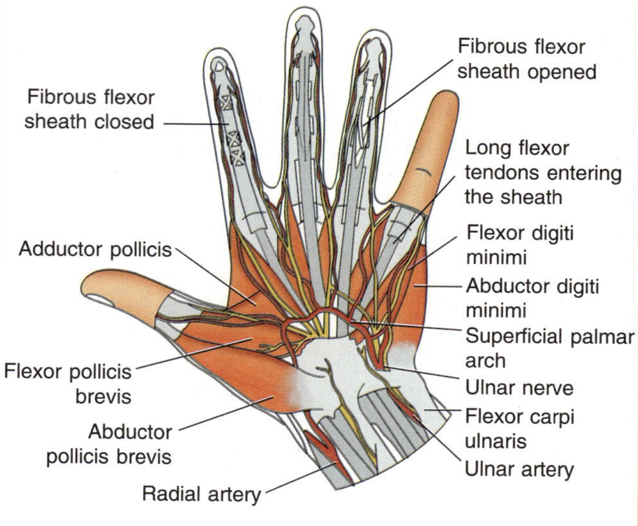

Inflammation of the tendons within the fibrous sheath is referred as '**Tenosynovitis**'. An infection from the little finger can spread into the ulnar bursa while an infection from the thumb can spread into the radial bursa. This in turn may spread into the fascial spaces of the hand (thenar and mid palmar spaces). Infections restricted to the digital synovial sheath are drained by two transverse incisions—one at the crease of distal interphalangeal joint and other at the distal palmar crease.

CASE-2

A 28-year-old woman, while working in the garden got a prick onto the anterior surface of the right index finger by a large thorn. Three days later the entire finger became swollen, red, and painful. On examination, the whole finger was found to be swollen and was held in semi flexed position. It was tender especially along the line of the flexor tendons. Flexion of the finger was difficult, and extension was limited by extreme pain. A small black dot over the anterior surface of the middle phalangeal region showed the site of entry of the thorn. With your knowledge of anatomy and assuming that the thorn was contaminated with infecting organisms, what is your diagnosis? If the diseased finger is left untreated, where is the infection likely to spread?

INTRINSIC MUSCLES OF THE HAND

The elevation, proximal to the thumb (lateral side of hand) is called **thenar eminence**. The underlying muscles produce this elevation. The muscles are (Figs 10.7 and 10.8)

1. Abductor pollicis brevis
2. Flexor pollicis brevis
3 Opponens pollicis
4. Adductor pollicis

All these muscles act on the thumb. They are all supplied by the **median nerve** except adductor pollicis, which is supplied by the **ulnar nerve**.

The elevation on medial side of the hand is called **hypothenar eminence**. It is produced by the underlying muscles (Figs 10.7 to 10.9).

Fig. 10.7 Fibrous flexor sheaths

Fibrous flexor sheath opened

Fibrous flexor sheath closed

Long flexor tendons entering the sheath

Flexor digiti minimi

Abductor digiti minimi

Superficial palmar arch

Ulnar nerve

Flexor carpi ulnaris

Ulnar artery

Adductor pollicis

Flexor pollicis brevis

Abductor pollicis brevis

Radial artery

SECTION 3

Table 10.1 Attachment of intrinsic muscles of the hand

Muscle	Origin	Insertion	Nerve supply	Actions
Thenar muscles Abductor pollicis brevis	Tubercle of scaphoid, trapezium, flexor retinaculum	Base of proximal phalanx of thumb	Median nerve	Abducts the thumb
Flexor pollicis brevis	Flexor retinaculum, trapezoid, capitate bones	Base of proximal phalanx of thumb	Median nerve	Flexes the thumb
Opponenspollicis	Flexor retinaculum	Lateral half of palmar surface of shaft of first metacarpal bone	Median nerve	Opposes thumb towards the fingers
Adductor pollicis (Fig.10.9)	Oblique head - bases of 2nd and 3rd meta-carpals Transverse head-shaft of 3rd meta-carpal	Base of proximal phalanx of thumb on its medial aspect	Ulnar nerve (deep branch)	Adduction of thumb
Hypothenar muscles Palmaris brevis	Flexor retinaculum	Skin of palm on medial side	Ulnar nerve (superficial branch)	Wrinkles the skin to improve grip
Abductor digiti minimi	Pisiform bone	Base of proximal phalanx of little finger	Ulnar nerve (deep branch)	Abducts little finger
Flexor digiti minimi	Flexor retinaculum	Base of proximal phalanx of little finger	Ulnar nerve (deep branch)	Flexes the little finger
Opponens digiti minimi	Flexor retinaculum	Medial border of 5th metacarpal	Ulnar nerve (deep branch)	Pulls the 5th metacarpal forwards as in cupping of palm

1. Palmaris brevis (lies under the skin)
2. Abductor digiti minimi
3. Flexor digiti minimi
4. Opponens digiti minimi

These muscles (except palmaris brevis) act on the little finger. They are supplied by **ulnar** nerve.

The attachments, specific nerve supply and actions are summarized in Table 10.1.

Lumbrical muscles

These are small worm like muscles, four in number, counted from lateral to medial side. They take origin from the tendon of flexor digitorum profundus. The first two are unipennate and the third and fourth are bipennate.

First lumbrical: It takes origin from the lateral side of the tendon of the flexor digitorum profundus of the index finger.

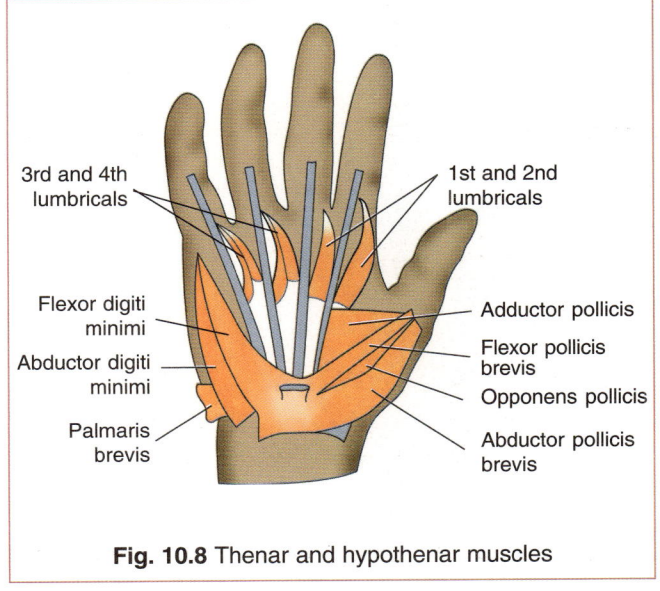

Fig. 10.8 Thenar and hypothenar muscles

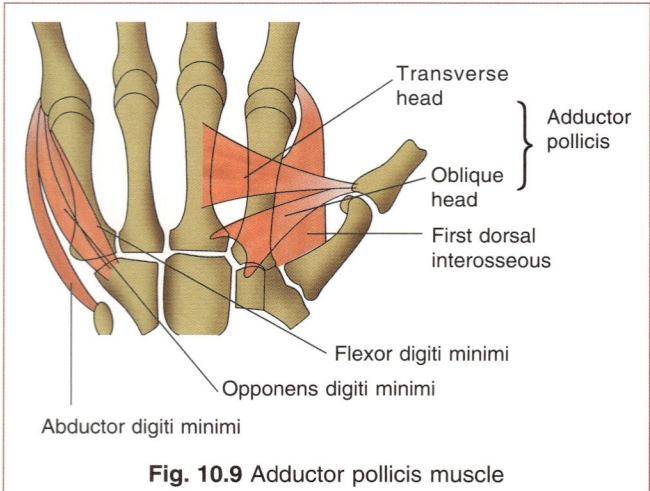

Fig. 10.9 Adductor pollicis muscle

It is inserted into the lateral side of the dorsal digital expansion of the index finger, through which it extends to dorsal aspect of the middle and distal phalanx (Fig.10.10).

Second lumbrical: It takes origin from the lateral side of the tendon of the flexor digitorum profundus of the middle finger. It is inserted into the lateral side of the dorsal digital expansion of the middle finger, through which it extends to dorsal aspect of the middle and distal phalanx.

Third lumbrical: It arises from the adjacent sides of profundus tendons for middle and ring fingers. It is inserted into the lateral side of the dorsal digital expansion of the ring finger, through which it extends to dorsal aspect of the middle and distal phalanx.

Fourth lumbrical: It arises from the adjacent sides of profundus tendons for ring and little fingers. It is inserted into the lateral side of the dorsal digital expansion of the little finger, through which it extends to dorsal aspect of the middle and distal phalanx.

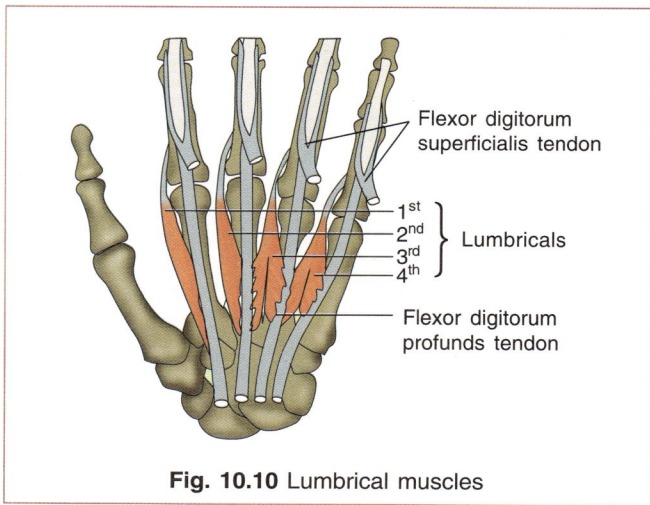

Fig. 10.10 Lumbrical muscles

Nerve supply: The first and second lumbricals are supplied by median nerve through their superficial surface. The third and the fourth are supplied by the deep branch of the ulnar nerve from their deep surface.

Actions: They flex the fingers at the metacarpophalangeal joints but extend the interphalangeal joints through dorsal digital expansion which is attached to the dorsal aspect of the middle and the distal phalanges.

They are mainly supplied by C8 and T1 fibres, hence in **Klumpke's paralysis** all the lumbricals are involved. But in case of an injury affecting ulnar nerve, among the lumbricals only third and fourth are involved resulting in partial claw hand.

Interosseous muscles (or interossei)

There are two groups. The superficial group is called **palmar interossei** and the deep group is called **dorsal interossei**. They are four each in number and counted from lateral to medial side. The palmar interossei are unipennate while dorsal interossei are bipennate muscles.

To understand the attachments of palmar and dorsal interossei, we need to look into their actions. The palmar interossei cause adduction of fingers (Remember PAD-means palmar interossei cause adduction), it means movements of the fingers towards the middle finger, because axis of the palm passes through the middle finger. The movement of the middle finger to either side consider as abduction, hence it does not receive any attachment of palmar interossei.

The dorsal interossi cause abduction of the fingers (Remember DAB-means dorsal interossei cause abduction), it means movement away from the middle finger. Since movement of middle finger on either side is considered as abduction, it receives two dorsal interossei. The thumb and the little fingers have separate abductors hence they do not receive dorsal interossei muscles.

First Palmar interossei: It arises from the medial side of the base of the first metacarpal bone. It is inserted into the proximal phalanx of the thumb on the medial side.

Second Palmar interossei: It arises from the medial side of the shaft of the second metacarpal bone. It is inserted into the proximal phalanx of the index finger and also into the dorsal digital expansion of the index finger (Fig.10.11).

Third Palmar interossei: It arises from the lateral side of the shaft of fourth metacarpal bone. It is inserted into the proximal phalanx of the ring finger and also into the dorsal digital expansion of the ring finger.

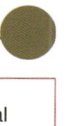

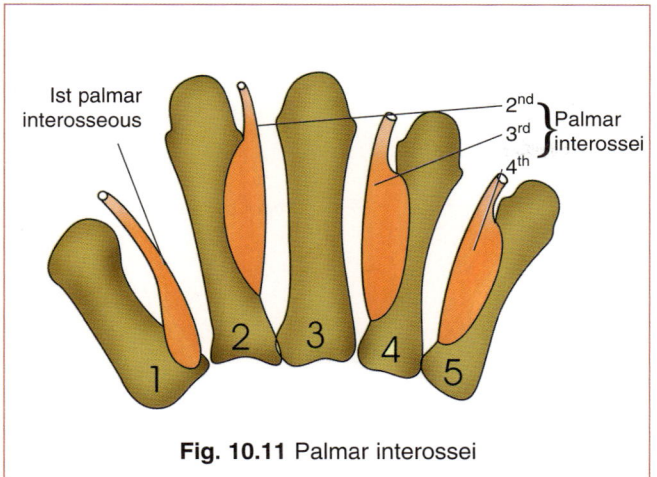

Fig. 10.11 Palmar interossei

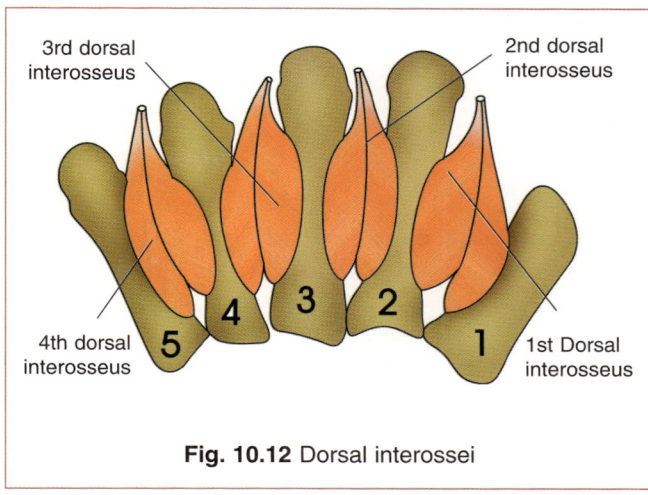

Fig. 10.12 Dorsal interossei

Fourth Palmar interossei: It arises from the lateral side of the shaft of fifth metacarpal bone. It is inserted into the proximal phalanx of the little finger and also into the dorsal digital expansion of the little finger (Fig.10.11).

Dorsal interossei being bipennate takes origin from the adjacent metacarpal bones (Fig.10.12).

First dorsal interossei: It takes origin from the shafts of the first and second metacarpal bones. It is inserted into the radial side of the proximal phalanx of the index finger and also into the dorsal digital expansion of the index finger. The gap between the two heads of the first dorsal interosseus transmits radial artery.

Second dorsal interossei: It takes origin from the shafts of the second and third metacarpal bones. It is inserted into the **radial** side of the proximal phalanx of the middle finger and also into the dorsal digital expansion of the middle finger.

Third dorsal interossei: It takes origin from the shafts of the third and fourth metacarpal bones. It is inserted into the **ulnar** side of the proximal phalanx of the middle finger and also into the dorsal digital expansion of the middle finger.

Fourth dorsal interossei: It takes origin from the shafts of the fourth and fifth metacarpal bones. It is inserted into the ulnar side of the proximal phalanx of the ring finger and also into the dorsal digital expansion of the ring finger.

Nerve supply: Both palmar and dorsal interossei are supplied by deep branch of the ulnar nerve.

Actions:

1. The palmar interossei are adductors of the fingers (moving the fingers towards the middle finger). They flex the metacarpophalangeal joint, but through dorsal digital expansion extend the middle and distal interphalangeal joints.

2. The dorsal interossei are abductors of the fingers (moving the fingers away from the middle finger). They flex the metacarpophalangeal joint, but through dorsal digital expansion extend the middle and distal interphalangeal joints.

All the interossei and lumbricals have a common action–flexion at metacarpophalangeal joint and extension at the interphalangeal joints. Hence paralysis of these muscles (injury to the ulnar nerve - T1 segment of the spinal cord) results in 'claw hand' (extension at metacarpophalangeal joint and flexion at the interphalangeal joint).

ARTERIAL ARCHES

The terminal branches of the ulnar and radial artery anastomose with each other in the form of superficial and deep palmar arches.

Superficial palmar arch

It is an arterial arch present on the superficial aspect of the palm.

Relations: It is present superficial to long flexor tendons and deep to the palmar aponeurosis.

Formation:

On medial side: The ulnar artery enters the palm superficial to the flexor retinaculum on the lateral side of the pisiform bone. Immediately the artery divides into superficial and deep branches. The superficial branch is the direct continuation of ulnar artery, which continues laterally to form the superficial palmar arch (contributing the arch on its medial 2/3rd).

On lateral side: The arch is contributed (lateral 1/3rd) by one of the following arteries (Fig.10.13).

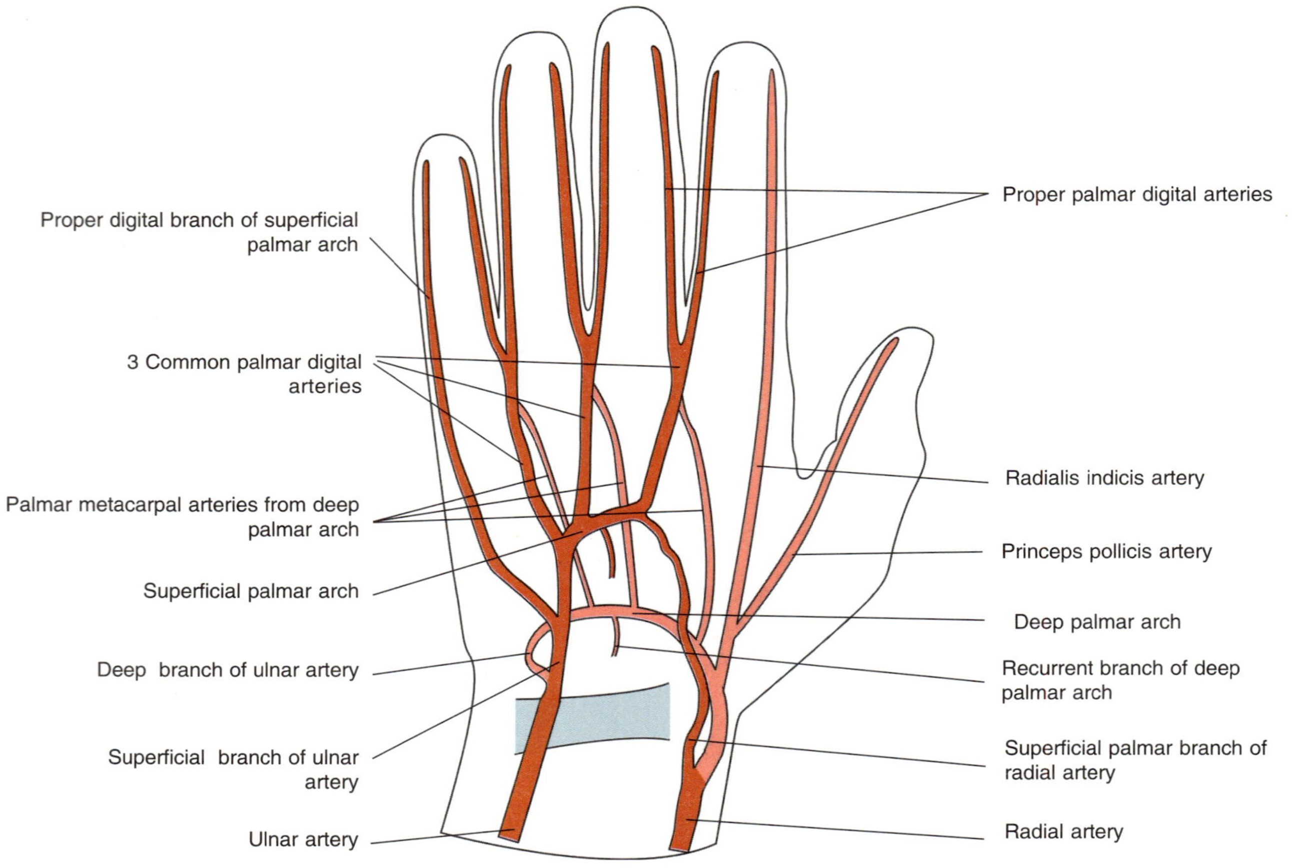

Proper digital branch of superficial palmar arch

Proper palmar digital arteries

3 Common palmar digital arteries

Palmar metacarpal arteries from deep palmar arch

Radialis indicis artery

Princeps pollicis artery

Superficial palmar arch

Deep palmar arch

Deep branch of ulnar artery

Recurrent branch of deep palmar arch

Superficial branch of ulnar artery

Superficial palmar branch of radial artery

Ulnar artery

Radial artery

Fig. 10.13 Palmar arches

1. Superficial palmar branch of the radial artery
2. Arteria princeps pollicis (branch of the radial artery)
3. Arteria radialis indicis (branch of the radial artery)
4. Arterial nervi mediana (median artery-branch from anterior interosseous artery accompanying median nerve)

Sometimes it is possible that the arch is incomplete without any contribution from above mentioned arteries.

Branches:

1. A proper digital artery to the medial side of the little finger
2. Three common palmar digital arteries: These branches arise from the convexity of the arch and proceed towards the second, third and the fourth web spaces where they divide into proper digital branches to the adjacent fingers.
3. Recurrent branch to palmar carpal arch

All these branches receives blood from palmar metacarpal arteries which are branches of deep palmar arch near the web space. In this way the superficial palmar arch is also connected with the deep palmar arch.

The superficial palmar arch does not supplies thumb and radial side of the index finger.

Surface marking: A convex line drawn at the level of distal palmar crease (a point from distal border of the thenar eminence in line with the cleft between the index and middle finger to a point lateral and distal to the pisiform bone).

Deep palmar arch

It is an arterial arch present deep to the long flexor tendons of the palm and proximal to the level of superficial palmar arch.

Formation:

On the lateral side: The radial artery after traversing the anatomical snuff box, enters the hand between the two heads of the first dorsal interossei muscle. It lies between the oblique and transverse head of the adductor pollicis muscle, where it continues to form deep palmar arch (contribution on the lateral $2/3^{rd}$).

On the medial side: The deep branch of the ulnar artery accompanied by the deep branch of the ulnar nerve passes between the abductor and flexor digiti minimi and then turns laterally below the hook of the hamate to join the radial artery to complete the deep palmar arch (Fig.10.13).

Branches:

1. Three palmar metacarpal arteries which join the common palmar digital arteries of the superficial palmar arch.

2. Three perforating branches pass backwards through 2nd to 4th interosseous space to anastomose with the dorsal metacarpal arteries.

3. Recurrent branch proceed backwards and take part in formation of palmar carpal arch.

Surface marking: A horizontal line drawn at the level of proximal palmar crease (horizontal line drawn just distal to the hook of the hamate about 1.2 cm proximal to the superficial arch).

The **radial artery** between the first dorsal interossei and the adductor pollicis muscle gives two branches (Fig.10.13).

1. **Arteria princeps pollicis:** It divides into 2 palmar digital branches to supply the two sides of the thumb.

2. **Arteria radialis indicis:** It supplies the radial side of the index finger.

> The superficial arch lies superficial, just deep to the palmar aponeurosis. Laceration of palm can cause severe bleeding. Bleeding can be controlled by compressing the brachial artery against humerus, not the radial or ulnar or both arteries (because of connection between palmar and dorsal arterial arches).

NERVES OF THE HAND

Median nerve in the hand

- The median nerve enters the hand deep to the flexor retinaculum through the carpal tunnel (Fig. 10.14).

- In the hand first it gives a '**recurrent**' branch which curves backwards at the distal border of the flexor retinaculum passes superficial to the tendon of the flexor pollicis longus and ends by supplying 3 thenar muscles – abductor pollicis brevis, flexor pollicis brevis and opponens pollicis.

- The main trunk soon divides into medial and lateral terminal branches.

- The lateral branch further divides into three proper palmar digital nerves, which supplies the skin of the both sides of the thumb and the radial side of the index finger. The branch to the index finger also supplies first **lumbrical**.

- The medial branch divides into two common palmar digital nerves, which passes distally deep to the superficial palmar arch.

- Among the two branches, the lateral branch supply second lumbrical and divides into proper digital branches at the second web space to supply the skin of the adjacent sides of index and middle fingers. The medial branch proceeds towards the third web space where it divides into proper digital branches to supply the skin of the adjacent sides of the middle and ring fingers. This branch often receives communicating branch from the ulnar nerve.

Summary of distribution of median nerve in the hand:

Motor distribution: It supplies 5 muscles—abductor pollicis brevis, flexor pollicis brevis, opponens pollicis, first and second lumbricals.

Sensory distribution: Skin of the palmar aspect of the lateral three and a half fingers including the skin of the dorsal surface of the same digits at the level of the middle and distal phalanx including the nail bed and also joints of those fingers.

> **Carpal tunnel syndrome**
>
> It occurs due to fluid retention in the carpal tunnel which may be due to infection and excessive exercise of the fingers cause swelling of the tendons/synovial sheaths. The myxedema, pregnancy or anterior dislocation of lunate bone also causes fluid retention and results in carpal tunnel syndrome. The signs and symptoms are gradual in onset.
>
> **Effects:**
> - At first it causes numbness, tingling and burning pain in lateral three and half fingers.

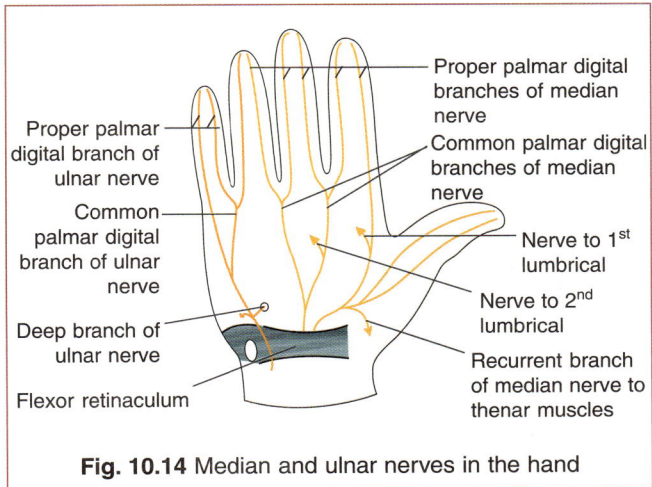

Fig. 10.14 Median and ulnar nerves in the hand

- Gradually there may be a loss of sensation in the same fingers in due course of time.

- Weakness of thenar muscles and flattening of thenar eminence, loss of motor function (loss of coordination and strength in the thumb- unable to **oppose the thumb**, difficulty in buttoning the shirt/blouse).

- Will lead to ape thumb deformity if left untreated.

- There is no sensory loss on the lateral part of the palm of the skin because this area is supplied by palmar cutaneous branch of the median nerve which arises in the forearm and enters the palm superficial to the flexor retinaculum.

  Surgical division of flexor retinaculum is one of the methods to relieve pressure on the median nerve in carpal tunnel.

CASE-3

A 32-year-old typist consults her physician, complaining that she feels tingling and slight pain in her right hand. The symptoms are localized to her thumb, index, middle and lateral side of her ring finger. The sensations are more intense at night or if she overworks. Recently, she has experienced some weakness while grasping the objects and also finds it more difficult to type. The movements of her right thumb are not as strong as before.

On examination, there is loss of power on certain movements of the thumb. She has impaired appreciation of light touch and pin pricks to the thumb, index, middle and lateral side of her ring finger, but sensation on her palm is not affected. Pressure and tapping over the flexor retinaculum causes tingling. After a complete examination, the patient is diagnosed with carpal tunnel syndrome. Using your knowledge of anatomy answer following questions.

1. What is Carpal tunnel? Where is it situated?
2. What movement of the thumb is greatly affected and how do you test the muscles involved in it?
3. How do you explain that major thumb movements are not affected in Carpal tunnel syndrome?
4. How do you explain the sensory deficit in the lateral 3½ fingers, but not on the lateral aspect of the palm?

Ulnar nerve in the hand

- The ulnar nerve is accompanied by ulnar vessels on its lateral side, passes superficial to the flexor retinaculum on the lateral side of the pisiform bone (Fig.10.14).

- It soon divides into superficial and deep branches.

Superficial terminal branch

- The superficial branch supplies Palmaris brevis muscle and then subdivides into two branches.

- A proper palmar digital branch to supply the skin of the medial side of little finger.

- A common palmar digital nerve proceeds towards the fourth web space where it divides into two proper digital nerves to supply the skin of the adjacent sides of the ring and little fingers.

- These digital branches in addition supplies skin of the dorsal aspect of the little and ring finger over the distal phalanx, nail beds and joints of those fingers.

Deep terminal branch

- It is accompanied by deep terminal branch of the ulnar artery passes deep between the origins of abductor and flexor digiti minimi, pierces the opponens digiti minimi.

- It then lodges in a groove below the hook of the hamate and follows the concavity of the deep palmar arch, deep to the long flexor tendons.

- It supplies
  1. Abductor digiti minimi
  2. Flexor digiti minimi
  3. Opponens digiti minimi
  4. Third and fourth lumbricals
  5. All the four palmar interossei
  6. All the four dorsal interossei
  7. Adductor pollicis
  8. Deep head of the flexor pollicis brevis
  9. Intercarpal and carpometacarpal joints

Injury to the ulnar nerve results in 'ulnar claw hand' in which there will be a hyperextension of metacarpophalangeal joint and hyperflexion at the interphalangeal joints. There will also be a sensory loss on the skin of the palmar aspect of the medial one and a half fingers.

CASE-4

A young girl while cleaning the glass pieces fell on the floor accidentally and cut her palmar aspect of the hand, which started to bleed severely. At the hospital the physician observed a laceration in front of her left wrist on the medial side. She had sensory loss over the palmar aspect of the medial one and a half fingers, but normal sensation at the back of these fingers. She was unable was unable to grip a piece of paper between her left index and middle fingers. All her long flexor tendons were intact.

1. Which nerve and artery got cut in the accident?
2. Why was the sensation on the dorsal aspect of the same finger intact?
3. Why was she not able to grip a piece of paper between index and little finger?

Ulnar bursa

It extends approximately 2.5-cm proximal to the flexor retinaculum. It encloses the tendons of flexor digitorum superficialis and profundus in a common sheath. Distally it continues with the digital synovial sheath of the little finger but not to the other fingers, where it ends as blind diverticula about half way along the 2nd, 3rd, 4th metacarpal bones (Fig.10.15).

Radial bursa

It extends about 2.5 cm proximal to the flexor retinaculum enclosing the tendon of the flexor pollicis longus. It continues with digital synovial sheath of the thumb enveloping the tendon up to its insertion (Fig.10.15).

FASCIAL SPACES OF THE HAND

These are potential spaces in the palm present deep to the long flexor tendons but superficial to the interossei muscles. This space is divided into a thenar space on the lateral side and the mid-palmar space on the medial side. These are potential sites where there is a possibility of accumulation of pus. The knowledge of anatomy of these spaces is important in understanding spreading of infection and also drainage of pus if required. The boundaries and extents of the mid-palmar and thenar spaces are tabulated in next page.

CASE-5

A 12-year-old boy, while playing with discarded building scraps caught his right hand on a rusty nail. A deep puncture wound occurred on the palm of the hand in front of the fourth metacarpal bone. Two days later, the wound became painful and tender and the back of the hand became swollen.

1. With your knowledge of anatomy, and assuming that the nail was contaminated with infecting organisms, which fascial space of the palm is likely to be infected?
2. Explain the fascial spaces of the hand with the help of a diagram with their communications.

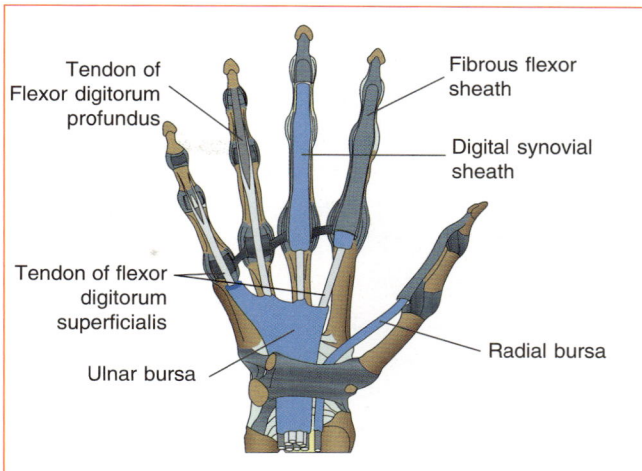

Fig. 10.15 Radial and ulnar bursa, digital synovial sheath

3. What are anatomical sites for putting incisions to drain the thenar and mid-palmar spaces?

CASE-6

A 34-year-old male patient visits hospital with a wound in his right index finger just above the meta-carpophalangeal joint. The patient related the wound to an injury that occurred about 10 days back while opening a tin can. Upon examination the index finger is swollen, as is the entire hand, particularly on the dorsum. The entire finger and hand are tender and was severe over the flexor tendon sheath, being most acute at proximal interphalangeal joint. Flexion of the index finger does not increase pain; but extension causes marked pain throughout the finger. There is no particular pain on the dorsum of the index finger. Axillary lymph nodes draining the injured side are markedly swollen. The patient has a temperature of 101°. This case was diagnosed as an infected wound of index finger characterised by inflammation of flexor sheath of index finger and metacarpophalangeal joint, lymph vessel and lymph node. The infection has secondarily spread to the thenar space. The physician opened the wound and passed a drainage tube through and across the dorsum between index and middle finger on the dorsum of the hand.

1. Which tendons are located in this fibrous flexor sheath?
2. What is the extent of fibrous flexor sheath from proximal to distal?
3. Why is the extension of the involved finger very painful as compared with its flexion?

Table-10.2: Palmar spaces, boundaries and extent		
	Mid-palmar space	**Thenar space**
Superficial	Palmar aponeurosis Superficial palmar arch Flexor tendons of medial 3 fingers	Palmar aponeurosis Superficial palmar arch Flexor tendons of index finger
Deep	Fascia covering the 3rd and 4th interosseous space	Fascia covering the adductor pollicis muscle
Medially	Medial palmar septum	Mid palmar septum
Laterally	Mid palmar septum	Lateral palmar septum
Proximally	Distal margin of the flexor retinaculum	Distal margin of the flexor retinaculum
Distally	Distal palmar crease and continues with 3rd and 4th web space	Distal palmar crease and continues with 1st web space
Surgical incision	Incision through 3rd or 4th web space	Incision through 1st web space along the radial side of the index finger

S E C T I O N 3

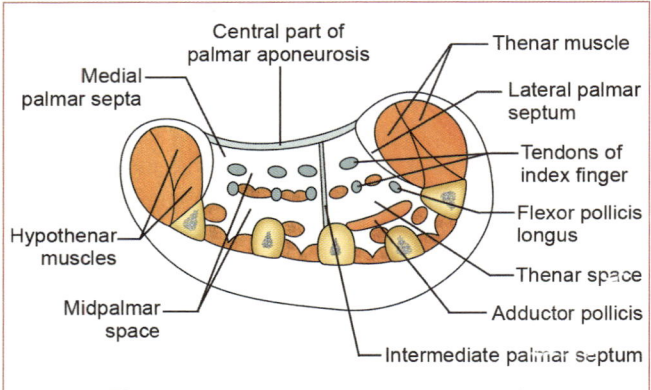

Fig. 10.16 Palmar spaces- coronal section

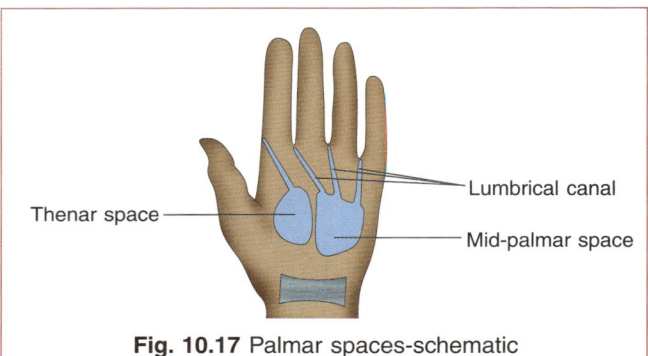

Fig. 10.17 Palmar spaces-schematic

4. Which are the deep spaces in the palm of the hand that are frequently affected and would localise infections?

5. Infection of which tendon sheath may lead to involvement of the thenar space most commonly, as in this case?

CASE-7

A 19-year-old woman visits her physician with complaints of severe pain and redness around the base of the nail of the right index finger. She stated that 3 days before she had trimmed the cuticle of her nail with scissors, following which the pain commenced very next day. On physical examination, the skin folds around the root of the nail were found to be swollen,

red, and extremely tender. The index finger was swollen and the dorsum of the hand was slightly edematous. Red streaks could be seen coursing up the front of the forearm. On examination of the infraclavicular fossa, some small, tender nodules could be palpated. The patient's temperature was high. From your knowledge of anatomy

1. Explain the cause for appearance of red streaks in front of the forearm.

2. What are these tender nodules in the infraclavicular fossa?

CASE-8

A 10-year-old boy, while climbing over the ruins of a building, slipped and caught his right hand between the railings and sustained an injury over the area of fourth metacarpal bone. Two days later the wound became

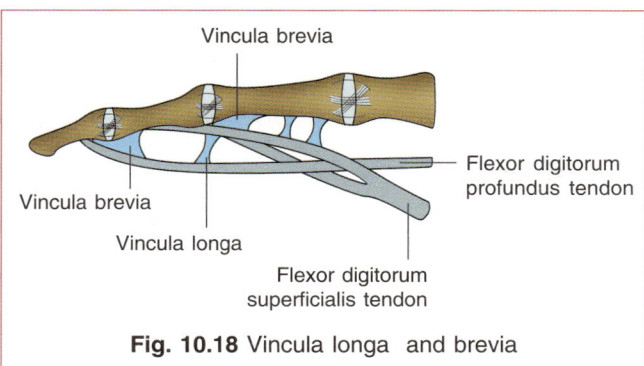

Fig. 10.18 Vincula longa and brevia

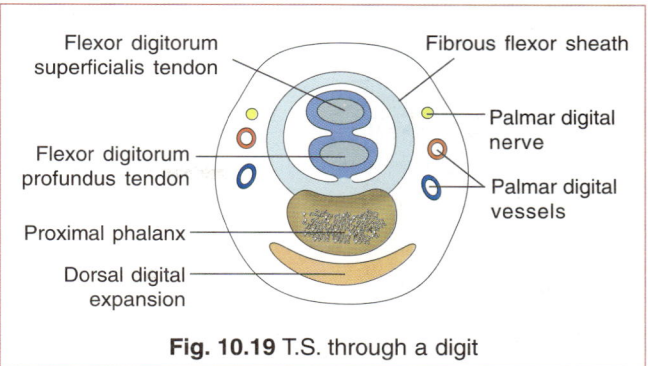

Fig. 10.19 T.S. through a digit

painful and tender and the back of the hand became swollen. With your knowledge of anatomy, and assuming that the nail was contaminated with infecting organisms what is your diagnosis (Figs 10.18 and 10.19)?

DIGITAL PULP SPACES

- These are spaces between the palmar skin and distal phalanx of all the fingers (Fig.10.20).
- It lies distal to the fibrous flexor sheath.
- Each pulp space is filled with fat and blood vessels.
- In each pulp space fibrous strands connect the skin to the periosteum of the distal phalanx dividing the pulp space into tight fat filled compartment.
- Infection of the pulp space is known as **whitlow**/felon which is characterised by severe throbbing pain.
- The pus from the pulp space is drained by an incision on the lateral side.
- The neglected case of whitlow can lead to avascular necrosis of the distal 4/5th of the terminal phalanx, which is due to the nature of blood supply to the distal phalanx.
- The distal 4/5th of the distal phalanx receives blood supply from the branches arising within the pulp space from the digital artery, while the proximal 1/5th of the distal phalanx receive blood supply from the branch which does not traverse the pulp space.

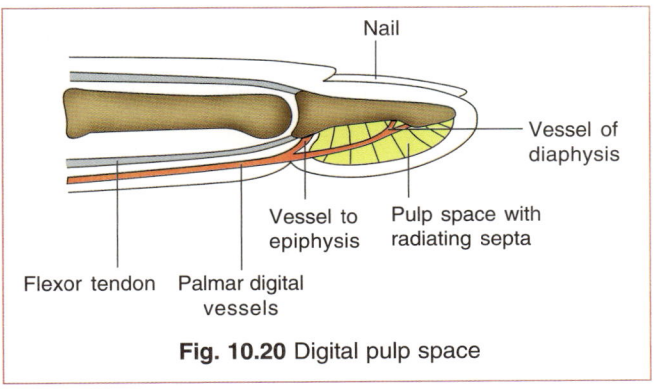

Fig. 10.20 Digital pulp space

CASE-9

A 7-year-old girl was playing with sewing machine when her mother was out of the room. When she started the machine, the point of the needle entered the pulp of the thumb of her left hand. After one and a half day, the child woke up in the night complaining of severe pain in her thumb. On examination the skin over the anterior surface of the terminal phalanx of the left thumb was found to be swollen, red, and extremely tender to touch. Over the centre of the pulp was a small area of yellow devitalized skin. This child had a pulp-space infection of the left thumb.

1. Explain the anatomy of the digital pulp space
2. What is the great danger of infections of this anatomical location?
3. What is the lymphatic drainage of this area?

DORSUM OF THE HAND

The skin of the dorsum is very thin. Deep to the skin is an aponeurotic layer formed by intertendinous connections. This aponeurotic layer divides this area into 2 spaces

1. Dorsal subcutaneous space
2. Dorsal subaponeurotic space

Due to the presence of these spaces on the dorsum and firmness of the skin of the palm, swelling appears in the dorsum from the infections in the palmar spaces.

The superficial fascia of the dorsum present irregular network of veins called 'dorsal venous arch' and also has cutaneous nerves supplying it.

Cutaneous innervation to the dorsum of the hand

1. The superficial terminal branch of the radial nerve supplies the skin of the lateral portion of the dorsum and also lateral 3½ fingers on their dorsal aspect.

2. The dorsal cutaneous branch of the ulnar nerve supplies the skin of the medial portion of the dorsum and the medial 1½ finger on their dorsal aspect.

The skin of the dorsal aspect of the digit from the distal interphalangeal joint to its tip is supplied by median nerve in the lateral 3½ fingers, while the medial 1½ fingers by ulnar nerve.

JOINTS OF THE HAND

Intercarpal joints

The individual carpal bones are connected to each other by plane synovial joints.

Midcarpal joint

It is the joint between proximal and distal rows of carpal bones.

First carpometacarpal joint (of the thumb)

- It is a saddle variety of synovial joint.
- It is the articulation between the trapezium and base of the first metacarpal bone (Fig.10.21).
- The joint permits flexion, extension, abduction, adduction and opposition movements.

Movements of the thumb and muscles producing them

Flexion: The palmar surface of the thumb moves across the palm towards the medial side, till the thumb comes in contact with the palm (Fig 10.22).

Muscles involved: Flexor pollicis brevis, opponens pollicis and flexor pollicis longus

Extension: The thumb moves away from the palm so that its dorsal surface comes to face the dorsum of the hand (Fig.10.22).

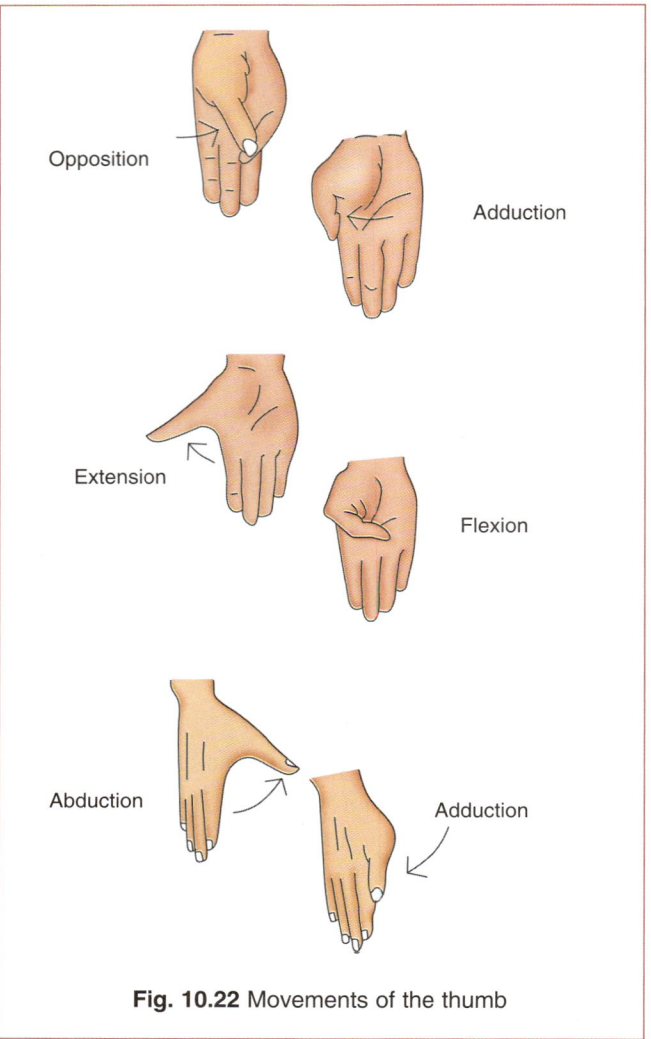

Fig. 10.22 Movements of the thumb

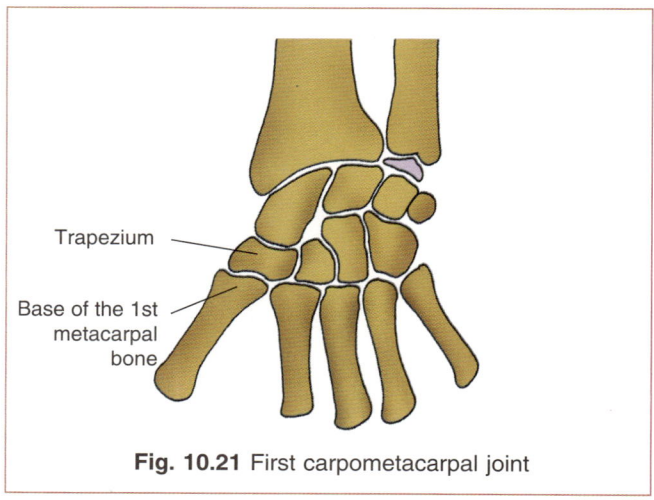

Fig. 10.21 First carpometacarpal joint

Muscles involved: Abductor pollicis longus, extensor pollicis brevis, extensor pollicis longus.

Abduction: The thumb moves away from the index finger at right angles to the plane of the palm (Fig.10.22).

Muscles involved: Abductor pollicis longus and abductor pollicis brevis.

Adduction: The thumb is brought back to the resting position (in contact with the index finger) (Fig.10.22)

Muscles involved: Adductor pollicis and first palmar interossei.

Opposition: The tip of the thumb is brought in contact with the base or tip of other fingers (Fig.10.22).

Muscles involved: Opponens pollicis

Metacarpophalangeal joints are ellipsoid variety of synovial joints. They permit flexion, extension, abduction and adduction.

Interphalangeal joints are hinge variety of synovial joints permitting flexion and extension.

SUMMARY OF THE MAJOR NERVES OF THE UPPER LIMB

Median nerve (C5, 6, 7, 8, T1)

Formation

The median nerve is formed by the union of two-nerve roots in the axilla (Fig. 10.23)

a. Medial root from the medial cord of the brachial plexus (C8, T1)

b. Lateral root from the lateral cord of the brachial plexus (C5, 6, 7)

Course

- It descends in the front of the arm and crosses the brachial artery from lateral to medial side and enters the cubital fossa.
- It leaves the cubital fossa between the two heads of pronator teres muscle and appears in the forearm.
- Median nerve descends between superficial and deep flexor muscles of forearm.
- It enters the palm by passing deep to the flexor retinaculum of the hand.

- It terminates in the palm by dividing into medial and lateral branches.

Branches and distribution

In the forearm

- Muscular branches to pronator teres, flexor carpi radialis, flexor digitorum superficialis, and palmaris longus muscles.
- Anterior interosseus branch supplies: lateral part of flexor digitorum profundus (tendons for the index and middle fingers), flexor pollicis longus, pronator quadratus.
- Palmar cutaneous branch supplies skin of the lateral part of the hand
- It also give articular and vascular branches
- **In the hand** it supplies skin of the lateral three and a half fingers, thenar muscles (abductor pollicis brevis, flexor pollicis brevis, opponens pollicis) first and second lumbricals.

To summarise: Median nerve supplies mainly flexor muscles of the forearm and few muscles of the hand acting on the thumb.

Compression of median nerve in the carpal tunnel leading to carpal tunnel syndrome is discussed before. If untreated leads to ape thumb deformity (Fig.10.24).

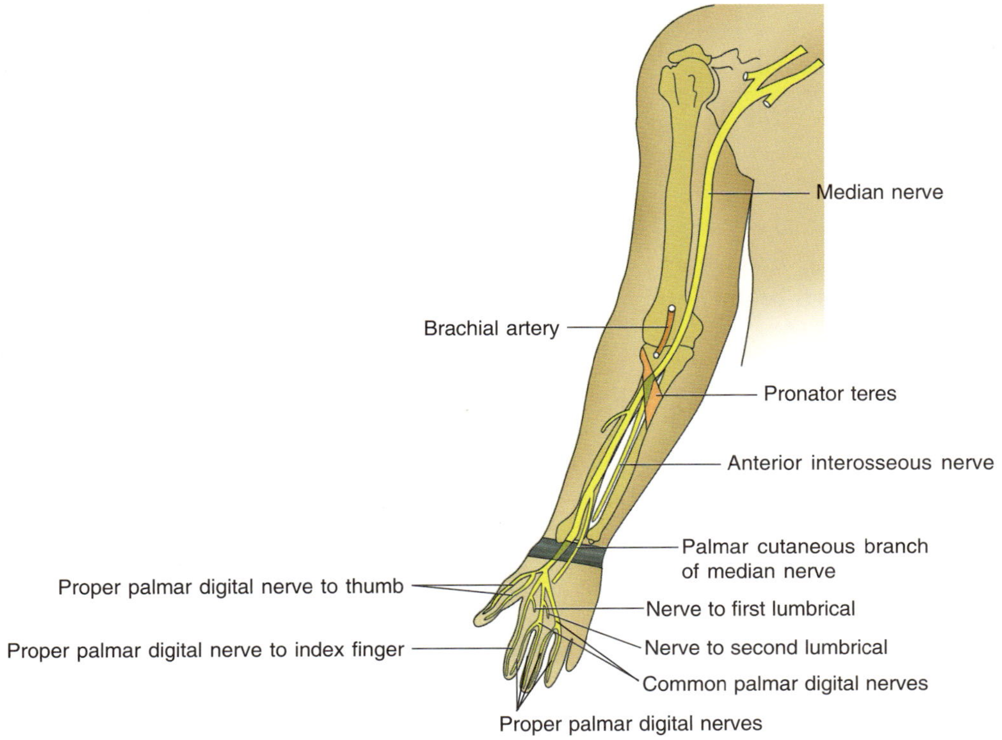

SECTION 3

Median nerve

Brachial artery

Pronator teres

Anterior interosseous nerve

Palmar cutaneous branch of median nerve

Proper palmar digital nerve to thumb

Nerve to first lumbrical

Proper palmar digital nerve to index finger

Nerve to second lumbrical

Common palmar digital nerves

Proper palmar digital nerves

Fig. 10.23 Median nerve-schematic

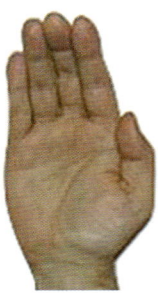

Fig. 10.24 Carpal tunnel syndrome

CASE-10

A 12-year-old boy running in a street carrying a bottle jar slipped and fell. The glass from the broken jar pierced the skin in front of his left hand. The wound was present at the level of proximal transverse crease. The palmaris longus tendon had been transected. The thumb was laterally rotated and adducted and the boy was unable to oppose his thumb to the other fingers. When he was asked to make a fist slowly, the flexion of the index and the middle finger lagged behind the ring and little fingers. There was diminished skin sensation over the lateral half of the palm of the hand and the palmar aspect of the lateral three and one-half fingers. There was also sensory loss of the skin of the distal part of the dorsal surface of the lateral three and one half fingers. Using your anatomical knowledge, name the structure or structures that has been damaged.

Ulnar nerve (C7, 8, T1)

Formation

The ulnar nerve is a branch of the medial cord of the brachial plexus. Occasionally ulnar nerve receives C7 fibres from the lateral root of the median nerve, which is believed to supply flexor carpi ulnaris muscle (Fig.10.25).

Course

- Ulnar nerve descends in the front of the arm on the medial side.
- At the middle of the arm it pierces the medial intermuscular septum and **passes posterior to the medial epicondyle of humerus.**
- The nerve enters the anterior compartment of the forearm by piercing the flexor carpi ulnaris muscle.
- In the forearm it is accompanied by ulnar vessels and together they enter the palm by passing superficial to the flexor retinaculum of the hand.
- In the palm it terminates by dividing into superficial and deep branches.

Branches and distribution

- Muscular branches in the forearm supply flexor carpi ulnaris and medial part of the flexor digitorum profundus (tendons for the ring and little fingers).

- Palmar cutaneous branch arises in the forearm enters the palm superficial to the flexor retinaculum. It supplies the skin of the palm on the medial side.

- Dorsal branch supplies the skin of the medial side of the dorsum of the hand and medial one and a half fingers on the dorsal aspect.

- The superficial terminal branch in the hand supplies palmaris brevis muscle and skin of the medial one and a half fingers on the palmar aspects.

- The deep branch supplies the following intrinsic muscles - abductor digiti minimi, flexor digiti minimi, opponens digiti minimi, adductor pollicis, third and fourth lumbricals, all the four palmar interossei, all the four dorsal interossei.

- Ulnar nerve also gives articular and vascular branches.

To summarise, the ulnar nerve mainly supplies intrinsic muscles of the hand and few flexor muscles of the forearm.

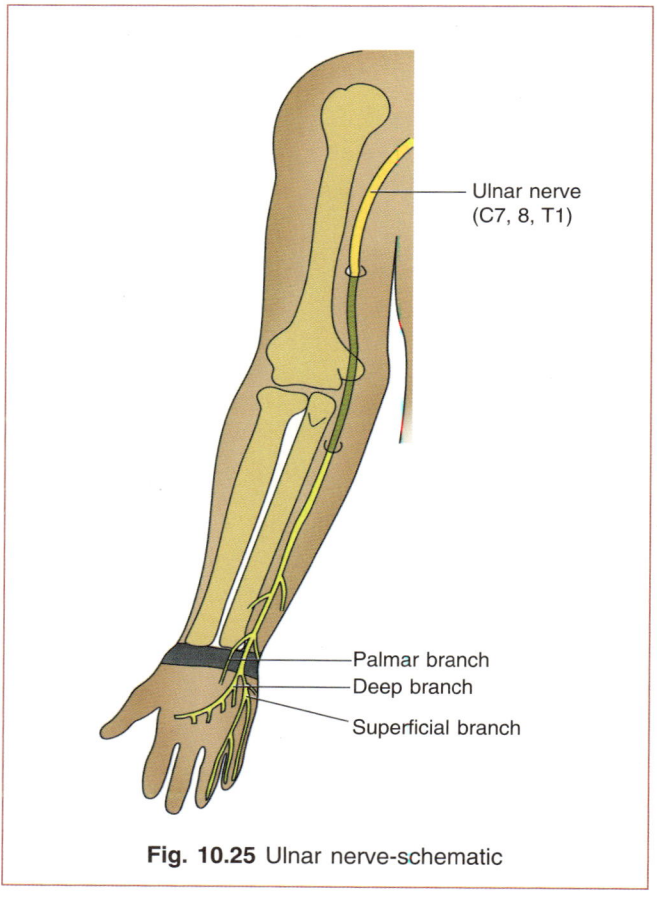

Ulnar nerve (C7, 8, T1)

Palmar branch
Deep branch
Superficial branch

Fig. 10.25 Ulnar nerve-schematic

SECTION 3

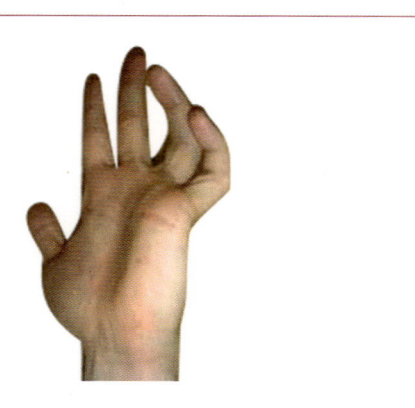

Fig. 10.26 Ulnar claw hand

An injury to the ulnar nerve leads to '**claw hand**' in which there will be a hyperextension of meta-carpophalangeal joint and hyperflexion at the inter-phalangeal joints due to paralysis of interossei, 3rd and 4th lumbricals. The index and middle finger is least affected because 1st and 2nd lumbricals are supplied by median nerve. There will also be a sensory loss on the skin over the hypothenar eminence and medial one and a half fingers on palmar surface (Fig. 10.26).

Radial nerve (C5, 6, 7, 8, T1)

Origin

The radial nerve is a branch from the posterior cord of the brachial plexus (Fig.10.27).

Course

- The radial nerve leaves the axilla by passing through the lower triangular space and enters the back of the arm
- It **descends in the radial groove (spiral) on the posterior aspect of the humerus** between lateral and medial heads of the triceps muscle. It is accompanied by profunda brachii artery.
- The radial nerve enters the front of the arm by piercing the lateral intermuscular septum and runs downwards between brachialis and brachioradialis muscles.
- It terminates in the cubital fossa by dividing into superficial and deep branches.
- The superficial branch descends along the radial (lateral) side of the forearm and enters the dorsum of the hand.
- The deep branch pierces the 'supinator muscle' and enters posterior compartment of the forearm as 'posterior interosseous nerve'.

S E C T I O N   3

Lateral
Posterior } Cords of brachial plexus
Medial

Radial nerve
Posterior cutaneous nerve of the arm
Branch to the long head of triceps
Branch to the medial head of triceps

Profunda brachii artery
Branch to the lateral head of triceps
Branch to the medial head of triceps
Posterior cutaneous branch of the forearm
Lower lateral cutaneous branch of the arm

Deep branch of radial nerve
(Posterior interosseous nerve)

Superficial branch of radial nerve

Radial artery

Dorsal digital branches of radial nerve

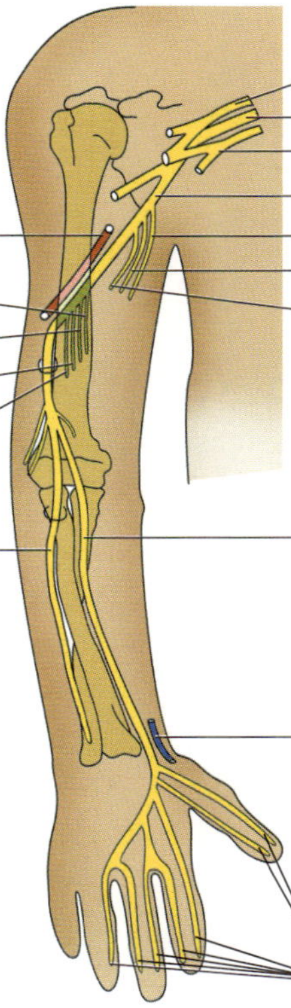

Fig. 10.27 Radial nerve-schematic

Branches and distribution

In the axilla

1. Muscular branches to long and medial head of the triceps.

2. Cutaneous branch – posterior cutaneous nerve of the arm.

In the spiral groove

1. **Muscular branche**s to lateral and medial head of the triceps.

2. Cutaneous branches - posterior cutaneous nerve of the forearm, and lower lateral cutaneous nerve of the arm.

In the front of the arm

It gives muscular branches to brachialis, brachioradialis and extensor carpi radialis longus.

Terminal branches

1. The superficial terminal branch supplies skin of the (lateral half) the dorsum of the hand and also dorsal aspect of the lateral three and a half fingers.

2. The deep terminal branch (posterior interosseous nerve) supplies muscles of the back of the forearm (extensor muscles). The muscles include

   i. Supinator

   ii. Extensor carpi radialis brevis

   iii. Extensor digitorum

   iv. Extensor digiti minimi

   v. Extensor indicis

   vi. Extensor carpi ulnaris

   vii. Abductor pollicis longus

   viii. Extensor pollicis brevis

To summarise, the radial nerve supplies all extensor muscles of arm and forearm. It also supplies skin of the back of the arm, forearm and lateral part of the dorsum of the hand.

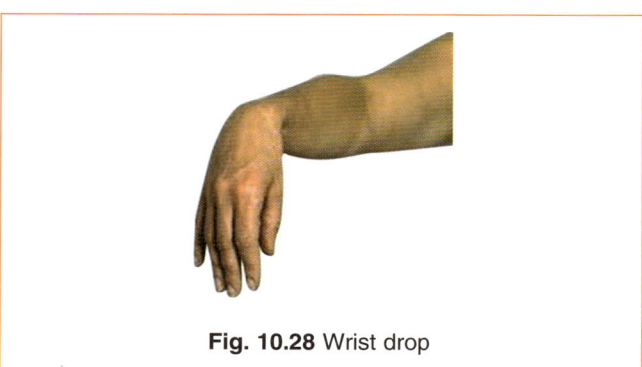

Fig. 10.28 Wrist drop

- Radial nerve may be injured in fracture of the humerus in the region of the spiral groove, which results in

Wrist drop

- Radial nerve can also be compressed by the pressure of a crutch in the axilla (crutch paralysis).

- Compression of the radial nerve against the spiral groove by placing the outstretched arm (as in sleeping) in an arm chair under drunken condition can lead to temporary 'Saturday night palsy'.

- **Injury to the radial nerve:** All the extensor muscles of the forearm are paralyzed and the patient will not able to extend the wrist. This condition is called '**wrist drop**'. Extension of the elbow is lost when the triceps is paralyzed (when the nerve is injured in the axilla). The sensory loss depends on the site of injury. If injured in the axilla, there will be a loss of cutaneous sensation at the back of the arm, forearm and lateral aspect of the dorsum of the hand (Fig. 10.28).

CASE-11

A 53-year-old woman fell down the stairs and dislocated her left shoulder joint. Several days after the dislocation had been reduced, it was noted that the patient had signs and symptoms indicative of radial nerve damage in the axilla.

1. Name the muscles that would be paralyzed and the area of skin that would show sensory loss.

2. Describe the deformity of the upper limb in a person with a long-standing radial nerve palsy following damage to the nerve in the axilla.

CASE-12

During examination of a 36-year-old patient it was noticed that he held his right forearm pronated and the wrist joint and the fingers flexed. He stated that he experienced difficulty in gripping objects in the hand with the wrist always in the flexed position. On examination of the upper arm, an old scar was seen crossing its posterior surface. On being questioned, the patient said that he had sustained a fracture of his arm when he was 12 years old, and this was followed by an operation some months later which his surgeons had considered to be unsuccessful.

1. Name the muscles that were paralyzed in this patient.

2. Which nerve was involved in this fracture?

3. Why was an operation necessary after the fracture and why was the operation a failure?

4. Why does the patient experience difficulty in holding objects in the hand?

Solution to the case studies

Case-1

The patient had **Dupuytren's contracture** involving the fibrosis of palmar aponeurosis at the base of the ring and little fingers of the left hand. The distal end of the aponeurosis gives four slips to the medial four fingers. Each slip is attached to the base of proximal phalanx and to the fibrous flexor sheath of each finger. Fibrous contracture of the slip to the ring finger resulted in permanent flexion of the metacarpophalangeal joint.

Case-2

This patient had acute suppurative (discharge of pus) **tenosynovitis** of the digital sheath of the index finger of the right hand, following the inoculation of pathogen into the sheath from the point of the thorn prick. In this condition, if the tension within the sheath is not relieved, it is likely to rupture at its proximal end, with discharge of pus into thenar fascial space. If the hand remains untreated, the infection of the thenar space may spread to the midpalmar space and may also spread upward into the forearm or downwards into the interval between the index and middle fingers. The early administration of antibiotics is the treatment of the choice.

Case-3

1. The carpal tunnel is an osseofascial space deep to the flexor retinaculum of the hand, which is bounded superficially by flexor retinaculum and on the deeper aspect by carpal bones. It contains the median nerve and tendons of flexor digitorum superficialis, profundus and flexor pollicis longus muscles.

2. Opposition movement of the thumb is greatly affected. The opponens pollicis pulls the thumb across the palm towards the base of the little finger. Ask the patient to do this against resistance.

3. The flexion of the thumb is possible because flexor pollicis longus is supplied by median nerve in the forearm and the deep head of the flexor pollicis brevis is supplied by deep branch of the ulnar nerve. The extension is possible because extensor pollicis longus is supplied by radial nerve. Though the abductor pollicis brevis is paralyzed, the abductor pollicis longus is intact which is supplied by radial nerve. The adduction is

possible because adductor pollicis and first palmar interossei are supplied by deep branch of the ulnar nerve.

4. The sensory deficit in the lateral 3½ fingers is because branches arise from the median nerve in the palm after passing through the carpal tunnel. However skin on the lateral aspect of the palm is supplied by palmar cutaneous branch of the median nerve in the forearm which passes superficial to the flexor retinaculum.

Case-4

1. The ulnar nerve and artery of the left hand were transected in front of the flexor retinaculum.

2. Skin on the dorsal aspect of the same finger receives branch from the dorsal cutaneous branch from the ulnar nerve which arises proximal to the flexor retinaculum

3. Inability to hold the piece of paper between index and the little finger is due to the involvement of the fourth palmar and dorsal interossei which are supplied by deep branch of the ulnar nerve.

Case-5

1. Mid-palmar space
2. Refer text
3. Refer text

Case-6

1. The tendons of the index finger are the flexor digitorum superficialis and flexor digitorum profundus.

2. The sheath ends proximally at the neck of the second metacarpal and distally at the base of the distal phalanx.

3. Extension causes stretching of flexor tendons, hence it is so painful. Spread of infection from proximal end of the tendons of the fingers to the palmar spaces of the hand is common because the flexor sheaths of second, third and fourth fingers begin at the level where the palmar space end.

4. The midpalmar space medially and the thenar space laterally are the spaces that lie deep to the flexor tendons in the palm. They are sometimes also called the medial and lateral deep palmar spaces.

5. Infection of the tendon sheath of the index finger may spread into the thenar space. Infection of tendon sheaths of the flexor pollicis longus (the radial bursa) may also spread into the thenar space. The reverse may happen with a primary infection of the thenar space breaking into the radial bursa.

Case-7

1. The patient had acute bacterial infection under the nail folds of the right index finger. The infection has spread

into the lymphatic vessels draining the area, and they themselves had become inflamed (lymphangitis). The red streaks were due to localized vasodilatation of blood vessels along the course of the lymphatic vessels in the forearm.

2. The lymphatic vessel from index finger follows the cephalic vein and drain into infraclavicular (deltopectoral) group of lymph nodes. Enlargement of these nodes causes swelling in the infraclavicular fossa.

Case-8

This patient had an acute infection of midpalmar space of the right hand. The infected nail penetrated through the skin and the palmar aponeurosis and inoculated the fascial space with pathogenic organisms. The lymphatic drainage of this area is into the network of lymphatic vessels present in the subcutaneous tissue on the dorsum of the hand. For this reason, edema of the loose skin on the back of the hand is common in infections of the palm.

Case-9

1. Refer text

2. The danger here is that the tension within the pulp space will rise and occlude the blood supply to the diaphysis of the terminal phalanx; osteomyelitis of the terminal phalanx may also occur. The presence of a small area of devitalized skin over the center of the pulp would suggest the presence of pus within the space and is pointing onto the surface.

3. The lymphatic drainage of the thumb is via vessels that accompany the cephalic vein and drain into the deltopectoral group of lymph nodes.

Case-10

The glass fragment has severed the median nerve as it lay between the tendons of flexor digitorum superficialis and flexor carpi radialis muscles and under cover of the palmaris longus tendon. The palmar cutaneous branch of the median nerve has also been severed.

Case-11

1. The muscles paralyzed would be triceps and extensor muscles present at the back of the forearm. The sensory loss would be in the posterior aspect of the arm, forearm, lower lateral aspect of the arm and the lateral part of the dorsum of the hand including dorsal aspect of the lateral three and a half fingers.

2. The wrist is held permanently in flexed position (wrist drop).

Case-12

1. The patient exhibited typical radial nerve palsy with wrist drop. The muscles involved are extensor muscles of the back of the forearm.

2. The radial nerve was presumably damaged in the spiral groove of the humerus when that bone was fractured, or was involved in the callus during repair process.

3. The surgeon probably waited to see if there was evidence of regeneration of the nerve fibres and then, because regeneration was delayed or absent, decided to explore the radial nerve in order to free it from the callus and approximate its proximal and distal ends. In any event, he was obviously unable to improve the situation, possibly damage to the radial nerve was excessive, and the nerve fibres never regenerated.

4. With the wrist held permanently in the flexed position, the long flexor muscles of the fingers are working at a mechanical disadvantage, and the fingers are unable to grip objects effectively (Try it on yourself).

MCQs

1. Loss of sensation from the tip of the index finger is indicative of injury to which nerve?
   A. Median
   B. Radial
   C. Ulnar
   D. Musculocutaneous

2. Compression of the median nerve in the carpal tunnel affects which muscle(s) in the hand?
   A. Adductor pollicis
   B. Palmar interossei
   C. Flexor pollicis longus
   D. Opponens pollicis

3. During an industrial accident, a sheet metal worker lacerates the anterior surface of his wrist at the junction of his wrist and hand. Examination reveals an intact hand functions, but the skin on the thumb side of his palm is numb. Branch of which nerve must have been severed?
   A. Median
   B. Radial
   C. Ulnar
   D. Anterior interosseous

4. In an industrial accident, the artery passing lateral to the pisiform bone was cut. Which is this artery?
   A. Radial
   B. Superficial palmar arch

SECTION 3

C. Superficial palmar branch of the radial artery

D. Ulnar

5. The extensor expansion of the ring finger receives tendons of

   A. 3rd palmar interossei, 4th dorsal interossei and 4th lumbricals

   B. 3rd palmar interossei, 4th dorsal interossei and 3rd lumbricals

   C. 2nd palmar interossei, 3rd dorsal interossei and 3rd lumbricals

   D. 3rd palmar interossei, 4th dorsal interossei and 2nd lumbricals

6. An injury to the recurrent branch of the median nerve distal to the flexor retinaculum would affect which movement of the thumb?

   A. Abduction

   B. Adduction

   C. Flexion of the distal phalanx

   D. Opposition

7. The main source of blood to the superficial palmar arterial arch is the:

   A. Radial artery

   B. Deep branch of the ulnar artery

   C. Ulnar artery

   D. Superficial palmar branch of the radial artery

8. The signs and symptoms of carpal tunnel syndrome may vary among patients, but they always result from compression of which structure in the carpal tunnel?

   A. Ulnar nerve

   B. Superficial radial nerve

   C. Radial nerve

   D. Median nerve

9. Which muscle tendon is enclosed within its own synovial sheath in the carpal tunnel?

   A. Flexor carpi ulnaris

   B. Flexor digitorum profundus to middle finger

   C. Flexor pollicis longus

   D. Flexor digitorum superficialis to ring finger

10. Which arterial vessel accompanies the deep branch of the ulnar nerve across the palm?

    A. Deep palmar arch

    B. Radial

    C. Ulnar

    D. Superficial palmar arch

11. The fourth dorsal interosseous muscle is innervated by the:

A. Superficial branch of the ulnar nerve

B. Recurrent (motor) branch of the median nerve

C. Dorsal branch of the ulnar nerve

D. Deep branch of the ulnar nerve

12. A patient sustained multiple deep lacerations on the palm of his hand and anterior surface of his wrist. During examination, the physician put a piece of paper between the patient's index and middle fingers and found that he was unable to squeeze them together with sufficient force to hold the paper. Which muscles are being tested?

    A. First dorsal and first palmar interosseous muscles

    B. Second dorsal and second palmar interosseous muscles

    C. First lumbrical and second dorsal interosseous muscles

    D. Second dorsal and first palmar interosseous muscles

13. A deep puncture wound in the palmar surface of the little finger near the proximal inter phalangeal joint might introduce infection into which synovial cavity:

    A. Bursa of flexor carpi ulnaris

    B. Fibrous digital sheath of fingers

    C. Radial bursa

    D. Ulnar bursa

14. After suffering a cut deep to the hypothenar eminence, the patient is unable to hold a sheet of paper between the second and third digits. The nerve most likely to be injured was:

    A. Radial

    B. Deep branch of ulnar

    C. Recurrent (motor) branch of median

    D. Superficial radial

15. Which movement of the thumb would be most affected by lesion of the median nerve in the cubital fossa?

    A. Flexion

    B. Abduction

    C. Adduction

    D. Extension

16. A medical student slips and falls on her outstretched hand. The intense pain forces her to go to the hospital. After X-rays of her wrist are taken, the radiologist says," You were lucky, there is no Colle's nor scaphoid fractures, but you have dislocated the middle carpal bone of the proximal row." Which bone was dislocated?

    A. Capitate

B. Scaphoid
C. Lunate
D. Trapezoid

17. A 28-year-old female patient had a tiny but exquisitely painful tumour under the nail of her index finger. In order to remove the mass which nerve needs to be blocked using anesthesia?
A. Ulnar
B. Median
C. Musculocutaneous
D. Superficial branch of radial

18. A patient presents to the emergency department after sustaining a laceration of the first web space of his hand. Which of the following structures is also likely to be injured?
A. Deep branch of radial nerve
B. Opponens pollicis
C. Radial artery
D. Recurrent branch of median nerve

19. You are examining a 34-year-old patient who has radial deviation of the hand at the wrist when he attempts to flex the wrist and altered sensation in the skin over the hypothenar eminence. What might account for these symptoms?
A. Fracture of the scaphoid bone
B. Fracture of the distal end of the radius
C. Anterior and inferior dislocation of the head of the humerus
D. Fracture of the medial epicondyle of the humerus

20. A 47-year-old female stenographer begins to develop pain and paresthesia in her right hand at night. The altered sensation is most evident on the palmar aspects of the index and middle fingers. What else do you expect to see in the patient?
A. Weakness in the ability to extend the thumb
B. Atrophy of the thenar eminence
C. Radial deviation of the hand at the wrist during wrist flexion
D. Inability to spread and oppose the fingers

21. A 28-year-old secretary develops pain and numbness in her thumb, index and middle fingers at night. Which of the following motor functions may also be weakened?
A. Adduction of the thumb
B. Extension of the thumb
C. Flexion of the index finger at the interphalangeal joints
D. Abduction of the thumb

22. A 32-year-old male presents weak abduction and adduction of his fingers but has no difficulty in flexing them. He has decreased sensation over the palmar surface of ring and little finger. These deficits most likely result from compression of which of the following nerves?
A. Median nerve in carpal tunnel
B. Median nerve at pronator teres
C. Ulnar nerve at pisiform bone
D. Ulnar nerve at medial epicondyle

23. If the medial epicondyle of the humerus is fractured and the nerve passing dorsal to it is injured, which muscle would be most affected?
A. Extensor carpi ulnaris
B. Extensor digitorum
C. Flexor carpi ulnaris
D. Flexor digitorum superficialis

24. A 24-year-old male presents with a fracture of the midshaft portion of the right humerus. Upon examination the physician determines that the patient has a wrist drop on the right side. Which nerve is involved?
A. Ulnar nerve
B. Median nerve
C. Musculocutaneous nerve
D. Radial nerve

25. A 36-year-old patient is examined by a physician. The patient has weakness of pronation and flexion at the index and middle fingers at the distal interphalangeal joints and an inability to form the letter '0' by touching the tip of the thumb to the tip of the index finger. There is no sensory deficit. Which nerve might have been compressed?
A. Recurrent branch of the median nerve
B. Deep branch of the radial nerve
C. Deep branch of the ulnar nerve
D. Anterior interosseous branch of the median nerve

26. A 56-year-old woman is diagnosed with an apical lung cancer that has invaded the inferior trunk of the brachial plexus. Which of the following muscle actions is most likely to show the greatest weakness after damage to this nerve?
A. Elbow flexion
B. Thumb and finger adduction
C. Wrist extension
D. Thumb extension

SECTION 3

27. You are observing a surgeon giving an incision in the web space between middle and ring finger to drain the pus accumulated in the hand. This incision indicates that the pus must have been collected in

A. Thenar space
B. Mid-palmar space
C. Pulp space
D. Ulnar bursa

Answers to MCQs

1. A
2. D
3. A
4. D
5. B
6. D
7. C
8. D
9. C
10. A
11. D
12. B
13. D
14. B
15. A
16. C
17. B
18. C
19. D
20. B
21. A
22. C
23. C
24. D
25. D
26. B
27. B

SECTION 3

Major questions

1. With the help of a neat labeled diagram describe the formation, branches and applied anatomy of the brachial plexus

2. Describe the shoulder joint under –type, subtype, bones articulating, structures stabilizing, nerve supply, movements and muscles producing them and applied anatomy

3. Write briefly on course, parts, major relations, branches and distribution of axillary artery

4. Describe the mammary gland under, location and extent, lymphatic drainage, blood supply and applied anatomy

5. Write briefly on attachments, nerve supply, actions of muscles attached to the scapula

6. Define pronation and supination. Give the attachments, nerve supply of the muscles causing them

7. Describe the radioulnar joints under, type, bones articulating, ligaments, movements, muscle producing them and applied anatomy

8. Name the fascial spaces of the hand. Describe the mid-palmar space and its applied anatomy

9. Describe the origin, root value, course, branches, distribution and applied anatomy of the median nerve

10. Describe the origin, root value, course, branches, distribution and applied anatomy of the radial nerve

11. Describe the origin, root value, course, branches, distribution and applied anatomy of the ulnar nerve

12. Describe the cubital fossa under – boundaries, contents and applied anatomy

13. Describe the elbow joint under – bones articulating, ligaments, movement and muscles producing them and applied anatomy

Write briefly on

1. Lymphatic drainage of the mammary gland
2. Serratus anterior muscle
3. Erb's point
4. Clavipectoral fascia
5. Deltoid muscle
6. Subacromial bursa
7. Rotator cuff
8. Abduction at the shoulder joint
9. Supraspinatus muscle
10. Quadrangular and triangular spaces
11. Radial nerve in the spiral groove
12. Axillary nerve
13. Pectoralis major muscle
14. Biceps brachii muscle
15. Musculocutaneous nerve
16. Median cubital vein
17. Radial collateral ligament of the elbow joint
18. Triceps muscle
19. Biceps brachii muscle
20. Radial bed (posterior relations of the radial artery)
21. Radial artery
22. Flexor retinaculum of the hand
23. Carpal tunnel
24. Pronator teres
25. Flexor digitorumprofundus
26. Superficial palmar arch
27. Deep palmar arch
28. Ulnar nerve in the hand
29. Median nerve in the hand
30. Thenar space
31. Mid-palmar space
32. Digital pulp space
33. Dorsal digital expansion of the fingers
34. Lumbricals of the hand
35. Adductor pollicis muscle
36. Anatomical snuff box
37. Cutaneous innervation to the hand
38. Posterior interosseus nerve
39. Supinator muscle
40. Anastomosis around the scapula
41. Anastomosis around the elbow
42. First carpo-metacarpal joint
43. Cephalic vein
44. Extensor retinaculum of wrist

SECTION 3

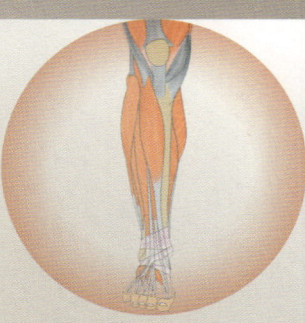

SECTION 4

Lower Limb

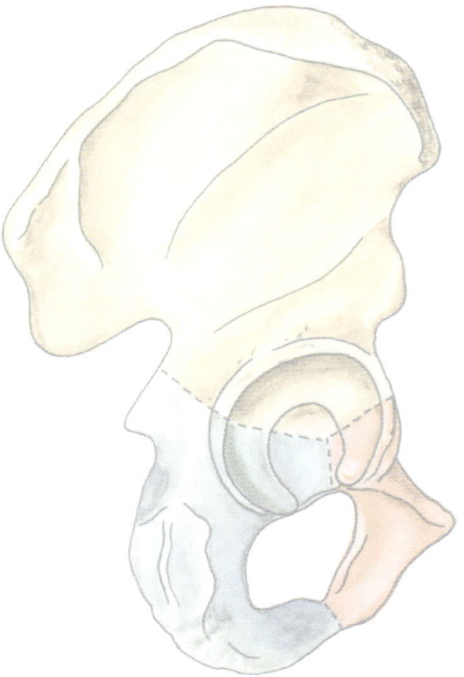

Osteology of the Lower Limb

11

- Hip bone
- Femur
- Patella
- Tibia
- Fibula
- Tarsal bones
- Metatarsals and phalanges

Objectives

- To list the bones forming the skeleton of the lower limb
- To explain the major parts, articulations, attachments, blood supply and clinical relevance of each of them

HIP BONE (INNOMINATE BONE)

It is an irregular bone forming the skeleton of the gluteal region (Figs 11.1 to 11.3).

It is made up of three parts:

1. Pubis
2. Ilium
3. Ischium

Pubis

It forms the anteroinferior part of the hip bone. It has body, superior and inferior ramus.

Body: It presents the following features:

- **Pubic crest:** It is a ridge along the upper border of the body of the pubis. It provides attachment to rectus abdominis muscle and conjoint tendon
- **Pubic tubercle:** It is the lateral end of the pubic crest. It provides attachment to the medial end of the inguinal ligament.

- **Pubic symphysis:** The right and left pubic bone meet in a median joint called pubic symphysis (a secondary cartilaginous joint).
- The body of the pubis presents anterior, posterior and medial surfaces.
- The anterior surface provides attachment to origin of muscles of the medial compartment namely gracilis, adductor longus, adductor brevis and obturator externus.
- The posterior surface is related to urinary bladder and this surface provides attachment to obturator internus and levator ani muscles.
- The medial surface articulates with medial surface of the opposite pubic bone to form pubic symphysis, a secondary cartilaginous joint.

Superior ramus: It extends from the body to the acetabulum. It presents:

- Pecten pubis (pectineal line): It extends from the pubic tubercle to iliopubic eminence. The pectineal ligament and lacunar ligament are attached to it. These ligaments are extensions of inguinal ligament.

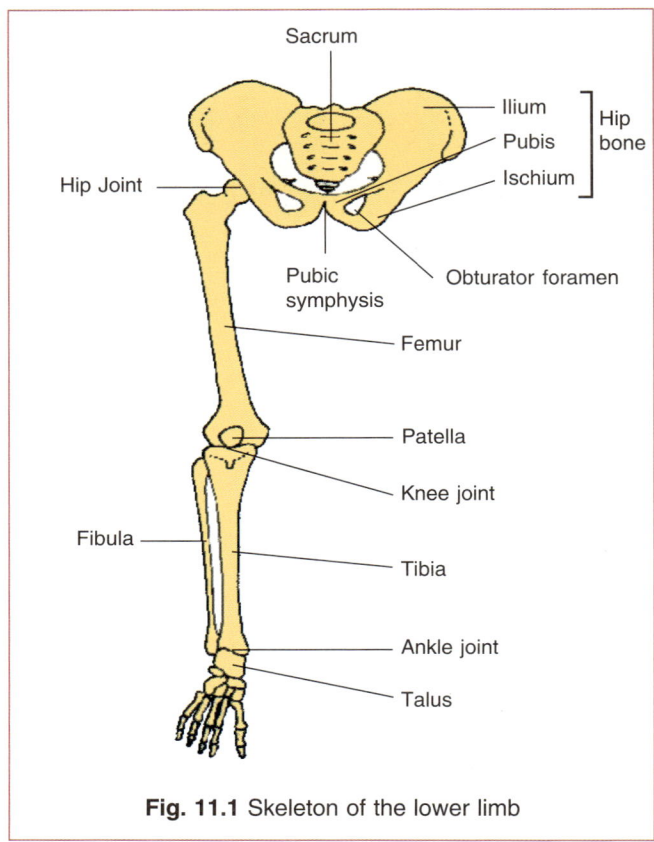

Fig. 11.1 Skeleton of the lower limb

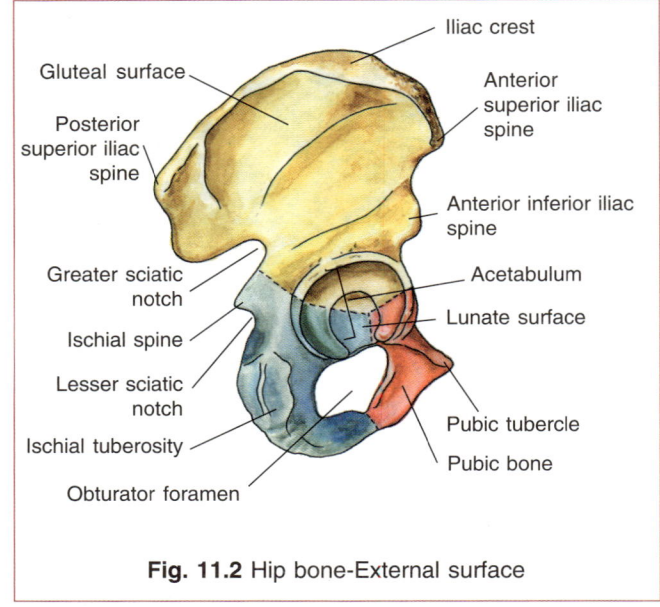

Fig. 11.2 Hip bone-External surface

- **Obturator crest:** It extends from the pubic tubercle to acetabular notch.

Inferior ramus: It extends from the body to ramus of the ischium. Together with ramus of the ischium it forms conjoint 'ischiopubic ramus'.

Ilium

It forms the upper expanded bony plate of hipbone. It has the following important features.

- **Iliac crest:** It is the upper border of the ilium. The highest point of the iliac crest is situated at the level of the spines of L4 vertebrae which is used to locate the interval between L3 and L4 spine during lumbar puncture. The anterior end of the iliac crest is called **anterior superior iliac spine** and the posterior end is called the **posterior superior iliac spine**. The anterior border of the ilium extends from the anterior superior iliac spine to the acetabulum. Its lowest part presents a prominence called anterior inferior iliac spine.

- The anterior superior iliac spine provides attachment to sartorius muscle and lateral end of the inguinal ligament. The anterior inferior iliac spine gives attachment to the straight head of the rectus femoris muscle and **iliofemoral ligament** of the hip joint.

- The posterior superior iliac spine is a dimple 4 cm lateral to the second sacral spine.

- The iliac crest is divided into anterior $2/3^{rd}$ and posterior $1/3^{rd}$.

- The posterior $1/3^{rd}$ provides attachment to gluteus maximus and erector spinae muscles.

- The anterior $2/3^{rd}$ of the iliac crest is divisible into an outer, an intermediate and inner lips. The outer lip provides attachment to external oblique abdominis, fascia lata and tensor fascia lata and latissimus dorsi muscles. The intermediate lip provides attachment to internal oblique muscles of the abdomen. The inner lip provides attachment to transversus abdominis muscles and also quadratus lumborum in the posterior part.

- Greater sciatic notch – It is the curved notch on the posterior border of ilium, just below the posterior inferior iliac spine. This notch is converted into greater sciatic foramen by two ligaments (sacrotuberous and sacrospinous ligaments). This foramen transmits nerves (sciatic nerve) and vessels to the lower limb.

- Ilium presents two surfaces.

1. **Outer gluteal surface**: It presents anterior, middle and posterior gluteal lines. The area behind the posterior gluteal line is for the origin of the gluteus maximus muscle. The area between anterior and posterior gluteal line provides attachment to gluteus medius muscle. The area between anterior and inferior gluteal line provides attachment to gluteus minimus muscle.

2. **Inner surface** presents iliac fossa in front and sacro-pelvic surface behind.

- Iliac fossa provides attachment to iliacus muscle. It forms false pelvis. Caecum with appendix is located in the right iliac fossa and sigmoid colon in the left iliac fossa.
- The sacropelvic surface presents 'auricular' (ear shaped) surface for the side of the sacrum to form sacroiliac joint.

Ischium

It forms the posteroinferior part of the hip bone. It consists of body and ramus. It presents an ischial spine and an ischial tuberosity.

- **Ischial tuberosity:** The lower end of the body forms 'ischial tuberosity'. The upper part of the ischial tuberosity provides origin to semimembranosus (on lateral side) and semitendinosus with long head of biceps femoris muscle (on medial side). The lower part provides origin to the hamstring part of the adductor magnus muscle.
- **Ischial spine:** The posterior border of the body of ischium presents spine like projection called 'ischial spine'. Above the ischial spine is the greater sciatic notch and below is the lesser sciatic notch. Lesser sciatic notch is also converted into a foramen by sacrotuberous and sacrospinous ligaments. The ischial spine provides attachment to sacrospinous ligament and coccygeus muscle.
- **Ramus of the ischium:** It arises from the lower part of the body and joins the inferior ramus of the pubis (conjoint ischiopubic ramus)
- **Acetabulum:** It is a cup shaped cavity on the lateral aspect of the hip bone. Its deficient lower margin is called the acetabular notch. Its lunate shaped articular surface articulates with the head of the femur to form the hip joint.
- **Obturator foramen:** It is a large gap in the hip bone. This foramen is closed by the obturator membrane. The medial margin of the foramen transmits obturator nerve and vessels. The margins of the foramen provides attachment to obturator externus on the outer aspect and the obturator internus on the inner aspects.

Ossification: The hip bone ossifies by 3 primary centres and 5 secondary centres.

The primary centres are for ilium appears during 2nd month, for ischium appears during 3rd month and for pubis at 4th month of intrauterine life.

Two secondary centres for iliac crest, two for acetabulum and one for ischial tuberosity appear during puberty. The ossification of the acetabulum is completed by 17 years and rest of the bone by 20–25 years.

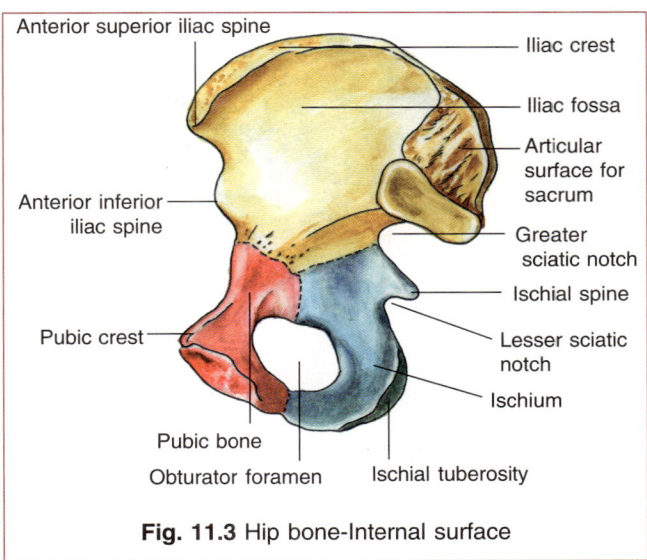

Fig. 11.3 Hip bone-Internal surface

Pelvic fractures affecting pubis can involve urinary bladder and urethra. For more clinical anatomy refer Chapter 42, bony pelvis.

FEMUR (THIGH BONE)

Femur is the longest and strongest bone of the body. It presents the following parts: upper end, shaft and lower end (Figs 11.4 and 11.5).

Upper end

- Head: It articulates with the acetabulum of the hip bone, to form hip joint.
- Fovea capitis is a pit below and behind the centre of head. Ligament of head of the femur (ligamentum teres) is attached to it. It transmits branches from obturator and medial circumflex iliac arteries to the head of the femur
- Neck: It connects the head with the shaft. It is about 5 cm in length. Its anterior surface and medial part of the posterior surface is intracapsular.

  Neck shaft angle: It is the angle between the lower border of the neck and medial border of the shaft. It is about 125° in adults and 160° in children. Its clinical relevance is explained in the hip joint.
- **Greater trochanter:** This is a large prominence at the upper part of the junction of the neck with the shaft.
- A ridge on the upper part of medial surface receives insertion of obturator internus, superior and inferior gemelli.
- Trochanteric fossa is a depression in the lower part of medial surface. It receives insertion of obturator externus.

SECTION 4

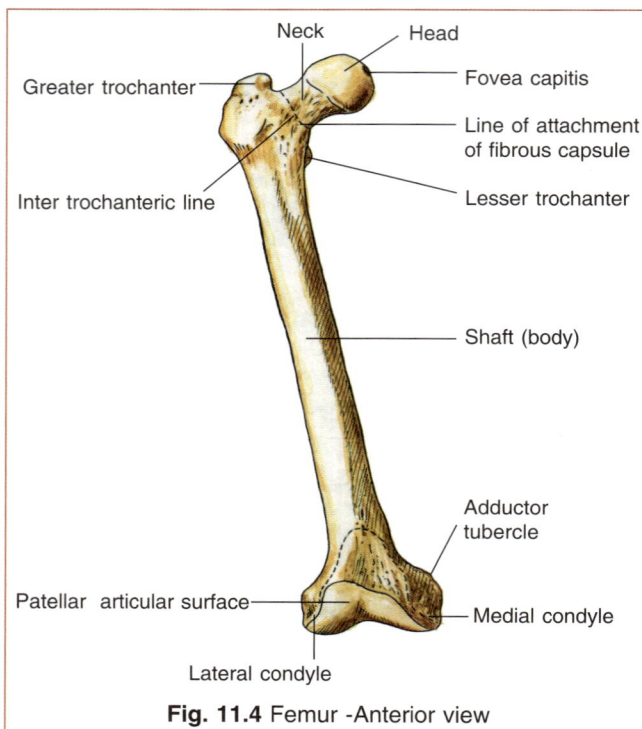

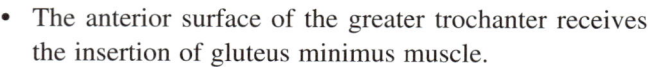

Fig. 11.4 Femur -Anterior view

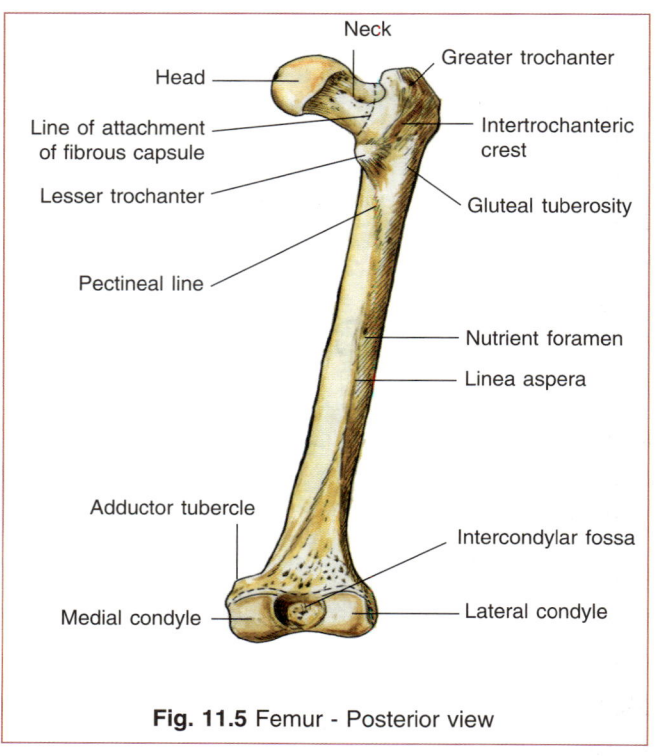

Fig. 11.5 Femur - Posterior view

- The anterior surface of the greater trochanter receives the insertion of gluteus minimus muscle.
- The lateral surface of the greater trochanter provides insertion to gluteus medius muscle. It is related to a bursa.
- Apex of greater trochanter receives insertion of piriformis muscle.
- **Lesser trochanter** is a conical eminence, present on the posteroinferior part of the neck. It receives the insertion of iliopsoas muscle.
- **Inter trochanteric crest**: It connects greater trochanter and lesser trochanter (junction between neck and shaft) posteriorly. **Quadrate tubercle** is an elevation in this crest that receives insertion of quadratus femoris muscle.
- **Intertrochanteric line:** It connects greater trochanter and lesser trochanter (junction between neck and shaft) anteriorly. The capsule of the hip joint is attached to this line.

Shaft

It is a cylindrical structure projected forward in the middle. It presents 3 borders (medial, lateral and posterior) and 3 surfaces (anterior, medial and lateral).

The posterior surface of the shaft presents a bony ridge called 'linea aspera' with medial and lateral lips. The medial lip of the linea aspera continues upwards as **spiral**

line and lateral lip as **gluteal tuberosity**. Below, the medial lip continues as medial supracondylar line and lateral lip as lateral supracondylar line. The triangular area between the medial and lateral supracondylar lines is called popliteal surface. It is related to popliteal vessels, the artery being nearer to the bone.

Major attachments:

The gluteal tuberosity provides insertion to 1/4th of the gluteus maximus muscle and the area lateral to it provides origin to vastus lateralis muscle.

The spiral line provides insertion to pectineus and area lateral to it for vastus medialis muscles.

The upper 3/4th of the anterior surface provides origin to vastus intermedius muscle and articularis genu in the lower part.

The medial surface is covered by vastus medialis muscle

Attachments to the linea aspera

The medial lip gives origin to vastus medialis muscle.

The area between the medial and the lateral lip provides insertion to adductor brevis in the upper part and the adductor longus in the lower part.

The area lateral to the attachment of adductor brevis and longus provides insertion to adductor magnus muscle.

The lateral lip provides origin to vastus lateralis muscle and to the short head of the biceps femoris in the lower part.

Lower end

- Condyles: The lower end of the femur is widely expanded to form two large condyles (medial and lateral). Posteriorly the two condyles are separated by a gap called intercondylar fossa.

Lateral condyle

- The lateral surface of the lateral condyle presents lateral epicondyle which is the highest point in this surface. It provides attachment to fibular collateral ligament. The area above and behind the lateral epicondyle provides origin to lateral head of the gastrocnemius muscle.

- A groove that lies below and behind the lateral epicondyle provides attachment to popliteus muscle in the anterior part. The posterior part of the groove is occupied by the tendon of the popliteus muscle (during full flexion of the knee joint)

- The medial surface of the lateral condyle provides attachment to anterior cruciate ligament.

Medial condyle

- The medial surface of the medial condyle presents 'medial epicondyle' which provides attachment to tibial collateral ligament of the knee joint.

- Above the medial epicondyle is a prominent tubercle called **adductor tubercle** which receives insertion of tendon of the adductor magnus muscle.

- The lateral surface of the medial condyle provides attachments to posterior cruciate ligament.

The condyle presents two articular surfaces.

1. The patellar surface articulates with the patella anteriorly (part of the knee joint). Its lateral part is extended higher up than the medial part to reciprocate with the articular surface of the patella.

2. The tibial surface on the inferior aspect articulates with the condyles of the tibia (the knee joint).

Angle of femoral torsion: In anatomical position the head and neck of the femur is placed forward when compared to the shaft and lower end of the femur. When the long axis of the head and neck of the femur (imaginary line passing through the centre of the head through neck and then greater trochanter) is superimposed with transverse axis of the condyles distally (when the femur is viewed along the long axis of the shaft), it makes an angle of about 12 to 15° in adults, but it is more in children.

Ossification: One primary centre for the shaft appears during 8th week of development. There are 4 secondary centres:

1. For lower end- it appears at 9 months of intrauterine life or day of birth.

2. For head- it appear during first year.

3. For greater trochanter- it appear during 3rd year.

4. For lesser trochanter- it appears during 13 years.

5. All the 3 secondary centres fuse with each other, which fuses with the shaft by 18 years. The lower epiphyses fuses with the shaft by 20 years

- The common site of fracture is at femur neck in old age and shaft in young age.

- The fracture of the neck may damage the blood vessels supplying neck and head of femur (neck is intracapsular). It may lead to necrosis of head.

- Medicolegal importance: The epiphyseal centre for the lower end of femur appears in the ninth month of intrauterine life just before birth. Hence its presence provides a proof for viability of the baby.

- In case of supracondylar fracture the distal segment is pulled backwards by gastrocnemius muscle which may injure the popliteal artery.

CASE-1

A 27-year-old man was admitted to the hospital following an automobile accident. Apart from other superficial injuries, he was found to have a fracture of the middle third of the right femur shaft. On examination, the right leg showed 2 inches (5 cm) of shortening when compared to normal side. A lateral radiograph showed overlapping of fragments with the distal fragment rotated backward. Using your knowledge of anatomy, can you explain the shortening of the right leg? Why was the distal fragment rotated posteriorly? What amount of force is necessary to restore the leg to its original length?

PATELLA (KNEE CAP)

The patella is the largest sesamoid bone in the body developed in the tendon of the quadriceps femoris muscle. It is situated in front of the lower end of femur, about 1 cm above the knee joint.

It has an apex, base, medial and lateral borders, anterior and posterior surfaces (Fig. 11.6).

- The base is directed upwards which receives insertion of rectus femoris in front and vastus intermedius behind.

- The apex of the patella is directed downwards and provides attachment to ligamentum patellae.

- The lateral border receives expansion from vastus lateralis muscle in the form of lateral patellar retinaculum
- The medial border receives expansion from the vastus medialis muscle in the form of medial patellar retinaculum and also few muscle fibres of vastus medialis muscle.
- Its anterior surface is separated from the skin by a prepatellar bursa
- The upper part of its posterior surface articulates with the femur. This articular area is divided into a large lateral facet for lateral condyle of the femur and a small medial area for the medial condyle of the femur.

Patella tends to be displaced laterally by an oblique and upward pull of quadriceps femoris muscle. However, this tendency is minimized by

1. Forward projection of lateral condyle of femur.
2. Insertion of vastus medialis extending to medial border.

The patella can be fractured by a direct blow. It is also possible that patella presents abnormal ossification resulting in two or three pieces of bones, which sometimes can be mistaken for patellar fracture.

TIBIA

Tibia is the medial and larger bone of the leg. It has the following important parts: upper end, shaft and lower end (Figs 11.7 and 11.8).

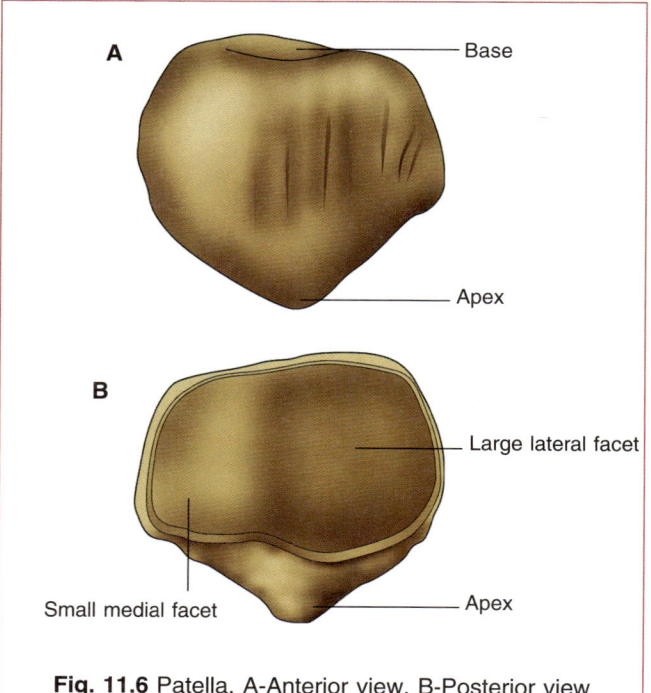

Fig. 11.6 Patella, A-Anterior view, B-Posterior view

Upper end

It is expanded to form two large condyles.

- **Medial condyle:** Its superior surface articulates with medial condyle of the femur (knee joint). A groove on the posterior aspect of the medial condyle receives the insertion of the semimembranosus muscle.
- **Lateral condyle:** Its superior surface articulates with lateral condyle of the femur (knee joint). Posteroinferiorly it presents a fibular facet for the head of the fibula (superior tibiofibular joint).
- **Intercondylar area:** It is the rough area between the superior articular surfaces of medial and lateral condyles. It provides attachment to cruciate ligaments and ends (horns) of menisci. The intercondylar area provides attachment to following structures from before backwards

  1. Anterior horn of the medial meniscus
  2. Anterior cruciate ligament
  3. Anterior horn of the lateral meniscus
  4. Posterior horn of the lateral meniscus
  5. Posterior horn of the medial meniscus
  6. Posterior cruciate ligament

  (It is usually remembered by a mnemonic – Medical College, Lucknow, Lucknow Medical College)

- The tibial tuberosity is a prominent elevation in the upper and anterior part of the tibia. It gives attachment to the ligamentum patellae.

Shaft

The shaft presents 3 borders (anterior, medial and lateral) and 3 surfaces (lateral, medial and posterior) (Figs 11.7 to 11.9).

- The anterior border extends from tibial tuberosity to anterior border of the medial malleolus. It is also called shin and provides attachment to superior extensor retinaculum in the lower part.
- The medial border extends from the medial condyle to the posterior border of the medial malleolus. It joins the soleal line at the junction of upper 1/3rd and lower 2/3rd.
- The lateral border extends from lateral condyle to anterior border of the fibular notch. It provides attachment to interosseus membrane.
- The medial surface is subcutaneous. Its upper part receives the insertions of sartorius, gracilis, semitendinosus muscles and tibial collateral ligament from before backwards. This surface is traversed by great saphenous vein.

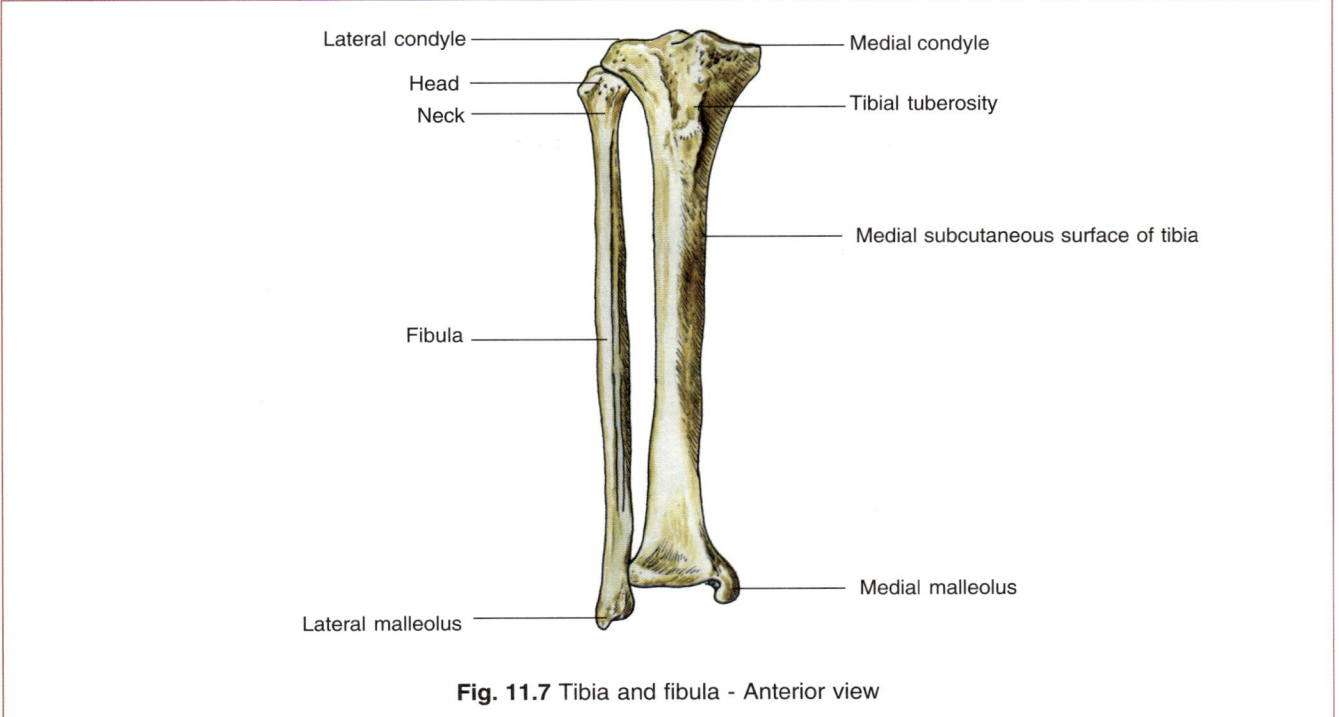

Lateral condyle

Head

Neck

Medial condyle

Tibial tuberosity

Medial subcutaneous surface of tibia

Fibula

Medial malleolus

Lateral malleolus

Fig. 11.7 Tibia and fibula - Anterior view

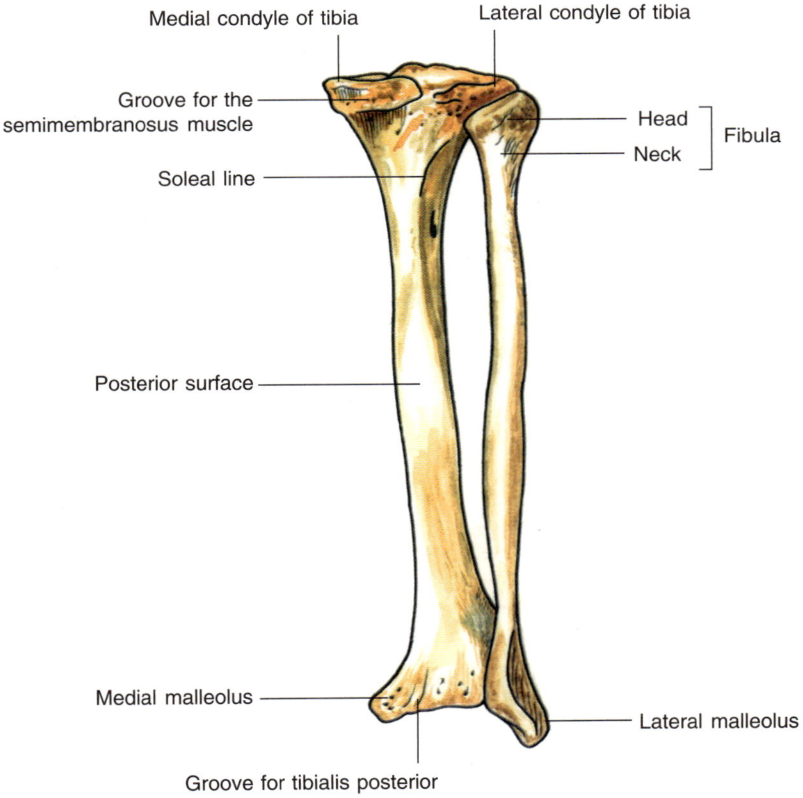

Medial condyle of tibia

Lateral condyle of tibia

Groove for the
semimembranosus muscle

Head

Neck

Fibula

Soleal line

Posterior surface

Medial malleolus

Lateral malleolus

Groove for tibialis posterior

Fig. 11.8 Tibia and Fibula - Posterior view

SECTION 4

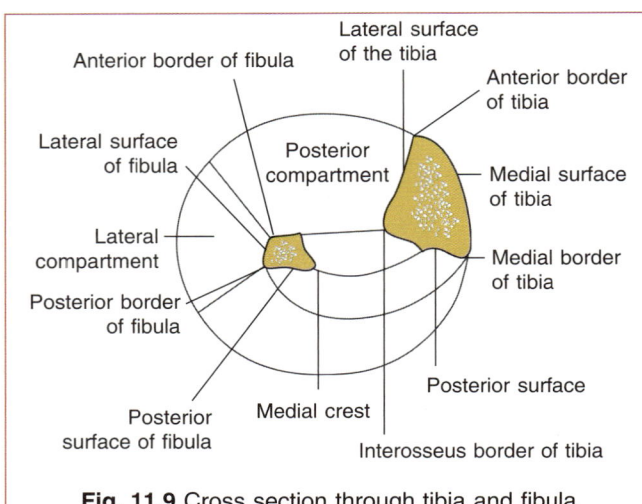

Fig. 11.9 Cross section through tibia and fibula

• The lateral surface provides origin to the tibialis anterior muscle in the upper 2/3rd. Its lower part is related to following structures from medial to lateral side-tibialis anterior, extensor hallucis longus, anterior tibial artery, deep peroneal nerve, extensor digitorum longus, peroneus tertius.

• The posterior surface presents an oblique ridge called soleal line, which provides origin to the soleus muscle. The triangular area above the soleal line receives the insertion of popliteus muscle. This surface presents nutrient foramen. The area below the soleal line is divided into medial and lateral parts. The medial part provides origin to flexor digitorum longus and tibialis posterior on the lateral side. The lower part of the posterior surface is related to following structures from before backwards-tibialis posterior, flexor digitorum longus, posterior tibial artery, tibial nerve and flexor hallucis longus.

Lower end

It presents 5 surfaces: anterior, medial, posterior, lateral and inferior.

Its lateral surface presents a triangular fibular notch. It is connected to the lower end of the fibula by an interosseus ligament (inferior tibiofibular joint).

Its medial surface continues with medial surface of the medial malleolus.

Its inferior surface articulates with the talus to form the ankle joint.

Medial malleolus

• It is a short, strong process, which projects down from the medial surface of the lower end of tibia.

• Its posterior surface presents a groove for the passage of the tendon of tibialis posterior muscle. Further behind

it provides attachment to the flexor retinaculum of the ankle.

• The lateral surface presents a facet for articulation with medial surface of the talus.

Ossification: One primary centre appears for the shaft at the age of the 8th week of intrauterine life. There are 2 secondary centres for upper and lower ends respectively. The centre for upper end appears at birth and fuses with shaft by 20 years, for the lower end it appears during 2nd year and fuses with the shaft by 18 years.

• Tibia is commonly fractured at the junction of the upper 2/3rd and lower 1/3rd of shaft. If the nutrient foramen is involved in fracture, nonunion of the fractured elements is possible due to involvement of nutrient artery.

• Upper end of the tibia is one of the commonest sites for acute osteomyelitis.

• In rickets (calcium deficiency) tibia is often involved leading to bowlegs. The outward curving of the tibia is referred as genu valgum and inward curving referred as genu varum.

• Bone grafts are easily obtained from the subcutaneous medial surface of the tibia.

• Inversion at the subtalar joint is associated with external rotation of talus. It can use to fracture of lateral malleolus but if it is a severe injury then involves fracture of medial malleolus followed by fracture of the posterior margin of the tibia. When it involves all 3 fractures it is referred as trimalleolar fracture but if it is involving only lateral and medial malleolus then called as **Pott's fracture**.

FIBULA

Fibula is the lateral bone of the leg. It has the following parts: upper end, shaft and lower end (Figs 11.7 to 11.9).

Upper end (head)

It is expanded in all directions.

• The superior surface bears an articular facet to articulate with the lateral condyle of the tibia (superior tibiofibular joint).

• The apex of the head is called as styloid process. It provides insertion to biceps femoris muscle in the form of the letter 'C'. The area within the hilum of the 'C' provides attachment to fibular collateral ligament.

• The constriction below the head is called the neck of the fibula. The common peroneal nerve winds round the neck.

Shaft

It is narrow elongated part, which connects the two ends. It presents 3 borders (anterior, posterior and medial) and 3 surfaces (medial, lateral and posterior)

- The anterior border splits inferiorly to enclose a triangular area. The anterior margin of this triangular area provides attachments to superior extensor retinaculum while posterior margin to superior peroneal retinaculum.

- The medial border is present very close to the anterior border lying just medial to it. It provides attachment to interosseus membrane.

- The medial surface is narrow present between anterior and medial borders. It provides attachment to extensor digitorum longus, extensor hallucis longus and peroneus tertius.

- The lateral surface is between anterior and posterior borders. It provides attachment to peroneus longus and brevis muscles.

- The posterior surface is between medial and posterior border. Its upper 2/3rd is divided into medial and lateral area by a sharp vertical ridge called 'medial crest'. It is related to peroneal artery and nerve to flexor hallucis longus. The area medial to the median crest gives origin to tibialis posterior and lateral area to flexor hallucis longus.

- The posterior surface presents a nutrient foramen and the nutrient artery is a branch from the peroneal artery.

- The lower part of the posterior surface provides attachment to anterior tibiofibular, interosseus tibiofibular and posterior tibiofibular ligaments.

Lower end (lateral malleolus)

It presents 4 surfaces: medial, lateral, anterior and posterior.
- Its medial surface articulates with the talus (ankle joint).
- The medial surface also presents a depression called the malleolar fossa. It provides attachment to posterior tibiofibular ligament and posterior talofibular ligament.
- The posterior surface presents groove for the passage of the tendons of peroneus longus and brevis muscles.

Ossification: One primary centre for the shaft appears during 8th week of intrauterine life. There are 2 secondary centres, one for upper end and another for lower end. The centre for upper end appears at 4 years and fuses with the shaft by 20 years. The secondary centre for the lower end appears during 2nd year and fuses with the shaft by 18 years. It **violates the law of ossification** because the lower

epiphyses (secondary centre appeared first for the lower end) fuse with the shaft before the upper epiphyses. Remember the law of union of ossification states that the centre (secondary) which appears first fuses last with the diaphysis and vice versa.

- The common peroneal nerve is commonly injured near the neck of the fibula.
- Fibula is the ideal spare bone for a bone graft.

TARSAL BONES

The skeleton of the foot is formed by tarsal bones. There are 7 tarsal bones arranged in two rows (Figs 11.10 and 11.11).

Proximal row presents
- Talus (above the calcaneum)
- Calcaneus

Distal row includes
- Medial cuneiform
- Intermediate cuneiform
- Lateral cuneiform
- Cuboid
- Navicular bone (it is interposed between the two rows).

Talus

- It articulates with tibia and fibula at ankle joint and with calcaneus and navicular at the subtalar joint.
- It has no muscular attachment.
- It presents head, neck and body.
- The head presents a convex anterior surface which articulated with concavity of the navicular bone. The inferior surface of the head presents 3 facets, the anterior and posterolateral are for calcaneus and the medial is for spring ligament.
- The undersurface of the neck is narrow and is called **sulcus tali**. It is in relation with sulcus calcanei of calcaneus to form **sinus tarsi**. The sinus tarsi presents interosseus talocalcaneal ligament and cervical ligament.
- The body presents 5 surfaces: Superior, inferior, medial, lateral and posterior. The upper surface is referred as trochlear articular surface which articulates with the under surface of the tibia. The inferior surface presents oval shaped facet for calcaneus. The medial surface presents comma shaped articular surface for articulation with the medial malleolus and provides attachment to deep part of the deltoid ligament, while lateral surface

209

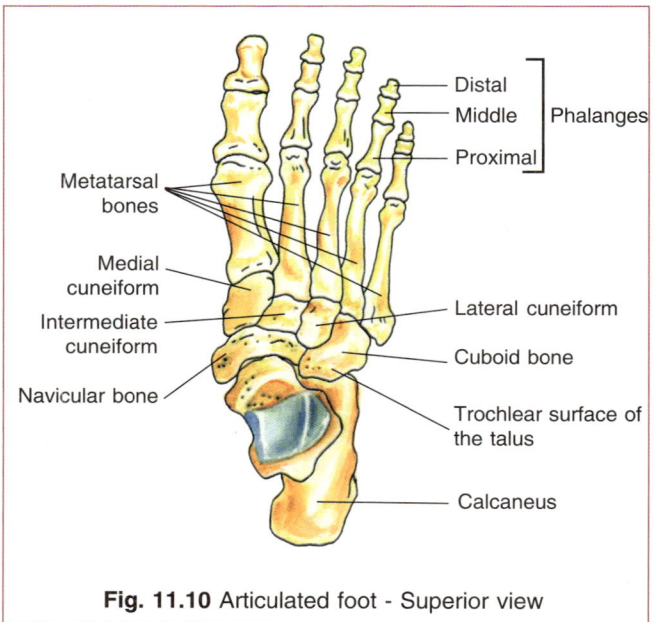

Fig. 11.10 Articulated foot - Superior view

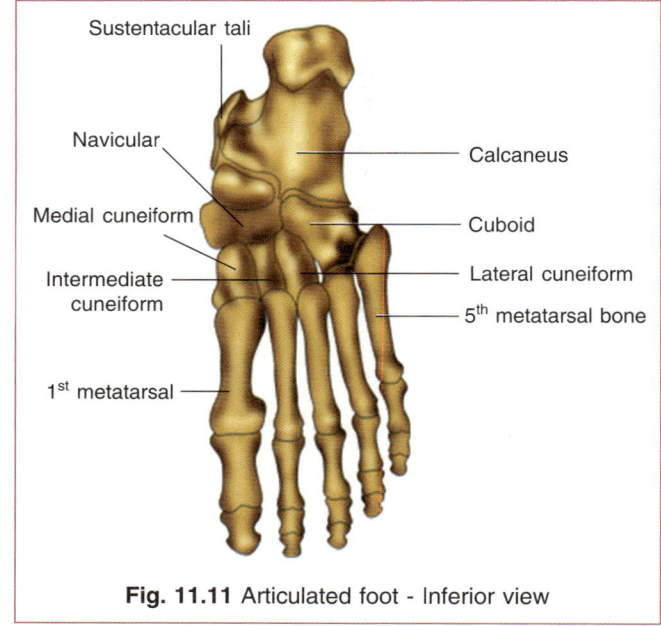

Fig. 11.11 Articulated foot - Inferior view

presents triangular shaped facet for articulation with the lateral malleolus. The posterior surface is grooved by tendon of flexor hallucis longus.

Forceful dorsiflexion may fracture the neck of the talus. The blood supply to the talus can be compared to the pattern of blood supply to scaphoid bone. The artery enters the bone through neck and proceeds backwards to the body. Fracture involving the neck can result in nonunion of the fractured elements and also avascular necrosis (Fig. 11.12).

Calcaneus

- It is the largest and strongest bone of the foot.
- It has 6 surfaces: anterior, posterior, superior, inferior, lateral and medial.

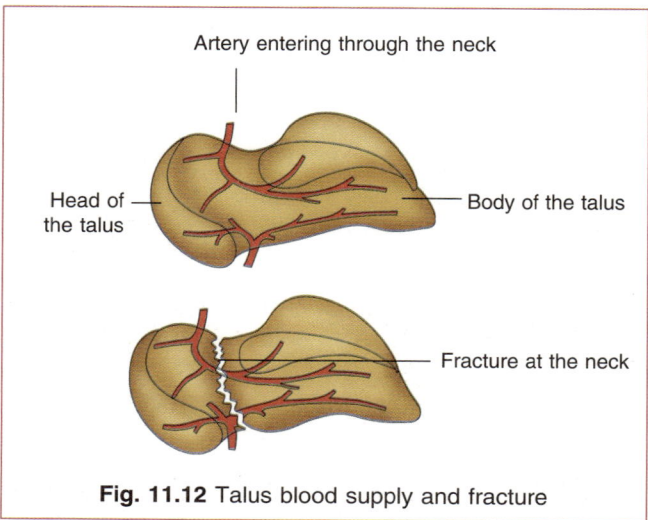

Fig. 11.12 Talus blood supply and fracture

- Anteriorly it articulates with cuboid.
- Its upper surface presents three facets for the articulation with talus of which the middle facet is situated over sustentaculum tali. Apart from that it has posterior and anterior non articular areas. The anterior non articular area presents 'sulcus calcanei with interosseus talocalcaneal ligament and cervical ligament on its medial side. On lateral side it provide attachment to stem of the inferior extensor retinaculum and origin of extensor digitorum brevis muscle.
- Its posterior part receives the insertion of tendocalcaneus in the middle while upper part is related to a bursa.
- The medial part of the calcaneus presents a bony projection called '**sustentaculum tali**'. It provides attachment to spring ligament, part of the deltoid ligament and few fibres of tibialis posterior muscle. The undersurface of the sustentaculum tali presents a groove for the passage of tendon of flexor hallucis longus.
- The lateral surface is subcutaneous in major part. It presents a small elevation in the anterior part called 'peroneal trochlea/tubercle', which separates the tendons of peroneus brevis above and peroneus longus below.
- The inferior (plantar) surface a small anterior tubercle and a posterior calcaneal tuberosity which is divided into the larger lateral and a smaller medial part. It provides attachment to plantar aponeurosis and muscles of the first layer of the sole and also long and short plantar ligaments.

Fracture of the calcaneus occurs when a person falls on his heals from a height.

Normally calcaneus ossifies from one centre which appears during 3rd month of IU life, but sometimes a secondary centre may appear for the posterior part at the age of 6–8 years. If present, it fuses with rest of the bone at the age of 16 years. Sometimes in a radiograph this could be mistaken for the fracture of the calcaneus in this age group.

Navicular bone

- Anteriorly it articulates with three cuneiform bones.
- Laterally it is connected to cuboid bone.
- Posteriorly it articulates with the head of talus.
- Tuberosity of the navicular bone is the projection on medial side. It receives insertion of tibialis posterior muscle.

  It is possible to have an accessory navicular bone in the foot.

Cuboid

- It is approximately cuboidal in shape.
- Anteriorly it articulates with the bases of 4th and 5th metatarsal bones.
- Posteriorly it articulates with calcaneum.
- Medially it articulates with lateral cuneiform bone and is connected with navicular bone (Fig. 11.13).
- The plantar surface of the cuboid presents a groove which is traversed by the tendon of peroneus longus muscle. The long plantar ligament converts this groove into a tunnel.

Cuneiform bones

- These are three wedge shaped bones named medial, intermediate and lateral cuneiform.

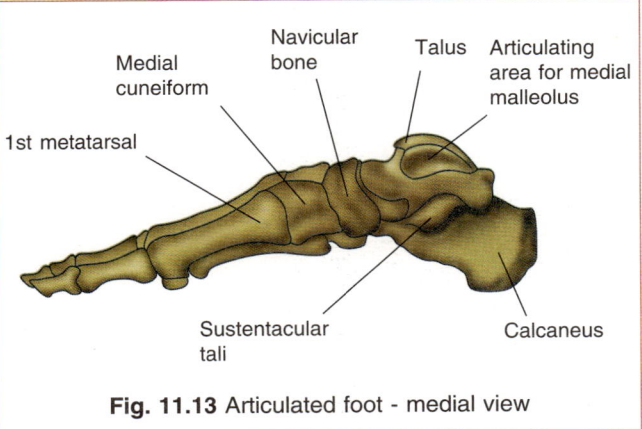

Fig. 11.13 Articulated foot - medial view

- The posterior end of each cuneiform articulates with navicular bone. Their anterior ends articulate with the bases of 1st, 2nd and 3rd metatarsal bones.
- Medial cuneiform bone receives the insertion of tibialis anterior and peroneus longus muscles.

Metatarsus

There are 5 metatarsal bones which are numbered from medial to lateral side. Proximally they articulate with the cuneiform and cuboid bones. Distally they articulate with the phalanges.

Fracture of the base of the 5th metatarsal is common.

Phalanges

There are 14 phalanges in each foot, 2 for the great toe and 3 for each of the other toes. These phalanges are smaller than the phalanges of the hand.

Solutions to the case studies

Case-1

The shortening of the leg was due to the distal fragment being pulled upwards and backwards by the hamstrings and the quadriceps femoris muscles. The backward rotation of the distal fragment was caused by the pull of the two heads of the gastrocnemius muscles. The muscles responsible for the shortening are very powerful, and prolonged traction to the distal fragment, using weights connected to a pin driven through the fragment which is required to obtain reduction of such a fracture.

MCQs

1. A building construction worker falls from a height and lands on his feet. Radiographs reveals a fracture of the sustentaculum tali. The muscle passing immediately beneath it that would be adversely affected is the:

   A. Tibialis anterior
   B. Tibialis posterior
   C. Peroneus longus
   D. Flexor hallucis longus

2. A deep laceration, 2 cm in length, immediately posterior to the medial malleolus, may injure any of the following *except*:

   A. Deep peroneal nerve
   B. Tibial nerve
   C. Tendon of tibialis posterior
   D. Tendon of flexor digitorum longus

3. An athlete complains of foot pain following one of his long running sessions. Upon examination, the physician

diagnoses tendinitis of the peroneus longus muscle. Because the tenderness is located deeply on the sole of the foot, it appears that the irritation occurred where the tendon grooves the under surface of the bone which is covered by long plantar ligament. Name the bone involved.

A. Medial cuneiform
B. Cuboid
C. Talus
D. Calcaneus

4. A patient has been diagnosed with bone cancer affecting the fibula that requires its removal. Which of the following muscles would be least affected following it's removal?

A. Biceps femoris
B. Extensor digitorum longus
C. Flexor digitorum longus
D. Flexor hallucis longus

5. Following are the muscles attached to the greater trochanter of the femur *except*

A. Piriformis
B. Obturator internus
C. Gluteus minimus
D. Gluteus maximus

6. The nerve which is likely to be damaged in the fracture affecting the neck of the fibula is

A. Tibial nerve
B. Common peroneal nerve
C. Sciatic nerve
D. Femoral nerve

7. The highest point of the iliac crest corresponds to the

A. disc between L1 and L2 vertebra
B. Spine of L3
C. disc between L3 and L4 vertebra
D. Spine of L4

Answers to MCQs

1. D
2. A
3. B
4. C
5. D
6. B
7. D

Thigh—Front, Medial and Back | 12

Objectives

- To explain the dermatomes, superficial veins and lymphatics of the lower limb.
- To explain the deep fascia of the thigh and its modifications.
- To know the cutaneous nerves, superficial arteries in front of the thigh.
- To explain the boundaries and contents of the femoral triangle.
- To explain the femoral sheath, canal, its contents and its clinical relevance
- To list the boundaries, contents and clinical relevance of adductor canal
- To explain the origin, course, termination and branches of femoral artery
- To explain the origin, course, branches, distribution and clinical relevance of femoral and obturator nerves
- To know the attachments, nerve supply and actions of muscles in front, medial compartment and back of the thigh.

CUTANEOUS NERVES OF THE THIGH AND DERMATOMES OF THE LOWER LIMB

The cutaneous innervation to the lower limb is derived from L1 to S3 segments with also contribution from T12 and S4 partly.

Cutaneous nerves in front of the thigh

The skin in front of the thigh is supplied by L1 to L3 segment of the spinal cord. The branches are derived from the lumbar plexus.

1. **Ilioinguinal nerve:** It is a branch from the lumbar plexus derived from ventral ramus of L1. It traverses the abdominal wall between internal oblique and transverses abdominis, pierces the internal oblique to enter the inguinal canal. It traverses the medial part of the inguinal canal, emerges through superficial inguinal ring. It supplies the upper and medial part of the front of thigh. In males it also supplies root of the penis, upper part of the scrotum and in female's mons pubis and upper part of labium majus (Fig. 12.1).

2. **Femoral branch of the genitofemoral nerve:** It is also a branch from the lumbar plexus derived from ventral ramus of L1 and L2 nerves. It arises as a common trunk called genitofemoral nerve which descends in relation to the psoas major muscle in the posterior abdominal wall to divide into genital and femoral branches. The genital branch enters the inguinal canal through deep inguinal ring supplying cremaster muscles. In males it supplies scrotum and in females labium majus. The femoral branch enters the lateral compartment of the femoral sheath lying usually in front of the femoral artery. It pierces the anterior wall of the femoral sheath, and fascia lata to supply the skin in front of the femoral triangle (Fig. 12.1).

3. **Anterior division of the obturator nerve:** The anterior division of the obturator nerve through subsartorial plexus supplies the skin of the medial side of the middle of thigh.

4. **Medial cutaneous nerves of the thigh:** It is a branch from the anterior division of the femoral nerve. Its

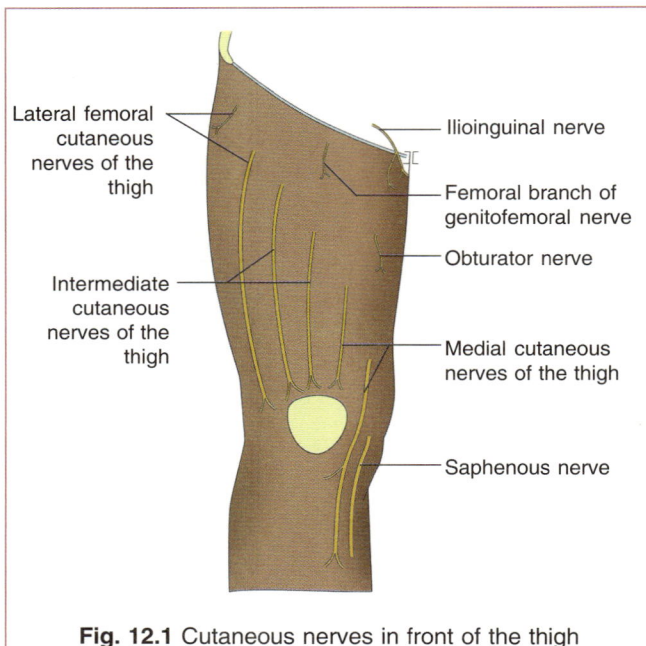

Fig. 12.1 Cutaneous nerves in front of the thigh

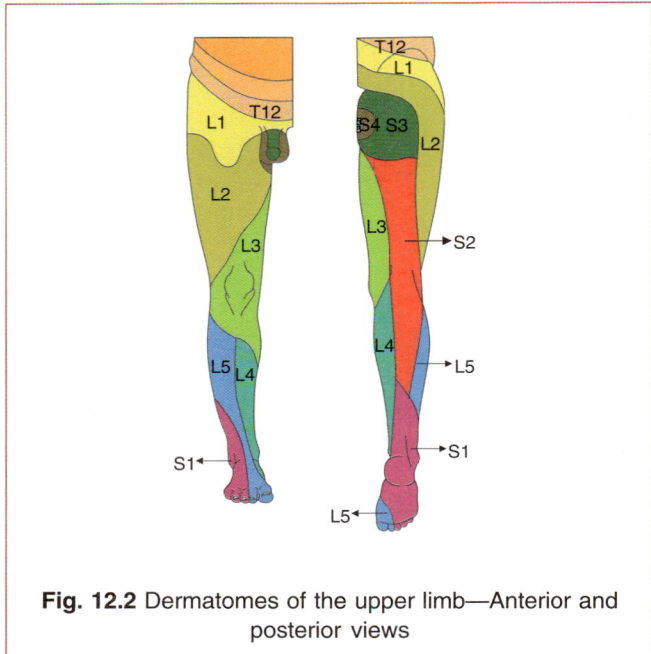

Fig. 12.2 Dermatomes of the upper limb—Anterior and posterior views

branches become superficial by piercing the fascia lata along the Sartorius muscle, supplies skin of the lower part of the front and medial side of the thigh.

5. **Intermediate cutaneous nerves of the thigh:** It is also a branch from the anterior division of the femoral nerve. Its branches pierce the fascia lata along the Sartorius muscle, little superior to the medial cutaneous branches. It supplies the skin of the lower part of the front of the thigh.

6. **Lateral cutaneous nerve of the thigh:** It is a branch from the lumbar plexus derived from L2 and L3 spinal nerves. It emerges from the lateral border of the psoas major muscle in the posterior abdominal wall, then crosses superficial to iliacus muscle. Medial to the anterior superior iliac spine it enters the thigh usually by passing deep to the inguinal ligament (sometimes pierces the ligament). In the thigh it divides into anterior and posterior branches. The anterior branch pierces the fascia lata about 10 cm below the anterior superior iliac spine. It supplies the skin of the lateral aspect of the front of the thigh. The posterior branch supplies the gluteal region, posterolateral aspect of the thigh.

Cutaneous nerve supply to the back of the thigh: The skin of the back of the thigh, the popliteal region and also the skin of the back of the upper part of the leg is supplied by posterior cutaneous nerve of the thigh. It is a branch from the sacral plexus derived from S1, S2 and S3 nerves. It also supplies the skin of the posteroinferior quadrant of the gluteal region.

The other cutaneous nerves supplying the lower limb are explained at appropriate chapter.

Dermatomes of the lower limb

The skin of the lower limb is supplied by L1 to S3 dermatomes with contribution from T12 and S4. There is a considerable overlapping of dermatomes; hence the area of sensory loss following damage to the spinal cord or nerve roots is less than the actual area of dermatome.

The central dermatomes-L4, L5 and S1 are represented only in the distal part of the limb and are buried proximally. The line along which the central dermatomes are buried is known as the axial line.

L1, L2 and L3 dermatomes:

The dermatomes in front of the thigh from above downwards are L1, L2 and L3. The L1 area involves skin below the inguinal ligament. The L2 area is below the L1 in front of the thigh, posterolateral aspect of the gluteal region and postural lateral aspect of the thigh. The L3 dermatome extends to posteromedial aspect of the thigh (Fig. 12.2).

L4 and L5 dermatomes:

The dermatome on the anteromedial and posteromedial side of the leg and medial side of the foot (both dorsum and plantar surface) L4, it includes the great toe.

The dermatome on the anterolateral and posterolateral side of the leg and middle part of the sole including plantar surface of the middle 3 toes is L5 (Fig. 12.2).

S1, S2 and S3 dermatomes:

The S1 dermatome involves the lateral border of the foot (both dorsum and plantar surface) including little toe and small strip of area along the posterolateral aspect of the ankle. (Thus sole is innervated by L4, L5 and S1 dermatomes.) The S2 dermatome involves the skin of the intermediate area on the back of the thigh and back of the upper $2/3^{rd}$ of the leg. The S3 dermatome involves lower portion of the gluteal region while S4 dermatome on the medial margin of the gluteal region (Fig. 12.2).

SUPERFICIAL VEINS OF THE LOWER LIMB

The superficial veins of the lower limb include great saphenous vein, small saphenous vein and irregular network of veins on the dorsum of the foot called 'dorsal venous arch'. The deeper veins accompany the arteries. Venous blood from the superficial veins is drained into deeper veins through perforating veins.

Great (long) saphenous vein

It is the longest superficial vein of the body. The term saphenous means easily seen, since the vein is superficial throughout its course it can be seen in most of the individuals.

Formation: It is formed by the union of medial end of the dorsal venous arch joining with the vein from the great toe (medial marginal vein).

Course:

- It ascends in front (about 2.5 cm) of the medial malleolus, superficial to the superior extensor retinaculum (Fig. 12.3).
- It ascends in relation to the lower $2/3^{rd}$ of the medial surface of the tibia. It is accompanied by saphenous nerve.
- Further the veins inclines posteriorly (one hand breadth posterior to the patella) to occupy posteromedial aspect of the knee.
- Then it ascends on the medial side of the thigh, where it is related to branches of medial cutaneous nerve of the thigh.

Termination: It passes through the saphenous opening after piercing the cribriform fascia and opens into femoral vein. The terminal part of the vein is accompanied by superficial inguinal lymph nodes.

Tributaries: There are many veins which drain into the great saphenous vein.

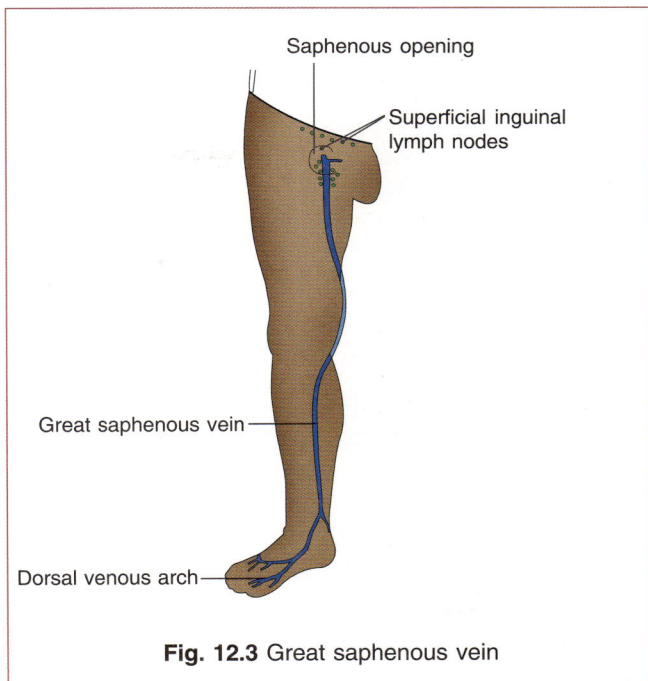

Fig. 12.3 Great saphenous vein

a. Posterior arch vein-from the posteromedial aspect of the calf

b. Anterior leg veins-ascends parallel to great saphenous vein in relation to the anterior aspect of the leg and opens into the great saphenous vein just below the knee.

c. There are many veins (anterolateral and posteromedial veins) opens into the great saphenous vein in the thigh.

d. Just before entering into the saphenous opening it receives 3 tributaries – superficial epigastric, superficial circumflex iliac and superficial external pudendal (corresponding to the superficial branches of the femoral artery).

e. Deep external pudendal vein draining blood from perineum also opens into the great saphenous vein.

A thoracoepigastric vein occasionally connects the superficial epigastric vein with lateral thoracic vein (a tributary of axillary vein). This communication will be useful for collateral circulation.

The great saphenous vein is connected with the deeper veins through many perforating veins. The perforating veins have valve and direct the blood from great saphenous to deeper veins.

  i. A perforating vein connected to femoral vein at the adductor canal

 ii. Couple of veins connected to posterior tibial vein just below the knee and also close to the medial border of the lower $2/3^{rd}$ of the tibia

iii. It is also connected with small saphenous vein

Valves of the great saphenous vein: There are about 10–12 valves present in the femoral vein. Of which the valve present just before the great saphenous vein's termination is called 'saphenofemoral valve'.

Venesection: In case of an emergency, when all the superficial veins are collapsed, venous cut down is performed through great saphenous vein just in front of the medial malleolus. The position of the vein is constant at this site, but care has to be taken to avoid damage to the saphenous nerve.

Varicose veins: Varicosity of the superficial veins of the lower limb is common in those who have to work in standing position for long periods. Age related structural changes in the valve are also responsible for varicosity. The varicose veins can cause inflammation of the affected part of the vein with pain, swelling and redness. The stagnation of venous blood causes change in the skin colour and leads to ulcers which can bleed.

Incompetence of the valves of the perforating veins or saphenofemoral vein cause varicosity of the great saphenous vein. A Trendelenburg test is performed to test whether valves of the perforating veins or the saphenofemoral valve are incompetent.

Testing: The patient is asked to lie down in supine position and the affected leg was raised to empty the blood in it. A tourniquet is applied in the upper part of the thigh to occlude the saphenous vein. The terminal part of the great saphenous vein can also be occluded manually by applying pressure through thumb (3 cm below and lateral to the pubic tubercle). Now the patient is asked to stand up. A slow filling of the great saphenous vein from below without releasing the pressure indicates the incompetency of valves of perforating vein. If the great saphenous vein is filled from above immediately after releasing the pressure at saphenofemoral junction indicates incompetency of saphenofemoral valve.

Great saphenous vein is often selected for coronary bypass surgeries in case of obstruction in coronary arteries. Due to the presence of valves, the vein has to be reversed while placing the graft.

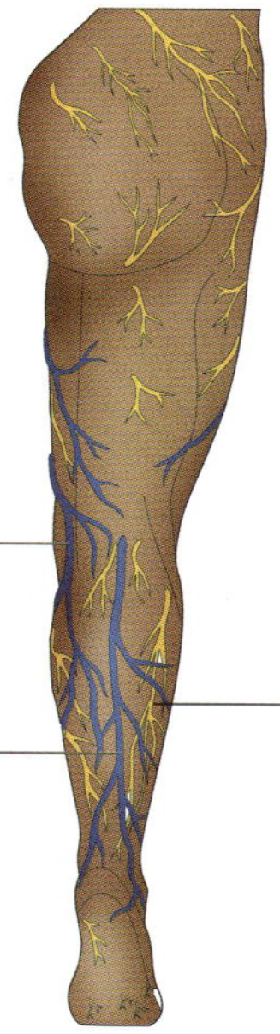

Small saphenous vein

Formation: It is formed by the union of the lateral end of the dorsal venous arch with a vein from the little toe (lateral marginal vein).

Course:

- It ascends posterior to the lateral malleolus where it is related to sural nerve.
- Thereafter the vein ascends along the middle of the back of the leg (Fig. 12.4).

Termination: At the back of the popliteal fossa it becomes deep by piercing the deep fascia and opens into popliteal vein. The terminal part of the vein is accompanied by few popliteal lymph nodes.

Venous pump of the leg: In standing position the venous return is against the gravity. Though the valves present in the superficial and deep veins allows unidirectional blood flow, the muscle contraction especially the calf muscles helps this cause. When the calf muscles contract the deep veins are compressed and the valves open up and the blood is propelled in upward direction. The soleus muscle contains many endothelial lined venous spaces and the contraction of this muscle squeeze the blood in upward direction. Hence soleus is often referred as peripheral heart. All the calf muscles together called 'venous pump'.

Fig. 12.4 Small saphenous vein

Great saphenous vein

Small saphenous vein

Sural nerve

CASE-1

A 49-year-old woman visited her physician complaining of a dull, aching pain in the lower part of both legs. She explains that this pain has been getting progressively worse since last one year and particularly bad at the end of a long day of standing at the working

SECTION 4

place. She also noticed that the skin along the medial side of the legs had started to become irritated. On examination, the patient was seen to have widespread varicose veins, extending from the lower part of the thigh to the dorsum of the foot in both legs. The skin showed marked discoloration over the medial malleoli and was dry and scaly. This patient had severe varicose veins of both legs, which required surgical treatment. On applying pressure over the varicose veins, it expanded further when the patient coughed.

1. Using your anatomical knowledge, name the vein involved in the present case.

2. What simple test must be performed before a radical venous operation is carried out?

3. Which important tributaries have to be ligated at operation?

4. Why did the varicose vein expanded on coughing?

5. Describe the so called "venous pump" of the leg.

LYMPHATIC DRAINAGE OF THE LOWER LIMB

Lymph nodes and lymph vessels of the lower limb can be divided into superficial and deep parts. The superficial lymph nodes are 'superficial inguinal lymph nodes'. The superficial lymph vessels accompany the great and small saphenous veins. The deep lymph nodes include deep inguinal and popliteal lymph nodes. The deep lymph vessels accompany the deeper veins and arteries.

Superficial inguinal lymph nodes

• They are located in the superficial fascia of the upper medial part of the thigh in relation to the terminal part of the great saphenous vein.

• The arrangement of the nodes resembles the letter 'T', with horizontal and vertical groups (Fig. 12.5).

• The horizontal group is located parallel and just below the inguinal ligament. The vertical group is present close to the terminal part of the great saphenous vein before piercing the cribriform fascia.

• The horizontal group is further divided into medial and lateral nodes. The medial nodes receive lymph from the external genitalia (except glans penis in males and clitoris in females), lower part of the anal canal, lower part of the vagina, terminal part of the male urethra and superolateral angle of the uterus.

• The lateral group receives lymph from superficial tissues of the gluteal region, adjoining part of the trunk.

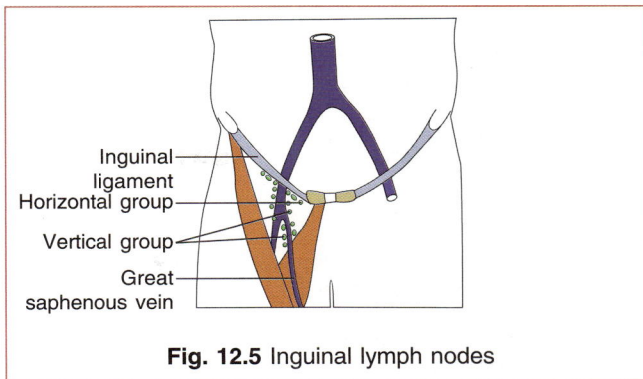

Fig. 12.5 Inguinal lymph nodes

• The horizontal group also receives lymph from superficial tissues of the anterior abdominal wall below the level of umbilicus (watershed line).

• The vertical group receives lymph from superficial tissue of the entire lower limb except the small saphenous area (heel, lateral part of the foot and posterolateral part of the leg.

Infection and inflammation are common in genital organs and examinations of these structures are important in enlargement of these nodes

Malignant melanoma usually affects the medial toes. It can spread through lymphatic vessels along the great saphenous vein and involves superficial inguinal lymph nodes. Hence in melanoma, the affected toe is amputated along with complete removal of superficial inguinal lymph nodes.

Elephantiasis of the lower limb occurs due to blockage of lymph vessels which results in massive edema. The lymphatic vessels are blocked by microfilarial parasites (Fig. 12.6).

Deep inguinal lymph nodes:

They are located medial to the femoral vein in the femoral triangle. It receives lymph from the deeper tissues of the entire lower limb, including lymph from popliteal nodes.

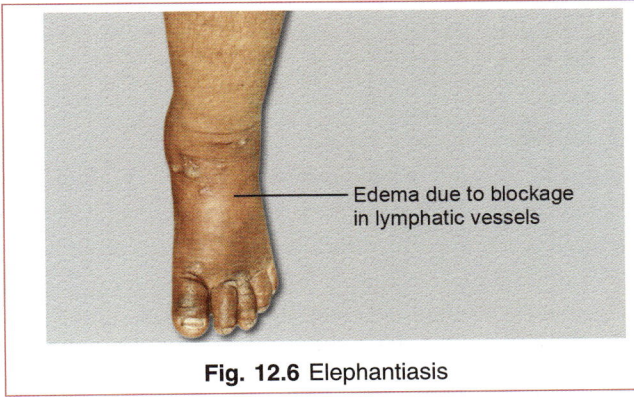

Fig. 12.6 Elephantiasis

Some of these nodes are within the femoral canal called 'Cloquet's' lymph nodes. These nodes receive lymph from glans penis in males and clitoris in females.

The efferent lymph vessels from inguinal lymph nodes drain into external iliac nodes.

Popliteal lymph nodes:

They are located in the popliteal fossa. The nodes present at the termination of the small saphenous vein receive lymph from sole, lateral border of the foot and posterolateral aspect of the leg. From these areas the lymph vessels follow the small saphenous vein. The deeper lymph nodes within the fossa receive lymph from deeper tissue of the leg and foot. The efferent vessels arising from popliteal nodes ends in deep inguinal lymph nodes

> Enlargement of the popliteal lymph nodes occur in infections of the heel which is common in diabetics.

CASE-2

A 47-year-old man visited his physician complaining of a lump in the groin. He had first noticed it three months ago, and it had gradually become larger. The lump was not causing any pain to the patient. On examination, a small discrete hard swelling was found about 2 inches (5 cm) below and lateral to the pubic tubercle on the front of the right thigh. Two smaller hard swellings were also found immediately below the other swelling. The patient's skin on the front and the back of the body was carefully examined from the level of umbilicus to the sole of the foot. The external genitalia were also carefully examined. Examination of the anal canal revealed nothing abnormal. The only abnormal lesion discovered was a small pigmented tumor beneath the nail of the right second toe.

1. What is the possible connection between the small painless mole on the second toe and the painless swellings in the groin?

2. Why did the physician examine such a wide area of the patient's body?

Fascia lata

The deep fascia in the body is best defined in the thigh and is called 'fascia lata'. It is very thick in the lateral part of the thigh where it forms iliotibial tract. It also presents an opening called saphenous opening. On its way for attachment with the iliac crest, the fascia lata splits twice to enclose 2 muscles tensor fasciae latae and gluteus maximus. Anterosuperiorly it is attached to the inguinal

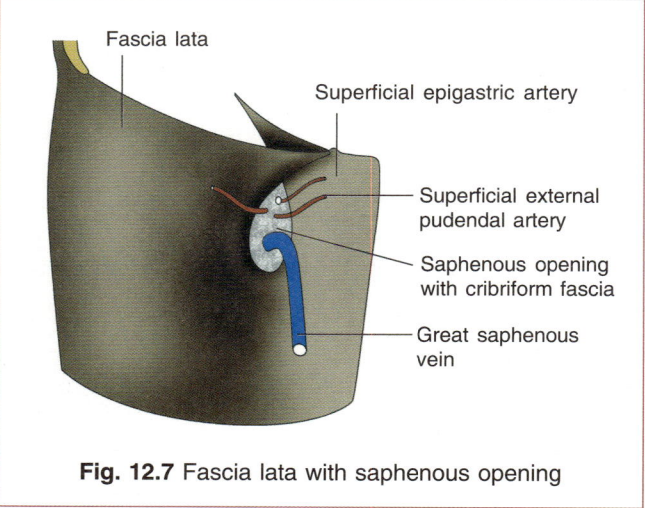

Fig. 12.7 Fascia lata with saphenous opening

ligament. It also sends intermuscular septa which are attached to the linea aspera and divides the thigh into 3 compartments-anterior, medial and posterior (Fig. 12.9). These fascia lata acts as a stocking to the thigh.

Saphenous opening: It is an oval opening in the fascia lata located about 3 cm below and lateral to the pubic tubercle. Its upper, lateral and lower margins are sharp and crescentic, but medial border is ill defined. The opening is covered by a thin fascia with many openings called 'cribriform fascia'. Following structures passes through the saphenous opening (Fig. 12.7).

a. Great saphenous vein

b. Superficial epigastric, superficial external pudendal arteries

c. Lymphatics connecting superficial and deep inguinal lymph nodes

d. Branches of medial cutaneous nerve of the thigh

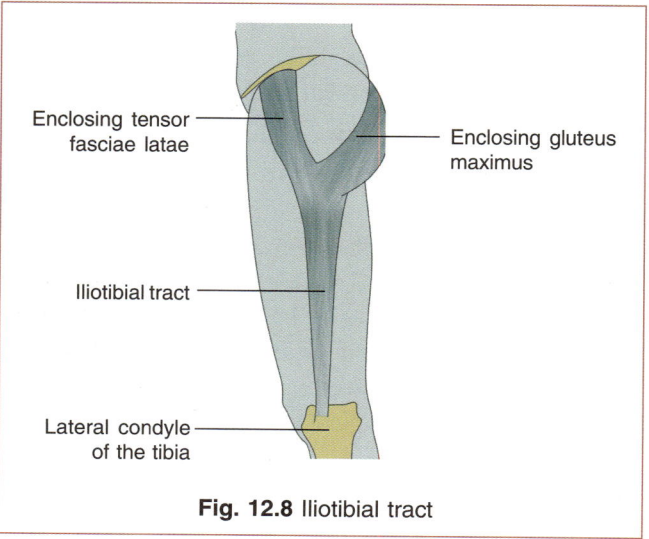

Fig. 12.8 Iliotibial tract

Iliotibial tract

- It is the lateral thick part of the fascia lata (Fig. 12.8).
- It is about 2.5 cm in width. Superiorly it splits into 2 layers to enclose the insertion of the tensor fasciae latae.
- Thereafter the superficial layer is attached to the iliac crest while the deep layer blends with the capsule of the hip joint. Posteriorly it receives the insertion of 3/4th of the gluteus maximus muscle.
- Inferiorly it is attached to the anterior surface of the lateral condyle of the tibia.
- Its inner surface continues as lateral intermuscular septum which is attached to the lateral lip of the linea aspera
- It stabilizes the knee in the extended position.

Subdivision of the thigh: The deep fascia sends intermuscular septa into the femur and divides the thigh into 3 compartments (Fig. 12.9).

1. **Anterior compartment**: It is mainly consists of quadriceps femoris muscle, but in the upper part presents iliopsoas muscle. The femoral artery and vein traverses this compartment. The nerve of the anterior compartment is the femoral nerve. The chief action of the quadriceps is extension of the knee joint.

2. **Medial compartment:** It consists of adductor muscles. They mainly cause adduction at the hip joint. They are supplied by obturator nerve.

3. **Posterior compartment:** It contains hamstring muscles and traversed by sciatic nerve. The sciatic nerve supplies hamstring muscles.

ANTERIOR COMPARTMENT OF THE THIGH

Muscles of the anterior (extensor) compartment of the thigh

The muscles in front of the thigh mainly extend the knee joint and this compartment is referred as extensor

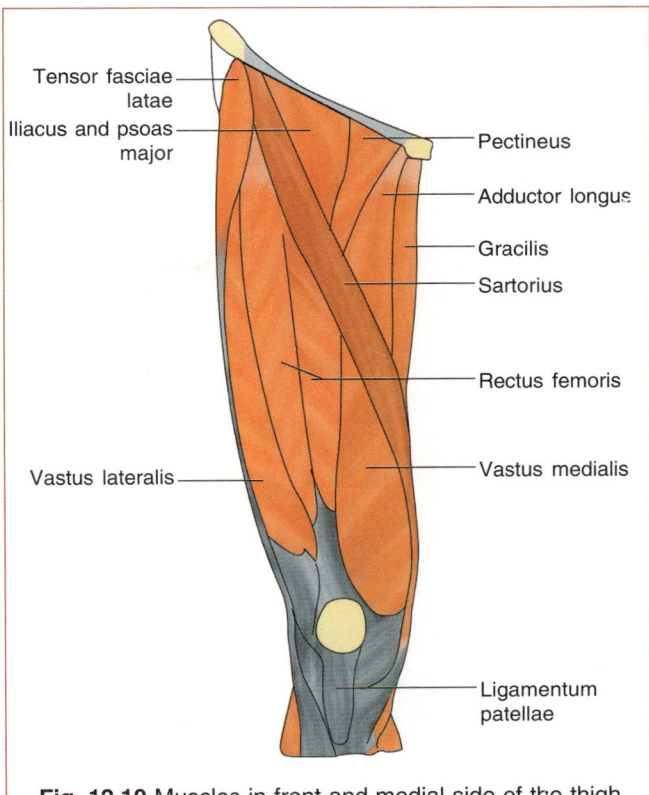

Fig. 12.10 Muscles in front and medial side of the thigh

compartment. The muscle is having 4 parts and called 'quadriceps femoris' (rectus femoris, vastus medialis, vastus intermedius and vastus lateralis). It is supplied by femoral nerve. The anterior compartment also includes muscles from the posterior abdominal wall and the iliac region. They are psoas major and iliacus. They end in the upper part of the thigh by getting inserted into the lesser trochanter. These muscles are the flexors of the hip joint. In addition it also

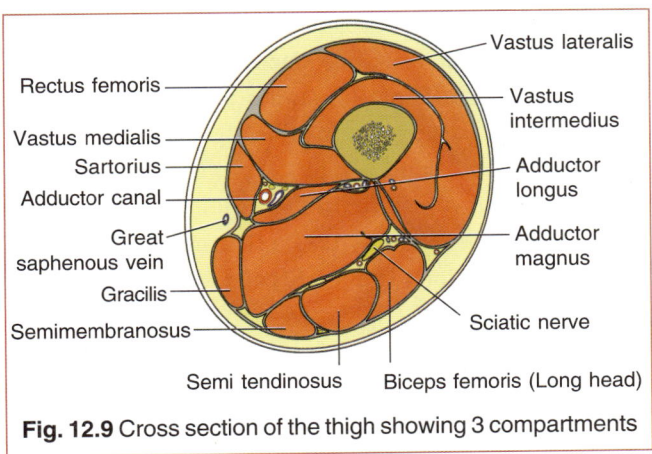

Fig. 12.9 Cross section of the thigh showing 3 compartments

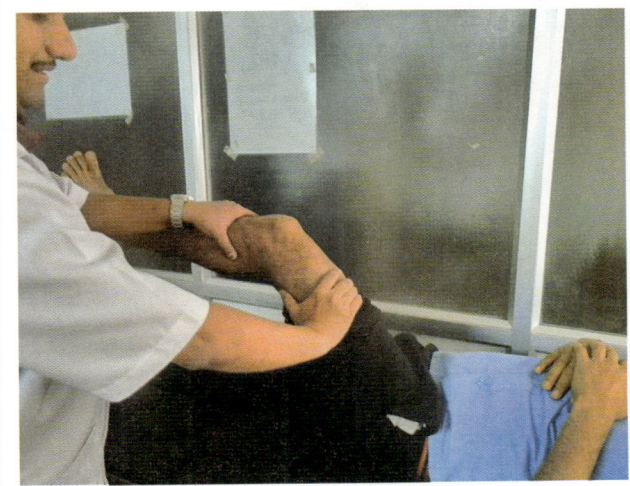

Fig. 12.11 Testing of quadriceps femoris muscle

Muscle	Origin	Insertion	Nerve supply	Actions
Rectus femoris	Straight head - upper half of anterior inferior iliac spine Reflected head- groove above the margin of aceta- bulum and capsule of hip joint	Base of patella anterior to vastusmedialis	Femoral nerve	Extensor of knee joint Flexor of hip joint
Vastus lateralis	Upper part of inter- trochanteric line Anterior and inferior borders of greater trochanter Lateral lip of gluteal tuberosity Upper half of lateral lip of linea aspera	Lateral 2/3rd of base and upper 1/3rd of lateral border of patella Capsule of knee joint	Femoral nerve	Extends the knee while standing, walking and running
Vastusmedialis	Lower part of inter- trochanteric line Spiral line Medial lip of linea aspera Upper 1/3rd of medial supracondylar line	Upper 2/3rd of the medial border and medial 1/3rd of the base of patella	Femoral nerve	Extends the knee joint prevents lateral displacement of patella rotates femur medially in locking of knee joint steadies the patella
Vastus intermedius	Upper 3/4th of ante- rior and lateral sur- face of femur shaft	Base of the patella	Femoral nerve	Extends the knee

Table 12.1 Quadriceps muscles

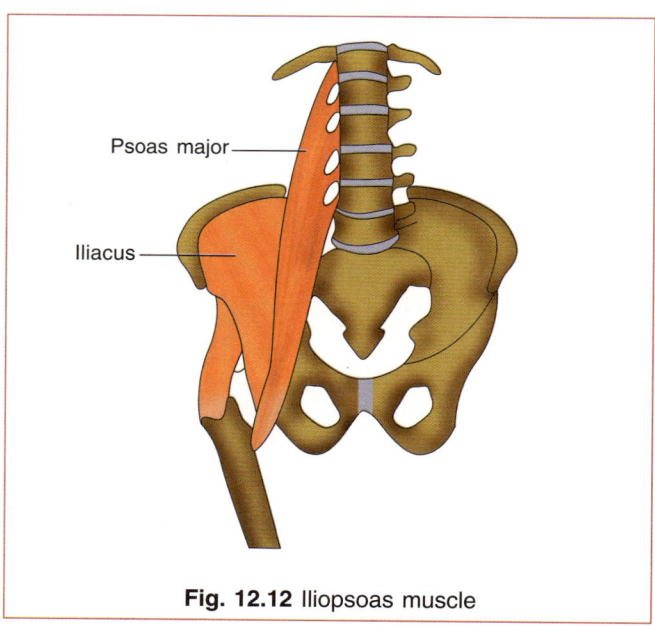

Fig. 12.12 Iliopsoas muscle

presents sartorius and tensor fasciae latae. The attachment, nerve supply and actions of quadriceps is discussed in Table 12.1 (Fig.12.10)

Iliopsoas muscle: It comprises two muscles namely psoas major and iliacus. The psoas major takes origin from the lumbar vertebral bodies while iliacus arises from iliac fossa of the ilium bone. The two muscles join together to form iliopsoas passes deep to the inguinal ligament and inserted into the lesser trochanter of the femur. The psoas is tendinous and fleshy fibres of iliacus join it. It contributes to the floor of the femoral triangle. The muscle is the chief flexor of the hip joint (Fig.12.12).

Sartorius muscle: The word sartor means tailor in latin. Tailor sits in both hip and knee flexed with thigh rotated laterally (Fig.12.10)

Origin: From anterior superior iliac spine

It descends downwards and laterally crossing in front of the thigh. It crosses superficial to quadriceps femoris muscle. It crosses posterior to the knee.

Insertion: It is inserted into upper part of the medial surface of the thigh (in front of the insertion of the gracilis and semitendinosus). At the insertion it is related to anserine bursa.

Nerve supply: Anterior division of the femoral nerve.

Actions: It causes flexion at both hip and knee joints and abductor of the hip joint.

Tensor fasciae latae: This muscle is located at the junction of the gluteal region and the thigh.

Origin: It takes origin from the anterior part of the iliac crest.

Insertion: It is inserted into the upper part of the iliotibial tract.

Nerve supply: Superior gluteal nerve.

Action: It abduct and medial rotator of the hip joint. Through the iliotibial tract it maintains the extended position of the knee joint.

Testing of Quadriceps femoris: The person is asked to lie down in supine position with knee partially flexed. Then he or she is asked to extend the knee when you are resisting this action, the normal muscle can be seen and felt easily (Fig.12.11).

Patellar tendon reflex: It tests the L2, L3 and L4 segment of the spinal cord or these spinal nerve roots forming femoral nerve. Tapping the ligamentum patellae with the knee hammer results in extension of the knee joint under normal circumstances. Both the afferent and efferent limb of the reflex is formed by femoral nerve.

Childhood immunizations are sometimes given via intramuscular injections into the quadriceps muscles especially vastus lateralis

---

Femoral triangle

It is a triangular depression in the upper part of the thigh. The base of the triangle is directed upwards and apex downwards (Figs 12.13 and 12.14).

Boundaries

Base: Inguinal ligament

Laterally: Medial border of sartorius

Medially: Medial border of adductor longus muscle

Apex: Meeting point of the medial and lateral borders (apex continues as adductor canal).

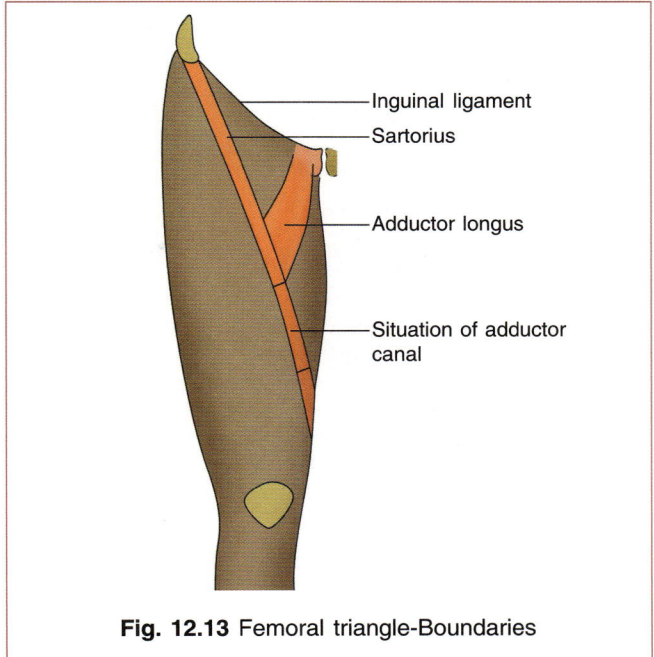

Fig. 12.13 Femoral triangle-Boundaries

- Inguinal ligament
- Sartorius
- Adductor longus
- Situation of adductor canal

Roof: Skin, Superficial fascia (with superficial inguinal lymph nodes, terminal part of the great saphenous vein, superficial arteries and cutaneous nerves).

Deep fascia (fascia lata) which shows an opening called 'saphenous opening'.

Floor: From medial to lateral side it is formed by Adductor longus, Pectineus, Iliopsoas muscles.

(Note: The interval between adductor longus and pectineus is traversed by profunda femoris vessels. The interval between pectineus and psoas is traversed by medial circumflex femoral artery. The interval between psoas and iliacus is occupied by femoral nerve)

Contents

1. Femoral artery and its branches
2. Femoral vein and its tributaries
3. Femoral nerve and its branches
4. Deep inguinal lymph nodes

Femoral sheath and femoral canal

It is a fascial sheath enclosing the proximal part of the femoral artery and vein. It extends from the level of the inguinal ligament and extends downwards for about 3 to 4 cm where it blends with the femoral vessels. It has anterior and posterior wall, which are connected by septa. The anterior wall of the sheath is derived from the fascia transversalis and the posterior layer by the fascia iliaca. The femoral nerve is outside the sheath because in the iliac fossa the nerve is deep to the fascia iliaca. The sheath is

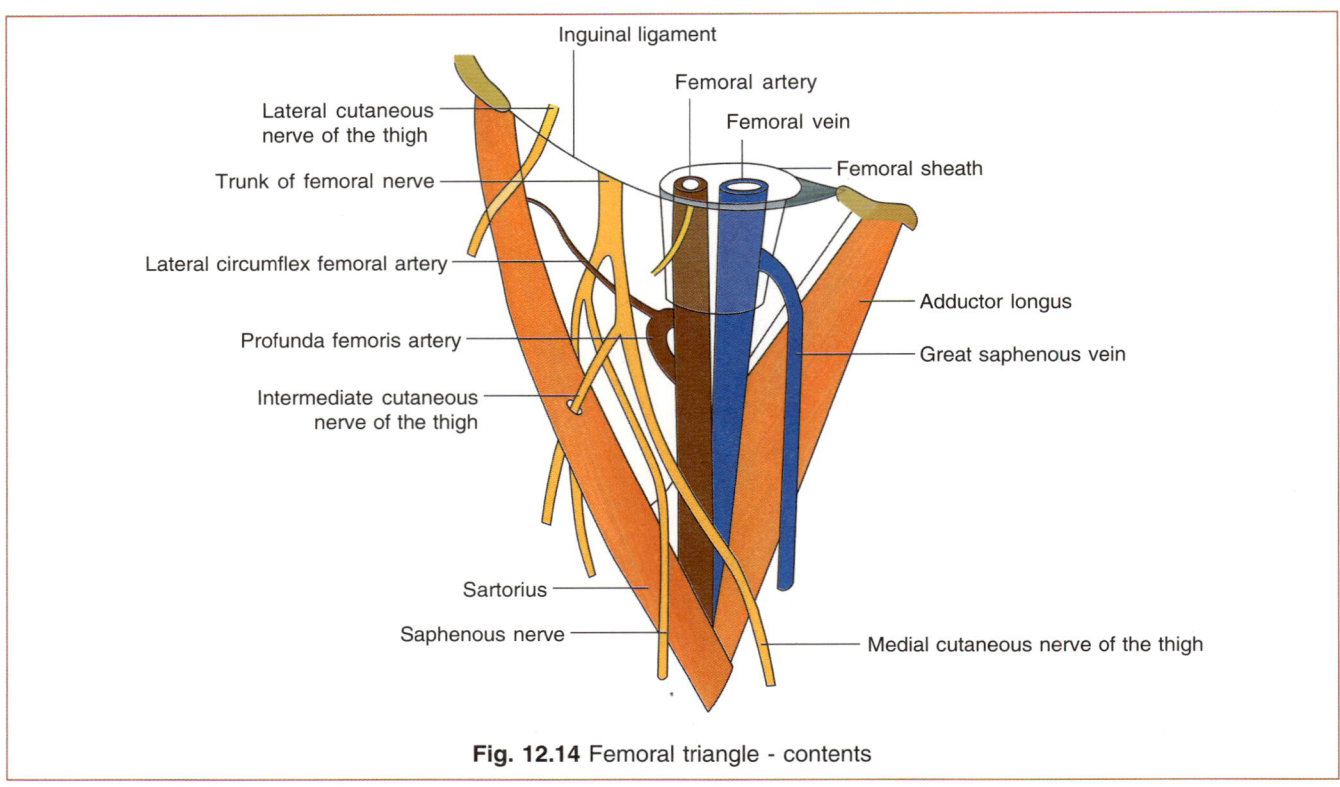

Fig. 12.14 Femoral triangle - contents

rudimentary at birth due to fetal flexed position, but extends below the inguinal ligament when the child starts extending the thigh. The femoral sheath protects the femoral vessels against the inguinal ligament during hip movement. The sheath is divided into three compartments (Figs 12.13 and 12.14).

1. Lateral arterial compartment encloses femoral artery and femoral branch of genitofemoral nerve.

2. Middle venous compartment encloses femoral vein.

3. Medial compartment is very short (1.25 cm long) and is called '*femoral canal*' (Fig. 12.15).

Femoral canal: It is the medial compartment of the femoral sheath. It is about 1.25 cm in length extending from the inguinal ligament. The lower end of the canal is anteriorly related to the saphenous opening. The canal is occupied by few deep inguinal lymph nodes. The upper part of the canal opens into abdominal cavity at femoral ring .

Femoral ring: It is the base of the femoral canal connecting the abdominal cavity with the femoral canal. The ring is closed by thin connective tissue called femoral septum with a depression facing upwards. The ring is wider in females due to the broader pelvis. The femoral hernia can occur through this canal and it is common in females. Femoral ring has the following boundaries

Anteriorly: Inguinal ligament

Posteriorly: Pectineus muscle with fascia covering it

Laterally: Separated from the femoral vein by a septum

Medially: Base of the Lacunar ligament, it is an extension of the inguinal ligament (from pubic tubercle to pectin pubis). It is triangular in shape with its apex attached to the pubic tubercle and concave base forms the medial boundary of the femoral ring. It has superior and inferior surfaces.

Femoral hernia: Hernia is an abnormal protrusion of the abdominal contents through weak areas in the body wall. Femoral ring is the week area in the lower part of the anterior abdominal wall. Hence it is possible that an intestinal loop with its peritoneal covering can

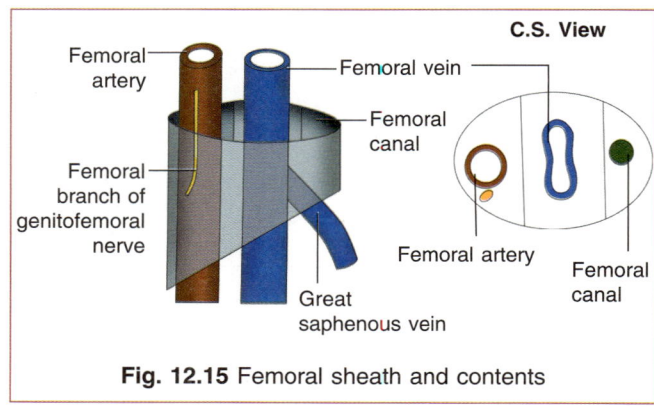

Fig. 12.15 Femoral sheath and contents

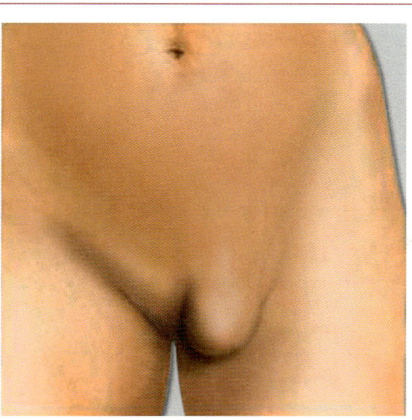

Fig. 12.16 Femoral hernia

protrude through this ring and enter the femoral canal with rise in the intra abdominal pressure. The intestinal loop is pushed downwards in the femoral canal and then forwards through saphenous opening. It (femoral hernia) appears as a swelling in the groin which is covered externally by skin. It is differentiated from inguinal hernia that it occupies below and lateral to the pubic tubercle, while inguinal hernia is related superolateral to the pubic tubercle. It is more common in females due to the wider femoral ring (Fig. 12.16).

It is possible to reduce the hernia manually by pushing the hernia mass backwards and upwards with thigh passively flexed. The complication of femoral hernia is when the neck of the hernia sac gets caught at the femoral ring and it leads to strangulation of intestinal loop. Strangulation cuts off the blood supply to the intestinal loop and it is fatal. In such cases the surgical reduction is done by cutting the lacunar ligament to make way back to the intestinal loop. While cutting the lacunar ligament, there is a possibility of involvement of abnormal obturator artery on the upper surface of the lacunar ligament causing bleeding. Abnormal obturator artery is the large pubic branch of the inferior epigastric artery replacing the obturator artery. If this artery is related lateral to the femoral ring, the possibility of its involvement is less.

CASE-3

A 48-year-old woman was seen in the emergency room complaining of abdominal pain and repeated vomiting. On questioning, the patient stated that the pain was severe and colicky in nature and most intense in the region of the umbilicus. On examination, the patient showed obvious signs of dehydration, namely, dry skin, dry tongue and sunken eyes. The abdomen showed no distension, but excessively loud bowel peristaltic sounds could be heard with the stethoscope. A small, tender, tense swelling was found in the front of the left thigh. When the patient was asked to cough, there was no expansion of the swelling. The swelling was located below and lateral to the left pubic tubercle. The patient said she had first noticed the swelling about three years ago and had increased in size since two days after coughing. Given that the patient has acute intestinal obstruction and using your knowledge of anatomy, what is your diagnosis?

Femoral artery

- It is the chief artery of the lower limb.

- Femoral artery is the continuation of the external iliac artery. It enters the thigh from behind the midinguinal point superficial to the tendon of psoas major muscle (Fig. 12.17).

- It descends from base to apex of the femoral triangle and then enters adductor canal. Finally it emerges from the adductor canal by passing through hiatus magnus (last opening in the adductor magnus muscle) to enter the popliteal fossa, where it continues as popliteal artery.

Relations of the artery in the femoral canal

In front: Skin, superficial fascia, fascia lata, anterior wall of the femoral sheath (in the upper part)

Behind: Posterior wall of the femoral sheath, tendon of the psoas major and hip joint.

Laterally: Femoral nerve

Medially: Femoral vein, but in the lower part of the triangle it inclines posterior to the artery

Relations in the adductor canal

The femoral vein is posterior to the artery in the upper part of the canal and lateral to it in the lower end of the canal

The saphenous nerve descends anterior to the artery from lateral to medial side.

Femoral artery gives three superficial and three deep branches. The superficial branches are (Fig. 12.17)

1. **Superficial epigastric artery:** It passes out through the saphenous opening and ascends upwards in the superficial fascia towards the umbilicus.

2. **Superficial circumflex iliac artery:** It passes out through the saphenous opening then proceeds laterally below the inguinal ligament towards anterior superior iliac spine.

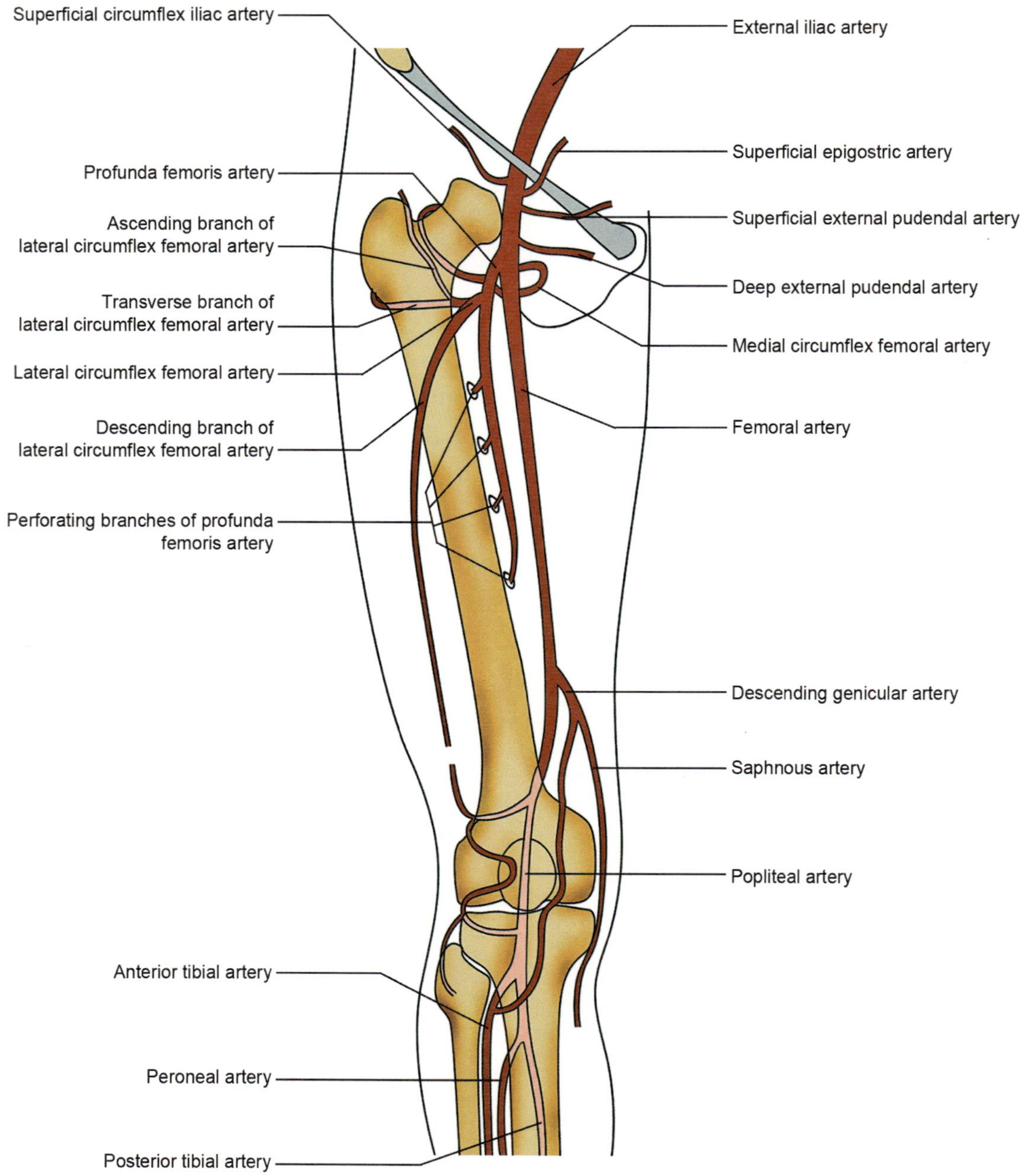

Superficial circumflex iliac artery

External iliac artery

Profunda femoris artery

Superficial epigostric artery

Ascending branch of
lateral circumflex femoral artery

Superficial external pudendal artery

Transverse branch of
lateral circumflex femoral artery

Deep external pudendal artery

Lateral circumflex femoral artery

Medial circumflex femoral artery

Descending branch of
lateral circumflex femoral artery

Femoral artery

Perforating branches of profunda
femoris artery

Descending genicular artery

Saphnous artery

Popliteal artery

Anterior tibial artery

Peroneal artery

Posterior tibial artery

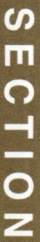

Fig. 12.17 Profunda femoris artery

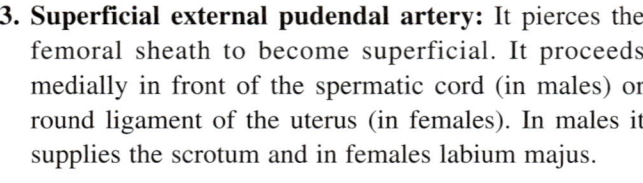

3. **Superficial external pudendal artery:** It pierces the femoral sheath to become superficial. It proceeds medially in front of the spermatic cord (in males) or round ligament of the uterus (in females). In males it supplies the scrotum and in females labium majus.

The deep branches include

4. **Profundafemoris artery**

5. **Deep external pudendal artery:** It pierces the fascia lata and passes medially behind the spermatic cord or round ligament of the uterus. It also supplies the scrotum or labium majus.

6. Muscular branches

Branches in the adductor canal

7. Muscular branches

8. **Descending genicular artery:** It arises from the distal part of the femoral artery and enters the substance of the vastus medialis muscle. It gives a saphenous branch which pierces the roof of the adductor canal and accompanies the saphenous nerve and take part in anastomoses around the knee joint.

> Femoral pulse: The pulsation of the femoral artery is felt at the midinguinal point (mid-point between the anterior superior iliac spine and the pubic symphysis) where the artery is against the tendon of psoas major muscle.
>
> Femoral artery is superficial in position in the upper part of the thigh and often selected for various procedures like angiographic studies (by injecting radiopaque dye through a catheter inserted to femoral artery) of abdominal, lower limb arteries and even coronary arteries.

Profunda femoris artery

It is the largest branch of the femoral artery supplies all the three compartments of the thigh (Fig.12.17).

Course:

- It arises from the lateral side of the femoral artery in the femoral triangle, about 3.5 cm below the inguinal ligament.

- It passes posterior to the femoral vessels, enter the interval between the pectineus and adductor longus.

- It further descends between adductor longus and brevis and then between adductor brevis and magnus.

- Finally it pierces the adductor magnus as fourth perforating branch.

Branches: It gives medial and lateral circumflex femoral arteries and also 3 perforating branches.

1. **Medial circumflex femoral artery:** It passes posteriorly between psoas and pectineus, and then between adductor brevis and obturator externus. Finally it appears in the interval between the upper border of the adductor magnus and lower border of the quadrates femoris muscle. It gives transverse branch for cruciate anastomosis and ascending branch for trochanteric anastomosis. The acetabular branch arising from medial circumflex femoral artery supplies head of the femur after passing through the head ligament of the femur.

2. **Lateral circumflex femoral artery:** It passes laterally between the anterior and posterior divisions of the femoral nerve, beneath the rectus femoris and Sartorius muscles. It gives ascending branch (for anastomosis around the anterior superior iliac spine) and transverse branch for cruciate anastomosis. The descending branch descends along the anterior border of the vastus lateralis and takes part in anastomosis around the knee.

3. **Perforating branches:** There are three perforating branches which perforates adductor magnus close to its insertion and enters the posterior compartment where all the perforating branches are connected to each other.

These anastomoses connects branches of internal iliac artery with popliteal artery.

> The profunda femoris artery is prone to injury in fracture of the shaft of the femur. The artery can also be involved in surgical procedures involving femur as the artery is closely related to the femur.

Femoral vein

The femoral vein is the continuation of the popliteal vein at the hiatus magnus (opening in the adductor magnus muscle). It ascends through adductor canal and then in the femoral triangle. Deep to the inguinal ligament it continues as external iliac vein. The vein crosses posterior to the femoral artery from lateral to medial side. It receives great saphenous vein and many other veins corresponding to the branches of the femoral artery.

> In infants and children femoral vein is selected for intravenous injections. It is also used to reach the right side of the heart (right atrium and right ventricle).

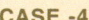

CASE -4

A 58-year-old woman was admitted to the hospital for cardiac catheterization in order to measure the pressures in the chambers of her heart. A catheter was inserted in her right femoral vein in the femoral triangle and floated through the iliac veins and the inferior vena cava to the right atrium, where diagnostic procedures were performed without any complications. Four hours after completion of the procedure, however, the patient began to feel the throbbing pain in her right groin. Over the course of the next hour, the pain worsened and she began to experience numbness and tingling in her right anteromedial side of the thigh and leg. On examination, her right leg felt cool and a mass was observed in the right groin. No pulses could be felt in the leg arteries. The patient was immediately taken up to surgery for exploration of the groin region.

1. Knowing the anatomy of the upper part of the thigh explain what are the risks associated with catheterization in this region?

2. What do you think caused the mass in the patient's groin?

3. How would you explain the numbness and absence of pulses in the arteries of the leg?

4. Why would the femoral vein be used for catheterization instead of vessels closer to the heart, like the external jugular, for instance?

Femoral nerve (L2, L3, L4)

Femoral nerve supplies muscles in the front of the thigh (Fig. 12.18). It mainly supplies the muscles of the anterior compartment of the thigh.

Origin: Femoral nerve arises from the lumbar plexus within the substance of psoas major muscle. It is formed by the dorsal divisions of ventral rami of second to fourth lumbar spinal nerves.

Course

1. After emerging from the psoas major muscle it descends in the posterior abdominal wall, the nerve lies in a groove between psoas and iliacus muscle.

2. The nerve enters, front of the thigh deep to the inguinal ligament lateral to the femoral vessels.

3. In the upper part of the thigh the nerve terminates by dividing into anterior and posterior divisions.

Branches and distribution

1. The **main trunk** in the abdomen gives muscular branches to iliacus and pectineus.

2. The **anterior division** provides one muscular and two cutaneous branches.
   • branch to sartorius muscle
   • medial cutaneous nerve of the thigh
   • intermediate cutaneous nerve of the thigh

3. The **posterior division** provides one cutaneous and four muscular branches.
   • Saphenous nerve: It supplies skin of the medial side of the leg and medial border of foot up to the ball of the big toe

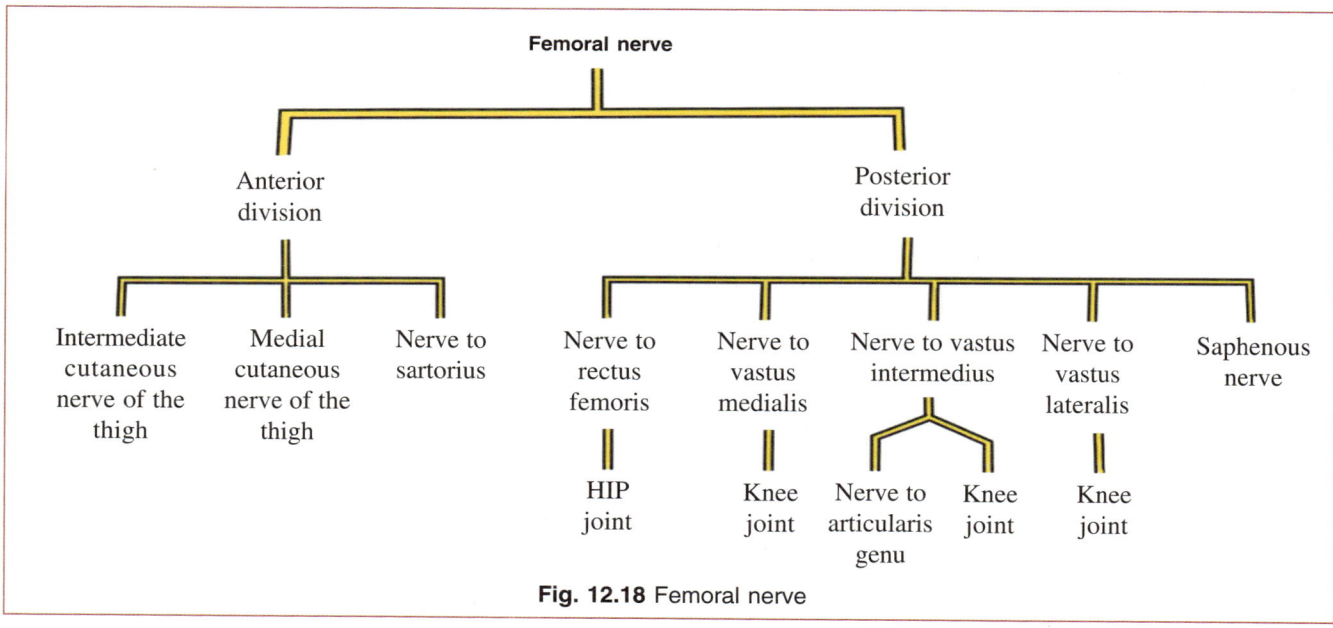

Fig. 12.18 Femoral nerve

S E C T I O N   4

Table 12.2 Muscles of medial compartment of thigh

Muscle	Origin	Insertion	Nerve supply	Actions
Adductor longus	Narrow tendon from front of body of pubis	Linea aspera in middle 1/3 between the vastus medialis and adductor brevis and magnus	Anterior division of obturator nerve	Adductors of thigh at hip joint
Adductor brevis	Anterior surface of body of pubis Outer surface of inferior ramus of pubis Outer surface of ramus of ischium	Line extending from lesser trochanter to linea aspera	Anterior or posterior division of obturator nerve	Adduction and flexion of hip joint
Adductor magnus	Inferolateral part of ischial tuberosity Ramus of ischium Lower part of inferior ramus of pubis	Medial margin of gluteal tuberosity Linea aspera Medial supracondylar line and adductor tubercle (Hamstring fibres)	Adductor part - posterior division of obturator nerve Hamstring part-tibial part of sciatic nerve	Adductor part - adduction of hip Hamstring part - Extension of hip joint
Gracilis	Medial margin of lower half of body of pubis. Inferior ramus of pubis Adjoining part of ramus of ischium	Upper part of medial surface of tibia behind Sartorius and in front of semitendinosus	Anterior division of obturator nerve	Flexor and medial rotator of thigh Weak adductor
Pectineus	Pectin pubis Upper half of pectineal surface of superior ramus of pubis Fascia covering pectineus	Line between lesser trochanter to linea aspera	Anterior fibres-femoral nerve Posterior fibres-anterior division of obturator nerve	Flexor and adductor of thigh

- Muscular branches supply rectus femoris, vastus medialis, and vastus intermedius and vastus lateralis muscles. The nerve supplying rectus femoris also supplies hip joint and the nerves supplying vasti muscle supply knee joint.

MEDIAL COMPARTMENT OF THE THIGH

The medial compartment mainly contains adductor muscles of the thigh and also obturator nerve and vessels and profunda femoris artery. The muscles are arranged in three strata. The superficial stratum contains pectineus, adductor longus and gracilis. The intermediate stratum contains adductor brevis andobturator externus. The deepest stratum contains adductor magnus muscle. All these muscles mainly cause adduction at the hip joint. They are all supplied by the obturator nerve. The attachments, specific nerve supply and actions are explained in Table 12.2 (Figs 12.19 and 12.20).

Adductor canal (Subsartorial canal/Hunter's canal)

It is an intermuscular space situated in the middle 1/3 of the medial part of the thigh. It connects the apex of the femoral triangle to popliteal fossa, at hiatus magnus (last opening in the adductor magnus muscle)

Boundaries: It is triangular in cross section with anterior, posterior and medial walls (Fig.12. 21).

SECTION 4

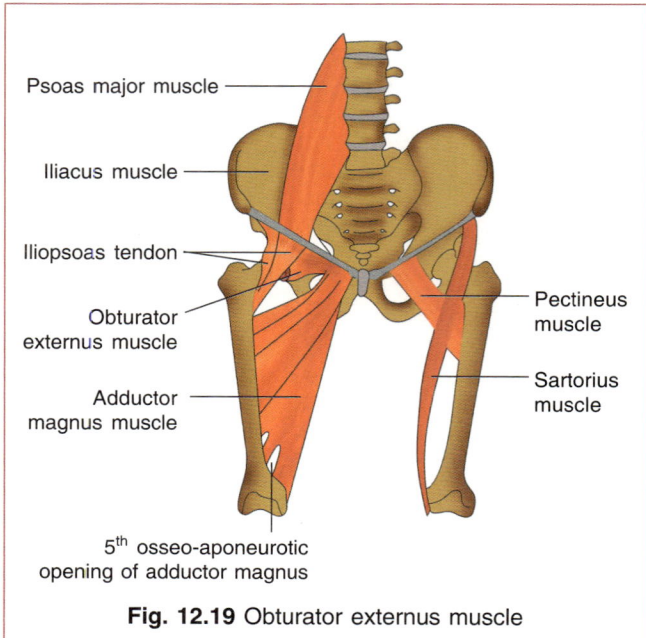

Psoas major muscle

Iliacus muscle

Iliopsoas tendon

Obturator externus muscle

Adductor magnus muscle

Pectineus muscle

Sartorius muscle

5th osseo-aponeurotic opening of adductor magnus

Fig. 12.19 Obturator externus muscle

Anteriorly: Vastus medialis

Posteriorly: Adductor longus above, Adductor magnus below

Medially (roof): A fibrous membrane connecting the anterior and posterior walls. Sartorius muscle is placed above this fibrous membrane.

Contents

1. Femoral artery with descending genicular branch

2. Femoral vein

3. Saphenous nerve: It is related lateral to the femoral artery in the upper part then crosses anterior to it and then pierces the fibrous roof to become superficial.

4. Nerve to vastus medialis: It is present only in the proximal part of the canal and ends by entering the substance of the vastus medialis muscle.

5. Posterior division of obturator nerve

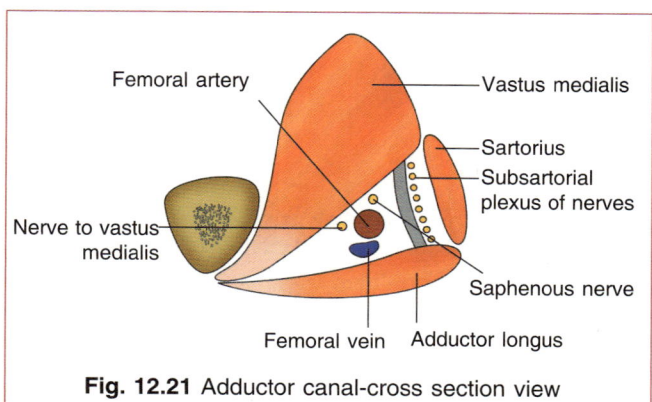

Femoral artery

Vastus medialis

Sartorius

Subsartorial plexus of nerves

Nerve to vastus medialis

Saphenous nerve

Femoral vein   Adductor longus

Fig. 12.21 Adductor canal-cross section view

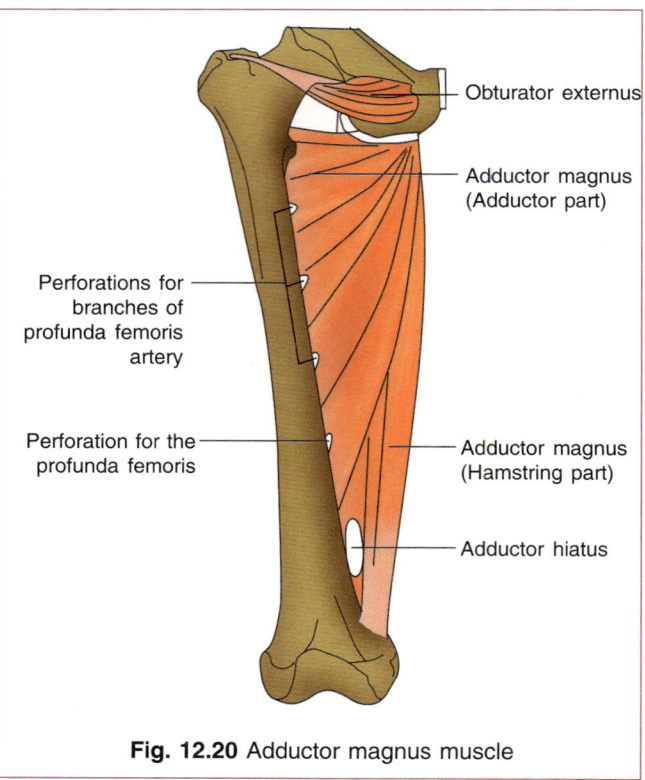

Obturator externus

Adductor magnus (Adductor part)

Perforations for branches of profunda femoris artery

Perforation for the profunda femoris

Adductor magnus (Hamstring part)

Adductor hiatus

Fig. 12.20 Adductor magnus muscle

In surgical dealing of popliteal aneurysm, the femoral artery is ligated in the adductor canal. Inspite of ligation blood enters the popliteal artery and arteries of the leg through anastomosis around the knee joint. The fibrous roof is incised to enter the canal.

Subsartorial plexus of nerves: It is a plexus of nerves located between the fibrous roof and Sartorius muscle. The plexus is formed by branches of anterior division of the obturator nerve, saphenous nerve and medial cutaneous nerve of the thigh. Through the plexus it supplies the skin of the medial side of thigh.

Obturator nerve (L2, L3, L4)

Obturator nerve supplies muscles of the medial compartment of the thigh.

Origin: It is a branch from the lumbar plexus formed by the ventral divisions of ventral rami of second, third and fourth lumbar spinal nerves.

Course

1. After emerging from the psoas major muscle it descends in the lateral pelvic wall. In females it is related to the ovary.

2. It enters the medial side of the thigh through obturator canal where it terminates by dividing into anterior and posterior divisions (Fig. 12.22). The anterior division

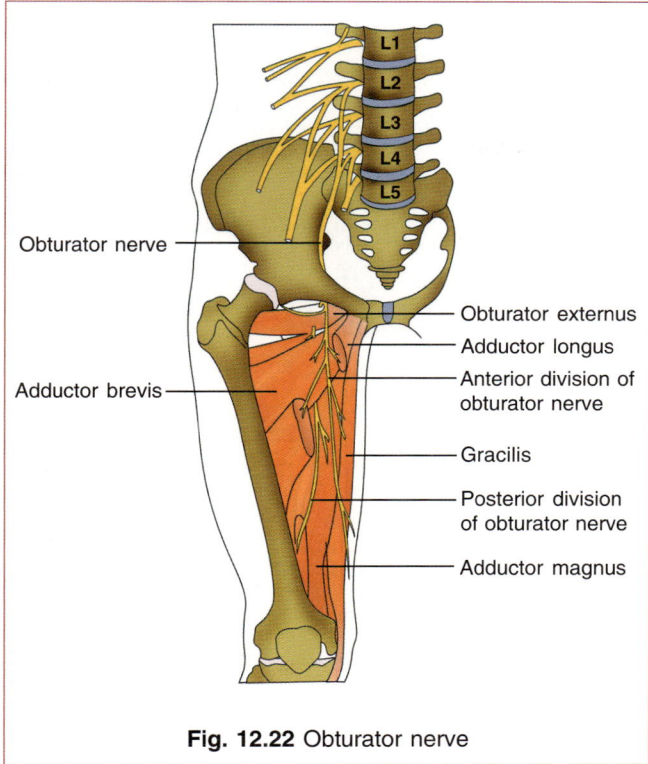

Fig. 12.22 Obturator nerve

descends posterior to adductor longus and anterior to adductor brevis. The posterior division pierces the obturator externus and descends in front of the adductor magnus, posterior to the adductor brevis muscle.

Branches and distribution

1. The **anterior, division** supplies gracilis, adductor longus, adductor brevis and pectineus muscles. It gives articular branch to the hip joint. It ends by contributing to subsartorial plexus.

2. The **posterior division** supplies obturator externus and part of the adductor magnus muscle. It accompanies the femoral artery, passes through hiatus magnus to follow the popliteal artery and curves forward at the back of the knee. It pierces the oblique popliteal ligament to supply the cruciate ligaments of the knee joint.

> In case of inflammation of ovary, there can be an involvement of obturator nerve which results in referred pain in hip and knee joint or medial side of the thigh.

Obturator artery: It is a branch from the anterior division of the internal iliac artery. It appears in the thigh along with the obturator nerve through the obturator canal. It ends by dividing into medial and lateral branches in the upper part of the thigh. The acetabular branch arising from lateral branch supplies head of the femur after traversing the head

ligament of the femur along with the branches of medial circumflex iliac artery. The branches of the artery in the pelvis are explained in the chapter pelvis.

Cruciate anastomosis: It is present at the upper border of the adductor magnus and lower border of quadratus femoris. The arteries involved are transverse branches of medial and lateral circumflex femoral arteries, descending branch from the inferior gluteal artery and ascending branch of the first perforating artery. This anastomosis provides connections between internal iliac artery with the branches of profunda femoris artery. All the perforating branches are connected to each other and the lower perforating branch is connected to anastomosis around the knee. This is helpful in collateral circulation.

Trochanteric anastomosis: It is located in the trochanteric fossa providing blood supply to the head and neck of the femur. The arteries involved are ascending branches of medial and lateral circumflex femoral arteries, branches from superior and inferior gluteal arteries.

POSTERIOR COMPARTMENT OF THE THIGH

The posterior compartment mainly contains muscles and sciatic nerve

Muscles of the back of the thigh

These groups of muscles are called *Hamstring muscles*. It includes semimembranosus, semitendinosus, long head of the biceps femoris and part of the adductor magnus (fibres arising from ischial tuberosity).

Characteristics of Hamstring muscles:

- All of them take origin from ischial tuberosity.
- **They act as flexors of knee and extensors of the hip joint (adductor magnus does not flex the knee).**
- All of them are supplied by the Sciatic nerve.
- They are inserted into either tibia or fibula except adductor magnus

Semimembranosus: The upper part of the muscle is membranous while its lower part is fleshy (Fig. 12.23).

Origin: It takes origin from the upper lateral part of the ischial tuberosity.

The muscle is crossed superficially by long head of the biceps femoris. The lower part forms the upper medial boundary of the popliteal fossa.

Insertion: It is inserted through a tendon on a groove on the posterior aspect of the medial condyle of the femur, deep to the tibial collateral ligament with a bursa close to

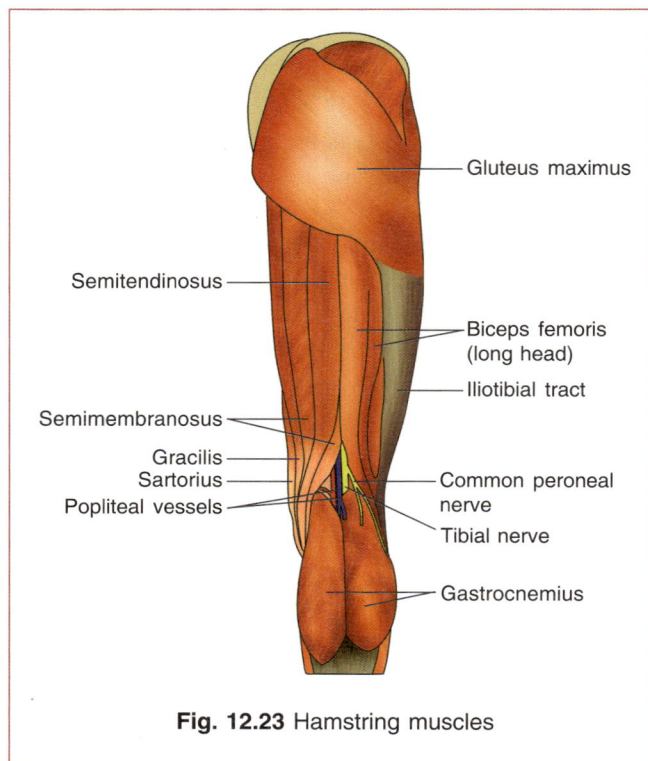

Fig. 12.23 Hamstring muscles

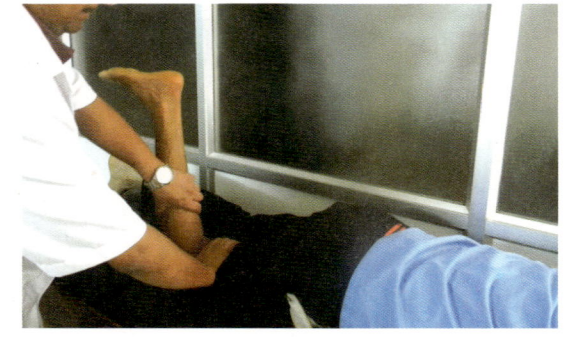

Fig. 12.25 Testing of Hamstring muscles

its insertion. From its insertion it gives tendinous expansions

i. Oblique popliteal ligament- which extends upwards and laterally at the back of the knee to get attached to the lateral condyle of the femur.

ii. Some fibres extend downwards covering popliteal muscle as fascia covering the popliteus muscle which is attached to the soleal line.

Nerve supply: Tibial component of the sciatic nerve

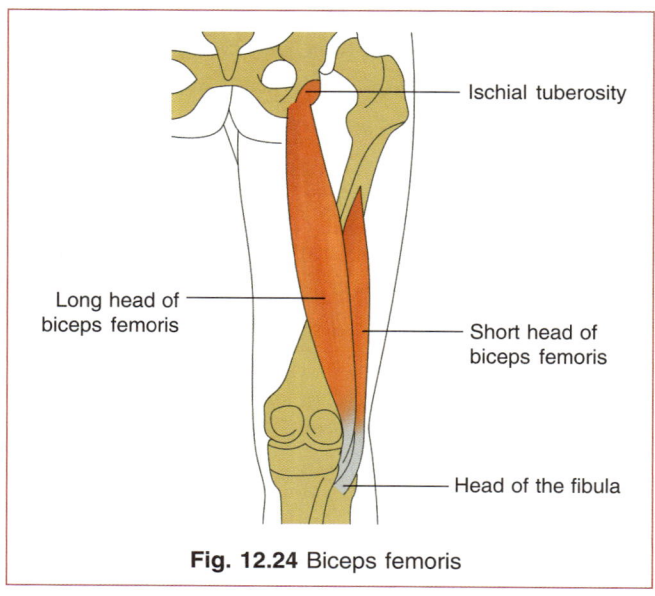

Fig. 12.24 Biceps femoris

Semitendinosus: It is fleshy in the upper part and becomes tendinous in the lower part which rests on the semimembranosus (Fig.12.23).

Origin: It takes origin from the lower medial part of the ischial tuberosity along with the long head of the biceps femoris. It passes behind the medial condyle of the femur.

Insertion: It is inserted into the upper part of the medial surface of the tibia (behind the sartorius and gracilis).

Nerve supply: Tibial component of the sciatic nerve.

Biceps femoris: It has 2 heads-long and short. Long head belongs to hamstring part but not the short head (Fig. 12.24).

Origin: The long head takes origin from lower medial part of the ischial tuberosity along with the semi-tendinosus. The short head from the lower part of the lateral lip of the linea aspera and upper 2/3rd of the lateral supracondylar line.

The long head passes downwards and laterally at the back of the thigh crossing superficial to the sciatic nerve, join with the short head on its deep surface.

Insertion: The 2 heads together forms a tendon which is inserted into head of the fibula in front of the styloid process. The 'C' shaped insertion encloses the fibular collateral ligament of the knee joint.

Testing of hamstring muscles: The person is asked to lie down in prone position with knee extended. He is asked to flex the knee against the resistance applied by the examiner (Fig. 12.25).

Hamstring pull: It is possible that the attachment of the hamstring muscle is torn from the ischial tuberosity in athletes. It results in severe pain.

Solution to the Case studies
Case-1

1. This patient had varicose veins of the great saphenous and small saphenous veins.

2. Before operating on these veins, it is a must to determine whether or not the deep veins of the leg, the venae comitantes, are patent. A person with deep vein thrombosis depends on the dilated superficial veins to return the blood in the leg to general circulation and deep vein thrombosis would be contraindication to operation.

3. The superficial epigastric, the superficial circumflex iliac, and the superficial external pudendal veins, together with the important perforating veins, must be ligated for a successful result to be lined. Large varicose veins possess incompetent valves. If the leg is raised above the level of the heart in a supine position, the varicose veins quickly empty. If the great saphenous vein is now occluded by digital pressure at the saphenous opening and the patient is asked to stand, when the digital pressure is removed, the veins fill from above and not from below, as they should normally.

4. With the patient standing, a cough will transmit a fluid thrill from the abdomen to the hand examining the veins, because the incompetent valves do not impede the passage of the pressure wave.

5. Refer text

Case-2

This patient had a malignant melanoma of the right second toe, which has spread by way of the lymphatics to involve the vertical group of superficial inguinal lymph nodes. The fact that the patient ignored the lump for three months worsened the prognosis. The treatment of choice is radical amputation of the toe and complete block dissection removal of all the inguinal lymph nodes on the rightside. The extensive physical examination was necessary because we know that the lymph from a wide area of the body drains into the inguinal lymph nodes.

Case-3

This patient had acute intestinal obstruction secondary to a strangulated left femoral hernia. When, two days before, the patient coughed, a loop of ileum was forced down into a preexisting femoral hernia sac. The unyielding nature of the femoral ring resulted in venous congestion of the intestine and later arterial occlusion. At this point, peristalsis ceased (paralytic ileus), and intestinal obstruction occurred.

Case-4

1. The risks of catheterization include damage to the femoral artery or vein leading to an internal hemorrhage, injury to the femoral nerve, needle introduction into the peritoneal cavity, and formation of an arteriovenous fistula.

2. The mass in the patient's groin was due to the formation of a hematoma. The hematoma could result from failure of the wound in the femoral vein to close, or more likely, due to a laceration of the femoral artery that occurred at some point during the procedure.

3. The numbness and absence of pulses in the leg arteries are most likely due to the compression of the neurovascular structures of the femoral triangle (femoral artery/vein/nerve) by the hematoma.

4. The femoral vessels have advantages over other possible locations for many procedures involving catheterization. First, the femoral vessels tend to be much larger than vessels in the arm or neck and allow a larger catheter. Second, they do not present the same risks as catheterization of the neck. Procedures in the neck require high skills because catheter can enter the pleural cavity causing pneumothorax, and, in the case of the carotid arteries, there is also the risk of thrombosis which can lead to a stroke. As a result, femoral catheterization is preferred for procedures (for example, angiographic studies) requiring access to the arterial circulation around the heart and the arch of the aorta (including arteries of the brain) and for procedures in the abdomen (venous and arterial). However, the trend in recent years, as physicians become more skilled in the techniques, the proximal locations for certain venous procedures (i e. internal jugular or subclavian venous catheterization) is used.

MCQs

1. A 65-year-old female visits hospital patient says that she has pain in her groin and upper thigh. Upon examination, you palpate a lump located below the inguinal ligament lateral to its attachment to the pubic tubercle. You suspect that this may be a hernia passing through the:

   A. Superficial inguinal ring
   B. Deep inguinal ring
   C. Obturator canal
   D. Femoral canal

2. The femoral canal contains

   A. Deep inguinal lymph node(s)
   B. Femoral artery
   C. Femoral nerve
   D. Femoral vein

3. Which movement would fail in case of paralysis of the quadriceps femoris muscle?

    A. Extension at the knee
    B. Flexion at the knee
    C. Extension at the hip
    D. Adduction at the hip

4. Which of the following structure does not pass deep to the inguinal ligament?

    A. Femoral artery
    B. Femoral nerve
    C. Psoas major muscle
    D. Round ligament of the uterus

5. When walking, the action of the iliopsoas muscle results in what movement at the hip joint?

    A. Abduction
    B. Adduction
    C. Extension
    D. Flexion

6. The pulsation of the femoral artery can be best felt at

    A. the apex of the femoral triangle
    B. the adductor canal
    C. the midinguinal point
    D. the popliteal fossa

7. If the femoral artery is occluded at the beginning of the adductor canal, which artery could help provide viability to the leg through collateral circulation?

    A. Medial circumflex femoral
    B. First perforating branch of the profunda femoris
    C. Descending genicular
    D. Descending branch of the lateral circumflex femoral

8. At which site could one expect to enter the femoral vein with a simple percutaneous (through the skin) introduction of an instrument?

    A. Lateral to the femoral arterial pulse
    B. Lateral to the pubic tubercle
    C. Medial to the femoral arterial pulse
    D. Medial to the pubic tubercle

9. Which of the following anterior thigh muscle must be retracted to expose the adductor canal and its contents?

    A. Adductor longus
    B. Gracilis

    C. Rectus femoris
    D. Sartorius

10. A serious complication of fractures of the femoral neck is avascular necrosis of the femoral head. This usually results from rupture of which artery?

    A. Deep circumflex iliac
    B. Descending branch of lateral circumflex femoral
    C. Medial circumflex femoral
    D. Second perforating branch of lateral circumflex

11. Following a penetrating injury to the left femoral triangle, a patient had difficulty in walking especially in extending the knee. This suggests paralysis of which muscle?

    A. Adductor magnus
    B. Biceps femoris
    C. Gluteus maximus
    D. Quadriceps femoris

12. An obturator hernia that compresses the obturator nerve in the obturator canal may affect the function of all of the following muscles *except*

    A. Adductor longus
    B. Gracilis
    C. Obturator externus
    D. Pectineus

13. Which of the following is not located within the adductor canal?

    A. Saphenous nerve
    B. Femoral artery
    C. Nerve to vastus medialis
    D. Profunda femoris artery

14. Inability to extend the knee and loss of cutaneous sensation over the anterior surface of the thigh would indicate a lesion or compression of the

    A. Obturator nerve
    B. Femoral nerve
    C. Sciatic nerve
    D. Tibial nerve

15. Following surgical opening of the adductor canal, a patient experienced a loss of cutaneous sensation of the medial side of the leg. Which nerve was cut?
    A. Saphenous
    B. Femoral
    C. Obturator
    D. Sural

16. The physiotherapist of a cricket team concerned about his main batsman who suffered "a pulled hamstring" while running. This result from a tearing of the origin of a hamstring muscle from

    A. Pubis
    B. Iliac crest
    C. Gluteal surface of the ilium
    D. Ischial tuberosity

17. In order to insert a cannula into the great saphenous vein ('saphenous cutdown) in a patient the surgeon decides to make an incision. To locate the great saphenous vein for the insertion of a cannula in which of the following locations should the incision be made?

    A. Anterior to the lateral malleolus
    B. Anterior to the medial malleolus
    C. Posterior to the lateral malleolus
    D. Posterior to the medial malleolus

18. What might you expect to see if the obturator nerve is damaged?

    A. Waddling gait
    B. Lateral swinging of the leg when walking
    C. Foot drop
    D. High stepping gait

19. A 54-year-old female patient has large varicose vein located on the posterior aspect of her calf. The vein involved in the present case is the

    A. great saphenous vein
    B. small saphenous vein
    C. femoral vein
    D. Posterior tibial

20. A needle biopsy of the sural nerve resulted in the formation of a hematoma. Which of the following veins closely adjacent to the nerve was accidently injured?

    A. Posterior tibial
    B. femoral
    C. greater saphenous
    D. small saphenous

Answers to MCQs

1. D
2. A
3. A
4. D
5. D
6. C
7. C
8. C
9. D
10. C
11. D
12. D
13. D
14. B
15. A
16. D
17. B
18. B
19. B
20. D

SECTION 4

Gluteal Region and Hip Joint

13

- Gluteal region
- Sciatic nerve
- Hip joint
- MCQs

Objectives

- To know the anatomical location for intramuscular injections in gluteal region
- To explain the attachment, nerve supply, actions of gluteal muscles and to list the structures present undercover of gluteus maximus muscle
- To explain the origin, course, relations, termination, branches, distribution and applied anatomy of sciatic nerve
- To explain the bones articulating, ligaments stabilizing, relations, movements occurring and muscles producing them in the hip joint

GLUTEAL REGION

Cutaneous nerves of the gluteal region

The skin of the gluteal region is supplied by L1, L2, L3, S1, S2 and S3 dermatomes. The nerves include both ventral and dorsal rami.

Upper part: From before back ward following nerves supply the skin

1. Lateral cutaneous branch of the subcostal nerve (T12)

2. Lateral cutaneous branch of the iliohypogastric nerve (L1)

3. Dorsal ramus of L1, L2 and L3 nerves.

Lower part: Recurrent gluteal branch from the posterior cutaneous nerve of the thigh around the lower border of the gluteus maximus muscle.

Medial part: Cutaneous branches from the dorsal rami of S1, S2 and S3 nerves.

Lateral part: Posterior branch of the lateral cutaneous nerve of the thigh.

Superficial fascia: It consists of abundant fat especially in females.

Deep fascia: It is the extension of the fascia lata. Superiorly it is attached to the iliac crest. It encloses the two muscles-tensor fasciae latae and gluteus maximus. Between them it forms a thick sheet called **gluteal aponeurosis** which covers the gluteus medius muscle.

Muscles of the Gluteal region

The bulkiest muscle of the body the gluteus maximus is the superficial muscle of this region. Deep to it are many muscles which act on the hip joint. The attachments, nerve supply and actions of these muscles are explained in Table 13.1.

Gluteus maximus (Fig. 13.1)

It is the bulkiest and more superficial muscle of this region.

Origin: Gluteal surface of the ilium behind the posterior gluteal line, posterior part of the iliac crest, gluteal aponeurosis, posterior surface of the lower part of the sacrum, coccyx, posterior layer of the thoracolumbar fascia and sacrotuberous ligament.

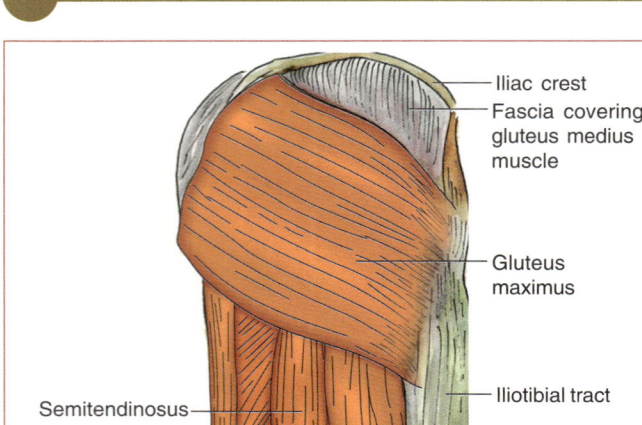

Fig. 13.1 Gluteus maximus muscle

The muscle fibres are directed downwards and laterally at angle of about 45°.

Insertion: Deep fibres of its lower half (1/4th of the muscle) is inserted into the gluteal tuberosity of the femur. The remaining muscle (3/4th) ends in aponeurosis which ends in the upper part of the iliotibial tract.

Nerve supply: Inferior gluteal nerve (L5, S1, S2)

Actions:

1. It is the main extensor of the hip joint which is required for running and climbing upstairs.

2. It is the abductor and lateral rotator of the hip joint

3. Through the ilio-tibial tract, it maintains the extended position of the knee joint.

Structures under cover of gluteus maximus muscle

There are plenty of structures present deep to the gluteus maximus, which includes muscles, bones, ligaments, nerves and vessels. The greater and lesser sciatic notches are converted into greater and lesser sciatic foramina by sacrotuberous and sacrospinous ligaments. Greater sciatic foramen allows the passage of piriformis muscle, which is a key structure under gluteus maximus. The greater sciatic foramen connects the pelvis and gluteal region allow the passage of nerves from sacral plexus and vessels from internal iliac arteries. The lesser sciatic notch connects the gluteal region with the perineum through pudendal canal. The foramen allows the passage of the obturator internus muscle and passage of pudendal nerve and internal pudendal vessels to perineum.

1. **Muscles:** Gluteus medius, Gluteus minimus, Piriformis, Obturator internus tendon, Superior and Inferior gemelli,

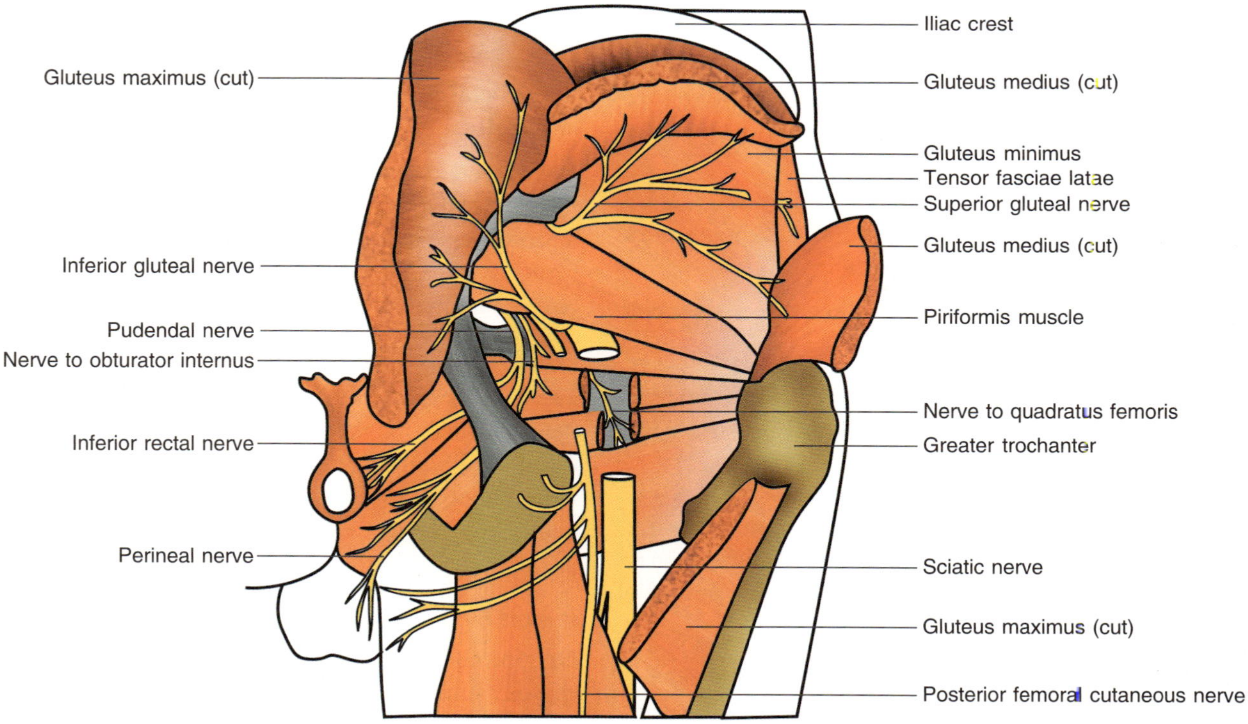

Fig. 13.2 Structures under cover of gluteus maximus muscle

Quadratus femoris and upper part of the adductor magnus muscles (Fig. 13.2).

2. **Bones and ligaments:** Ilium, sacrum, coccyx, ischial tuberosity, greater trochanter, sacrotuberous and sacrospinous ligaments.

3. **Nerves and Vessels:**

Emerging above the piriformis: Superior gluteal nerve and vessels (passes between gluteus medius and minimus)

Emerging below the piriformis:

  i. Inferior gluteal nerve and vessels

  ii. Sciatic nerve

 iii. Posterior cutaneous nerve of the thigh

 iv. Pudendal nerve

  v. Nerve to obturator internus

 vi. Nerve to quadratus femoris muscle

vii. Internal pudendal vessels.

4. **Bursae:** Trochanteric bursa (between gluteus maximus and greater trochanter), ischial bursa (between g.maximus and ischial tuberosity) and gluteo-femoral bursa (between V. lateralis and G. maximus)

Gluteus medius

Origin: Gluteal surface of the ilium between the posterior and anterior gluteal line of the hip bone. The muscle passes downwards, forwards and laterally.

Insertion: It is inserted into the lateral surface of the greater trochanter of the femur

Nerve supply: Superior gluteal nerve

Gluteus minimus

Origin: Gluteal surface of the ilium between anterior and inferior gluteal line of the hip bone

Insertion: It is inserted into the anterior surface of the greater trochanter.

Nerve supply: Superior gluteal nerve

Actions of Gluteus medius and minimus:

1. Abductors of the hip joint.

2. Anterior fibres of both muscles act as medial rotators of the hip joint. These two actions are exerted when its attachment to the greater trochanter is acting as insertion.

3. When its attachment to the hip bone acts as insertion, it tends to pull the hip bone towards the femur, which is required to raise the opposite hip. Hence it prevents the unsupported side of the pelvis from sagging downwards during locomotion, e.g. when right foot is off the ground

the right anterior superior iliac spine is raised by left gluteus medius and minimus muscle (Fig. 13.4). If these muscles (of left side) are paralysed the right side of the pelvis drops. This is called Trendelenberg's sign and the person walks with a lurching gait.

Intramuscular injections: Intramuscular injections are often preferred in the gluteal region. The gluteal muscle provides a large surface area for absorption of drugs. The superolateral quadrant is safe site for intramuscular injection. An injection, little below and behind the anterior superior iliac spine involves following structures successively-skin, superficial fascia, deep fascia and gluteus medius. Injecting superomedial quadrant, endanger the superior gluteal nerve and inferomedial quadrant, endanger the sciatic nerve and also inferior gluteal nerves and vessels (Fig. 13.3).

Trendelenburg's test: When both feet are supporting the body weight, the anterior superior iliac spine of two sides lies in the same horizontal plane. When right foot is supporting body weight, the left foot is raised by opposite (right) gluteus medius and minimus muscles. If the right gluteus medius and minimus are paralysed, the unsupported left side of the pelvis drops indicating positive Trendelenburg's test (Fig. 13.5).

CASE-1

Following a major abdominal surgery, a patient was given a course of antibiotics through intramuscular route. The nurse was instructed to give the injections into the buttock. After few days, the patient started to experience numbness and a tingling sensation in the anterior and lateral sides of the right leg and dorsum of the foot. He also stated that his right leg felt heavy and that his right foot tends to catch on steps. On examination, there was evidence of impaired skin sensation on the anterior and lateral sides of the right leg and dorsum of the right foot. The patient was holding his foot in plantar flexed and slightly inverted

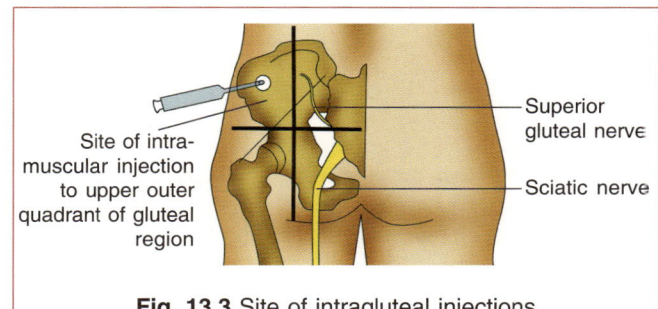

Fig. 13.3 Site of intragluteal injections

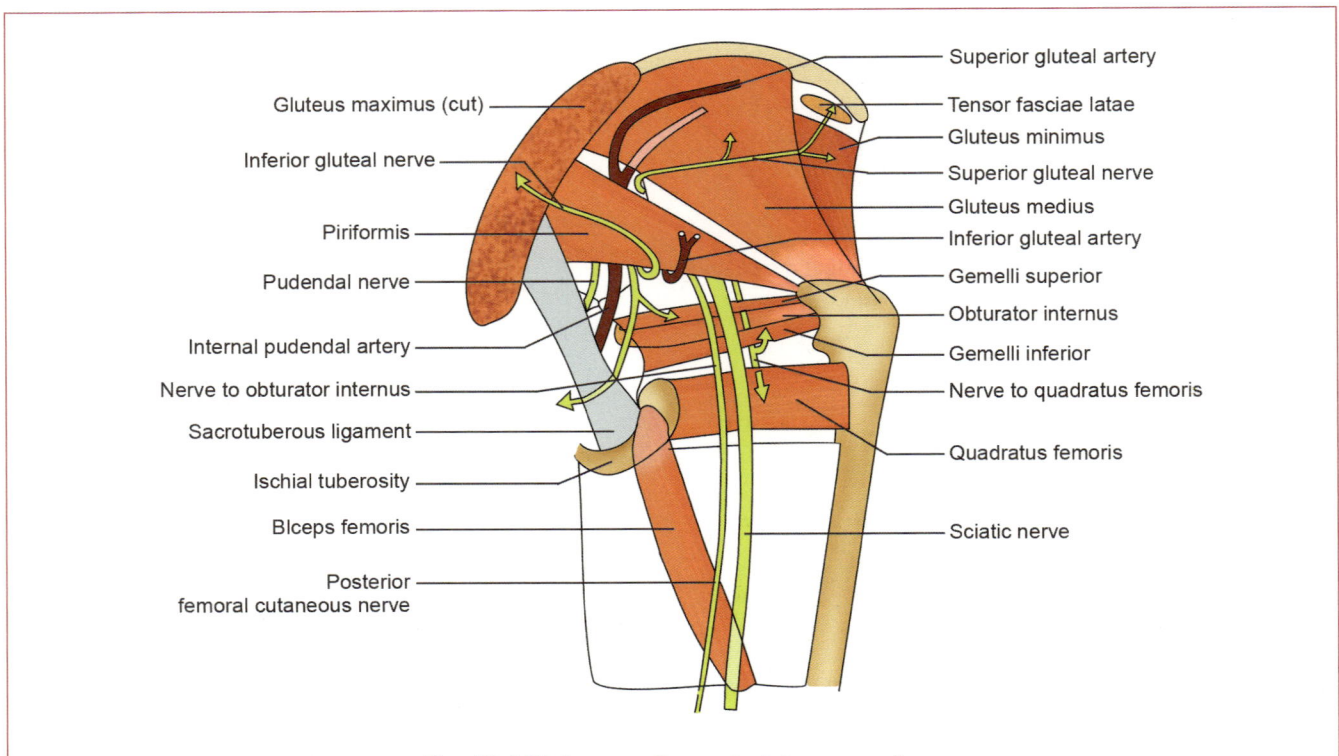

Fig. 13.4 Gluteus medius and minimus muscles

position. On comparing the relative strength of the plantar flexors and dorsiflexors of the ankle joint on both legs, it was found that dorsiflexion of the right ankle was weaker than normal. The evertor muscles were also weaker than normal. Using your knowledge of anatomy, explain the patient's signs and symptoms. What precautions should a nurse be taking when giving intramuscular injections into the buttock?

Superior gluteal nerve (L4,L5,S1): It is a branch of the sacral plexus, appears in the gluteal region by passing above the piriformis. The nerve passes between gluteus medius and minimus muscles. It supplies gluteus medius and minimus muscles. In addition it also supplies tensor fasciae latae.

Inferior gluteal nerve (L5,S1,S2): It is a branch of the sacral plexus, appears in the gluteal region by passing below the piriformis. It curves upwards and supplies gluteus maximus muscle from its undersurface.

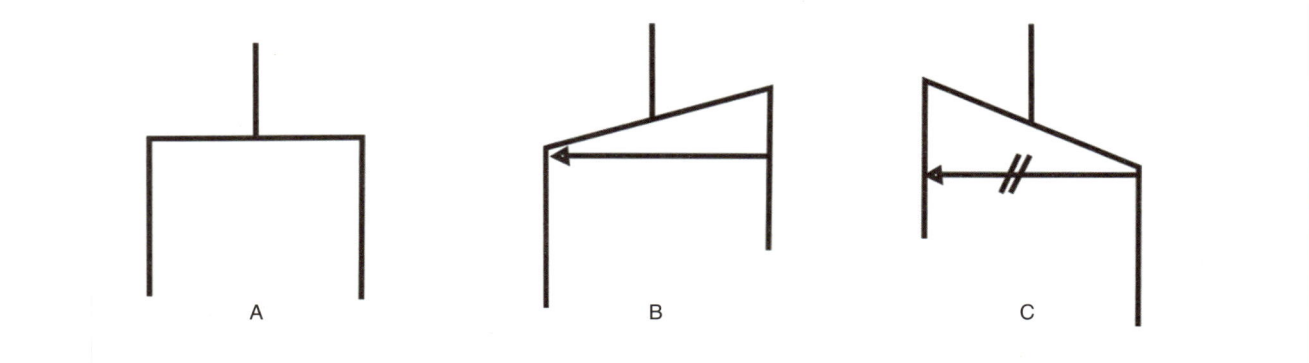

A - When both feet are supporting the body weight horizontal level of pelvis is maintained
B - When right foot is supporting the body weight, left side of the pelvis is raised by right gluteus medius and minimus muscle
C - If the right gluteus medius and minimus are paralysed, the unsupported left side of pelvis sags (positive Trendelenburg's sign)

Fig. 13.5 Trendelenburg's sign

Table 13.1: Muscles under cover of Gluteus maximus

Name of the muscles	Origin	Insertion	Nerve supply	Actions
Piriformis: It arises from the pelvis, passes through greater sciatic foramen to reach gluteal region	Ventral surface of the sacrum (between ventral sacral foramina, capsule of the sacro-iliac joint and upper margin of the greater sciatic notch	Apex of the greater trochanter of the femur	S1 and S2 nerves	Lateral rotator of the hip joint
Superior gemellus	Spine of the ischium	The two gemulli and tendon of the obturator internus join together to form a tricipital tendon. It crosses the posterior aspect of the neck of the femur, inserted into medial surface of the greater trochanter above and in front of the trochanteric fossa	Nerve to obturator internus	Lateral rotator of the hip joint
Inferior gemellus	Lower margin of the lesser sciatic notch and upper part of the ischial tuberosity		Nerve to obturator internus	Lateral rotator of the hip joint
Obturator internus It forms the lateral wall of the pelvis	Inner surface of the obturator membrane, adjoining pelvic surface of the ischium and ischiopubic ramus		Nerve to quadrates femoris	Lateral rotator of the hip joint
Quadratus femoris	External surface of the ischial tuberosity	Quadrate tubercle near the middle of the inter-trochanteric crest	Nerve to quadrates femoris	Lateral rotator of the hip joint

Nerve to obturator internus (L5, S1, S2): It is a branch of the sacral plexus, appears in the gluteal region by passing below the piriformis. It also winds around the ischial spine to enter the lesser sciatic foramen. It supplies obturator internus and also superior gemellus muscles.

Nerve to quadratus femoris (L4, L5, S1): It is a branch from the sacral plexus, appears in the gluteal region below the piriformis and sciatic nerve. It descends deep (anterior) to the tendon of the obturator internus and two gemelli muscles. It supplies quadrates femoris and inferior gemellus.

Pudendal nerve (S2, S3, S4): It is a branch from the sacral plexus. It appears in the gluteal region by passing below the piriformis muscle. It winds around the ischial spine (rather more medially around the sacrospinous ligament) and enters the lesser sciatic foramen along with the internal pudendal vessels, then proceeds in the pudendal canal. It has both motor and sensory nerve supply in the perineal region. It is explained in the chapter pelvis.

Posterior cutaneous nerve of the thigh (S1, S2, S3): It appears below the piriformis, superficial or medial to the sciatic nerve. It accompanies the sciatic nerve, descends in the back of the thigh. It pierces the deep fascia in the popliteal region to become superficial. It further descends in the superficial fascia to supply the skin of the back of the upper part of the leg. It gives many cutaneous branches which supplies the skin of the lower part of the gluteal region and the back of the thigh. Its perineal branch supplies the posterior part of the scrotum or labium majus.

Superior gluteal artery: It is a branch from the posterior division of the internal iliac artery. It appears in the gluteal region above the piriformis along with the superior gluteal nerve. It passes between the gluteus medius and minimus muscles. Its branches take part in trochanteric anastomosis and also anastomosis around the anterior superior iliac spine.

Inferior gluteal artery: It is a branch from the anterior division of the internal iliac artery. It appears in the gluteal region below the piriformis. It provides major blood supply to the gluteus maximus, its branches take part in trochanteric and cruciate anastomosis. Arteria nervi ischiadic accompanies and supplies the sciatic nerve.

Internal pudendal artery: It is a branch from the anterior division of the internal iliac artery. It appears below the piriformis through the greater sciatic foramen. It winds around the ischial spine to enter the lesser sciatic foramen along with the pudendal nerve. It traverses the pudendal canal and supplies external genitalia and perineum region.

SCIATIC NERVE

It is the thickest nerve of the body, about 2 cm broad and supplies majority of the muscles of lower limb through its branches (Fig.13.6).

Origin

It arises from the sacral plexus and it has tibial and peroneal components.

a. **Tibial component** is derived from ventral divisions of ventral rami of L4, L5, S1, S2 and S3 nerves.

b. **Peroneal component** is derived from dorsal divisions of ventral rami of L4, L5, S1 and S2 nerves.

Course

1. From the pelvis, the sciatic nerve enters the gluteal region through the greater sciatic foramen below the piriformis muscle. Its nerve roots are related to posterolateral aspect of the rectum.

2. It is possible that sometimes there will be early division of sciatic nerve into tibial and common peroneal nerve. In such case the tibial nerve passes below the piriformis while common peroneal nerve pierces the piriformis muscle.

3. In the gluteal region it passes deep to the gluteus maximus, mid-way between greater trochanter of the femur and the ischial tuberosity.

4. It descends in the gluteal region successively resting on superior and inferior gemelli, obturator internus tendon and quadrates femoris muscles. These muscles separate the posterior aspect of the hip joint from sciatic nerve.

5. In the back of the thigh the nerve lies on adductor magnus muscle and is crossed superficially by the long head of the biceps femoris muscle.

6. In the interval between the lower border of the gluteus maximus muscle and the long head of the biceps femoris muscle, the sciatic nerve is superficial and is related to skin and fascia.

4. Sciatic nerve terminates in the superior angle of the popliteal fossa by dividing into tibial and common peroneal nerves.

Branches and distribution

1. Muscular branches supply all the hamstring muscles - Semimembranosus, Semitendinosus, Long head of biceps femoris and Adductor magnus (partly). These branches are derived from tibial component. All these

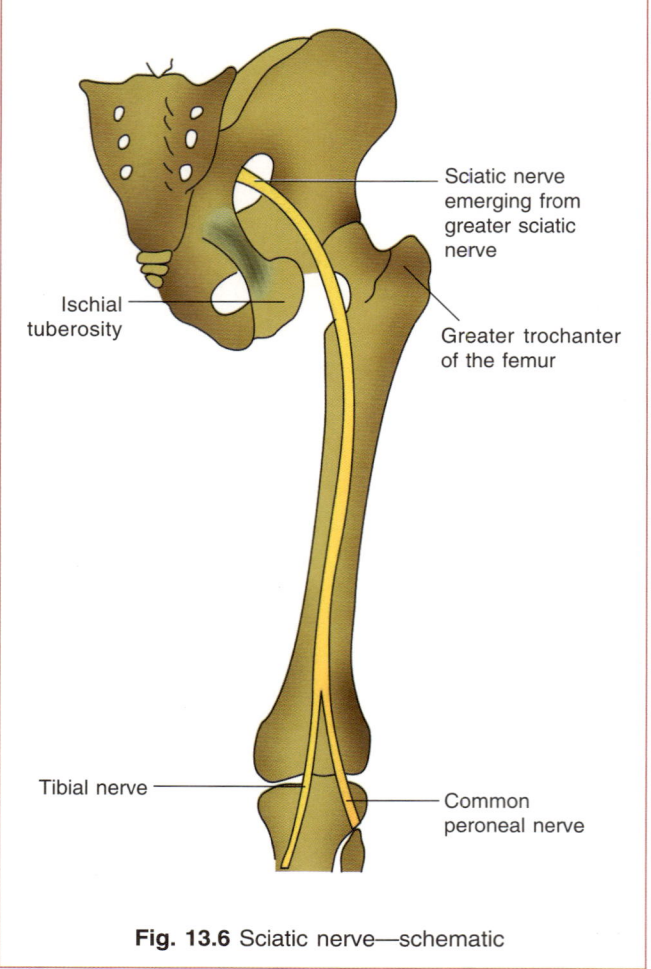

Fig. 13.6 Sciatic nerve—schematic

branches arise from the medial side of the sciatic nerve. The short head of the biceps femoris is supplied by the peroneal component of the sciatic nerve.

2. Articular branches to the hip joint.

Injury to the sciatic nerve as in posterior dislocation or fracture of the hip causes paralysis of all the muscles below the knee (with foot drop).

Sciatica: It is caused by prolapse of the intervertebral disc which compresses the lower lumbar and upper sacral nerve roots or causes pressure on the sacral plexus. The patient experiences radiating pain down the posterior aspect of the thigh, posterior and lateral side of the leg and lateral part of the foot. The disc prolapsed between L4 and L5 vertebra involves L5 nerve which is manifested by numbness in the **medial 3 toes and difficulty in dorsiflexion**. The disc prolapsed between L5 and S1 involves S1 nerve which is manifested by numbness in the **lateral border of the foot and difficulty in plantar flexion.**

Sleeping foot: It is due to temporary compression of the sciatic nerve against the femur, at the lower border of gluteus maximus, when a person sits on the hard edge of a chair for a long time.

The motor effect of injury to sciatic nerve (posterior dislocation) is paralysis of the muscles of posterior compartment of the thigh and of the leg and foot. There is a sensory loss below the knee except for femoral area

HIP JOINT

Type

It is a ball and socket variety of synovial joint.

Bones taking part

Head of the femur articulating with lunate surface of the acetabulum (of hip bone). The acetabulum presents a notch below called acetabular notch. The articulating surfaces are covered by hyaline cartilage (Figs 13.7 and 13.8).

Structures stabilizing the joint

1. **Capsular ligament (fibrous capsule):** Structurally, it is made of collagen and elastic fibres. Inferomedial part of the fibrous capsule is weakest and is stretched during abduction.

   Attachment: It is attached to the inter-trochanteric line of the femur in front and medial part of the inter-trochanteric crest behind. Hence the neck of the femur is intra capsular and is covered by synovial membrane. Some part of the fibrous capsule is reflected towards the neck as retinacular fibres, which carry blood vessels to the neck and head of the femur.

Medially the fibrous capsule is attached close to the acetabular margin and also blends with transverse acetabular ligament.

Synovial membrane: It lines the inner surface of the fibrous capsule, acetabular labrum and intra-capsular part of the neck of femur. The synovial membrane also invests the ligament of the head of the femur.

2. **Acetabular labrum:** It is a fibro-cartilaginous rim attached to the acetabular margin. It deepens the socket and holds the femoral head tightly.

3. **Transverse acetabular ligament:** It extends across the acetabular notch. Thus the acetabular notch is converted into a foramen through which blood vessels and nerves enter the joint.

4. **Ligament of the head of the femur (ligamentum teres femoris):** It is triangular in shape with its apex attached to the fovea capitis of the femoral head and by its base to transverse acetabular ligament. This ligament is stretched in adduction of semiflexed hip. It transmits blood vessels into the head of femur.

5. **Iliofemoral ligament (ligament of Bigelow):** It is one of the strongest ligaments of the body. It is triangular in shape with its apex attached to the anterior inferior iliac spine of the hip bone. The base is attached to the intertrochanteric line. It prevents the hyperextension of hip joint (Fig.13.8).

6. **Pubofemoral ligament:** It is the thickening of the fibrous capsule on inferomedial aspect. It is attached above to the iliopubic eminence and obturator crest. Below it blends with medial part of the iliofemoral ligament (Fig.13.8). The psoas bursa communicate with the joint cavity through the interval between iliofemoral and pubofemoral ligaments.

7. **Ischiofemoral ligament:** It covers the joint posteriorly. It is attached to the ischium close to the acetabular

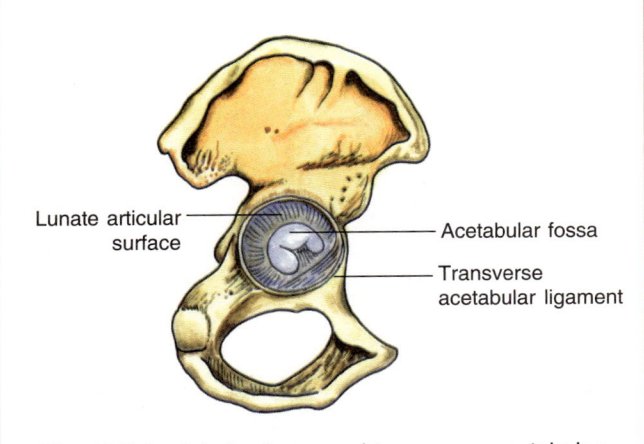

Fig. 13.7 Acetabular fossa and transverse acetabular ligament

Lunate articular surface
Acetabular fossa
Transverse acetabular ligament

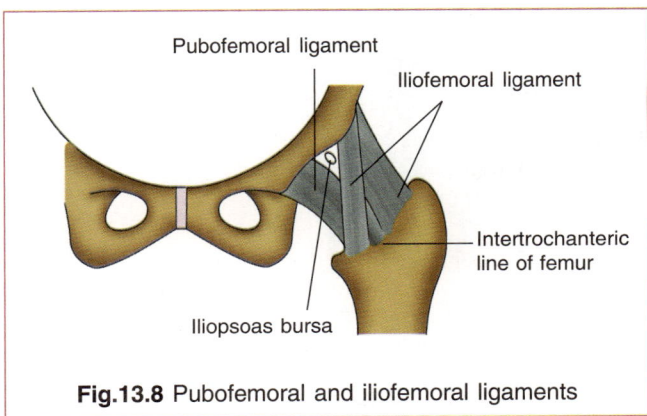

Fig.13.8 Pubofemoral and iliofemoral ligaments

Pubofemoral ligament
Iliofemoral ligament
Intertrochanteric line of femur
Iliopsoas bursa

SECTION 4

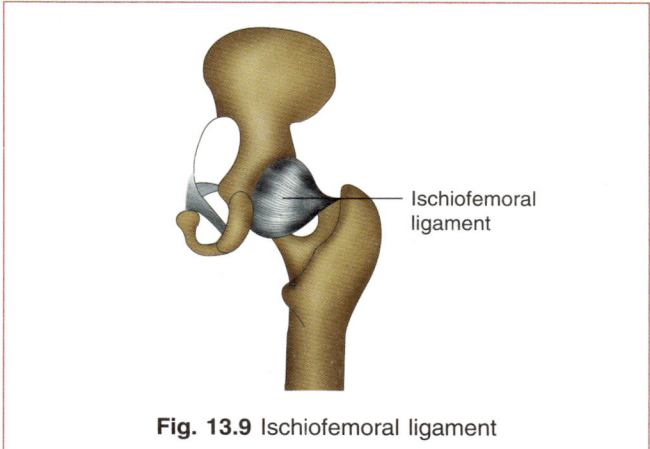

Fig. 13.9 Ischiofemoral ligament

margin. The twisted fibres pass behind the neck and are attached to the greater trochanter of the femur but most of the fibres are continuous with the inner circular fibres of the fibrous capsule (zona orbicularis) (Fig. 13.9).

Arterial supply

The area of the femoral head around the fovea is supplied by acetabular branch of obturator artery and medial circumflex femoral artery. The rest of the head and neck receives blood from arterial circle around the capsular ligament (medial circumflex femoral is the chief source). The retinacular arteries from this vascular ring, pierce the capsule and run along the neck of the femur to supply it and the head. The arterial supply of the head and neck is solely dependent on the retinacular arteries. In the rupture of these arteries (in intracapsular fracture of the neck of the femur) the head of the femur undergoes avascular necrosis. The hip joint is also supplied by branches from superior and inferior gluteal arteries (Fig. 13.10).

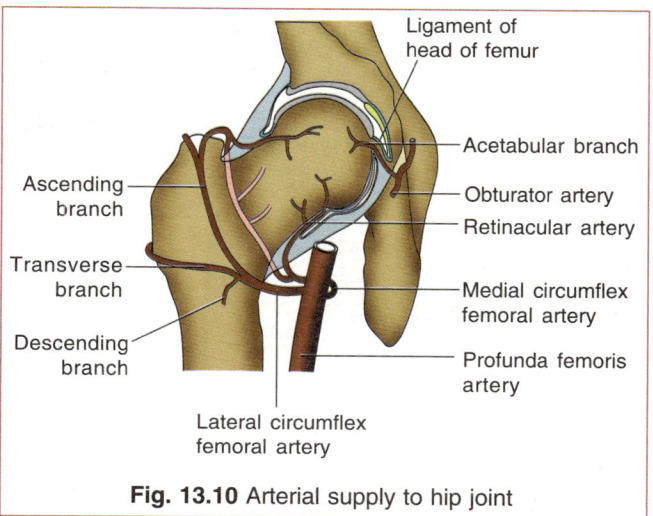

Fig. 13.10 Arterial supply to hip joint

Nerve supply

The hip joint is supplied by femoral (branch supplying rectus femoris), anterior division of obturator nerve and nerve to quadratus femoris. Accessory obturator nerve if present may supply the hip joint. L2 and L3 nerve roots or spinal segments regulate flexion while L3 and L4 extension.

Movements and muscles producing them

Flexion: Psoas major and iliacus, pectineus, sartorius, rectus femoris.

Extension: Gluteus maximus and hamstring muscles. Gluteus maximus helps in raising the trunk from sitting position or in climbing upstairs. Hamstring muscles maintain extension in normal standing and walking.

Adduction: Adductor longus, brevis and magnus, gracilis and pectineus.

Abduction: Gluteus medius and minimus and tensor fasciae latae.

Medial rotation: Mainly by anterior fibres of gluteus medius and minimus with tensor fasciae latae.

Lateral rotation: Obturator internus and externus, superior and inferior gemelli, quadratus femoris, piriformis, gluteus maximus and sartorius.

Relations of the joint

In front: Iliopsoas, straight head of the rectus femoris and lateral part of the pectineus muscles occupies immediately in front of the joint. Further in front are femoral nerve (between iliacus and psoas), femoral artery (opposite to psoas tenson) and femoral vein.

Behind: Piriformis, obturator externus, gemelli, obturator internus, quadrates femoris muscles separate hip joint from sciatic nerve.

Above: Reflected head of the rectus femoris and medial part of the gluteus minimus

Below: Pectineus and obturator externus

- **Dislocation of hip joint** is more common on posterior aspect. The sciatic nerve may be injured in this dislocation.

  The fracture of the neck of femur

- It is very common in elderly due to osteoporotic changes in the neck.

- Postmenopausal women who develop osteoporosis, are more prone to this fracture on trauma. This fracture is of 2 types.

SECTION 4

• **Intracapsular:** In this retinacular arteries are injured leading to delay in healing or non-union of fracture. Its serious complication is avascular necrosis of head of the femur with resultant loss of function of hip joint. In intracapsular fracture, the affected limb is shortened and held in characteristic laterally rotated position with toes pointing laterally. The anatomical explanation of this is as follows. Since the head of femur separates from the shaft (carrying the trochanter) in intracapsular fracture, the shaft can rotate independent of the head. The gluteus maximus and short lateral rotator muscles rotate the femur laterally. The psoas major becomes a lateral rotator after fracture due to the axis of action (Fig. 13.11).

Extracapsular fracture of neck (example-intertrochanteric fracture). Here the retinacular arteries are saved, hence healing is faster.

• Diseases of the hip may cause referred pain in the knee joint.

Shenton's line: By joining the medial margin of the femoral neck and the inferior margin of the superior ramus of pubis, a smoothly curved Shenton's line is demarcated. Fracture of neck or dislocation of hip joint distorts this line.

Neck-shaft angle (angle of inclination): The normal neck-shaft angle is 125° in adult and 160° in children. When there is increase in angle it is called coxa valga. It is found in congenital dislocation of the hip joint. Coxa valga limits the adduction movement of the hip joint (Fig. 13.12).

If the angle is reduced it is called coxa vara. It is seen in fracture of neck of femur and it limits the abduction at the hip joint.

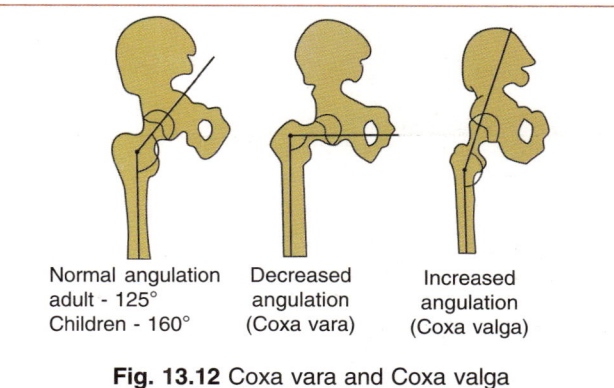

| Normal angulation adult - 125° Children - 160° | Decreased angulation (Coxa vara) | Increased angulation (Coxa valga) |

Fig. 13.12 Coxa vara and Coxa valga

Congenital Hip Dislocation

• Girls are affected more often than boys.

• About 60% of the affected children are first sibling, suggesting unstretched uterine and abdominal walls that limit foetal movement.

• If it is not detected the child's hip may develop incorrectly and is evident when the child begins to walk.

• If one hip is affected the child will have a limp and lurch (sways on one side to clear the opposite foot of the ground) and if it is bilateral dislocation then there will be a waddling gait (Fig. 13.13).

Galeazzi test: It is also known as the Alli's sign, is used in the diagnosis of congenital dislocation of the hip. It is performed by flexing an infant's knees in the supine position so that the ankles touch the buttocks. If the knees are not at same level then the test is positive, indicating a potential congenital hip malformation.

Ortolani maneuver: Gently abducting the infant's thigh with the examiner's thumb while placing anterior pressure on the greater trochanter using index finger. A distinctive 'clunk', is heard indicating the

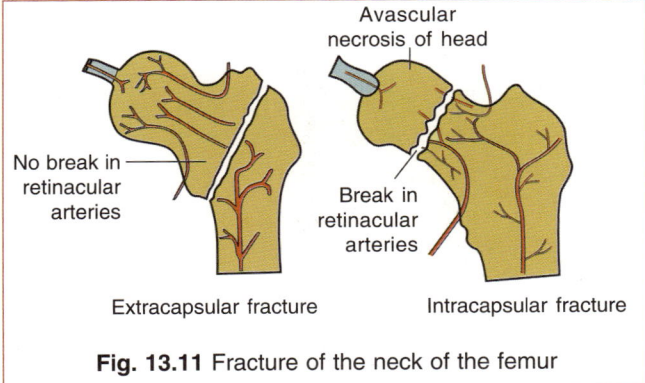

Fig. 13.11 Fracture of the neck of the femur

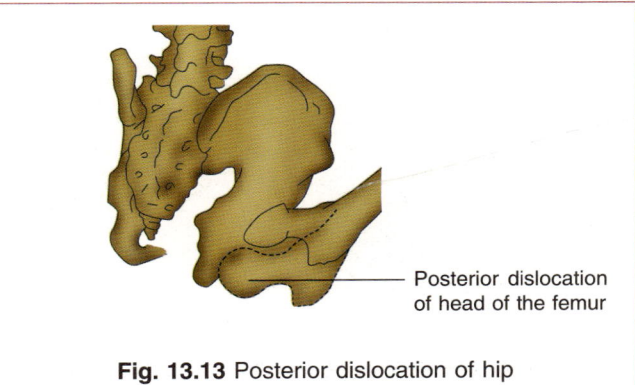

Fig. 13.13 Posterior dislocation of hip

relocation of head anteriorly into the acetabulum. This test usually follows Barlow's maneuver.

Barlow's maneuver: Gently adducting the hip of infant and applying light pressure on the knee and directing the force posteriorly. If the hip is dislocatable - that is if the hip can be popped out of socket in this test then it is considered positive. This is an examination that is performed to screen out for hip dysplasia in new born.

Acquired dislocation: Uncommon, In posterior dislocation the sciatic nerve may be injured.

Complications of Hip dislocations include deep venous thrombosis (DVT), sciatic nerve injury, avascular necrosis, vascular injury, recurrent dislocation, arthritis and chronic pain.

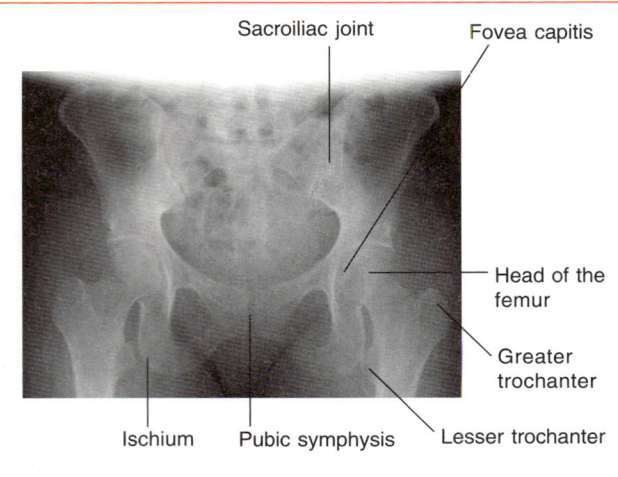

Fig. 13.14 Normal radiograph of the hip joint

CASE-2

A 5-year-old girl was brought to the orthopedic clinic with complaints of dipping gait on walking. The history revealed that she started to walk late and that she always had a slight limp on the "left" side. On observing her walk, it was seen that her pelvis sagged down on the left side. When the girl was asked to stand on her left leg and raise the opposite leg off the ground, the pelvis on the unsupported side was lifted above the horizontal. When she was asked to stand on her right leg and raise the left leg off the ground, the pelvis on the unsupported side lifted down below the horizontal. With the patient standing upright on both legs, the top of the greater trochanter on the right side was situated above a line drawn between the anterior superior iliac spine and the ischial tuberosity. On the left side the greater trochanter was normally placed on this line. Radiological examination of the right hip joint showed that Shenton's line was not intact. Using your anatomical knowledge, make a diagnosis. What is the anatomical basis the Trendelenburg's sign?

CASE-3

On a routine anteroposterior X-ray examination of a patient's right hip joint, the long axis of the neck of the femur was found to be at an angle of 160 degrees with the long axis of the femoral shaft. Is this angle normal in a 5-year-old child and in a 35-year-old man? What is the clinical condition called in which the angle is smaller than normal? Which movement of the hip joint is limited by this condition (Fig. 13.14)?

CASE-4

Fractures of the neck of the femur in the adult commonly result in avascular necrosis of part of the femoral head. Can you explain this on anatomical grounds? Trochanteric fractures are never accompanied by avascular necrosis. Why?

CASE-5

A 37-year-old male was picked up by his wife at his office. He gets into the passenger seat of their car and turns to get the safety belt as his wife begins to exit the parking lot. Another vehicle entering the lot strikes their vehicle head on and he is thrown forward by the sudden deceleration. His left knee strikes the dashboard violently, and he feels a painful pop in his left hip. After shifting to the hospital he is noted to have great pain in the left hip region. Compared to his right leg, he is noted to have a shortened left leg which is adducted and medially rotated. There is a painful mass in the lateral gluteal region.

1. What is the most likely diagnosis?

2. What are the structures involved in this injury?

3. Which clinically important structure is at potential risk?

4. Describe the anatomy of the hip joint including the proximal femur, joint capsule, ligament and acetabulum.

Solutions to the case studies:

Case-1

This patient sustained damage to the right sciatic nerve as a result of administration of an intramuscular injection into the right buttock at a wrong site. On questioning, the nurse showed the site where she gave the injections; it overlies the course of the sciatic nerve. The problem was compounded by the fact that the patient received intramuscular injections into the same site, in the same buttock, each day for three weeks. The common peroneal component of the sciatic nerve was damaged resulting in the loss of skin sensation in the areas normally supplied by the lateral cutaneous nerve of the leg and the superficial peroneal nerve. The muscles of the anterior and lateral compartments of leg were partially paralyzed. The unopposed planter flexors and invertors of the foot caused the patient to hold his foot in plantar flexed and inverted (equinovarus). Intramuscular injections should be restricted to the upper lateral quadrant of the buttock and alternate buttocks or other sites for injections should be used when there are multiple injections extending for many weeks.

Case-2

This little girl had a congenital dislocation of the right hip joint. The left hip joint was normal. When she stood on the right leg and lifted the left leg off the ground, the right hip joint could not act normally as a fulcrum for the pelvis and the contracting gluteus medius and minimus muscles. In fact, the right femoral head was not situated in the acetabulum, lad ridden up onto the gluteal surface of the ilium, due to a failure of the upper border of the acetabulum to develop adequately. As a consequence of this, the gluteus medius and minimus muscles on the right side could not tilt the pelvis, and it sagged downward on the unsupported side.

Case-3

This angle is within normal limits in a 5-year-old. It is too great in a 35-year-old man; the condition is called coxa valga, in which adduction of the hip joint is limited. When the angle of the femoral neck is smaller than normal (coxa vara), abduction of the hip joint is limited.

Case-4

The femoral head receives its blood supply from two sources: (1) a small arteries that runs with the head ligament of the femur (2) a large amount of blood supply is from the medial circumflex femoral artery, branches of which ascend the femoral neck beneath the synovial membrane. Fracture of the femoral neck may deprive the blood supply to the femoral head partly or completely from source 2, and avascular necrosis will occur. The blood supply to the trochanter is profuse so that both fractured fragments of this region will have an adequate blood supply.

Case-5

1. Posterior dislocation of the hip joint
2. Posterior part of the capsule, ischiofemoral ligament, gemelli, obturator internus tendon and quadrates femoris muscles
3. Sciatic nerve
4. Refer text

MCQs

1. In a patient who has a posterior dislocation of the hip, which of the following ligamentous structures would be torn?

   A. Pubofemoral ligament
   B. Iliofemoral ligament
   C. Ischiofemoral ligament
   D. Lacunar ligament

2. A 55-year-old man has dislocated his right hip. The physician is concerned about the integrity of the joint's blood supply. Which of the following artery is the main source of blood supply to the hip joint?

   A. Lateral circumflex femoral
   B. Medial circumflex femoral
   C. Superficial circumflex iliac
   D. Deep circumflex iliac

3. During recovery from a gunshot wound of the right pelvis, the patient notices a lurch in his gait. When he lifts his left foot off the ground, his pelvis dips down on the left side. The nerve that appears to have been injured is the:

   A. Right superior gluteal nerve
   B. Right inferior gluteal nerve
   C. Sciatic nerve
   D. Femoral nerve

4. Which muscle passes through the lesser sciatic foramen?

   A. Gluteus minimus
   B. Obturator internus
   C. Piriformis
   D. Obturator externus

5. In order to avoid injury to the sciatic nerve, intramuscular injections should be given in which quadrant of the buttock?

   A. Upper medial
   B. Upper lateral
   C. Lower medial
   D. Lower lateral

S E C T I O N 4

6. As a patient with paralysis of gluteus medius and minimus muscles on the left side attempts to stand on the left limb only, the right side of the pelvis typically:

   A. Drops
   B. Elevates
   C. Rotates laterally
   D. Rotates medially

7. After suffering a deep stab wound in the medial upper quadrant of the right buttock, the patient was found walking with difficult. The basic problem was that, during stepping, her left hip sagged down as soon as the left foot was lifted off the ground to swing forward. What nerve was damaged?

   A. Femoral
   B. Inferior gluteal
   C. Obturator
   D. Superior gluteal

8. An elderly patient complains of difficulty in walking up stairs. Tests by her doctor reveals weakness in extension of her hip but no change in hip flexion or flexion and extension of the knee. Based upon these results, what muscle is not functioning normally?

   A. Adductor magnus
   B. Gluteus maximus
   C. Gluteus medius
   D. Iliopsoas

9. Weakness in climbing stairs or jumping would indicate a lesion of which nerve?
   A. Tibial
   B. Superior gluteal
   C. Inferior gluteal
   D. Obturator

10. Of the branches of the internal iliac artery, the one which exits from the greater sciatic foramen superior to the piriformis muscle is the:

    A. Iliolumbar artery
    B. Internal pudendal artery
    C. Lateral sacral artery
    D. Superior gluteal artery

11. An elderly woman who suffers from osteoporosis falls and "breaks her hip." The orthopedic surgeon recommends that the proximal part of the femur be replaced with a prosthesis as she is likely to suffer from avascular necrosis of the head of the femur. Which artery that is supplying the neck and head of the femur might have lacerated by the fracture?

    A. Inferior gluteal artery
    B. Medial circumflex femoral artery

C. Pudendal artery
D. Profunda femoral artery

12. On examination it was shown that when a patient stands with her left lower extremity supporting her weight, the right side of her pelvis drops. This sign may be caused by a lesion of which of the following nerves?

    A. Left superior gluteal
    B. Right superior gluteal
    C. Left inferior gluteal
    D. Right superior gluteal

13. An 8-year-old boy is brought to the pediatrician by his mother. She states that for the past week, the child had a limp in his left leg that seems to be getting worse. Initially, he did not complain of pain, but now he has pain in his left anterior thigh. On examination, he has a gait with decreased abduction at the left hip. An X-ray shows flattening of the femoral head and an irregular appearance of the capital-femoral epiphysis compared to the right side. A disruption of blood supply from which of the following vessels has occurred?

    A. Inferior gluteal artery
    B. Femoral artery
    C. Lateral circumflex femoral artery
    D. Medial circumflex femoral artery

14. A fifty-year-old man has been a construction worker since he was 18 years of age. For the past five years, he had been suffering from chronic back pain. The solutions suggested by his physician seemed to have been of less help. Now he is experiencing difficulty in extending his left thigh and flexing his knee. He also has pain in the posterior thigh, the lateral leg, and foot. Which of the fallowing nerves is the most likely a source of his problems?

    A. Femoral nerve
    B. Inferior gluteal nerve
    C. Obturator nerve
    D. Sciatic nerve

Answers to MCQs

1. C	6. A	11. B
2. B	7. D	12. A
3. A	8. B	13. D
4. B	9. C	14. D
5. B	10. D	

Popliteal Fossa and Knee Joint | 14

- Popliteal fossa
- Knee joint
- MCQs

Objectives

- To list the boundaries and contents of the popliteal fossa
- To explain the branches and distribution of tibial and common peroneal nerves in the popliteal fossa
- To explain the extent, branches and relations of popliteal artery
- To explain the bones articulating, ligaments stabilizing, movements occurring and muscles producing them in the knee joint
- To explain the applied anatomy of the knee joint

POPLITEAL FOSSA

It is a diamond shaped space behind the knee occupying the lower 1/3rd of femur, the back of the knee joint and the upper part of the tibia.

Boundaries

- Superomedially: Semimembranosus and semitendinosus muscles.
- Superolaterally: Biceps femoris muscle.
- Inferomedially: Medial head of gastrocnemius muscle.
- Inferolaterally: Lateral head of gastrocnemius and plantaris muscles (Fig. 14.1).

Roof: Skin, superficial and deep fascia. The superficial fascia is traversed by small saphenous vein, terminal part of the posterior cutaneous nerve of thigh and sural communicating nerve. The deep fascia is called as popliteal fascia.

Floor: From above downwards (Fig. 14.2)

1. Popliteal surface of the femur

2. Posterior aspect of the capsule of the knee joint.

3. Popliteus muscle with the fascia covering it.

Contents

1. Popliteal artery and its branches.

2. Popliteal vein and its tributaries.

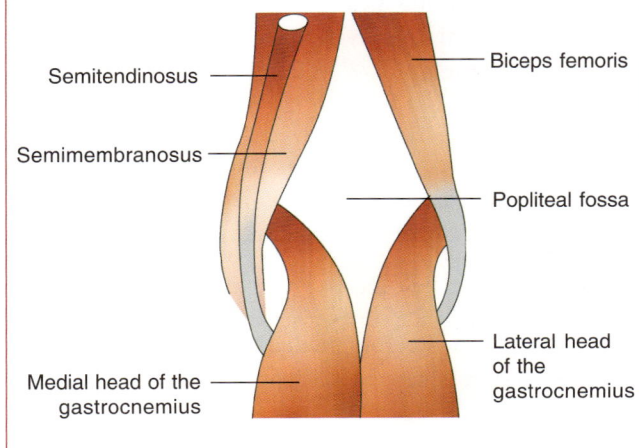

Fig. 14.1 Boundaries and roof of the popliteal fossa

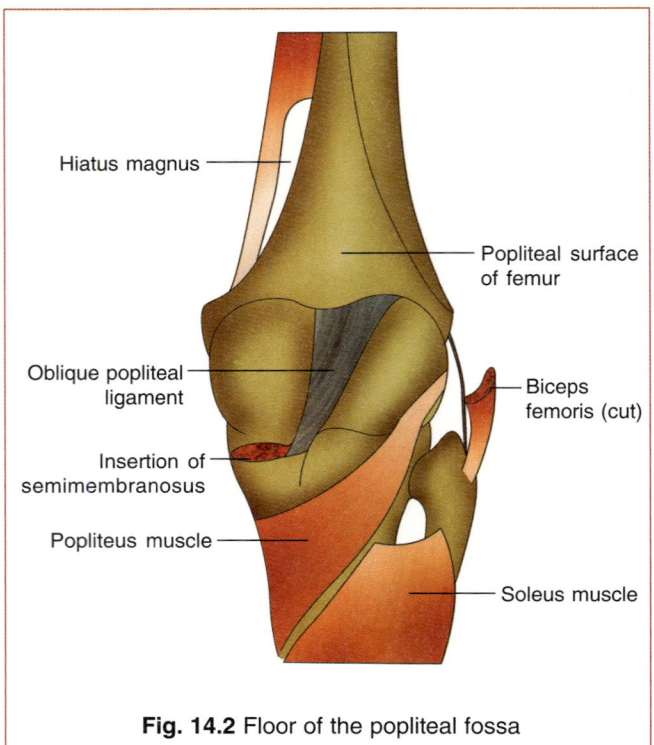

Hiatus magnus

Popliteal surface
of femur

Oblique popliteal
ligament

Biceps
femoris (cut)

Insertion of
semimembranosus

Popliteus muscle

Soleus muscle

Fig. 14.2 Floor of the popliteal fossa

3. Tibial nerve and its branches.

4. Common peroneal nerve and its branches.

5. Lymph nodes and fat.

Popliteal artery

Origin: It is the continuation of the femoral artery. It begins at the level of hiatus magnus (fifth opening in the adductor magnus muscle (Fig. 14.3).

It is the deepest structure in the popliteal fossa in contact with the popliteal surface of the femur and the capsule of the knee joint. It is about 20 cm in length.

Termination: It terminates by dividing into anterior tibial and posterior tibial arteries at the level of lower border of the popliteus muscle.

Relations:

• The popliteal vein accompanies the artery. In the upper part the vein is posterolateral to the artery, in the middle part posterior (superficial) and in the lower part medial to the artery (Fig. 14.3).

• The tibial nerve descends vertically downwards crossing the artery from lateral to medial side. In the middle part of the fossa it is separated from the popliteal artery by popliteal vein.

• The anterior (deep) relations of the artery from above downwards includes: popliteal surface of the femur,

oblique popliteal ligament and the fascia covering the popliteus muscle.

• The posterior relation includes gastrocnemius muscles in the lower part.

Branches: The popliteal artery gives cutaneous, muscular and genicular branches. The 5 genicular branches supply the knee joint and also take part in anastomosis around the knee joint which connects the distal part of the femoral artery with the arteries of the leg. The genicular branches include superior medial, inferior medial, superior lateral, inferior lateral and middle genicular. The middle genicular pierces the oblique popliteal ligament.

> Popliteal pulse: Among the arteries of the lower limb, it is difficult to feel the pulse of the popliteal artery as it is the deepest content of the fossa. However the pulse can be felt when the knee is flexed and the finger tips of both hands are placed in the fossa firmly with the thumbs resting on the patella.
>
> Popliteal aneurysm can compress the popliteal vein which results in edema of the leg. The aneurysm presents as a midline swelling in the fossa with prominent pulse.

Tibial nerve in the popliteal fossa

It is one of the terminal branches of the sciatic nerve given at the superior angle of the popliteal fossa. It is derived from ventral division of anterior primary rami of L4, L5, S1, S2 and S3 nerves. It is the most superficial content of the popliteal fossa, descends vertically downwards from superior angle to the inferior angle of the fossa. The popliteal vein and artery are related anterior (deep) to it. It gives muscular, cutaneous and genicular branches in the popliteal fossa.

Muscular branches:

1. To medial head of the gastrocnemius

2. To the lateral head of the gastrocnemius

3. To soleus

4. To plantaris

5. Nerve to popliteus

All these branches arise from the lateral side of the tibial nerve except the branch to the medial head of the gastrocnemius. The remaining branches descends superficial to the plantaris while nerve to popliteus passes deep to the plantaris (Fig. 14.3).

The nerve to popliteus in addition to popliteus muscle also supplies superior and inferior tibiofibular joints, interosseus

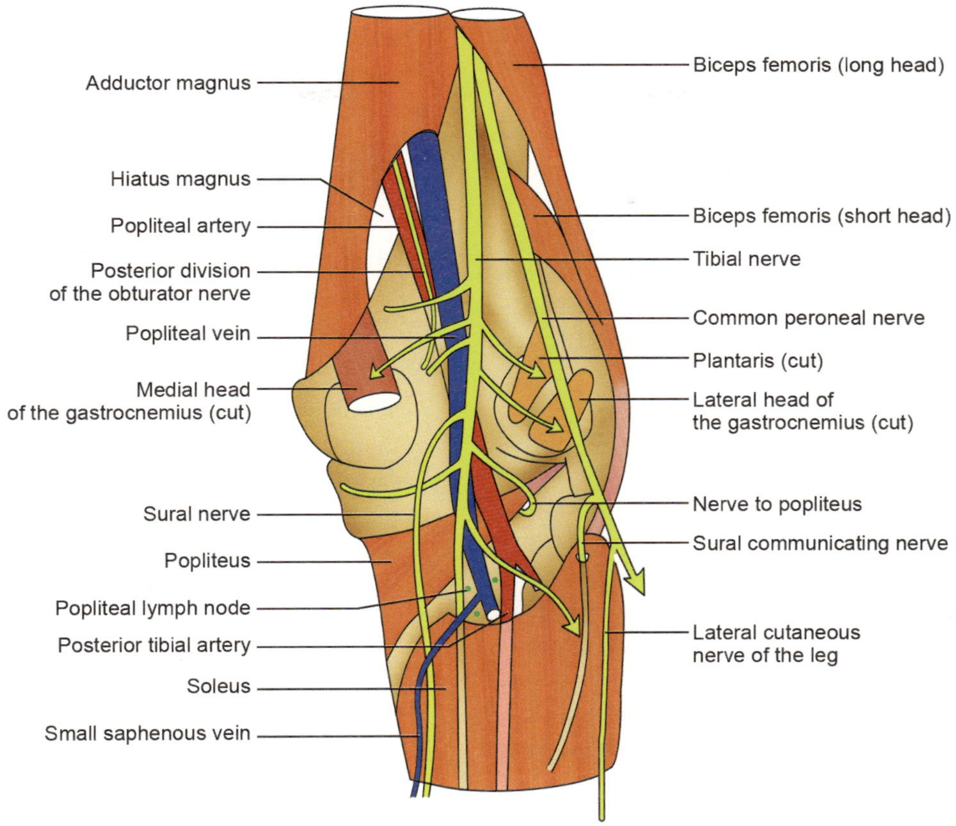

Adductor magnus

Hiatus magnus

Popliteal artery

Posterior division
of the obturator nerve

Popliteal vein

Medial head
of the gastrocnemius (cut)

Sural nerve

Popliteus

Popliteal lymph node

Posterior tibial artery

Soleus

Small saphenous vein

Biceps femoris (long head)

Biceps femoris (short head)

Tibial nerve

Common peroneal nerve

Plantaris (cut)

Lateral head of
the gastrocnemius (cut)

Nerve to popliteus

Sural communicating nerve

Lateral cutaneous
nerve of the leg

Fig. 14.3 Contents of the popliteal fossa

membrane, tibialis posterior muscle and a medullary branch to the tibia.

Genicular (articular) branches: It gives 3 genicular branches-superior medial, inferior medial and middle genicular. The middle genicular pierces the oblique popliteal ligament to supply the interior of the knee joint.

Cutaneous branch: Tibial nerve gives one cutaneous branch called 'sural' nerve.

Sural nerve: It is a cutaneous nerve arises from the medial aspect of the tibial nerve. It pierces the roof and becomes superficial. It is joined by the sural communicating nerve (a branch from the common peroneal nerve). It descends in the posterolateral aspect of the leg, behind the lateral malleolus, where it is accompanied by the small saphenous vein. It supplies the skin of the lower part of the leg (posterolateral aspect) and lateral border of the foot.

Common peroneal nerve in the popliteal fossa

Origin: It is one of the terminal branches of the sciatic nerve given at the level of superior angle of the popliteal fossa. It is derived from dorsal division of anterior primary rami of L4, L5, S1 and S2 nerves.

Course:

It descends obliquely (downwards and laterally) parallel to the tendon of biceps femoris muscle. At the lateral angle of the fossa, it passes superficial to the plantaris and lateral head of the gastrocnemius muscle to reach the back of the head of the fibula (Fig. 14.3).

Termination: It curves forward on the lateral side of the neck of the fibula, deep to the peroneus longus muscle. It ends by dividing into superficial and deep peroneal nerves.

Branches: It gives cutaneous and genicular branches (Note: Common peroneal nerve does not give any muscular branch in the popliteal fossa).

Cutaneous branches:

1. Sural communicating branch: It arises from the common peroneal nerve opposite to the head of the fibula. It descends superficial to the lateral head of the gastrocnemius and joins the sural nerve.

2. Lateral cutaneous nerve of the leg (of calf): It supplies the skin of the front and back of the leg along the lateral border.

SECTION 4

249

Genicular (articular) branches: It gives 3 genicular branches: superior lateral, inferior lateral and recurrent genicular.

Popliteal vein

It is formed by the union of venae comitantes accompanying the anterior and posterior tibial arteries. It ascends in the popliteal fossa superficial to the popliteal artery but deep to the tibial nerve. It continues as femoral vein at the hiatus magnus. The tributaries of the popliteal vein correspond to the branches of popliteal artery.

Popliteal lymph nodes

They are located in the popliteal fossa from roof to the floor. They can be classified into superficial, intermediate and deep groups. The nodes present in the roof (superficial nodes) are related to terminal part of the small saphenous vein. It receives lymph from superficial tissue (skin and fasciae) along the lateral border of the foot, sole and posterolateral aspect of the leg. The intermediate group is located along the popliteal vein, receives lymph from deeper tissue of the foot and leg. The deep nodes are located close to the knee joint capsule receiving lymph from the knee joint.

> Infections and inflammations affecting the sole and lateral border of the foot can lead to enlargement of the popliteal nodes present in the roof. Enlargement of the deeper nodes may compress the nerves and vessels of the fossa.

KNEE JOINT

Type

It is a modified hinge variety of the synovial joint. It is also a complex (by the presence of menisci) and compound (more than two bones taking part) joint.

The articulation between the condyles of femur and tibia is a **condylar** variety of synovial joint. The articulation between femur and patella is a **saddle** variety of synovial joint (Fig. 14.4).

Bones taking part

Condyles of the femur articulate with condyles of tibia. The patellar articular surface of the femur articulates with posterior surface of the patella.

Structures stabilizing

Structurally, knee joint is a weak joint, however, it is stabilised by number of factors of which cruciate and collateral ligaments are important.

1. **Capsular ligament (Fibrous capsule):**

   The fibrous capsule is absent in the anterior aspect, where it is replaced by tendon of the quadriceps femoris muscle, patella and ligamentum patellae (from above downwards).

   On the lateral side the capsule extends between vastus lateralis and lateral margin of the patella and ligamentum patellae as lateral patellar retinaculum. On the medial side the capsule extends between vastus medialis and medial margin of the patella and ligamentum patellae as medial patellar retinaculum.

   Femoral attachment: It is attached to the articular margin of the femur (intercondylar line), however, it is absent in the anterior aspect. The attachment encloses the origin of the popliteus muscle.

   Tibial attachment: Anteriorly it is attached to the margins of the condyles extending up to the tibial tuberosity. Posteriorly, it is attached to intercondylar ridge. The part of the fibrous capsule attached from the peripheral margins of the menisci to the articular margins of tibial condyle is called coronary ligament.

   Synovial membrane: The investment of the synovial membrane is complex. It is absent on the inner aspect of the patella. Above the patella it extends upwards as 'suprapatellar bursa'. Below the patella it is separated from the ligamentum patellae by fat (infrapatellar pad of fat). Posteriorly, it is reflected forward by the cruciate ligaments (Fig. 14.6).

2. **Ligamentum patellae**

   It is an extension of the tendon of quadriceps femoris muscle. It extends from the apex of patella to the tuberosity of tibia. It is used for eliciting patellar reflex or knee jerk by tapping this ligament with a knee hammer.

3. **Tibial collateral (medial) ligament:**

   It is a strong ligament stabilizing the knee from medial side. Above it is attached to the medial epicondyle of the femur. Below it divides into superficial and deep parts. The superficial part is attached to the upper part of the medial surface of the tibia. Its lower part is crossed superficially by Sartorius, gracilis and semitendinosus muscles. The deep part of the ligament is attached to the medial condyle of the tibia. The tibial collateral ligament is attached to the peripheral margin of the medial meniscus. Tibial collateral ligament represents the detached part of the adductor magnus muscle (Fig. 14.4).

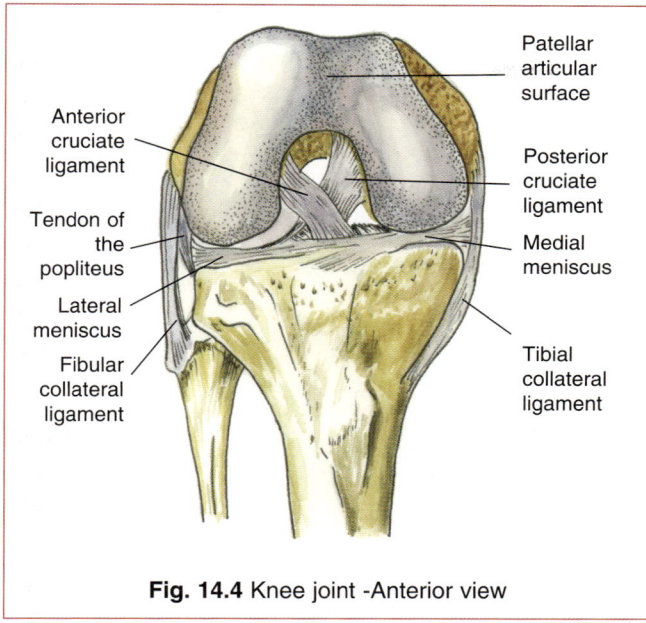

Fig. 14.4 Knee joint -Anterior view

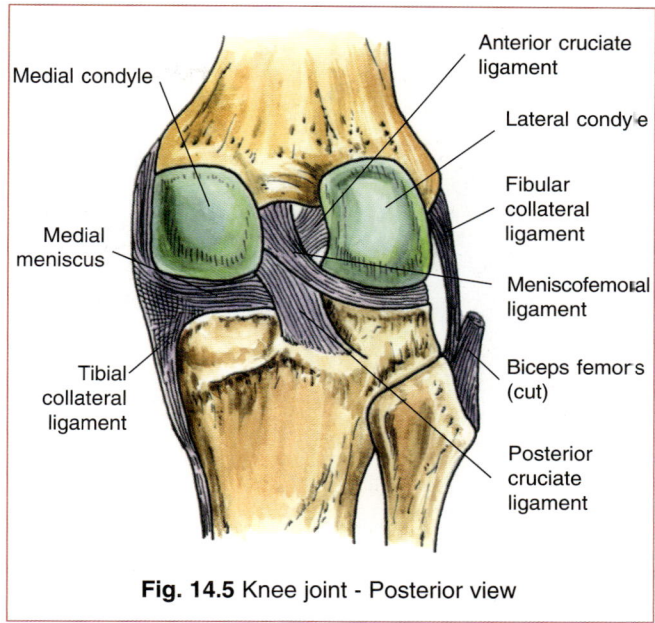

Fig. 14.5 Knee joint - Posterior view

4. Fibular collateral (lateral) ligament:

Above it is attached to the lateral epicondyle of the femur. Below it is attached to the apex of the fibula. It is separated from the lateral meniscus by the tendon of popliteus and part of the fibrous capsule. Morphologically it is derived from detached part of peroneus longus muscle (Figs 14.4 and 14.5).

5. Oblique popliteal ligament:

It is an extension from the tendon of semimembranosus muscle. It thickens the posterior aspect of the fibrous capsule and is attached to the lateral condyle of the femur. It is pierced by middle genicular nerve and vessels and also posterior division of the obturator nerve.

6. Arcuate popliteal ligament:

It is a 'Y' shaped ligament with its stem attached to the head of the fibula. Its posterior band arches superficial to tendon of popliteus and attached to the lateral condyle of the tibia. The anterior band passes deep to the fibular collateral ligament and is attached to the lateral condyle of the femur (Fig.14.8).

Intra articular structures

The intra articular structures include anterior and posterior cruciate ligaments, medial and lateral menisci, meniscofemoral ligament and tendon of popliteus.

7. Cruciate ligaments

These are two strong fibrous ligaments connecting the femur and tibia. The anterior and posterior cruciate ligaments cross each other like the letter X. They are

named anterior and posterior on the basis of their attachments to the tibia (Figs 14.5 to 14.7).

a. **Anterior cruciate ligament (ACL):** It extends from the anterior part of the intercondylar area of the tibia. It passes upwards, backwards and laterally and is attached to medial surface of lateral condyle of femur. It is stretched during extension of the knee joint. It prevents the forward displacement of tibial condyles on femur (or posterior dislocation of femur on tibia).

b. **Posterior cruciate ligament (PCL):** It extends from the posterior part of the intercondylar area of the tibia. It passes upwards, forwards and medially and is attached

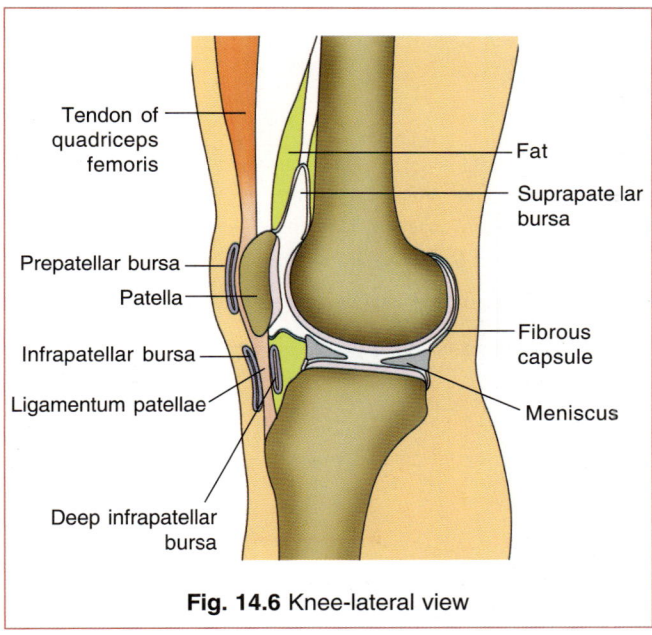

Fig. 14.6 Knee-lateral view

SECTION 4

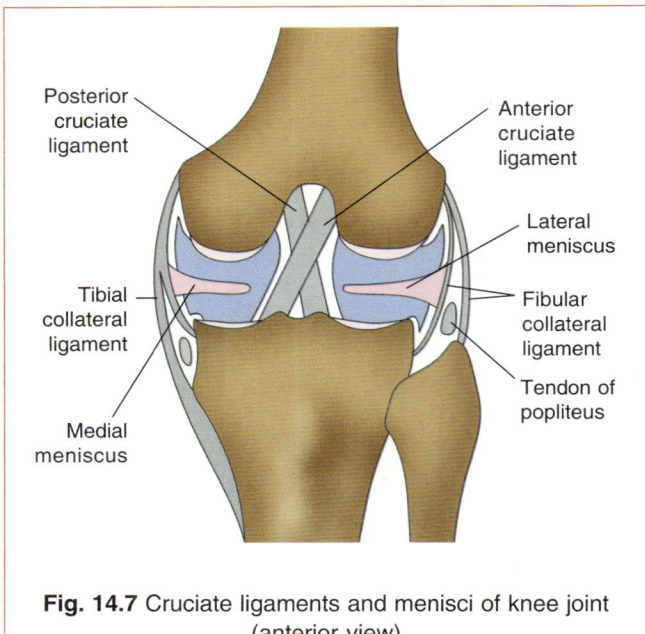

Fig. 14.7 Cruciate ligaments and menisci of knee joint (anterior view)

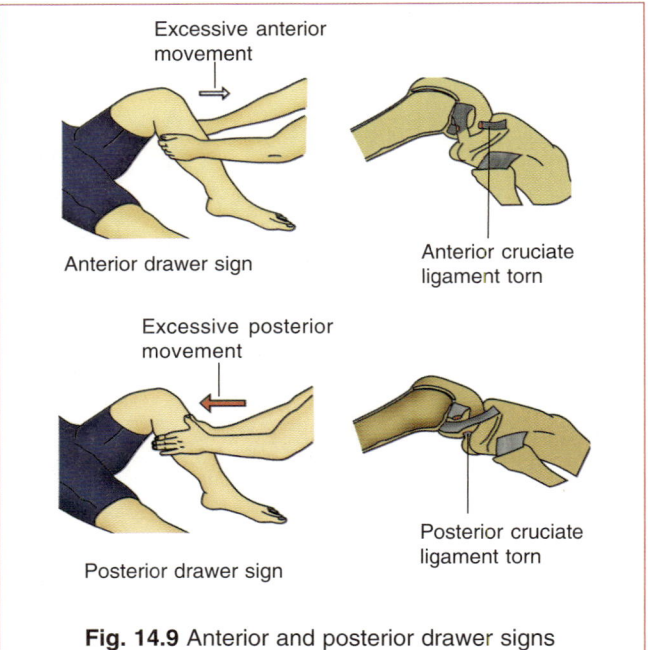

Fig. 14.9 Anterior and posterior drawer signs

to the lateral surface of the medial condyle of femur. It is stretched during flexion of the knee joint. It prevents the backward displacement of tibial condyles on femur (or anterior dislocation of femur on tibia).

Both ligaments are covered by synovial membrane on their anterior aspect.

Anterior cruciate ligament is more prone for injury (in hyperextension or anterior dislocation of the tibia). It causes severe pain and the swelling of the knee joint.

Drawer sign: It is a test to evaluate the integrity of the cruciate ligaments. The person is in supine position with hip and knee in flexed position. The examiner firmly grasp the leg with both hands with thumbs placed on the patella. If there is excessive forward (anterior) movement of the leg (tibia), it indicates injury to the anterior cruciate ligament and is called anterior drawer sign. If there is an excessive backward (posterior) movement of the leg, it indicates the injury

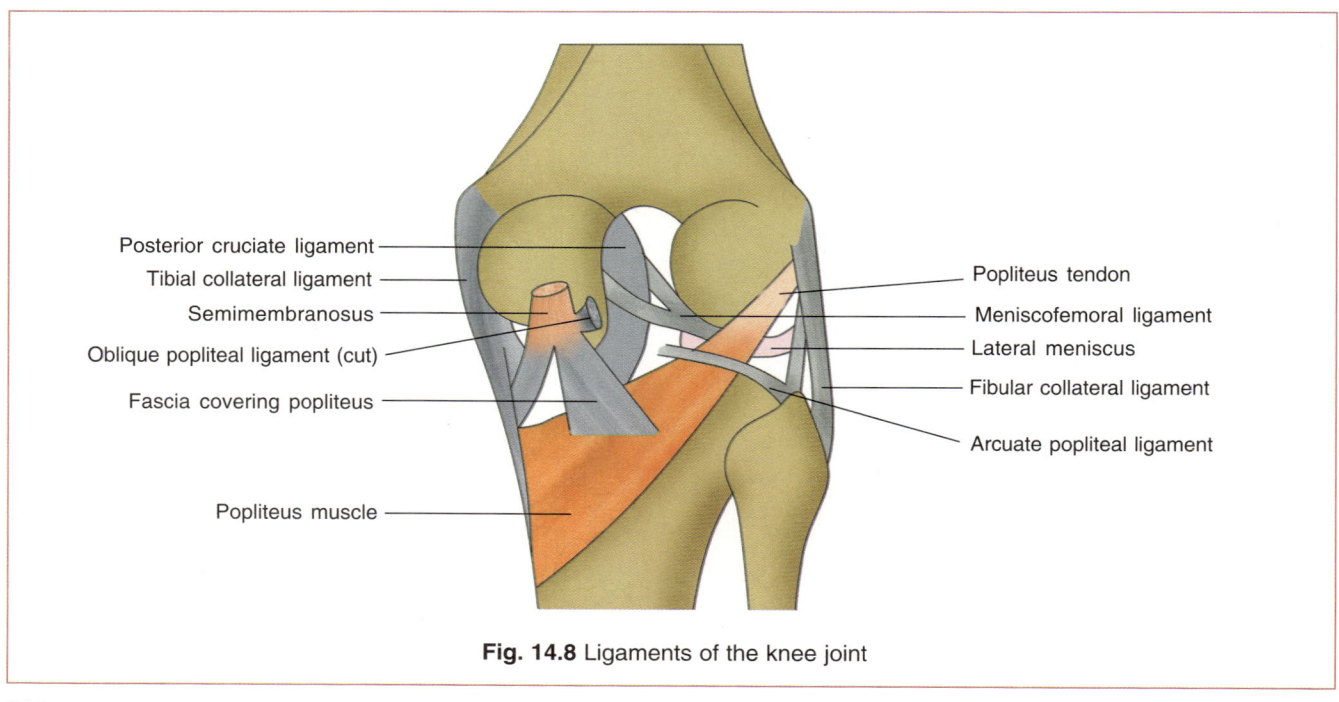

Fig. 14.8 Ligaments of the knee joint

SECTION 4

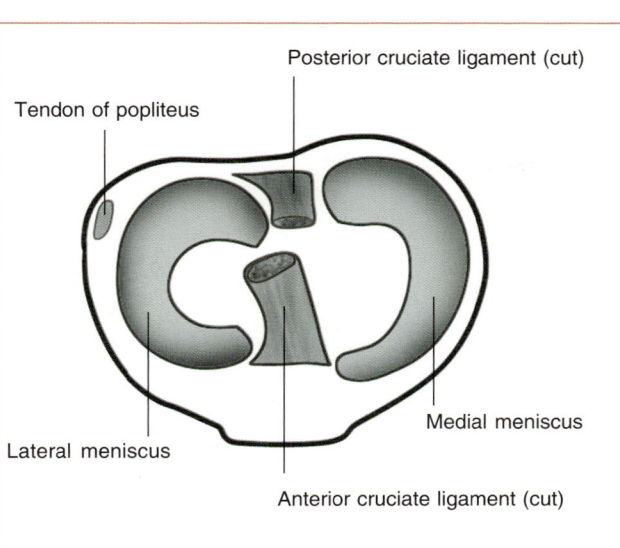

Fig. 14.10 Menisci of the knee joint

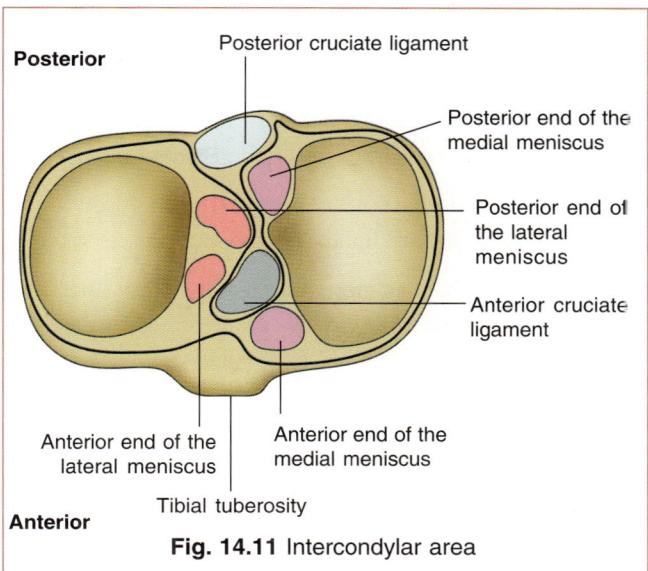

Fig. 14.11 Intercondylar area

to posterior cruciate ligament and is called posterior drawer sign (Fig. 14.9).

8. Menisci (Semilunar cartilages):

Menisci are fibrocartilaginous structures, which deepens the articular surfaces of tibia.

Each meniscus presents anterior and posterior ends, upper and lower surfaces, medial and lateral margins.

The outer margin is thick and inner margin is free. The upper surface is concave for femur and lower surface is flat and articulates with the tibial condyles (Fig. 14.10).

a. Medial meniscus: It is semilunar in shape. The anterior ends of the medial and lateral menisci are connected by '**transverse ligament**'. The peripheral margin of the medial meniscus is attached to tibial collateral ligament. This makes the medial meniscus less mobile and more prone for injuries.

b. Lateral meniscus: It is circular in shape. The anterior and posterior ends of the lateral meniscus are attached to the intercondylar area of the tibia. The peripheral margin of the meniscus is not attached to the fibular collateral ligament or fibrous capsule unlike medial meniscus. The tendon of the popliteus passes between the lateral meniscus and fibular collateral ligament. Some fibres of popliteus is attached to the posterior horn of the lateral meniscus, which pulls the meniscus backwards when femur is rotated laterally which prevents the crushing of meniscus during flexion of the knee joint. In this way popliteus protects the lateral meniscus.

The posterior end of the lateral meniscus is connected with medial condyle of the femur by two-meniscofemoral

ligaments. The anterior and posterior meniscofemoral ligaments passes anterior and posterior to the posterior cruciate ligaments respectively. The tendon of the popliteus is attached to the lateral meniscus, which pulls the meniscus backwards and prevents its injury.

Functions of menisci

* They deepen the tibial articular surfaces.
* They act as shock absorbers to protect the articular cartilages.
* They flush the synovial fluid to provide nutrition to the articular cartilages.

Meniscal tears:

* A sudden blow on the lateral side of a flexed weight-bearing knee can cause rupture of the tibial collateral ligament with a concomitant tear in the medial meniscus.

* The bucket handle rupture of the medial meniscus is common in football player.

* During extension of knee the femoral condyles first roll forwards and then spin forward on the upper surface of the menisci.

* The anterior horn of the medial meniscus is the last part to receive medial femoral condyle

* Since the anterior horn of the medial meniscus is the site of rotation of medial condyle of femur during locking and unlocking, it undergoes wear and tear.

* A sudden blow on the lateral side of a flexed weight-bearing knee can cause rupture of the tibial collateral

ligament with a concomitant tear in the medial meniscus

- On rupture of medial meniscus, the knee gets locked in the flexed position and swollen due to synovitis.

- Medial meniscus is less mobile (firmly fused with the tibial collateral ligament) and more prone to tear.

- Lateral miniscus is more mobile, since few fibers of popliteus are attached to the posterior horn of lateral miniscus, the muscle pulls the meniscus back if the femur is rotated laterally

- A combination of injury to the tibial collateral ligaments, medial meniscus and anterior cruciate ligament is called 'unhappy triad' of knee joint.

- Rupture of anterior cruciate ligament may occur if the knee is forcibly hyperextended

Bursae related to the knee joint

There are many bursae around the knee joint. Some of the important bursae are explained below (Fig. 14.6).

Bursae related in the anterior aspect:

1. **Subcutaneous prepatellar bursa:** The prepatellar bursa is located between the patella and the overlying skin and prepatellar tendon. It is lined by synovial membrane and contains very little fluid. Its function is to diminish friction and ensure maximal range of motion at the knee.

   Chronic trauma from repeated kneeling is one cause of prepatellar bursitis, also called "**housemaid's knee.**" It is common in roofers, plumbers and carpet layers.

   Symptoms of prepatellar bursitis include knee pain, swelling, redness and Inability to flex the knee on the affected side. The symptoms are usually relieved by rest. Physical examination reveals tenderness to palpation, erythema, crepitance, and fluctuant edema over the lower pole of the patella.

2. Subcutaneous infrapatellar bursa: It is present between the ligamentum patellae and the skin. Inflammation of this bursa gives rise to Clergyman's knee.

3. Deep infrapatellar bursa: It is located behind the ligamentum patellae and in front of the upper end of the tibia.

4. Supra patellar bursa: It is present behind the lower end of the quadriceps femoris and in front of the femoral shaft. It communicates with the joint cavity.

Bursae related to the lateral aspect:

5. Between the joint capsule and the lateral head of the gastrocnemius.

6. Between fibular collateral ligament and biceps femoris tendon

7. Between tendon of the popliteus and fibular collateral ligament

Bursae related to the medial aspect:

8. Between the medial head of the gastrocnemius and the joint capsule (Brodies bursa)

9. Between tibial collateral ligament and 3 muscles crossing it (Sartorius, gracilis and semitendinosus) and this bursa is called 'ansarine' bursa

10. Between the insertion of semimembranosus and the medial condyle of the tibia. Inflammation of this bursa may produce a fluctuant swelling (Baker's cyst) in the popliteal fossa.

Relations of the knee joint

Anteriorly: Lower part of the quadriceps femoris muscle, patella and ligamentum patella

Posteriorly: Popliteal vessels, tibial nerve

Posteromedially: Semimembranosus, Tendons of sartorisus, gracilis and semitendinosus

Posterolaterally: Tendon of the biceps femoris and common peroneal nerve

Arterial supply

Knee joint is supplied by many genicular arteries derived from popliteal, femoral, anterior and posterior tibial arteries.

Nerve supply

a. Femoral nerve supplying vasti muscles also supply knee joint.

b. Genicular branches of tibial, common peroneal and posterior division of obturator nerves.

   L3 and L4 regulate the extension and L5 and S1 regulates the flexion of knee joint.

Movements and Muscles producing them

1. **Flexion:** Hamstring muscles (Biceps femoris, Semitendinosus, Semimembranosus) assisted by gracilis, sartorius and popliteus muscle.

2. **Extension:** Quadriceps femoris and tensor fascia latae.

3. **Rotation** of knee occurs below the menisci and this range of movement is very less.

S E C T I O N 4

In the process of extension of the knee joint, the lateral condyle of the femur comes in contact with lateral condyle of the tibia before the medial condyles. This is because of larger anteroposterior diameter of the medial condyle of the femur. At the terminal stages of extension still small surface of the medial femoral condyle will not make contact with tibia. To achieve full congruity between the articular surface of the medial condyles of femur and tibia, the femur rotates medially on the tibia (or the tibia rotates laterally on the femur). This conjunct rotation occurs automatically during flexion and extension

a. Medial rotation: Semitendinosus, semimembranosus and popliteus.

b. Lateral rotation: Biceps femoris.

4. **Locking of the knee**: It is defined as medial rotation of femur on tibia during the final stages of extension (last 30°) of the knee, when the foot is on the ground. It is lateral rotation of the tibia when the foot is off the ground. When the knee is locked all the ligaments are stretched. It is an asset to the knee joint because knee can be held in extended position without any muscular contraction. A person is able to stand for hours together without strain to the quadriceps femoris when the knee joint is locked.

5. **Unlocking of the knee**: It is defined as '**lateral rotation of femur on tibia during initial stages of flexion of the knee joint when the foot is on the ground**. It is medial rotation of tibia when the foot is off the ground. **Popliteus muscle unlocks** the knee by initiating flexion and further flexion is brought by hamstring muscles.

The natural tendency of displacement of patella is on the lateral side but it is prevented by –

a. Raised lateral margin of the patellar articular surface of the femur.

b. Insertion of the vastus medialis extends further below when compared to the insertion of the vastus lateralis on the lateral margin of the patella.

CASE-1

A 68-year-old woman with a long history of diabetes has been suffering from worsening numbness and pain in the right leg and foot. She was admitted to the hospital as a case of peripheral vascular disease with neuropathy. The examining physician found that both the dorsalis pedis pulse and the popliteal pulsations were weak. Neurological examination revealed an area of skin over the lateral aspect of the right leg was numb. The physician recommended doing arteriography to assess the extent of vascular occlusion.

1. What are the contents of the popliteal fossa?

2. Where would you feel the pulsation of the popliteal artery? Why was it weak in this case?

3. How do you explain the presence of an abnormal sensation of the lateral aspect of the right leg? Which cutaneous nerve is most likely involved?

CASE-2

A 52-year-old house made visits hospital with a painful swelling in front of the lower part of the left knee. While taking the history she revealed that her work involves cleaning the floor area bending her knee for most of the time. Using your knowledge of anatomy, what is the diagnosis?

CASE-3

A medical student, while playing football collided with another player and fell to the ground. As he fell, the right knee, which was taking the weight of his body, was partially flexed, the femur was rotated medially, and the leg abducted on the thigh. A sudden pain was felt in the right knee joint, and he was unable to extend it. When examined by a physician an hour later, the student was still unable to extend the knee, which was by now greatly swollen. Severe local tenderness was felt along the medial side of the joint line. What is the diagnosis? Why was the knee locked? Why was the swelling of the knee so excessive over the front of the joint?

CASE-4

Following a severe automobile accident, a 27-year-old woman was found to have an unstable right knee joint. On examination under an anesthetic, it was possible to pull the tibia forward excessively on the femur. The patient's knee joint was fixed in plaster for three months, and vigorous physiotherapy was carried out on her quadriceps femoris muscle. What structure was damaged in the knee joint? Why was it necessary to have physiotherapy on the quadriceps femoris muscle?

CASE-5

A 19-year-old student was hit on the posterolateral side of his right knee by an opponent player while playing a foot ball match. At the time of impact, the student's right foot was firmly planted (weight bearing). The leg was severely abducted by the blow, and the knee buckled and the student collapsed to the ground in severe pain. A stretcher was required to remove him from the play ground. He was then shifted to the hospital where the knee was thoroughly examined. Severe pain was localized to the medial side of the right knee, and drawer test was positive. The student underwent surgery and he was unable to return to the playing field until the following season.

1. Based on the information given, which ligaments were probably injured?
2. What other structures may also be injured?
3. What is the drawer test?
4. Why does a blow on the lateral side of the knee usually produce a more serious injury than a blow to the medial side?

Solutions to the case studies:

Case-1

1. Refer text
2. Pulsation can be felt on deep palpation in the popliteal fossa with the leg slightly flexed. Weak popliteal artery pulsation in this case is due to obstructive vascular disease that happens due to atherosclerosis in patients with diabetes.
3. Patients with poorly managed diabetes may have peripheral neuropathy characterized by abnormal sensation along the cutaneous distribution of the affected nerve. The cutaneous nerve affected in this case is the lateral cutaneous nerve of the leg.

Case-2

On examination this patient was found to have a swelling in front of her ligamentum patellae on the left side. Repeated unaccustomed trauma to the subcutaneous infrapatellar bursa had produced an inflammatory response in the bursa which resulted in an excessive production of fluid, hence the swelling.

Case-3

As the student fell, the medial meniscus was drawn laterally within the knee joint. The sudden movement of knee joint, which occurred on striking the ground, resulted in the relatively immobile medial meniscus torn between the medial femoral and tibial condyles. The meniscus split along part of its length, and the detached portion became jammed, like a wedge, between the articular surfaces, limiting further extension, i.e. locking the joint. The

tenderness was experienced over the torn medial meniscus. The trauma stimulated an excessive production of synovial fluid, which filled the joint cavity and the supra patellar bursa. The distension of the latter was responsible for the large amount of swelling seen in front of the joint.

Case-4

In this patient the anterior cruciate ligament in the right knee has been ruptured. The strength of the knee joint depends primarily on the tone of the quadriceps femoris muscle and secondarily on the ligaments. Operative union of torn cruciate ligaments is unsatisfactory. The loss of this ligament can be compensated by developing the tone of the quadriceps muscle.

Case-5

1. The medial collateral ligament and the anterior cruciate ligament were involved in this case. The localized pain medially suggests a medial collateral ligament injury and the positive drawer test indicates a ruptured anterior cruciate ligament.
2. The medial meniscus is probably also damaged because it is attached to the medial collateral ligament. Undue stress from a blow to the lateral side of the knee usually results in tearing of both the medial collateral ligament and the medial meniscus.
3. The drawer test involves firmly grasping the leg with both hands just below the knee with the thumbs on the tibial tuberosity. With the knee flexed, the examiner pushes and pulls the leg in a line parallel to the long axis of the femur. Excessive mobility anteriorly indicates a ruptured anterior cruciate ligament, while excessive posterior movement suggests a ruptured posterior cruciate ligament.
4. Because the medial collateral ligament and the medial meniscus are attached, these structures are frequently injured together as a result of a blow to the lateral side of the knee. The same is not true for blows to the medial side of the knee. In this case, only the lateral collateral ligament is usually injured. The lateral collateral ligament and the lateral meniscus are not attached to each other, but are separated by the tendon of the popliteus muscle.

MCQs

1. Your patient has sustained an external force to the knee. Which of the following ligaments has prevented abduction of the leg at the knee?
   A. Anterior cruciate
   B. Posterior cruciate

C. Fibular collateral

D. Tibial collateral

2. In this same patient, which of the following ligaments prevented posterior displacement of the tibia on the femur?

A. Oblique popliteal

B. Anterior cruciate

C. Posterior cruciate

D. Lateral collateral

3. You have examined a patient and found that there is weakness in flexing the knee. This indicates a lesion of which of the following nerves?

A. Sciatic

B. Femoral

C. Obturator

D. Saphenous

4. A 26-year-old woman is bitten by a stray cat. She ignored the wound which became erythematous and swollen five days later. The woman further ignored the signs of infection until she developed a swollen and tender lymph node in his popliteal fossa. An infected skin lesion in which of the following sites would most likely to cause lymphadenopathy in this region?

A. Medial side of the dorsum of the foot

B. Lateral side of the dorsum of the foot

C. Medial side of the leg below the knee

D. Medial side of the thigh

5. When the femur is fractured, the broken distal end often turns posteriorly to enter the popliteal fossa due to muscle traction. Because of its position deep in the fossa, which structure is most vulnerable to laceration?

A. Common peroneal nerve

B. Small saphenous vein

C. Popliteal artery

D. Tibial nerve

6. During surgical repair of a popliteal artery aneurysm, ligation of the femoral artery at mid-thigh would not interrupt supply to the hamstring muscles because the

A. Genicular anastomosis ensures blood supply to the posterior thigh

B. Cruciate anastomosis ensures blood supply to the posterior thigh

C. Perforating branches of the deep femoral artery supply the posterior thigh

D. Obturator artery supplies the posterior thigh

7. An athlete has a knee injury, and the doctor performs a "drawer test" by pulling and pushing on the leg with the knee flexed. If the leg translates anteriorly, i.e. "gives" or moves anteriorly when the leg is pulled anteriorly, which joint structure is most likely to have been injured?

A. Anterior cruciate ligament

B. Lateral collateral ligament

C. Medial collateral ligament

D. Posterior cruciate ligament

8. One of the menisci of the knee is often injured in a sprain of the knee because the:

A. Anterior cruciate ligament is attached to the medial meniscus

B. Lateral collateral ligament is attached to the lateral meniscus

C. Medial collateral ligament is attached to the medial meniscus

D. Posterior cruciate ligament is attached to the lateral meniscus

9. A young man involved in a head-on automobile collision had his flexed knee hit the dashboard of the car. He was later found to have a major instability of the knee, where his tibia could be moved posteriorly relative to the femur. What ligament was likely damaged?

A. Lateral collateral ligament

B. Medial collateral ligament

C. Anterior cruciate ligament

D. Posterior cruciate ligament

10. A 47-year-old gardener visits the hospital with knee pain. He reports that he spends hours on his knees while gardening. Which of the following bursae do you expect to be mostly affected in this patient?

A. Suprapatellar bursa

B. Prepatellar bursa

C Anserine bursa

D. Semimembranous (popliteal) bursa

11. An 18-year-old boy receives a powerful blow to the lateral aspect of his knee. He is unable to walk and complains of excruciating pain in the knee. The knee is swollen and can be passively displaced anteriorly as well as passively abducted. Based on these symptoms, the physician determines that the boy has injured two of the ligaments in his knee. One of his damaged ligaments prevents excessive abduction of the knee.

SECTION 4

257

The other ligament which is damaged prevents which of the following actions?

A. Excessive adduction of the knee
B. Hyperextension of the knee
C. Hyperflexion of the knee
D. Lateral rotation of the knee

Answers to MCQs

1. D
2. B
3. A
4. B
5. C
6. A
7. A
8. A
9. D
10. B
11. B

Leg—Anterior and Lateral Compartments and Dorsum of the Foot

15

- Anterior compartment of the leg
- Dorsum of the foot
- Lateral compartment of the leg
- MCQs

Objectives

- To explain the attachments of superior and inferior extensor retinacula of the ankle and to identify the structures passing superficial and deep to them.
- To explain the attachments of superior and inferior peroneal retinacula of the ankle and to identify the structures passing superficial and deep to them.
- To know the attachments of the muscles of the anterior and lateral compartments of the leg, their nerve supply and actions.
- To explain the course and distribution and clinical relevance of common peroneal nerve and its branches
- To explain the course and branches of anterior tibial and dorsalis pedis arteries
- To explain the cutaneous innervations of the dorsum of the foot

ANTERIOR COMPARTMENT OF THE LEG

Cutaneous nerve supply to the front of the leg

The skin of the front of the leg is innervated by L4 and L5 dermatomes. Following nerves supply the skin in front of the leg.

1. Infrapatellar nerve
2. Lateral cutaneous nerve of the leg
3. Saphenous nerve
4. Superficial peroneal nerve

Contents of the anterior compartment

It is also called extensor compartment. It has 4 muscles namely-tibialis anterior, extensor hallucis longus, extensor digitorum longus and peroneus tertius. The nerve of this compartment is deep peroneal nerve which supplies all these muscles. All these muscles mainly cause dorsiflexion at the ankle joint. The artery of the compartment is the anterior tibial artery (Fig. 15.1).

The deep fascia in this region forms 2 retinacula in front of the ankle -superior and inferior extensor retinacula. The superior retinacula is present in front of the ankle at the lower part of the leg and the inferior on the dorsum of the foot.

Superior extensor retinaculum

It is thick deep fascia present in front of the ankle. It holds the extensor tendons in their position during movement of the joint.

Attachments:

Medially: Lower part of the anterior border of the tibia

Laterally: Lower part of the anterior surface of the fibula

Structures passing superficial to the retinaculum:

1. Great saphenous vein
2. Saphenous nerve
3. Superficial peroneal nerve

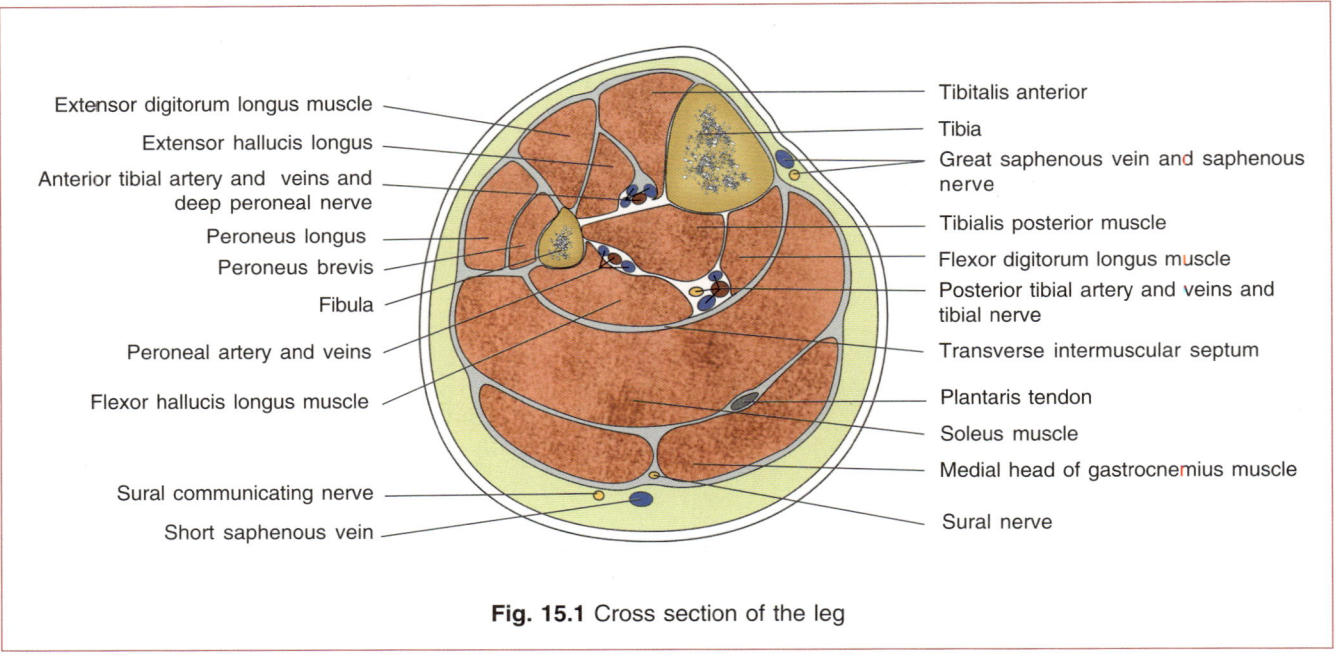

Extensor digitorum longus muscle

Extensor hallucis longus

Anterior tibial artery and veins and deep peroneal nerve

Peroneus longus

Peroneus brevis

Fibula

Peroneal artery and veins

Flexor hallucis longus muscle

Sural communicating nerve

Short saphenous vein

Tibitalis anterior

Tibia

Great saphenous vein and saphenous nerve

Tibialis posterior muscle

Flexor digitorum longus muscle

Posterior tibial artery and veins and tibial nerve

Transverse intermuscular septum

Plantaris tendon

Soleus muscle

Medial head of gastrocnemius muscle

Sural nerve

Fig. 15.1 Cross section of the leg

Structures passing deep to the retinacula (Fig. 15.2)

Following structures passes from medial to lateral side

1. Tibialis anterior
2. Extensor hallucis longus
3. Anterior tibial vessels
4. Deep peroneal nerve
5. Extensor digitorum longus
6. Peroneus tertius

The tendons of these muscle has separate synovial sheath which allows frictionless movement.

Inferior extensor retinaculum

It is a thick modified deep fascia present on the dorsum of the foot. It is 'Y' shaped with the stem of the 'Y' present on the lateral side.

Attachments:

The stem is attached to the upper surface of the calcaneus in its anterior part.

Medially the upper band is attached to the medial malleolus and the lower band passes to the medial margin of the foot and continues with deep fascia of the sole (plantar aponeurosis).

The relations of the retinaculum (structures passing superficial and deep) is similar to the superior extensor retinaculum except for anterior tibial artery, it is **dorsalis pedis artery** (dorsalis pedis artery is the continuation of the anterior tibial artery).

Muscles of the anterior compartment

The attachments, nerve supply and actions of the anterior compartment muscles are explained in Table 15.1

Shin splints: It is a condition results from injury to the tibialis anterior muscle. It is common in people who are not used to exercise regularly.

Anterior compartment syndrome: This also results from excessive usage of leg muscle as in severe exercise or long distance running. It leads to swelling in the muscles of the leg especially in the anterior compartment where muscles are tightly held by deep fascia. The muscular swelling may compress the veins

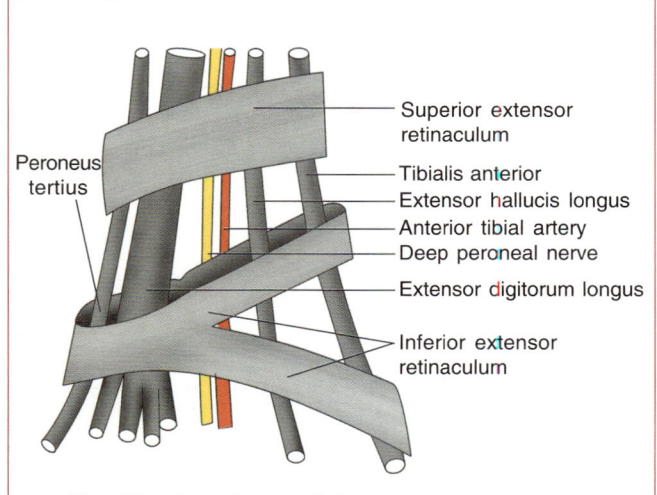

Peroneus tertius

Superior extensor retinaculum

Tibialis anterior

Extensor hallucis longus

Anterior tibial artery

Deep peroneal nerve

Extensor digitorum longus

Inferior extensor retinaculum

Fig. 15.2 Superior and inferior extensor retinacula

Table 15.1 Muscles of anterior compartment of leg

Muscle	Origin	Insertion	Nerve supply	Actions
Tibialis anterior	Lateral condyle of tibia. Upper 2/3rd of lateral surface of shaft of tibia Adjoining interosseous membrane	Inferomedial surface of medial cuneiform and adjoining part of base of the first metatarsal	Deep peroneal nerve	Dorsiflexor and invertor of foot Maintains medial longitudinal arch of foot
Extensor hallucis longus	Posterior part of middle 2/4th of medial surface of shaft of fibula. Upper part of interosseous membrane	Dorsal surface of base of distal phalanx of great toe	Deep peroneal nerve	Dorsiflexes the foot and extends the metatarsophalangeal, proximal and distal interphalangeal joints of great toe
Extensor digitorum longus	Lateral condyle of tibia Upper ¼ and anterior half of middle 2/4th of medial surface of shaft of fibula Upper part of interosseous membrane	Divides into four tendons for lateral four toes Tendons of 2nd, 3rd, 4th digits are joined by tendon of extensor digitorum brevis laterally which together forms the dorsal digital expansion and gets inserted to bases of middle and distal phalanx	Deep peroneal nerve	Dorsiflexes the foot and extends the metatarsophalangeal, proximal and distal interphalangeal joints of 2nd to 5th toes
Peroneus tertius	Lower 1/4th of medial surface of shaft of fibula Adjoining interosseous membrane	Medial part of dorsal surface of base of 5th metatarsal	Deep peroneal nerve	Dorsiflexor and evertor of foot
Extensor digitorum brevis	Anterior part of superior surface of calcaneum	Divided into 4 tendons for medial 4 toes. The first tendon (extensor hallucis brevis) is inserted to dorsal surface of base of proximal phalanx of great toe Lateral three tendons joins the lateral side of tendons of extensor digitorum longus and thereby to dorsal digital expansion of 2nd, 3rd, 4th toes.	Lateral terminal branch of deep peroneal nerve	First tendon extends the great toe at metatarsophalangeal joint, while the latter three extends 2nd, 3rd, 4th digits at metatarsophalangeal joints and interphalangeal joints

which cause accumulation of the fluid in this compartment. The increased pressure in this compartment can compress deep peroneal nerve and anterior tibial artery. Arterial compression can cause gangrene of the foot. To relieve the pressure the deep fascia of the leg is cut along the whole length of the anterior compartment. Fracture of the tibia with bleeding inside can also cause anterior compartment syndrome (Fig. 15.3).

CASE-1

A 16-year-old girl decides to participate in a long distance running event. She started practice and after a couple of days of workout, she started to have pain in the anterior portion of her left leg. Her coach ignored this pain and insisted the girl to keep running. As the workout continued, the pain worsened and the girl was forced to stop the running practice. The pain continued to get worse overnight, so she was taken into the hospital. On examination, the physician found the leg to be red and swollen. The anterior aspect of the leg was very sensitive to palpation and felt hard and warmer than other parts of the leg. Dorsiflexion of the foot and toes was severely limited. The dorsalis pedis pulse was weak, and also a sensory loss was noted between the first and second toes. The patient was taken to surgery and the fascia over the anterolateral aspect of the leg was incised to relieve the pressure in the anterior compartment of her leg.

1. What do you think happened to the girl's leg in this case?

2. This condition is called anterior compartment syndrome of the leg. What about the anatomy of the anterior compartment of the leg makes it susceptible to this type of injury?

3. How do you explain the sensory loss on the foot? Which muscle outside the anterior compartment could you test to see if there has been any motor loss as well?

4. Suppose that the pressure in the anterior compartment of the leg was sufficient to stop blood flow through the anterior tibial artery. How would you explain the presence of a weak pulse in the dorsalis pedis artery?

Anterior tibial artery

• It is the one of the terminal branches of the popliteal artery given at the level of the lower border of the popliteus muscle (Fig. 15.4)

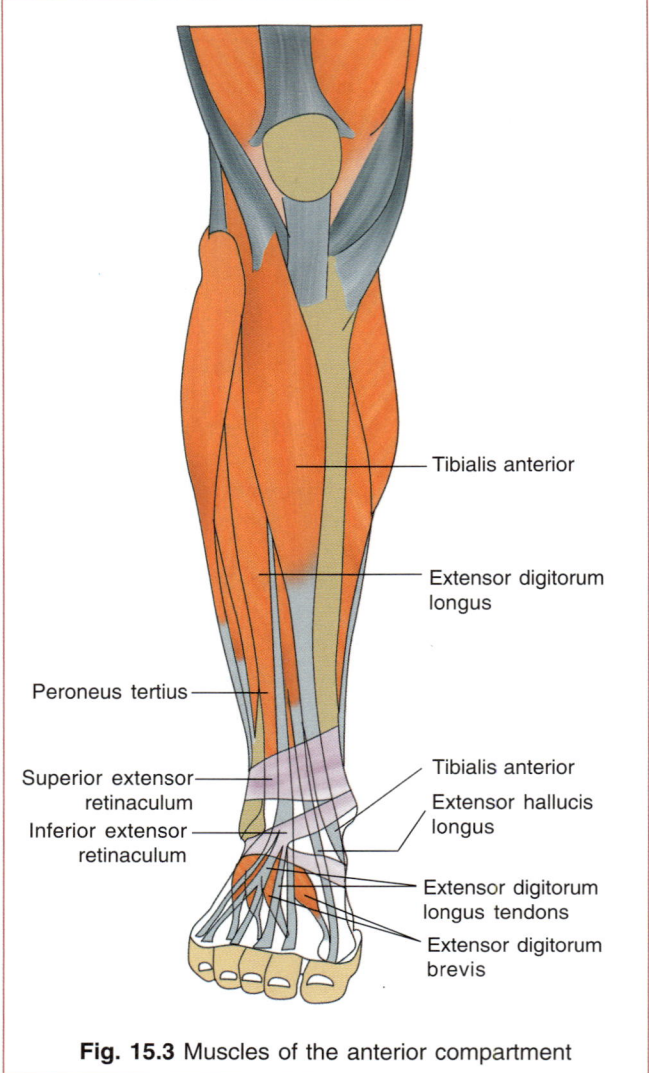

Fig. 15.3 Muscles of the anterior compartment

• It is the main artery supplying anterior compartment and dorsum of the foot

• Its terminal part is connected with posterior tibial artery.

• It enters the anterior compartment through an opening in the upper part of interosseous membrane.

• In its course, the artery lies between tibialis anterior and extensor digitorum longus in the upper part, between tibialis anterior and extensor hallucis longus in the middle and between extensor hallucis longus and extensor digitorum longus in the lower part.

• It is accompanied by deep peroneal nerve that lies lateral to it in the upper and lower third, while anterior to it in the middle third of the leg.

• It is accompanied by a pair of veins.

• At the midpoint of the two malleoli, the anterior tibial artery continues as dorsalis pedis artery.

Branches

- Muscular branches to the muscles of the anterior compartment

- Anastomotic branches: It includes anterior and posterior tibial recurrent arteries which take part in anastomoses around the knee.

- Medial malleolar artery: It passes medially towards medial malleolus to anastomose with branches of posterior tibial and medial plantar arteries.

- Lateral malleolar artery: It passes laterally towards lateral malleolus and anastomoses with the perforating branches of posterior tibial and branches of lateral tarsal artery.

Inadequate blood supply to the leg is characterized by pain in the leg while walking and its disappearance after rest. This is referred as intermittent claudication. While walking the muscles demand more blood supply and insufficient supply causes pain. Atherosclerosis, diabetes and hypertension are the causes for narrowing of the arteries which results in insufficient arterial supply. It can cause gangrene of the toes and foot.

Sympathetic fibres to the blood vessels of the lower limb: It is derived from lateral horn cells of the T10 to L2 segment of the spinal cord. The preganglionic fibres passes out through ventral rami of the respective spinal nerves and reach lumbar and sacral sympathetic ganglia via white rami communicantes. The post ganglionic fibres enter the nerves of the lumbar and sacral plexus through grey rami communicantes. Surgical or chemical lumbar sympathectomy may be indicated in arterial disease of the lower limb.

CASE-2

A 66-year-old man was admitted to the hospital suffering from severe intermittent claudication of the left leg. He could walk about 50 yards before the cramp-like pain in his calf muscles forced him to rest. On examination, his femoral pulses were found to be normal in both legs. The popliteal, dorsalis pedis, and posterior tibial arteries were present in the right leg, but completely absent in the left leg. Angiography revealed a normal right femoral artery, but the artery on the left was completely blocked at the level of the adductor tubercle. Other blocks were seen at different levels lower down the arterial tree. In view of the extensive arteriosclerosis involving many areas of the main arterial supply, it was decided that a venous grafting operation would not be performed. Instead, an attempt

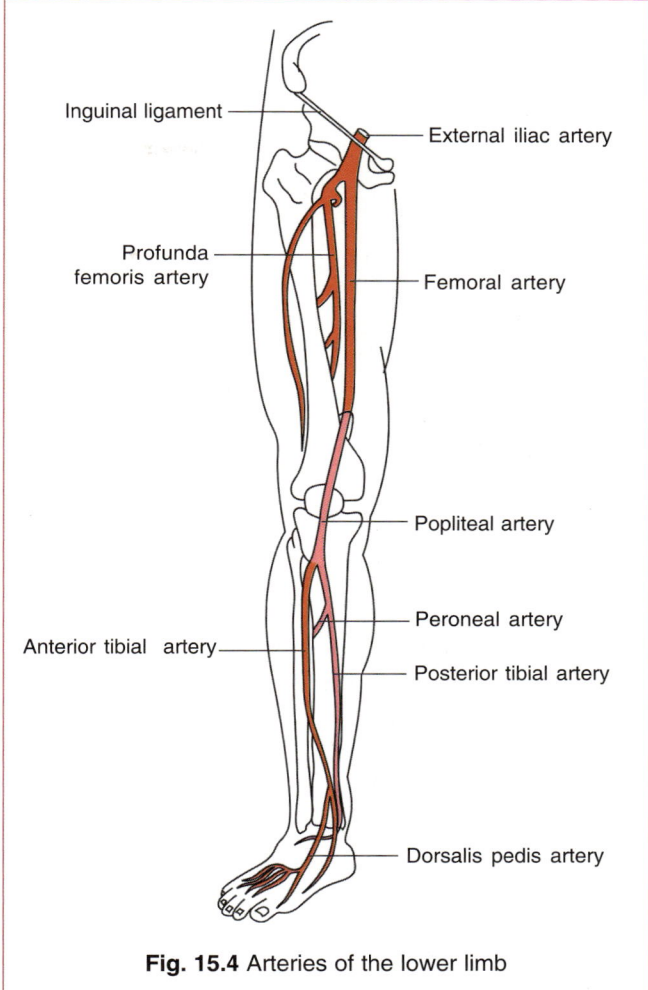

Fig. 15.4 Arteries of the lower limb

would be made to increase the blood flow through the collateral circulation.

1. Where would you palpate the femoral, popliteal, dorsalis pedis, and posterior tibial arteries?

2. How is it possible to increase the blood flow through the collateral circulation?

3. How does blood reach the distal part of the leg in the presence of a block in the femoral artery at the opening in the adductor magnus?

4. What is the sympathetic innervation to the arteries of the lower limb?

Deep peroneal nerve: It is explained separately under the heading common peroneal nerve.

DORSUM OF THE FOOT

Dorsal venous arch: It is an irregular network of veins present at the dorsum of the foot. It receives most of the blood from the plantar surface through perforating veins.

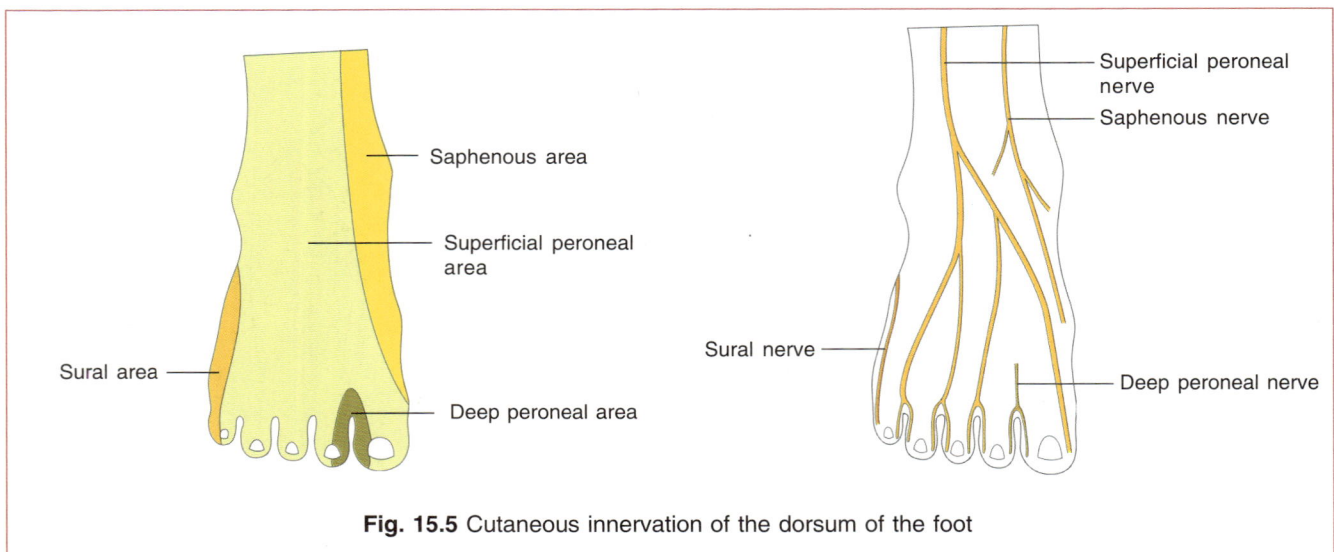

Fig. 15.5 Cutaneous innervation of the dorsum of the foot

The great saphenous vein arises from the medial side of the arch, while small saphenous vein from the lateral side.

Cutaneous nerve supply to the dorsum of the foot

1. Superficial peroneal nerve: It supplies the major portion of the dorsum with 3 exceptions - medial border up to the level of the head of the first metatarsal bone (ball of the great toe), lateral border of the foot and the cleft between great toe and second toe (Fig. 15.5).

2. Deep peroneal nerve: It supplies the cleft between great toe and the second toe (Note: Medial border of the great toe is supplied by superficial peroneal nerve).

3. Saphenous nerve: It supplies medial border of the foot up to the level of the head of the first metatarsal bone.

4. Sural nerve: It supplies the lateral margin of the foot including lateral border of the little toe.

   Knowledge of the cutaneous nerve supply of the dorsum is important in differentiating the nerve lesions involving branches of peroneal nerve.

Muscle of the dorsum: The dorsum of the foot resents a muscle called extensor digitorum brevis. It is explained in Table 15.1.

Dorsalis pedis artery

• It is the continuation of the anterior tibial artery at the midpoint between the 2 malleoli.

• It passes forwards along the medial side of the dorsum to reach the proximal end of the first intermetatarsal space.

• Here the artery enters the sole to form the plantar arch by joining with lateral plantar artery.

Branches

1. Lateral tarsal artery: It arises opposite to the navicular bone, passes laterally and takes part in lateral malleolar anastomosis.

2. Medial tarsal arteries: They are 2 to 3 in number passes towards the medial malleolus to take part in medial malleolar anastomosis.

3. First dorsal metatarsal artery: It passes towards the cleft between great toe and the second toe where it gives digital branches.

4. Arcuate artery: It arises opposite to the intermediate cuneiform bone, passes laterally across the bases of metatarsal bones. It gives second to fourth metatarsal arteries. Each artery passes forwards towards the clefts between the toes where it gives digital branches. Each dorsal metatarsal artery is connected with the arteries of the sole through proximal and distal perforating arteries. In this way the terminal end of the anterior and posterior tibial artery are connected.

Dorsalis pedis artery pulse: It is felt in front of the ankle lateral to the tendon of extensor hallucis longus against the tarsal bone. Reduced dorsalis pedis artery indicates an arterial occlusion in the proximal arterial tree. It is also to be remembered that in some individuals the dorsalis pedis artery may be replaced by perforating branch of the peroneal artery (Fig. 15.6).

LATERAL COMPARTMENT

It presents 2 muscles namely- peroneus longus and brevis. Both these muscles are supplied by superficial peroneal nerve. Its main function is eversion at the subtalar joint.

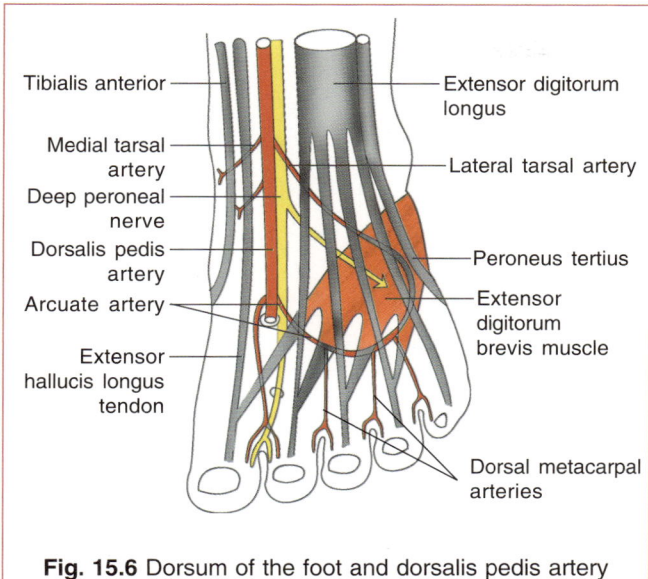

Fig. 15.6 Dorsum of the foot and dorsalis pedis artery

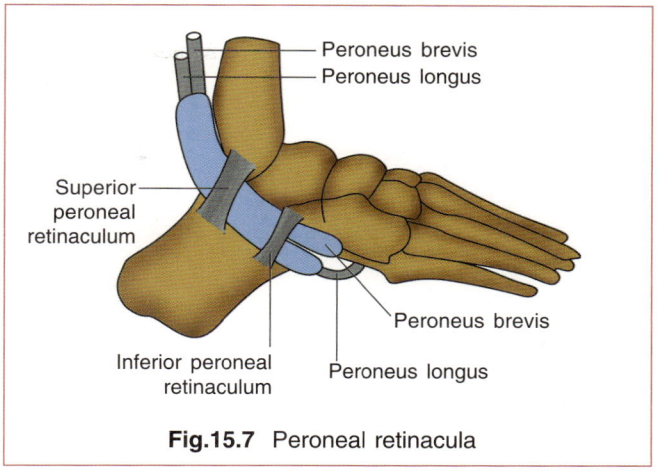

Fig.15.7 Peroneal retinacula

These muscles while crossing lateral to the ankle passes deep to the peroneal retinacula. The attachments, nerve supply and actions are explained in Table 15.2.

Peroneal retinacula

These are modified deep fascia present lateral to the ankle. It hold the tendons of the lateral compartment muscles during the movement of the ankle joint.

Superior peroneal retinaculum: It extends from lateral malleolus to the lateral surface of the calcaneus. The tendon of the peroneus longus and brevis are enclosed in with a common synovial sheath, where tendon of peroneus longus is superficial (Fig. 15.7).

Inferior peroneal retinaculum: Above it is attached to the anterior part of the superior surface of the calcaneus where it becomes continues with the stem of the inferior extensor retinaculum and below the lateral surface of the calcaneus. The tendon of the peroneus brevis with its separate synovial sheath occupies the upper compartment beneath the retinaculum, while tendon of the peroneus longus in the lower compartment with its synovial sheath. A peroneal trochlea or tubercle separates the two tendons.

Common peroneal nerve

Origin and root value: It is one of the terminal branches of the sciatic nerve given at the level of the superior angle of the popliteal fossa. Its root value is L4, L5, S1, and S2.

Course:

• It descends parallel and medial to the tendon of the biceps femoris muscle in the popliteal fossa.

Table 15.2: Lateral compartment of leg (Peroneal compartment) (Fig. 15.8)				
Muscle	*Origin*	*Insertion*	*Nerve supply*	*Actions*
Peroneus longus	Head of fibula Upper 1/3rd and posterior half of middle 1/3rd of lateral surface of fibula	Passes deep to peroneal retinaculum, runs in the tunnel of cuboid and inserted to Lateral side of base of first metatarsal Adjoining medial cuneiform	Superficial peroneal nerve	Evertor of foot off the ground Maintains the medial longitudinal and transverse arches of foot acting as a sling
Peroneus brevis	Anterior half of middle 1/3rd and lower 1/3rd of lateral surface of fibula	Passes deep to peroneal retinacula and is inserted to lateral side of base of 5th metatarsal	Superficial peroneal nerve	Evertor of foot

S E C T I O N 4

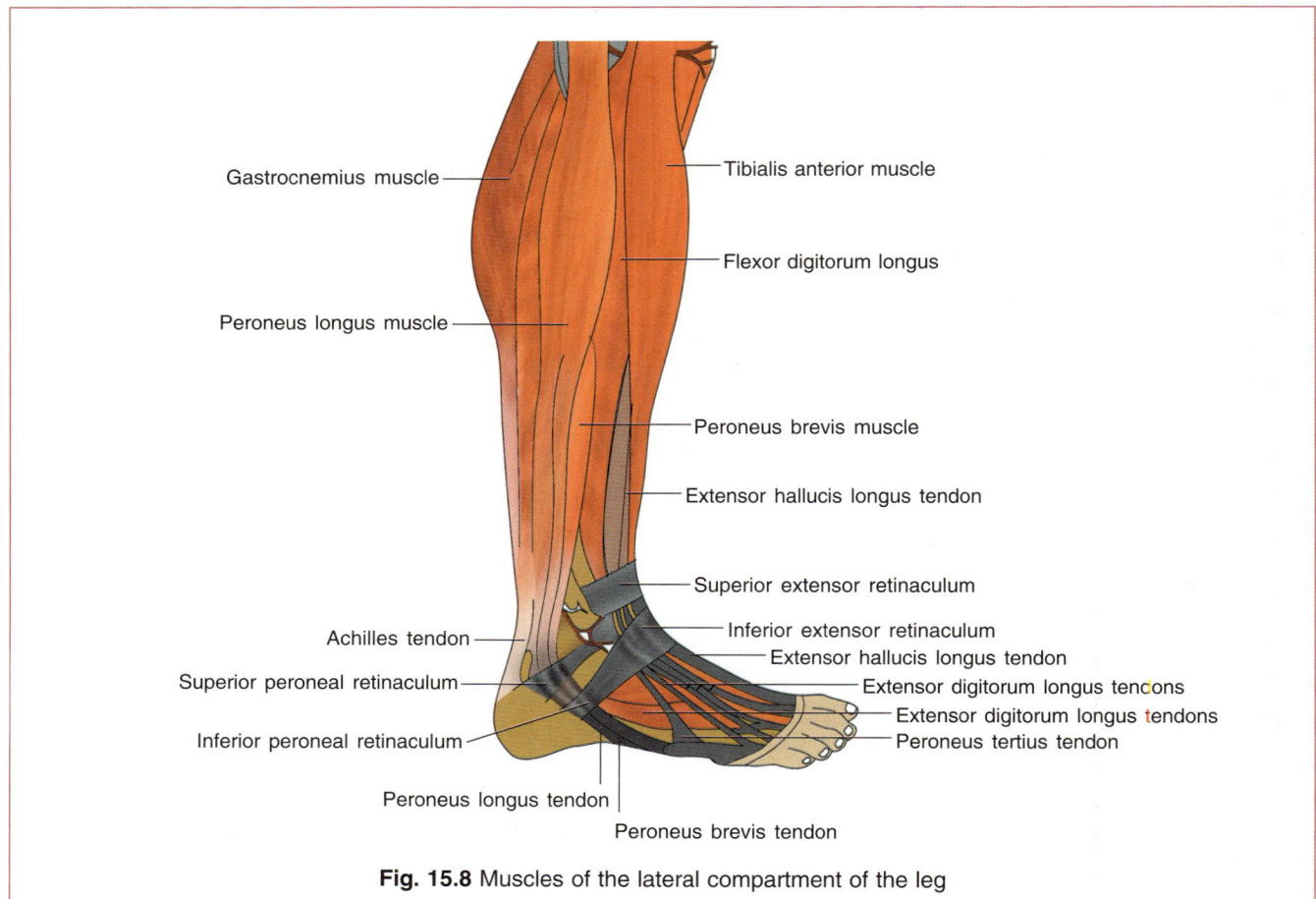

Fig. 15.8 Muscles of the lateral compartment of the leg

- At the lateral angle of the popliteal fossa it descends superficial to the lateral head of the gastrocnemius muscle.

- The nerve curves on the lateral side of the neck of the fibula (where it can be rolled against the bone) to enter the substance of peroneus longus muscle.

- Finally it divides into superficial and deep peroneal nerves.

Branches in the popliteal fossa

Cutaneous branches

1. **Sural communicating nerve:** It arise medial to the head of the fibula. It joins the sural nerve after crossing superficial to the lateral head of the gastrocnemius muscle.

2. **Lateral cutaneous nerve of the leg (nerve of calf):** It supplies the skin of the upper lateral part of the leg (L5 and S1 dermatome)

Genicular branches: They are classified into superior lateral, inferior lateral and recurrent genicular branches. They supply the knee joint.

Terminal branches: The superficial peroneal nerve and the deep peroneal nerve.

Superficial peroneal nerve

It is one of the terminal branches of the common peroneal nerve given at the level of the neck of the fibula, deep to the peroneus longus muscle (Fig. 15.9).

Course

- It descends between peroneus longus and brevis muscles

- At the junction of upper 2/3rd and lower 1/3rd of the leg, the nerve pierces the deep fascia and becomes superficial.

- It divides into medial and lateral branches, both of which descends superficial to the superior and inferior extensor retinacula.

Cutaneous distribution: It supplies the skin of the

- Lower part of the leg

- Major portion of the dorsum of the foot except for the area supplied by saphenous, deep peroneal and sural nerves

SECTION 4

Motor distribution: It supplies two muscles

1. Peroneus longus
2. Peroneus brevis

Deep peroneal nerve (nervus hesitans)

It is one of the terminal branches of the common peroneal nerve given at the level of the neck of the fibula. It is also referred as anterior tibial nerve (Fig. 15.10).

Course:

- It appears in the anterior compartment of the leg after piercing the anterior intermuscular septum.
- In the proximal part of the leg the nerve descends between tibialis anterior and extensor digitorum longus muscles.
- In the middle part of the leg it descends between tibialis anterior and extensor hallucis longus muscles.
- In the distal part of the leg it descends between extensor digitorum longus and extensor hallucis longus.
- Throughout its course in the leg the nerve lies lateral to the anterior tibial vessels except in the middle where the nerve lies in front of the vessels.
- It descends deep to the superior and inferior extensor retinacula of the ankle to enter the dorsum of the foot.

- Deep to the inferior extensor retinaculum it is accompanied by dorsalis pedis artery on its medial side.
- At the dorsum of the foot it divides into medial and lateral terminal branches
- The lateral terminal branch passes laterally deep to the extensor digitorum brevis and ends in a pseudoganglion. It supplies extensor digitorum brevis, tarsal and metatarsophalangeal joints of middle three toes.
- The medial terminal branch supply the skin of the adjacent sides of great and second toes. In addition, it also supplies first metatarsophalangeal joint.

Cutaneous distribution:

It supplies the skin of the first interdigital cleft (between great toe and second toe)

Motor distribution: It supplies following muscles
Muscles of the anterior compartment of the leg

   1. Tibialis anterior

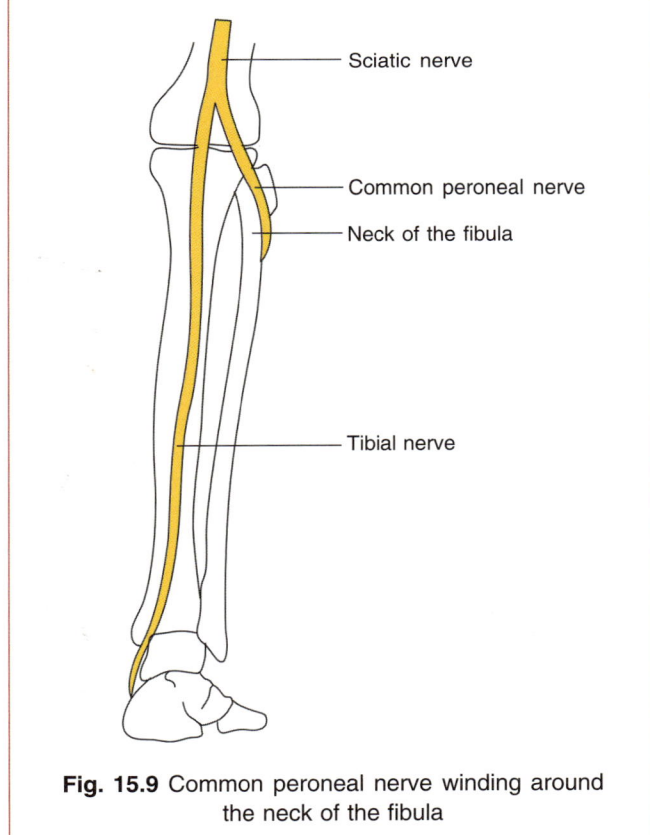

Fig. 15.9 Common peroneal nerve winding around the neck of the fibula

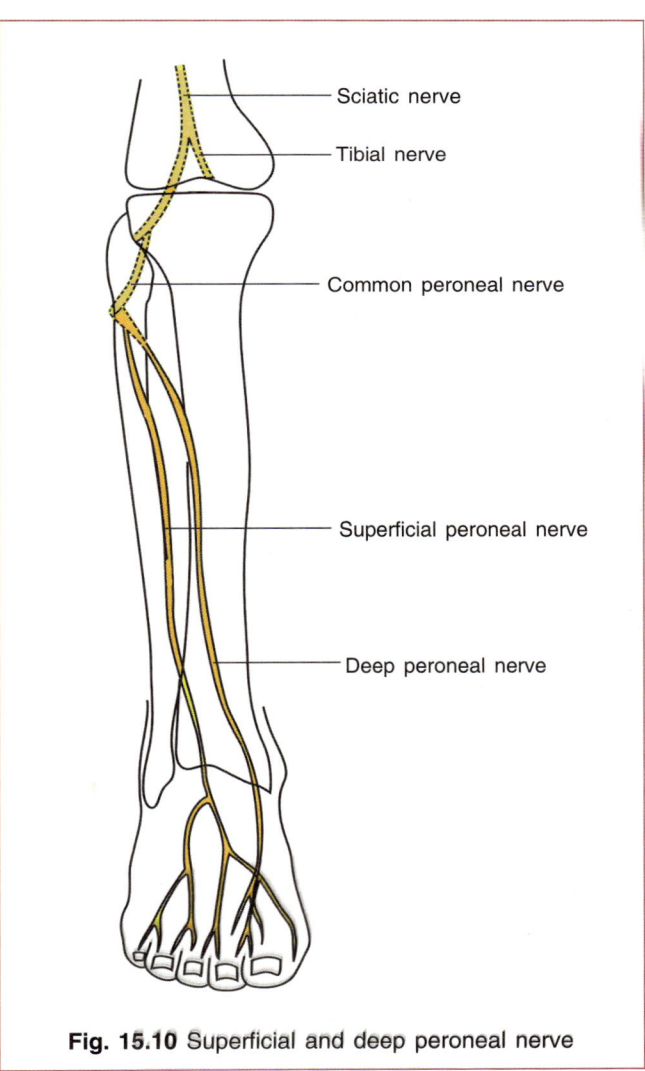

Fig. 15.10 Superficial and deep peroneal nerve

2. Extensor hallucis longus

3. Extensor digitorum

4. Peroneus tertius

Muscle on the dorsum of the foot

5. Extensor digitorum brevis

The lateral terminal branch supply second dorsal interossei, while medial terminal branch supplies first dorsal interossei.

Genicular branches

It supplies tarsal and tarso-metatarsal joints of medial 4 toes.

Injury to the common peroneal nerve: It is more vulnerable to injury compared to the tibial nerve as it lies superficial against the head of the fibula before winding around the neck of the fibula. A tight plaster cast can also compress the common peroneal nerve.

Motor manifestation: Injury to the common peroneal nerve results in paralysis of dorsiflexors of the ankle joint (muscles of the anterior compartment through its deep peroneal nerve) and evertors of the foot (peroneus longus and brevis through superficial peroneal nerve). This results in foot drop. In this deformity the foot is inverted and plantar flexed. This deformity is referred as talipes equinovarus and the patient walks on toes.

Sensory loss: The sensory manifestation depends on site of nerve injury. The common site of nerve injury is at the level of the neck of the fibula. Hence lateral cutaneous nerve of the leg and peroneal communicating nerves are spared. There will be a sensory loss on most

of the dorsum of the foot except at the medial border up to the ball of the great toes (saphenous nerve), lateral border of the foot (sural branch of the tibial nerve).

Deep peroneal nerve entrapment: Injury or compression of the deep peroneal nerve results from anterior compartment syndrome. It is common in runners and dancers. Excessive use of the anterior compartment muscles results in swelling of the muscle which interferes with venous return causing edema in the anterior compartment. The pressure is released by an incision to the deep fascia along the whole length of the anterior compartment.

Motor manifestation: The muscles of the anterior compartment are paralyzed with disability to dorsiflex at the ankle joint. This results in foot drop. The patient walks on tips of the toes on the affected side.

Sensory manifestation: Loss of cutaneous sensation in the first interdigital cleft.

Superficial peroneal nerve entrapment: It can occur in chronic ankle sprain.

Motor manifestation: It results in weakness in eversion of the foot.

Sensory manifestation: It involves the lower part of the anterior aspect of the leg, major portion of the dorsum of the foot except for saphenous and sural areas.

Disc prolapsed and nerve injury of the lower limb: The major part of the lower limb is supplied by sciatic

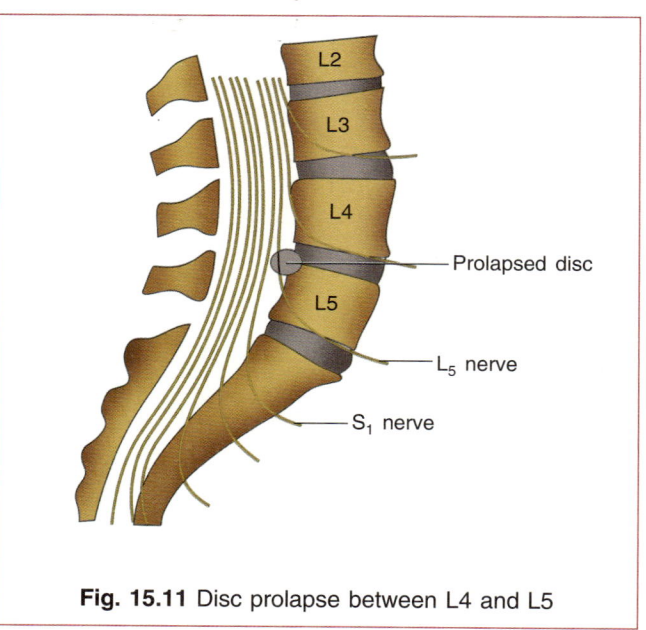

Fig. 15.11 Disc prolapse between L4 and L5

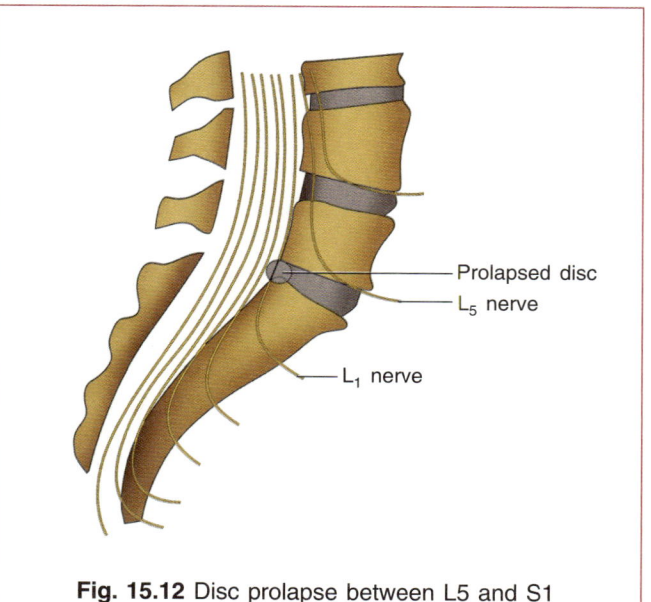

Fig. 15.12 Disc prolapse between L5 and S1

nerve with its terminal branches-tibial and common peroneal branches.

Sciatic nerve is a composite of L4,L5, S1, S2 and S3 spinal nerves. A herniated intervertebral disc (disc prolapsed) can involve some of these nerve roots and have manifestation in the lower limb. The disc prolapsed is common in lower lumbar region. A disc prolapsed between L4 and L5 vertebra can compress 5th lumbar spinal nerve (Fig. 15.11). Similarly a disc prolapsed between L5 and S1 vertebra can compress 1st sacral spinal nerve.

Remember the intervertebral foramen between L4 and L5 vertebra allow the passage of L4 spinal nerve and the intervertebral foramen between L5 and S1 vertebra allow the passage of L5 spinal nerve. The nerve emerging between the vertebrae and the nerve likely to be injured is different. This is because the vertical length of the intervertebral foramen in the lumbar region increases lower down, hence the L4 and L5 nerve passes through the upper part of the intervertebral foramen and escapes from injury.

The 2 nerve roots commonly involved in disc prolapsed and their clinical manifestations are explained in Table 15.3. This knowledge is important is assessing the nerve roots involved in disc prolapsed.

A 23-year-old football player was taken to the emergency room after receiving a blow to the left leg that resulted in severe pain and inability to stand up. The attending physician was able to locate a very painful area just below the knee and suspected a fracture to the fibula. He ordered a plain AP and lateral X-ray of the leg and knee (Fig. 15.3). A clear spiral fracture in the left fibular neck and a cracked tibial shaft were shown on the X-ray. The patient was given

Table 15.3: Disc prolapsed and their clinical manifestations

A herniated disc between L4 and L5 would compress 5th lumbar spinal nerve root	A herniated disc between L5 and S1 would compress 1st sacral spinal nerve root
Pain over the hip, lateral part of the thigh and leg	Pain over the hip, posterolateral part of the thigh and leg to heel
Numbness in the medial 3 toes	Numbness in the posterior part of the calf and lateral border of the heel
Difficulty in dorsiflexion at the ankle, difficulty in walking on heel and foot drop may occur	Difficulty in plantarflexion at the ankle, difficulty in walking on toes
Muscular atrophy is minor	Muscular atrophy of gastrocnemius and soleus and ankle jerk diminished or absent

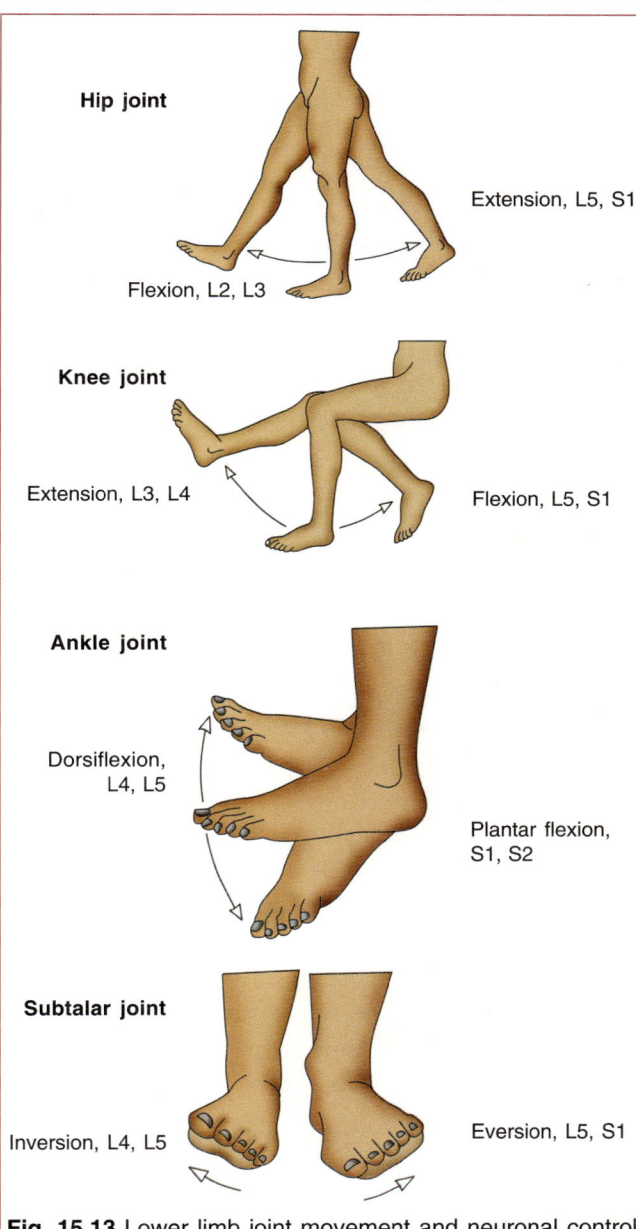

Hip joint — Extension, L5, S1 — Flexion, L2, L3

Knee joint — Extension, L3, L4 — Flexion, L5, S1

Ankle joint — Dorsiflexion, L4, L5 — Plantar flexion, S1, S2

Subtalar joint — Inversion, L4, L5 — Eversion, L5, S1

Fig. 15.13 Lower limb joint movement and neuronal control

SECTION 4

analgesics, and a thorough neurological examination was done. No signs of nerve injury were detected. A plaster cast was applied, and the patient was discharged.

1. Which nerve is most likely to be injured in such incidents?

2. What would the doctor look for to confirm nerve injury?

3. Which of the two injured leg bones was the primary factor in the patient's inability to walk and why?

4. What problems may be encountered in tibial fractures?

Solutions to the case studies:

Case-1

1. Presumably, the heavy exercise of caused them to swell. The swelling of the muscles reduced the blood flow to the region, causing ischemia or impaired venous return further causing more swelling, leading to pain.

2. The walls of the anterior compartment of the leg are primarily bone or relatively unyielding fascia, and as a result, injured muscles that begin to swell have no space to expand into. The swelling causes an increase in intracompartmental pressure and results in further pain and injury.

3. The sensory loss on the foot occurs in the region of distribution of the deep peroneal nerve (between the great and 2nd toes), suggesting that this nerve has been damaged. The cause of this damage is most likely compression of the nerve as the pressure in the anterior compartment increases. The integrity of the deep peroneal nerve could also be tested by examining the action of the extensor digitorum brevis muscle on the dorsum of the foot. Paralysis of this muscle would indicate deep peroneal nerve injury. The muscles of the anterior compartment in an injury like this would not be good indicators of deep peroneal nerve injury because their apparent paralysis may be a direct result of increased pressure in the anterior compartment; however, paralysis of the extensor digitorum brevis of the foot, which is outside the anterior compartment, would confirm a nerve injury.

4. The presence of a weak pulse in the dorsalis pedis artery would be the result of collateral circulation from branches of the posterior tibial artery or the perforating branch of the peroneal artery.

Case-2

1. The femoral artery can be palpated at the midinguinal point, i.e. midway between the anterior superior iliac spine and symphysis pubis. The popliteal artery is felt deep in the popliteal fossa, with the deep fascia relaxed and the knee joint flexed. The dorsalis pedis artery is felt on the front of the ankle, between the tendons of the extensor hallucis longus and the extensor digitorum longus. The posterior tibial artery can be felt behind the medial malleolus.

2. Dilatation of the collateral arteries can be obtained by preganglionic lumbar sympathectomy provided that the arteries are free of disease.

3. The muscular and genicular branches of the femoral artery, the perforating branches of the profunda femoris, and the muscular and genicular branches of the popliteal artery anastomose with one another.

4. Refer text

Case-3

1. Common peroneal nerve

2. There is loss of eversion and dorsiflexion of the foot. Foot-drop is the usual result of this injury, but this cannot be confirmed very early after the accident or when the patient is still having pain on walking. Tendon reflexes will be weak or absent. There is loss of sensation on the anterolateral aspect of the leg and the dorsum of the foot.

3. The tibia, since it is the principal weight-bearing bone of the leg.

4. Non union is common if the fracture crosses the nutrient canal (due to damage to the nutrient artery). Since the tibia has a relatively poor blood supply, tibial fractures take longer to heal, sometimes up to 6 months.

MCQs

1. A 32-year-old male was brought to the hospital with a deep cut on the dorsum of his ankle. As you inspect the wound and test for functional and sensory deficits, you find that no tendons have been cut, but the dorsalis pedis artery and the accompanying nerve have been cut. You would expect to find:

   A. club foot
   B. foot drop
   C. inability to extend the big toe
   D. numbness between the first and second toes

2. The most usual site for feeling the pulsations of the dorsalis pedis artery in the foot is:

A. Just behind the medial malleolus
B. Just lateral to the tendon of extensor hallucis longus
C. Behind the lateral malleolus
D. In the second dorsal metatarsal space

3. A patient with a fracture to the left upper tibia was treated with a plaster cast. A few days later he started to develop progressive numbness over the dorsum of the foot and weakness in dorsiflexion. The cast was quickly changed and the signs were attributed to nerve compression. The compressed nerve was most likely the:

A. Tibial
B. Obturator
C. Femoral
D. Common peroneal

4. A long distance runner complained of swelling and pain of his shin. At physical examination, skin testing showed normal cutaneous sensation of the leg. However, muscular strength tests showed marked weakness of dorsiflexion and impaired inversion of the foot. Which nerve serves the muscles involved?

A. Common peroneal
B. Deep peroneal
C. Sciatic
D. Superficial peroneal

5. Your patient was struck by a car's bumper as she crossed the street, and her fibular neck is broken. After the bone has healed, she has "foot drop", i. e. she cannot dorsiflex her foot, and so it flops onto the ground during walking. Denervation (paralysis) of which of the following muscles would be associated with foot drop?

A. Peroneus longus
B. Tibialis anterior
C. Tibialis posterior
D. Peroneus brevis

6. A pedestrian is struck by a car, and his fibular neck is fractured. There is no indication of foot drop, but he cannot evert his foot and the dorsum of his foot is numb. This apparent nerve lesion would affect which of the following muscles?

A. Tibialis posterior
B. Tibialis anterior
C. Peroneus tertius
D. Peroneus longus

7. The most likely finding resulting from this anterior compartment syndrome is:

A. numbness on the dorsum of the foot
B. inability to evert the foot
C. foot drop
D. inability to plantar flexes the foot

8. A college cross-country runner begins to experience leg and foot pain during and after training for the upcoming season. The pain radiates from the anterolateral leg into the dorsal aspect of the foot. Dorsiflexion and extension of the toes are performed only with pain. The leg appears to be swollen in the area of the pain. Which of the following arteries may have been compressed by the swelling?

A. Popliteal artery
B. Anterior tibial artery
C. Posterior tibial artery
D. Peroneal artery

9. You are examining a patient who had a disc prolapse. He has difficulty in walking on the tip of the toes, numbness in the lateral border of the foot, pain over the hip, posterolateral part of the thigh and leg to heel. There was muscular atrophy of the gastrocnemius. Using your knowledge of anatomy what spinal nerve might have injured by the prolapsed disc in this patient.

A. 4th lumbar nerve root
B. 5th lumbar nerve root
C. 1st sacral nerve root
D. 3rd lumbar nerve root

Answers to MCQs
1. D
2. B
3. D
4. B
5. B
6. D
7. C
8. B
9. C

SECTION 4

Back of the Leg, Sole, Ankle Joint and Arches of Foot

16

- Back of the leg
- Sole
- Ankle joint
- Joints of the foot
- Arches of foot
- MCQs

Objectives:

- To name the muscles of the back of the leg, to know their attachment, nerve supply and actions
- To explain the attachment of the flexor retinaculum of the ankle and to identify the structures passing deep to it
- To explain the branches and distribution of tibial nerve and posterior tibial artery and related applied anatomy
- To explain the cutaneous innervations of the sole and its applied anatomy
- To explain the attachment and clinical relevance of plantar aponeurosis
- To list the structures in various layers of the sole and to know the distribution of medial and lateral plantar nerves
- To explain the plantar arch formation and its branches
- To explain the bones articulating, structures stabilizing, movements occurring and muscles producing them in ankle and subtalar joints
- To know the common injuries affecting ankle and subtalar joints
- To explain the formation, maintenance and significance of arches of foot and to discuss major foot deformities

BACK OF THE LEG

Cutaneous nerve supply to the back of the leg

The skin of the back of the leg is innervated by L4 , L5 and S1 dermatomes. Following nerves supply the skin of the back of the leg.

1. Posterior cutaneous nerve of the thigh
2. Branches from the saphenous nerve
3. Sural nerve
4. Lateral cutaneous nerve of the leg

Flexor retinaculum of the ankle

It is a thick modified deep fascia present behind the medial malleolus. It holds the deep muscles of the back of the leg that are entering the sole during movement of the ankle joint (Fig. 16.1).

Attachments:

Anteriorly: Posterior border of the medial malleolus

Posteriorly: Medial tubercle of the calcaneum. Septa arising from the under surface of the retinaculum divides the area

deep to it into 4 compartments. Following structures passes through each compartment from anterior to posterior.

1. Tibialis posterior tendon
2. Flexor digitorum longus tendon
3. Posterior tibial vessels and tibial nerve
4. Flexor hallucis longus tendon

The retinaculum is pierced by medial calcanean vessels and nerves supplying heel area.

Muscles of the back of the leg

These muscles are often called the calf muscles. They are arranged in superficial and deep groups. They are all supplied by **tibial nerve**. They cause mainly plantar flexion at the ankle joint.

The attachments, nerve supply and actions of the muscles are explained in Tables 16.1 and 16.2.

- Soleus and Gastrocnemius together form a tendon called **tendocalcaneus**, which extends in the lower part of the posterior aspect of the leg. Inferiorly it is attached

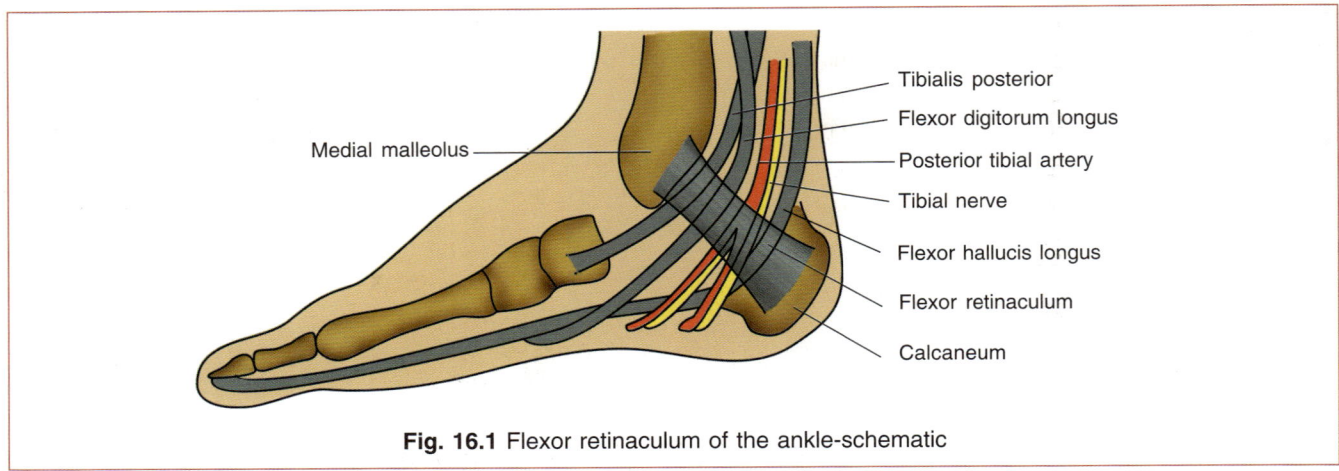

Fig. 16.1 Flexor retinaculum of the ankle-schematic

the middle one third of the posterior surface of the calcaneus (Figs 16.1 and 16.3).

- Both soleus and gastrocnemius are involved in walking movement. The soleus overcomes the inertia of the body weight (initiates the walking movement). Gastrocnemius further increases the speed of walking.

- The substance of the soleus muscle presents many venous spaces. Contraction of the muscle helps in venous return. Hence soleus is called as '**peripheral heart**'.

The ankle jerk or Achillis tendon reflex: On tapping the tendon with knee hammer, there is reflex contraction of gastrocnemius with resultant plantar

flexion of the foot. The nerve responsible for this is tibial nerve and the spinal centre is S1 segment. In paralysis of gastrocnemius or involvement of S1 segment the patient will not be able to stand on the toes and there will be loss of ankle jerk (Fig. 16.4)

Popliteus

It takes origin by a tendon from the lateral condyle of the femur within the joint cavity. It passes through the knee joint cavity. The tendon passes downwards and medially between the fibular collateral ligament and the lateral meniscus. It comes out from the fibrous capsule of the joint and is inserted into popliteal surface of the tibia above the soleal line. It is supplied by tibial nerve. Popliteus initiates

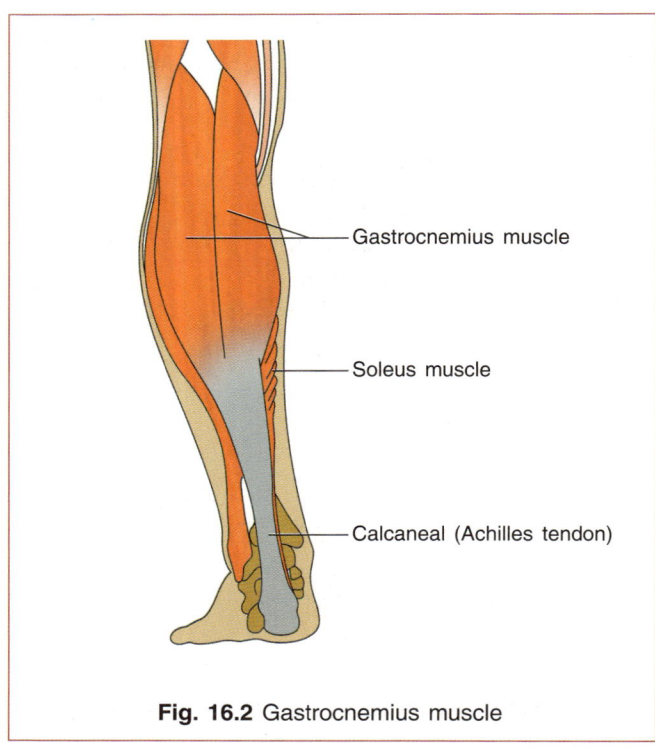

Fig. 16.2 Gastrocnemius muscle

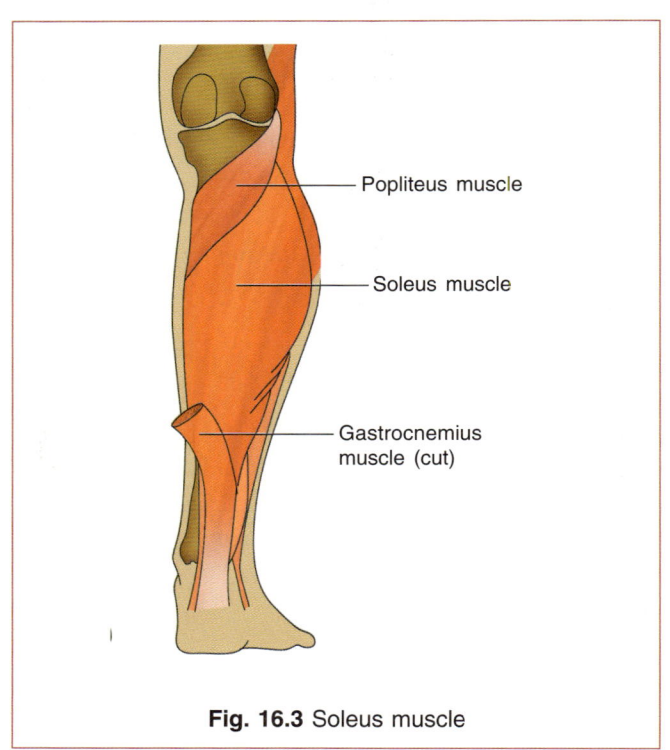

Fig. 16.3 Soleus muscle

Table 16.1 Muscles of anterior compartment of leg

Muscle	Origin	Insertion	Nerve supply	Actions
Gastrocnemius	Medial head- arises as broad flat tendon-postero superior depression on medial condyle of femur behind adductor tubercle Part of popliteal surface of femur Capsule of knee joint Lateral head-lateral surface of lateral condyle of femur Lateral supracondylar line Capsule of knee joint	Fuses with tendon of soleus to form tendoachilles and inserted to middle 1/3rd of posterior surface of calcaneum	Tibial nerve	Gastrocnemius and soleus are strong plantar flexors of foot at ankle joint along with soleus in running and walking Gastrocnemius is also a flexor of knee joint Soleus is more powerful than gastrocnemius while the latter is fast in action Soleus acts as powergear while gastrocnemius acts as top gear of a car
Soleus	Back of head of the fibula and upper ¼ of posterior surface of shaft of fibula, soleal line and middle 1/3rd of medial border of shaft of tibia. Tendinous soleal arch between tibia and fibula	Refer gastrocnemius insertion	Tibial nerve	Refer gastrocnemius
Plantaris	Lower part of lateral supracondylar line of femur	Tendon is thin, runs medial to tendo-achilles and inserted to posterior surface of calcaneum Plantar aponeurosis is its degenerated tendon	Tibial nerve	Rudimentary Used in tendon transplants

the flexion at knee joint (unlocking). Some of its fibres are attached to the lateral meniscus which pulls the lateral meniscus backward and prevents its injury during initiation of flexion.

CASE-1

A 34-year-old man suspected of having a neurological disorder was asked to cross his knees and relax while ligamentum patella was tapped briskly with a small knee hammer. The process was repeated on the opposite

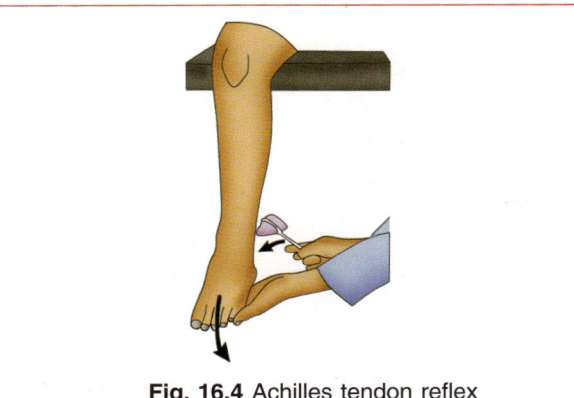

Fig. 16.4 Achilles tendon reflex

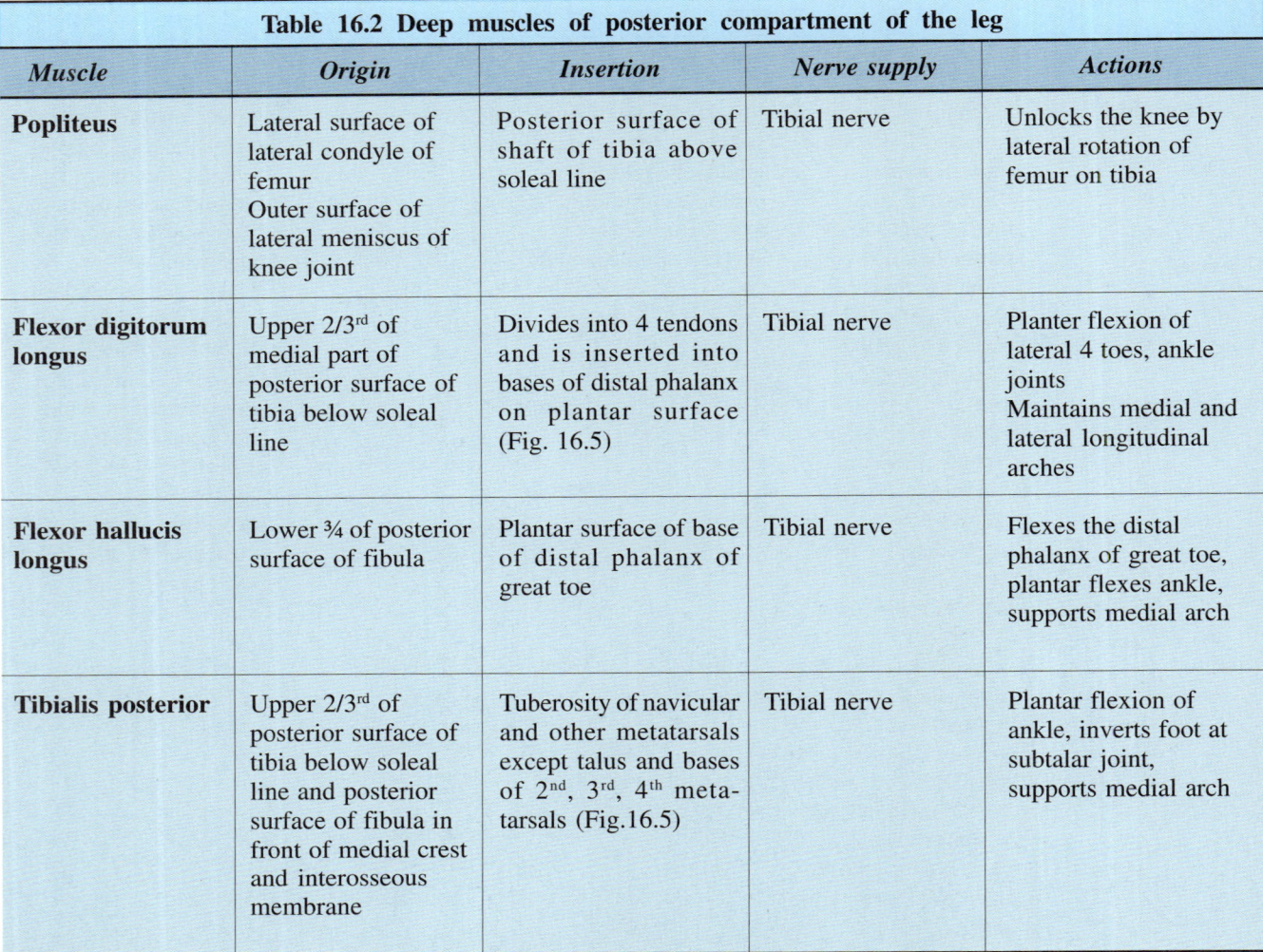

Table 16.2 Deep muscles of posterior compartment of the leg

Muscle	Origin	Insertion	Nerve supply	Actions
Popliteus	Lateral surface of lateral condyle of femur Outer surface of lateral meniscus of knee joint	Posterior surface of shaft of tibia above soleal line	Tibial nerve	Unlocks the knee by lateral rotation of femur on tibia
Flexor digitorum longus	Upper 2/3rd of medial part of posterior surface of tibia below soleal line	Divides into 4 tendons and is inserted into bases of distal phalanx on plantar surface (Fig. 16.5)	Tibial nerve	Planter flexion of lateral 4 toes, ankle joints Maintains medial and lateral longitudinal arches
Flexor hallucis longus	Lower ¾ of posterior surface of fibula	Plantar surface of base of distal phalanx of great toe	Tibial nerve	Flexes the distal phalanx of great toe, plantar flexes ankle, supports medial arch
Tibialis posterior	Upper 2/3rd of posterior surface of tibia below soleal line and posterior surface of fibula in front of medial crest and interosseous membrane	Tuberosity of navicular and other metatarsals except talus and bases of 2nd, 3rd, 4th metatarsals (Fig.16.5)	Tibial nerve	Plantar flexion of ankle, inverts foot at subtalar joint, supports medial arch

leg. The patient was then asked to kneel on a chair, and the examiner gently held his foot, the tendocalcaneus was tapped briskly with a hammer. This was repeated on the opposite side. Finally, the patient was asked to lie flat on his back, and a sharp, pointed instrument was drawn steadily along the lateral border of the sole of the foot (Babinski test). What are the anatomical reasons for performing (1) the knee jerk, (2) the ankle jerk, and (3) the Babinski test?

Tibial nerve

Origin and root value: It is one of the terminal branches of the sciatic nerve given at the level of the superior angle of the popliteal fossa. It is derived from ventral division of L4, L5, S1, S2 and S3.

Course:

• It descends vertically downwards in the popliteal fossa from the superior angle to the inferior angle. In the upper part of the fossa the nerve lies superficial and lateral to the popliteal vessels while in the lower part of the fossa it lies superficial and medial to the vessels.

• At the lower margin of the popliteal muscles, it enters the posterior compartment by descending deep to the tendinous arch of origin of the soleus.

• The nerve descends deep to the soleus along with the posterior tibial vessels between flexor hallucis longus and flexor digitorum longus muscles.

• The nerve descends medial to the posterior tibial vessels in the upper part and lateral to it in the lower part.

• Deep to the flexor retinaculum it ends by dividing into medial and lateral plantar nerves which enter the sole of the foot.

Branches and distribution

Motor distribution

In the popliteal fossa: In the popliteal fossa it gives following muscular branches.

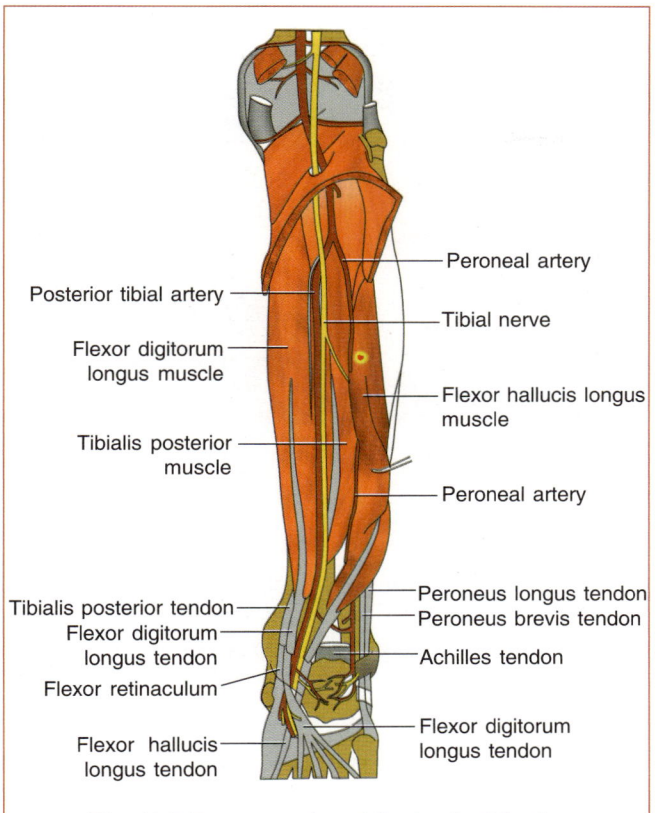

Posterior tibial artery

Flexor digitorum longus muscle

Tibialis posterior muscle

Tibialis posterior tendon

Flexor digitorum longus tendon

Flexor retinaculum

Flexor hallucis longus tendon

Peroneal artery

Tibial nerve

Flexor hallucis longus muscle

Peroneal artery

Peroneus longus tendon
Peroneus brevis tendon

Achilles tendon

Flexor digitorum longus tendon

Fig. 16.5 Deep muscles of the back of the leg

1. To medial head of the gastrocnemius
2. To lateral head of the gastrocnemius
3. To the plantaris
4. To soleus
5. Nerve to popliteus

Except the nerve to medial head of the gastrocnemius, rest of the branch arises from the lateral side of the tibial nerve. The nerve to popliteus descends deep to the plantaris muscle then winds around the lower border of the muscle to supply it from its anterior surface. This branch also supplies superior and inferior tibio-fibular joints, branch to tibia, interosseus membrane and tibialis posterior muscle.

In the back of the leg: In the posterior compartment of the leg it supplies following muscles

1. Tibialis posterior
2. Flexor digitorum longus
3. Flexor hallucis longus
4. Soleus

Cutaneous distribution

In the popliteal fossa:

1. Sural nerve: It arises from the medial side. It descends downwards and pierces the deep fascia of the leg to

become superficial. It supplies the skin of the posterolateral aspect of the leg, lateral border of the foot including the lateral margin of the little toe. The terminal part of the nerve near the lateral malleolus is accompanied by small saphenous vein. It is joined by sural communicating branch from the common peroneal nerve. It is often used for nerve grafting due its superficial position.

In the back of the leg:

Medial calcanean branch: It pierces the flexor retinaculum and supplies the skin of the heel.

Articular branches: It supplies ankle joint.

Injury to the tibial nerve is rare due its safe position. However injury to the tibial nerve results in dorsiflexion of the ankle joint and inversion at the subtalar joint. This deformity is referred as talipes calcaneovalgus. There will also be a sensory loss in sural area and heel.

Posterior tibial artery

- It is the larger terminal branch of popliteal artery given at the level of lower border of popliteus muscle.
- It passes deep to gastrocnemius and soleus to enter the posterior compartment of leg.
- In the lower third of the leg the artery lies along the medial border of tendoachilles.
- At the ankle it passes deep to the flexor retinaculum between flexor digitorum longus laterally and flexor hallucis longus medially accompanied by a pair of venae commitantes.
- It terminates by dividing into medial and lateral plantar nerves deep to flexor retinaculum.

Branches

- Muscular branches
- Peroneal artery
- Nutrient artery to tibia
- Anastomotic branches include circumflex fibular branch which take part in knee anastomoses, communicating branch joins similar branch from the peroneal artery, malleolar branch which takes part in medial malleolar anastomoses and calcaneal branch.
- The terminal branches are medial and lateral plantar arteries.

Peroneal artery

- It begins 2.5 cm below the lower border of popliteus muscle. It descends along the medial crest of the fibula accompanied by nerve to flexor hallucis longus.

- It passes behind the inferior tibio-fibular joint.
- It terminates by dividing into numerous lateral calcaneal branches.
- It supplies the anterior and lateral compartments of leg.

Branches

1. Muscular branches
2. Nutrient artery to fibula
3. Anastomotic branches

- Large perforating branch pierces the lower part of the interosseus membrane and joins the lateral mallolar network. The perforating branch of the peroneal artery may replace the dorsalis pedis artery.
- Communicating branch with posterior tibial artery
- Calcaneal branch which take part in lateral malleolar network.

SOLE

Cutaneous nerve supply to the sole

1. The heel area is supplied by medial calcanean branch of the tibial nerve (Fig. 16.6).
2. Medial part of the sole and also medial three and a half toes is supplied by medial plantar nerve.
3. Lateral part of the sole and also lateral three and a half of the toes is supplied by lateral plantar nerve.

   The heel area and the lateral part of the sole is S1 dermatome. The medial part of the sole is L4 dermatome, while the intermediate area of the sole is L5 dermatome.

Plantar reflex: The lateral aspect of the sole (S1 dermatome) of the foot is stroked with a blunt object (Fig. 16.7). Flexion of the toes is a normal response.

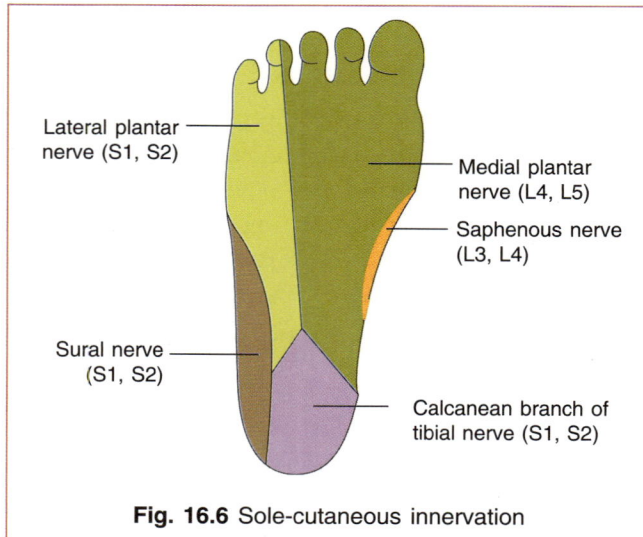

Fig. 16.6 Sole-cutaneous innervation

Lateral plantar nerve (S1, S2)
Medial plantar nerve (L4, L5)
Saphenous nerve (L3, L4)
Sural nerve (S1, S2)
Calcanean branch of tibial nerve (S1, S2)

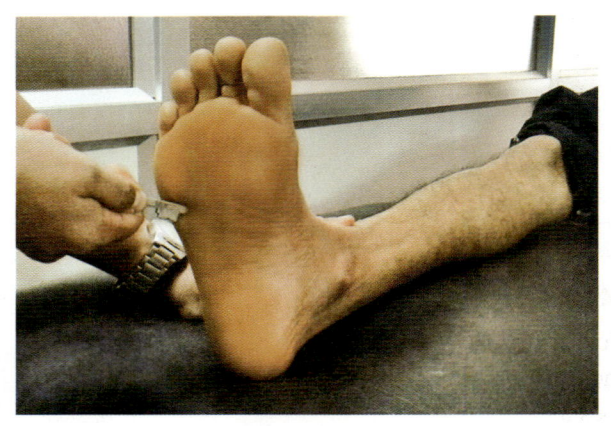

Fig. 16.7 Plantar reflex

Slight fanning of the lateral 4 toes and dorsiflexion of the great toe is an abnormal response (Babinski sign). It indicates brain injury (Upper motor neuron) or cerebral disease, but considered normal in infants.

Plantar aponeurosis

The deep fascia of the sole is thick in the central part forming plantar aponeurosis. The plantar aponeurosis is triangular in shape with its apex directed proximally and the base distally. The apex is attached to the medial tubercle of the calcaneus. The base divides into 5 slips near the heads of the metatarsals (Fig. 16.8). The interval between the slips allows the passage of the digital nerves and vessels. Each slip divides into superficial and deep slip. The superficial slip is attached to the skin and the deep slip blends with fibrous flexor sheaths and also with deep transverse metatarsal ligaments.

The plantar aponeurosis provides protection to the deeper structure. It also contributes to the maintenance of the arch.

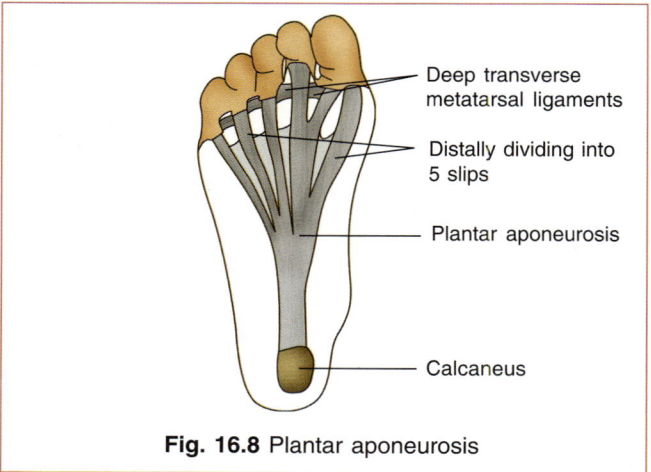

Deep transverse metatarsal ligaments
Distally dividing into 5 slips
Plantar aponeurosis
Calcaneus

Fig. 16.8 Plantar aponeurosis

SECTION 4

Plantar fascitis: It occurs due to straining and inflammation of plantar aponeurosis. It is characterized by pain over heel and medial aspect of foot, which increases with passive extension of great toe and by dorsiflexion of ankle joint. It results from running and high-impact aerobics (most common hind-foot problem in runners).

Muscles of the sole

Foot is an organ of support and locomotion. Accordingly, the muscles of the foot (sole) are modified to steady the toes and to maintain the arches of foot.

There are 18 intrinsic muscles in the sole. Structures of the sole is explained in many layers (Tables 16.3 to 16.6).

First layer has 3 muscles (Fig.16.9)

1. Flexor digitorum brevis

2. Abductor hallucis

3. Abductor digiti minimi

Second layer has 5 muscles: Flexor digitorum accessorius, 4 lumbricals and also tendons of flexor digitorum longus and Flexor hallucis longus (Fig.16.10).

Third layer has 3 muscles (Fig. 16.11)

• Flexor hallucis brevis

• Flexor digiti minimi

• Adductor hallucis

Fourth layer has 7 muscles (Fig. 16.12)

• Three (3) plantar interossei

• Four (4) dorsal interossei

This layer also presents tendons of tibialis posterior and peroneus longus.

These muscles are supplied by medial and lateral plantar nerves (terminal branches of tibial nerve).

Medial plantar artery

It is the small terminal branch of posterior tibial artery that lies along the medial border of foot (Fig. 16.13).

Branches: It gives following branches.

• Cutaneous branches

• Muscular branches

• First to third plantar digital arteries that anastomose with plantar metatarsal arteries (branches from plantar arch).

Table 16.3 Muscles of first layer of sole				
Muscle	*Origin*	*Insertion*	*Nerve supply*	*Actions*
Flexor digitorum brevis	Medial tubercle of calcaneum Plantar aponeurosis	Divides into four tendons for lateral 4 toes. Each tendon splits into two and gets inserted to sides of middle phalanx of lateral four toes	Medial plantar nerve	Flexion of toes at proximal interphalangeal joint and metatarsophalangeal joints
Abductor hallucis	Medial and lateral intermuscular septum Medial tubercle of calcaneum Lateral intermuscular septum, deep fascia	Medial side of base of proximal phalanx of great toe	Medial plantar nerve	Abduction of great toe
Abductor digiti minimi	Medial and lateral tubercles of calcaneum Lateral intermuscular septum, deep fascia	Lateral side of base of proximal phalanx of little toe	Trunk of lateral plantar nerve	Abduction of little toe

Muscle	Origin	Insertion	Nerve supply	Actions
Flexor digitorum accessorius (Quadratus plantae)	Medial head-medial surface of calcaneum Lateral head-calcaneum in front of lateral tubercle	Lateral side of tendon of flexor digitorum longus	Lateral plantar nerve	It straightens the oblique pull of action of the flexor digitorum longus on the lateral four toes
Lumbricals	Arises from 4 tendons of flexor digitorum longus 1st lumbrical is unipennate arises from medial side of tendon, while other 3 are bipennate arising from adjacent sides of 1st, 2nd, 3rd, 4th, tendons	Each tendon pass forwards on medial side of the metatarsophalangeal joints of the lateral 4 toes, then inserted into the extensor expansion on the dorsal side	First lumbrical is supplied by medial plantar and the remaining by lateral plantar nerve	They maintain the extension of the toes at the interphalangeal joint which prevents buckling of the toes during walking

Table 16.4 Muscles and tendons of second layer of sole

S E C T I O N   4

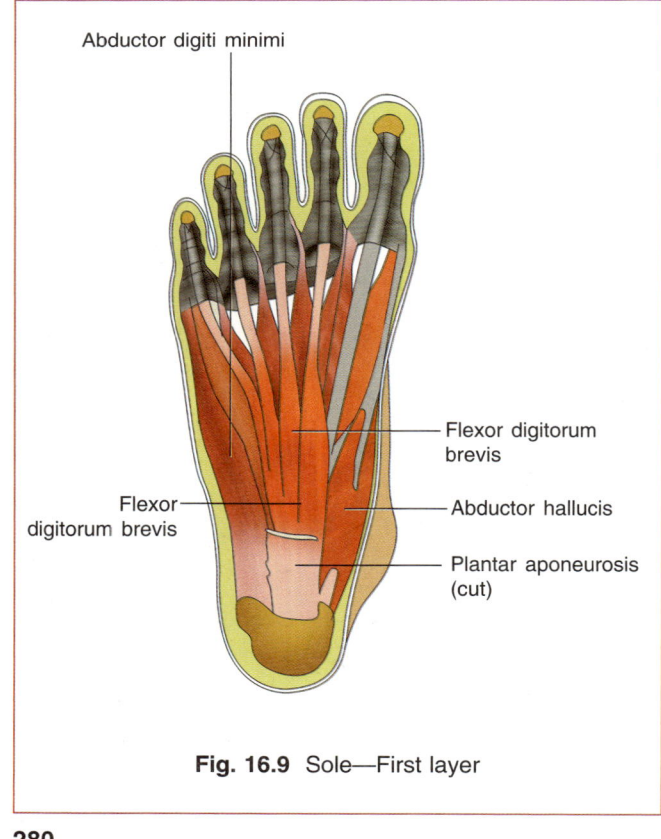

Abductor digiti minimi

Flexor digitorum brevis

Flexor digitorum brevis

Flexor digitorum brevis

Abductor hallucis

Plantar aponeurosis (cut)

Fig. 16.9 Sole—First layer

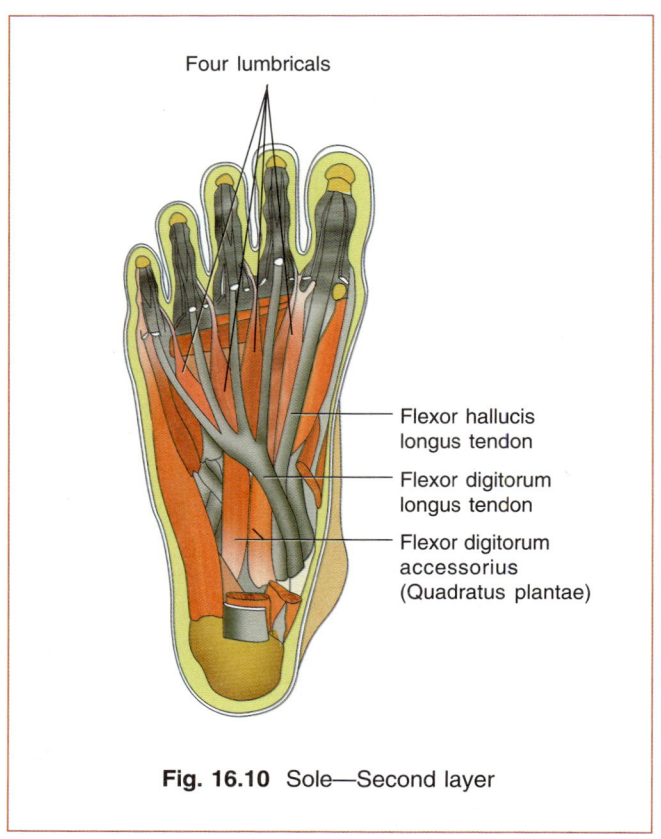

Four lumbricals

Flexor hallucis longus tendon

Flexor digitorum longus tendon

Flexor digitorum accessorius (Quadratus plantae)

Fig. 16.10 Sole—Second layer

Table 16.5 Muscles of the third layer of sole

Muscle	Origin	Insertion	Nerve supply	Actions
Flexor hallucis brevis	Arises by two limbs Lateral limb-plantar surface of cuboid behind the groove for peroneus longus and adjoining lateral cuneiform Medial limb-continuation of tendon of tibialis posterior	Splits into two tendons and gets inserted to corresponding sides of proximal phalanx of great toe	Medial plantar nerve	Flexes the proximal phalanx at metatarsophalangeal joint
Adductor hallucis	Oblique head- bases of 2nd, 3rd, 4th metatarsals Sheath of tendon of peroneus longus Transverse head-deep metatarsal ligaments, plantar ligaments of metatarsophalangeal joints of 3rd, 4th, 5th toes	Lateral side of base of proximal phalanx of great toe	Deep branch of lateral plantar nerve	Adductor of great toe Maintains transverse arch
Flexor digiti minimi brevis	Base of 5th metatarsal and sheath of peroneus longus	Lateral side of base of proximal phalanx of little toe	Superficial branch of lateral plantar nerve	Flexes the little toe at metatarsophalangeal joints

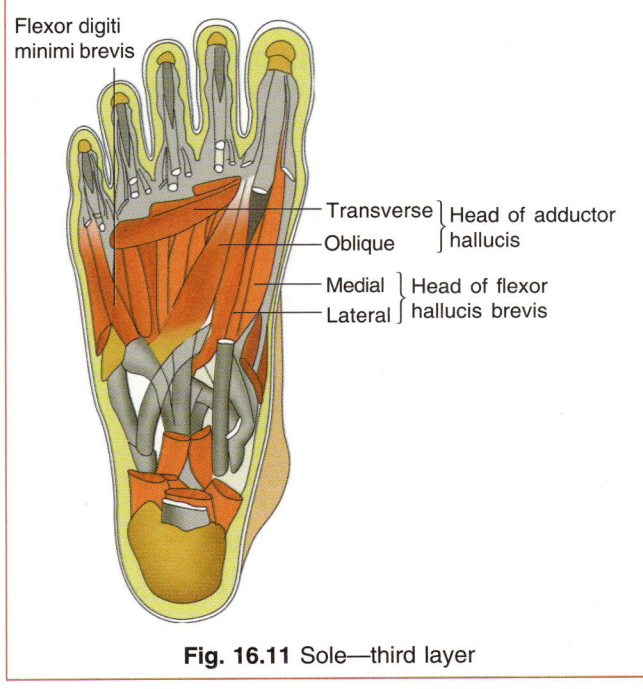

Fig. 16.11 Sole—third layer

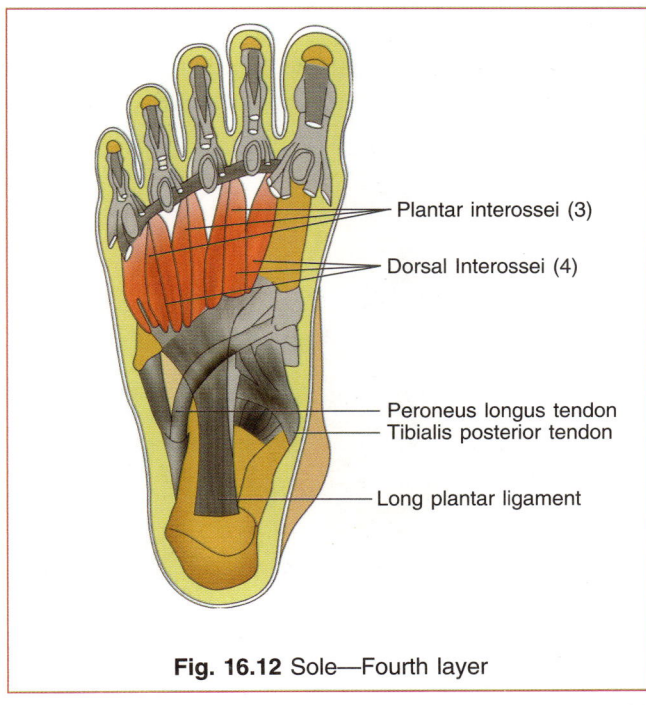

Fig. 16.12 Sole—Fourth layer

SECTION 4

Table 16.6 Muscles and tendons in the fourth layer of sole				
Muscle	*Origin*	*Insertion*	*Nerve supply*	*Actions*
Plantar interossei (3)	Bases and adjoining medial sides of 3rd, 4th, and 5th meta-tarsals	Bases of proximal phalanges on medial side and thereby to dorsal digital expansion	1st and 2nd -lateral plantar nerve (deep) 3rd - lateral plantar nerve	Adductor of 3rd, 4th, 5th toes towards axis Flexes metatarsophalangeal joints and extends the interphalangeal joints of lateral three digits
Dorsal interossei (4)	Adjacent sides of metatarsals	Bases of proximal phalanx and dorsal digital expansion 1st - medial side of 2nd toe 2nd - lateral side of 2nd toe 3rd - lateral side of 3rd toe 4th - lateral side of 4th toe	1st, 2nd, 3rd-lateral plantar nerve (deep) 4th - lateral plantar nerve	Abducts the toes away from axis of 2nd toe 1st and 2nd causes both medial and lateral abduction of 2nd toe

Lateral plantar artery

It is the larger terminal branch of posterior tibial artery. It continues as plantar arch (Fig. 16.13).

Branches: It gives following branches

- Muscular branches.
- Cutaneous branches.
- Anastomotic branches that anastomose with arteries of dorsum of foot along the lateral border.
- Calcaneal branch to the heel.

Plantar arch

It occupies the plane between the third and fourth layers of the sole. It is formed by direct continuation of the lateral

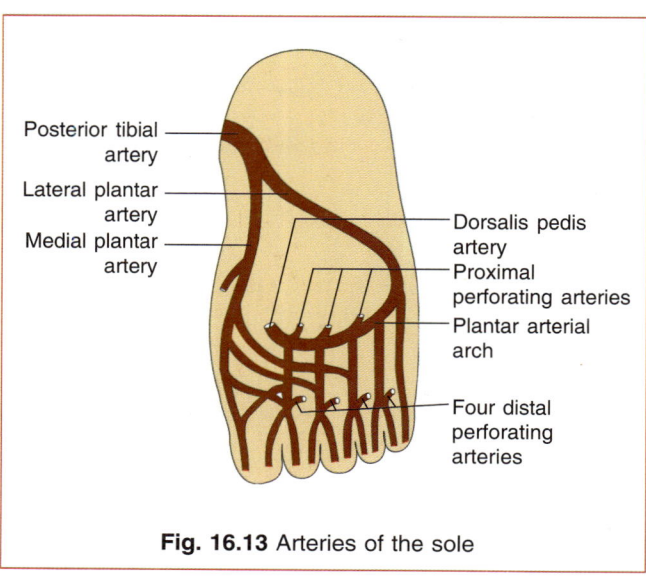

Fig. 16.13 Arteries of the sole

Labels:
- Posterior tibial artery
- Lateral plantar artery
- Medial plantar artery
- Dorsalis pedis artery
- Proximal perforating arteries
- Plantar arterial arch
- Four distal perforating arteries

plantar artery. On the medial side it is completed by dorsalis pedis artery. It extends from the base of the fifth metatarsal bone to the proximal part of the first intermetatarsal space.

Branches:

Four plantar metatarsal arteries: Each artery passes distally into the interdigital spaces where it divides into proper digital branches. The distal end of each plantar metatarsal artery gives off distal perforating artery which joins the distal part of the corresponding dorsal metatarsal artery.

Three proximal perforating branches: It passes through the second, third and fourth intermetatarsal spaces and connected with dorsal metatarsal arteries which are branches of arcuate artery

Medial plantar nerve

It is the larger terminal branch of the tibial nerve given deep to the flexor retinaculum of the ankle (Fig. 16.14)

Muscular branches: The main trunk gives branches to abductor hallucis and flexor digitorum brevis. Its digital branch supplies flexor hallucis brevis and first lumbricals.

Cutaneous branches: The main trunk supplies the skin of the medial side of the sole. It gives proper digital branch to the medial side of the great toe and 3 common plantar digital nerves which supplies medial three and a half digits including the nail bed on the dorsal side.

Lateral plantar nerve

It is the smaller terminal branch of the tibial nerve given deep to the flexor retinaculum of the ankle (Fig. 16.14).

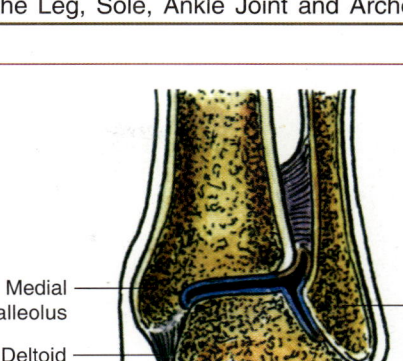

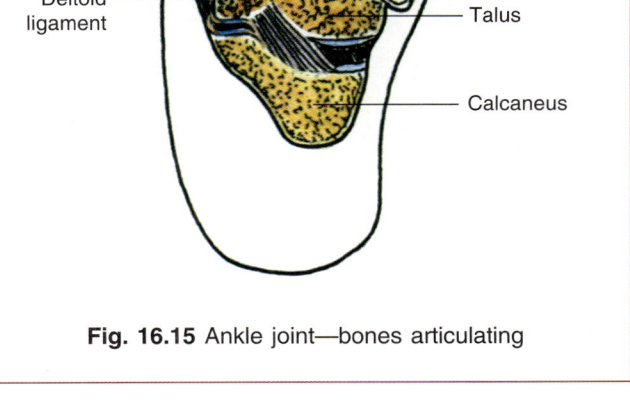

Fig. 16.14 Nerves of the sole

Branches: The main trunk ends by dividing into superficial and deep branches. The main trunk supplies flexor digitorum accessories and abductor digiti minimi and the skin of the lateral side of the sole.

The **superficial branch** supplies 3 muscles namely- flexor digitorum brevis, third plantar and fourth dorsal interossei and the skin of the lateral one and a half digits.

The **deep branch** supplies 9 muscles namely: second, third, fourth lumbricals, adductor hallucis, first, second and third dorsal interossei, first and second plantar interossei.

ANKLE JOINT

Type
It is a hinge variety of synovial joint.

Articulating bones
From above: Inferior end of the tibia with medial malleolus, lateral malleolus of fibula and inferior transverse tibio-fibular ligament.

From below: Superior surface of the body of the talus. (Fig. 16.15)

The ankle joint is more stable when the foot is dorsiflexed, because during this movement the anterior wider part of the trochlea of talus comes in grip between the malleoli. During plantar flexion the joint is relatively weak because

Fig. 16.15 Ankle joint—bones articulating

the narrower posterior part of the trochlea does not fill the socket.

Structures stabilizing
1. **Fibrous capsule (Capsular ligament):**

   It is attached to articular margins but anteroinferiorly it extends up to the neck of the talus (for allowing dosiflexion). The synovial membrane lines the fibrous capsule.

2. **Deltoid (medial collateral) ligament:**

   It is a strong triangular shaped ligament. Its apex is attached to the medial malleolus of tibia. It has a superficial and a deep part (Fig.16.16).

Superficial part: It consists of following ligaments
1. Tibio-navicular – to the tuberosity of the navicular bone
2. Tibio-calcaneal – to the whole length of the sustanculum tali
3. Posterior tibio-talar – to the medial surface of the talus

Deep part: It consists of **anterior tibiotalar ligament** which is attached to the anterior part of the medial surface of the talus.

3. **Lateral (fibular collateral) ligament:**

   It consists of three bands, which extend from the lateral malleolus to talus and calcaneum. It has been explained in three parts namely (Fig. 16.17).

   • Anterior talo-fibular ligament – to the neck of the talus

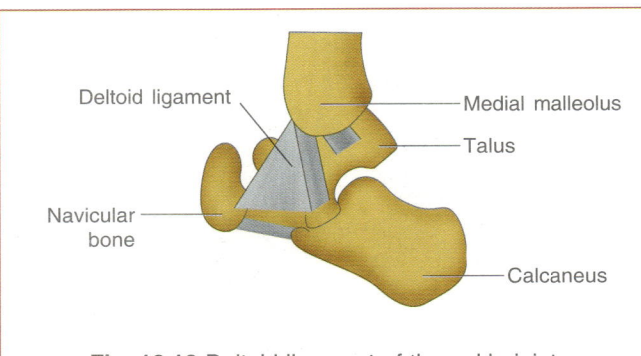

Fig. 16.16 Deltoid ligament of the ankle joint

- Posterior talo-fibular ligament – it extends from the lower part of the malleolar fossa of the fibula to the lateral tubercle of the talus

- Calcaneo-fibular ligament – to the tubercle on the lateral surface of the calcaneus

Arterial supply: The joint is supplied by anterior and posterior tibial arteries.

Nerve supply: The joint is supplied by deep peroneal and tibial nerves.

Movements and muscles producing them

1. **Dorsiflexion:** The forefoot is raised and the angle between front of the leg and dorsum of the foot is diminished.

   Muscles involved: Tibialis anterior, extensor digitorum longus, extensor hallucis longus and peroneus tertius.

2. **Plantar flexion:** The forefoot is depressed and the angle between the leg and foot is increased.

   Muscles involved: Gastrocnemius, soleus, tibialis posterior, flexor hallucis longus, flexor digitorum longus, peroneus longus and peroneus brevis.

- Ankle joint is most frequently injured. Injury occurs in plantar flexed position of the foot. The lateral

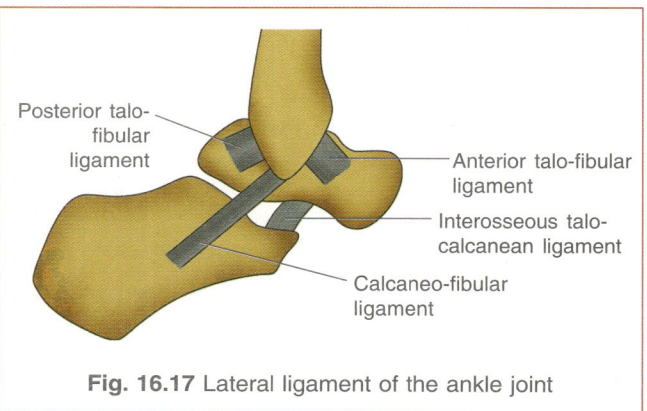

Fig. 16.17 Lateral ligament of the ankle joint

ligament is more often injured compared to the medial. The anterior talofibular ligament is the most common of the lateral ligaments to be injured. A sprained ankle results due to tear of anterior talofibular and calcaneofibular ligament, when the foot is twisted in lateral direction (inversion injury).

- In forcible eversion of foot the deltoid ligament may be torn. At times, the deltoid ligament pulls the medial malleolus thereby causing avulsion fracture of the medial malleolus.

Pott's fracture (fracture dislocation of ankle): It is caused by forcible eversion leading to horizontal fracture of medial malleolus and oblique fracture of shaft of fibula and also lateral malleolus. It occurs when the foot is caught in the rabbit hole in the ground and the foot is forcibly everted. If the tibia is carried anteriorly, the posterior margin of the distal end of the tibia is also broken by the talus producing 'trimalleolar fracture' (Fig.16.18).

CASE-2

A 17-year-old girl while running in an uneven mud road stumbled and over inverted her left foot. Later she was examined in the hospital by an orthopaedician. The lateral side of the ankle was tender and swollen. Movements of the ankle were restricted, especially when the foot was inverted. Careful, gentle palpation demonstrated a small area of great tenderness below and in front of the lateral malleolus. The X-ray examination of the ankle joint was normal. What is this case is likely to be? In which joints do eversion and inversion of the foot take place?

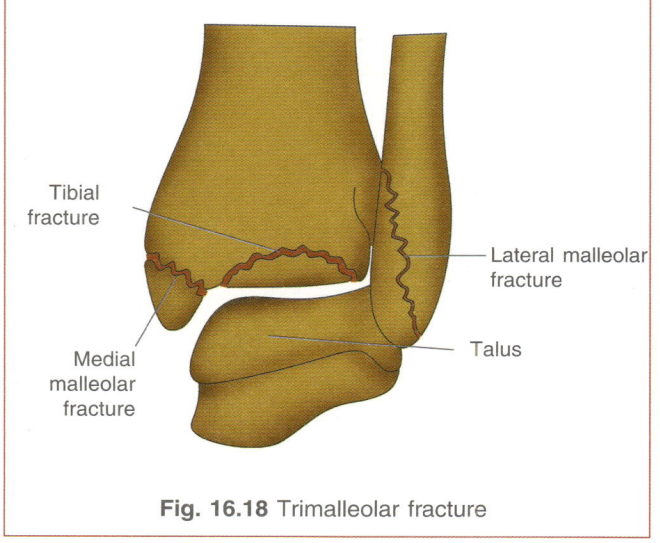

Fig. 16.18 Trimalleolar fracture

CASE-3

A 27-year-old man while running for a cross country race, his left foot was caught in a rabbit hole. As he fell, left foot was violently rotated laterally and over-everted. On attempting to stand, he found he could place no weight on his left foot. He was taken into the hospital and was examined by an orthopaedician. The left ankle was considerably swollen, especially on the lateral side. The left heel appeared to be unduly prominent. Anteroposterior and lateral radiographs of the ankle showed a fracture of the medial and lateral malleolus and a fracture of the lower end of the tibia. The tibia was displaced forward on the talus. The diagnosis of severe fracture dislocation of the ankle joint was made.

1. Is ankle joint normally a stable joint? If so, what does its stability depend upon?

2. What is the type of fracture called if it involves the lateral and medial malleoli-transverse, oblique, or spiral?

Tibiofibular joints

1. **Superior tibiofibular joint:** It is a plane synovial joint. The head of the fibula articulates with lateral condyle of tibia.

2. **Inferior tibiofibular joint:** It is a syndesmosis variety of fibrous joint. The lower ends of tibia and fibula are connected by a strong interosseous ligament.

JOINTS OF THE FOOT

Subtalar joint (Talocalcanean joint)

The talus and calcaneum are connected by two strong joints-talocalcaneonavicular joint and talocalcaneal joints.

Talocalcaneonavicular joint

Type: It is a ball and socket variety of synovial joint.

Bones taking parts: The head of the talus articulates with the calcaneo-navicular socket (formed by calcaneum and navicular bone).

Structures stabilizing: The two bones are connected by fibrous capsule, interosseus talocalcaneal ligament, spring ligament and medial part of the bifurcate ligament.

Interosseus talocalcaneal ligament: It occupies the sinus tarsi. It stretches between sulcus tali to sulcus calcanei. The ligament separates the talocalcaneonavicular and posterior talocalcanean joint. It becomes stretched in eversion and limits this movement.

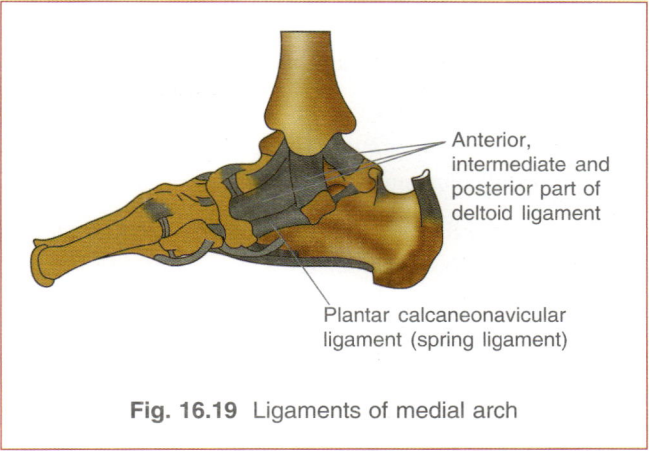

Fig. 16.19 Ligaments of medial arch

Spring ligament (plantar calcaneonavicular ligament): It extends from the anterior margin of the sustentaculum tali to the plantar surface of the navicular bone. The head of the talus directly rests on the upper surface of the spring ligament, separated by a fibrocartilage. This ligament is the key structure in maintaining the medial longitudinal arch (Fig. 16.19).

Bifurcate ligament: It is a 'Y' shaped ligament. Its stem is attached to the anterolateral part of the sulcus calcanei. The medial limb is attached to navicular bone and the lateral limb to the cuboid bone.

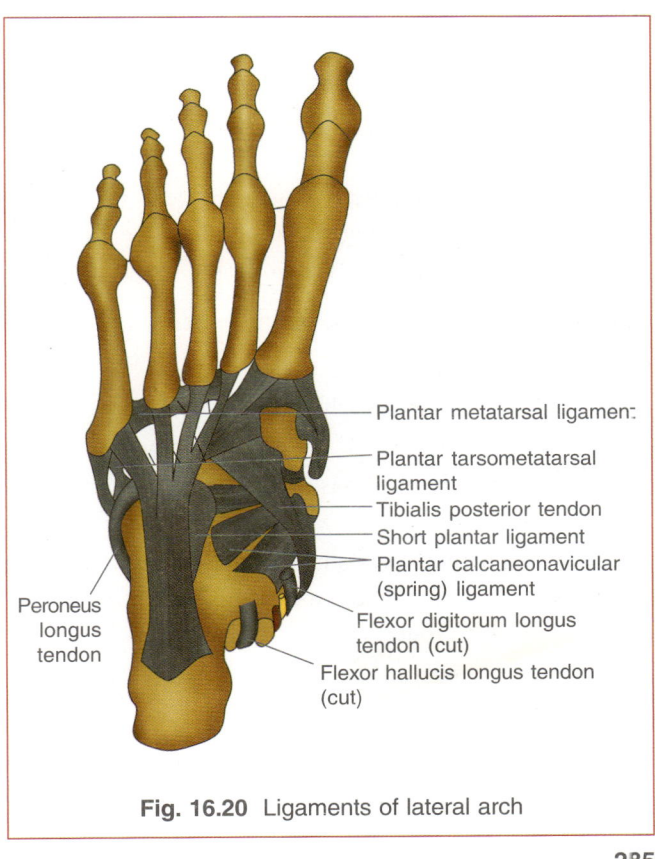

Fig. 16.20 Ligaments of lateral arch

Talocalcanean joint

Type: It is a plane synovial joint

Bones taking parts: It is the articulation between the inferior surface of the talus and middle part of the superior surface of the calcaneum.

Structures stabilizing: The joint is stabilized by fibrous capsule, interosseus talocalcaneal ligament and cervical ligament.

Cervical ligament: It is present lateral to the sinus tarsi. It extends from the upper surface of the calcaneus to the tubercle present on the inferolateral aspect of the neck of the talus. It becomes stretched in inversion and limits this movement.

Calcaneocuboid joint

It is a saddle joint between calcaneus and cuboid. The bones are connected by fibrous capsule, lateral limb of the bifurcate ligament, long and short plantar ligaments.

Long plantar ligament: Posteriorly it is attached to the plantar surface of the calcaneus and anteriorly into the bases of the middle three metatarsals and also to the distal lip on the groove present on the **plantar surface of the cuboid bone**. It converts the groove on the plantar surface of the cuboid bone into a tunnel for the passage of the tendon of the peroneus longus muscle. It is one of the structure maintains the longitudinal arch of the foot (Fig.16.20). Morphologically it represents the divorced tendon of the gastrocnemius.

Short plantar ligament: It is present deep to the long plantar ligament extending from anterior tubercle of the calcaneus to the plantar surface of the cuboid (Fig. 16.20).

Movements and muscles producing them:

Inversion:

- It is the movement in which the medial border of the foot is raised

- The degree of inversion is greater when the foot is off the ground

- It is a combination of adduction and lateral rotation of forefoot with plantar flexion at ankle joint, when the foot is off the ground

- When the foot is on the ground, it is only the lateral rotation of the forefoot

Muscles causing inversion: Tibialis anterior and Tibialis posterior assisted by flexor hallucis longus and flexor digitorum longus.

Eversion

- It is the movement in which the lateral border of the foot is raised.

- The degree of inversion is greater when the foot is off the ground.

- It is a combination of abduction and medial rotation of forefoot with dorsiflexion at ankle joint, when the foot is off the ground

- When the foot is on the ground, it is only the medial rotation of the forefoot

Muscles causing eversion: Peroneus longus and Peroneus brevis assisted by peroneus tertius.

ARCHES OF THE FOOT

Human foot is designed to perform two basic functions:

- It acts as a flexible platform to support the body weight and to adapt into the uneven surfaces.

- It acts as a lever to propel the body forward during locomotion.

- To perform these functions the foot is designed in the form of elastic arches.

- This is possible because the foot is made of many small bones connected by many synovial joints.

Functions of arches of foot

- Proportional distribution of body weight.

- Arched foot acts as a segmented lever through series of joints, and thus made pliable to adapt it to uneven surfaces.

- Plantar concavity of the arch protects the nerves and vessels of the sole.

- Arched foot acts as a shock absorber and helps in jumping movement.

Elastic arches are classified into longitudinal and transverse arches.

Longitudinal arches

When the foot is on the ground only the anterior (heads of the metatarsals) and posterior (calcaneus) parts rest on the ground forming a convex arch directed upwards. This longitudinal arch is divided into medial and lateral arches. The medial arch is higher than lateral arch (Figs 16.21 and 16.22).

Each arch is made up of anterior and posterior ends, summit, anterior and posterior pillars and a main joint which are given in Table 16.7.

Table 16.7 Formation of longitudinal arch		
	Medial longitudinal arch	**Lateral longitudinal arch**
Anterior end	Heads of the medial 3 metatarsals	Heads of the 4th and 5th metatarsals
Posterior end	Medial tubercle of the calcaneus	Lateral tubercle of the calcaneus
Summit	Trochlear (upper) surface of the talus	Facet on the superior surface of the calcaneus
Anterior pillar	Shafts of the medial 3 metatarsals	Shafts of 4th and 5th metatarsals
Posterior pillar	Medial part of the calcaneus	Lateral part of the calcaneus
Main joint of the arch	Talo-calcaneonavicular joint	Calcaneocuboid joint

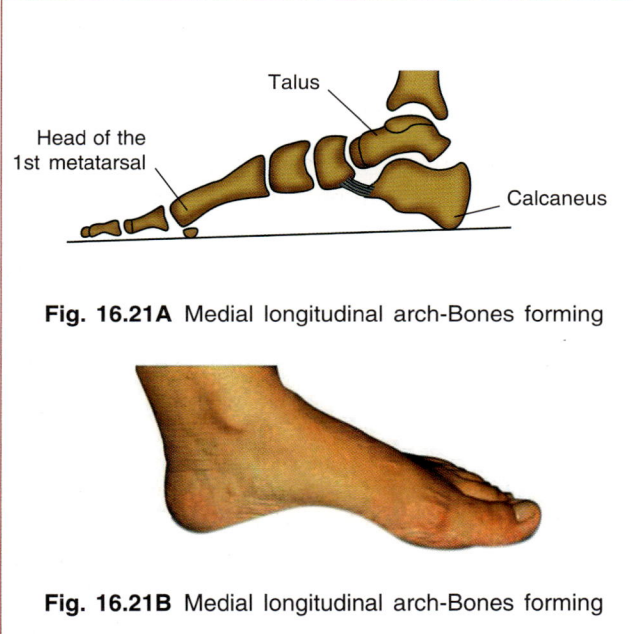

Fig. 16.21A Medial longitudinal arch-Bones forming

Fig. 16.21B Medial longitudinal arch-Bones forming

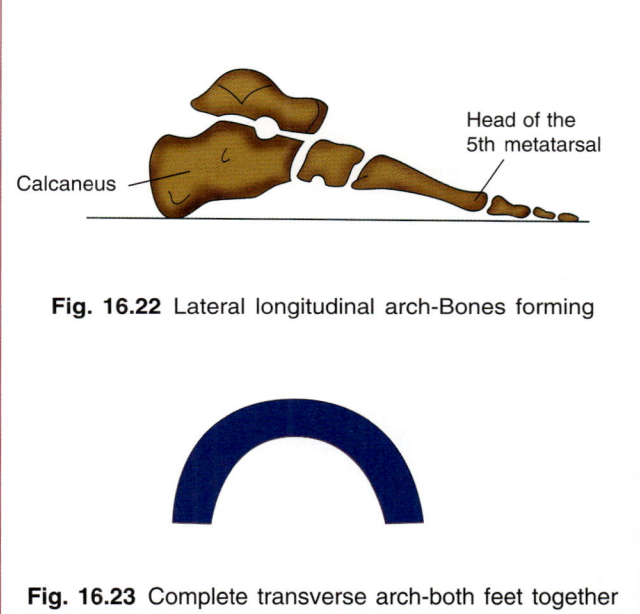

Fig. 16.22 Lateral longitudinal arch-Bones forming

Fig. 16.23 Complete transverse arch-both feet together

Transverse arch

Foot also presents anterior and posterior transverse arches. The anterior end of the transverse arch is formed by heads of the metatarsals and posteriorly by the base of the metatarsals. A complete transverse arch is formed when medial borders of both feet are approximated (Fig. 16.23).

Maintenance (mechanisms) of arches of foot
(Table 16.8)

There are many structural and mechanical factors that are responsible for maintenance of arches of the foot. An arched foot is often compared to an arched bridge made up of stones and engineering devices which take care of the stability of a stoned bridge. Following are the important facts about the stability of the bridge or arched foot (Fig. 16.24).

1. **Shape of the bones:** If the bones are cuboidal or rectangular, it is not possible to form an arched foot.

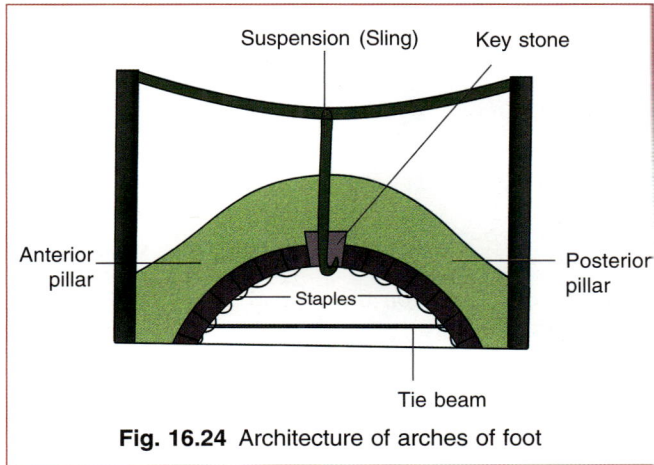

Fig. 16.24 Architecture of arches of foot

Table 16.8 Maintenance of arches of foot

Factors responsible for maintenance	Medial longitudinal arch	Lateral longitudinal arch
Shape of the bones	Sustentaculum tali hold up the talus. Rounded head of talus is 'key stone'	Calcanean angle of the cuboid
Intersegmental ties	Spring ligament, Long plantar ligament and dorsal ligaments	Long and short plantar ligaments, dorsal ligaments
Tie beams	Medial part of the plantar aponeurosis, Medial part of the flexor digitorum brevis and longus, Abductor hallucis, Flexor hallucis longus and brevis	Lateral part of the plantar aponeurosis, Lateral part of the flexor digitorum brevis and longus, Abductor digiti minimi, Flexor digiti minimi brevis
Sling support)	Tibialis anterior, superficial fibres of deltoid ligament and, Tibialis posterior muscles	Peroneus longus, brevis and tertius muscles

The bones contributing to the arch must be wedge shaped with their thin edges face inferiorly. Especially the bones occupying the centre of the arch act as a key bone (stone) (Fig. 16.25).

2. **The inferior edges of the bones are tied together (Intersegmental ties):** The plantar surface of the bones involved in the arch are connected by many strong ligaments which act like metal staples connecting the undersurface of the stones in an arched bridge.

3. **The use of tie beams:** A structure usually a long tendon connecting the anterior and posterior ends of the arch act as a tie beam which prevents separation of the pillars and consequent sagging of arch (Fig. 16.26).

4. **A suspension bridge (Sling support):** The convexity of the arch is maintained by upward pull of the summit by muscles that act as a suspension bridge.

Maintenance of the transverse arch

Shape of the bone: Wedge shaped 3 cuneiforms and bases of middle 3 metatarsals

Intersegmental ties: Deep transverse ligaments, Dorsal interossei and Adductor hallucis muscle

Tie beams: Tendon of peroneus longus muscle

Sling support: Tendon of Peroneus brevis and tertius on lateral side, Tendon of tibialis anterior on medial side

Pes planus (flat foot): It is a term referring to a flat foot. Abnormal distribution of the body weight on to the arch causes flat foot. Predisposing factors for pes planus includes rapid increase in body weight, loss of tone in leg muscles from prolonged standing, faulty foot-wear and bad walking style. A pes planus can

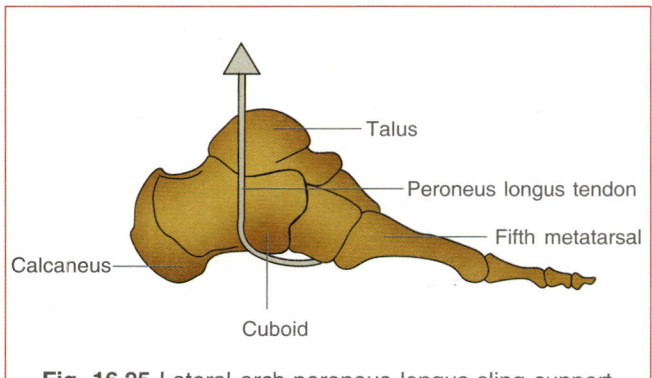
Fig. 16.25 Lateral arch-peroneus longus-sling support

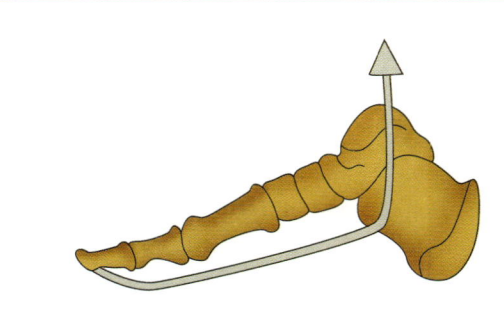
Fig. 16.26 Medial arch-Flexor hallucis longus-tie beam

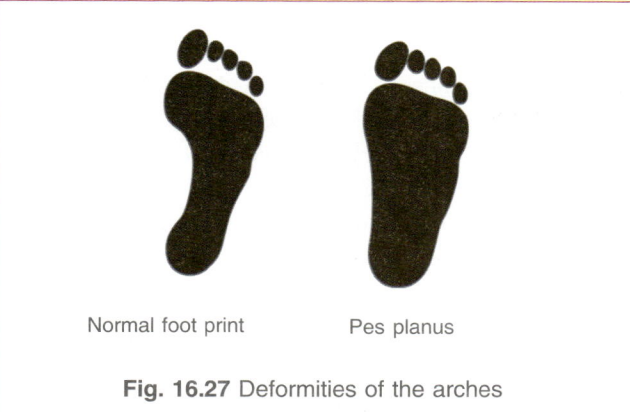

Normal foot print   Pes planus

Fig. 16.27 Deformities of the arches

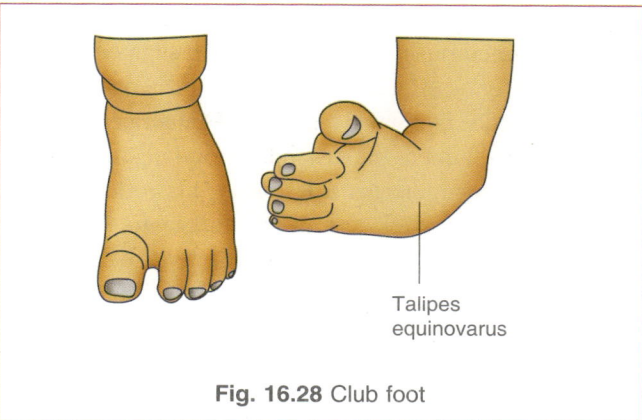

Talipes
equinovarus

Fig. 16.28 Club foot

cause shuffling gait, trauma, osteoarthritis and metatarsalgia (Fig.16.27).

Pes cavus: It is a condition with exaggeration of arches of foot. Toes are dorsiflexed at the metacarpophalangeal joint and plantar flexed at interphalangeal joint. This is due to atrophy of lumbrical and interossei muscles. These conditions are often associated with spina bifida and poliomyelitis.

Rocker bottom feet: The plantar concavity is replaced by convexity. This is found in babies born with trisomy 18 (Edward syndrome).

Claw foot: In this condition toes are dorsiflexed at metatarsophalangeal joints and plantar flexed at interphalangeal joints.

Hammer toe: The metatarsophalangeal and distal interphalangeal joints are hyper extended but proximal interphalangeal joint is acutely flexed. It usually affects second and third toes due to involvement of lumbrical muscles.

Talipes equinus: In this condition the person walks on the forefoot with raised heel. It is also a feature of nerve injury affecting deep peroneal nerve. The talipes equines is further classified into

a) **Talipes equino varus:** In this condition the foot is inverted and adducted. The patient walks on the outer border of the foot. This is the commonest deformity of the foot (foot is inverted, adducted and plantar flexed) and referred as 'club foot' (Fig. 16.28).

b) **Talipes equino valgus:** In this condition foot is everted and abducted. The patient walks on the inner border of the foot.

Talipes calcaneus: In this condition the person walks on heel with raised forefoot. This is also a feature of

nerve injury affecting the tibial nerve. The talipes equinovalgus is also classified into talipes calcaneovarus and valgus.

Hallux valgus: This is a condition in which the great toe is adducted (lateral deviation) at the metatarsophalangeal joint. It is common in women. The prominence of head of first metatarsal rubs on the shoe, giving rise to a hard lump (bunion) on its medial side (Fig. 16.29).

CASE-4

A 17-year-old girl decided to work as a waitress to take care of herself after sudden loss of her parents. She had never done this type of work before. After working for eight hours a day for a week, she found that her feet were swollen and painful. Using your anatomical knowledge, explain the underlying cause for her discomfort.

Solutions to the case studies

Case-1

The knee jerk depends on the integrity of (1) the afferent neuron, which extends from the stretch receptors in the ligamentum patellae to the spinal cord via the femoral nerve

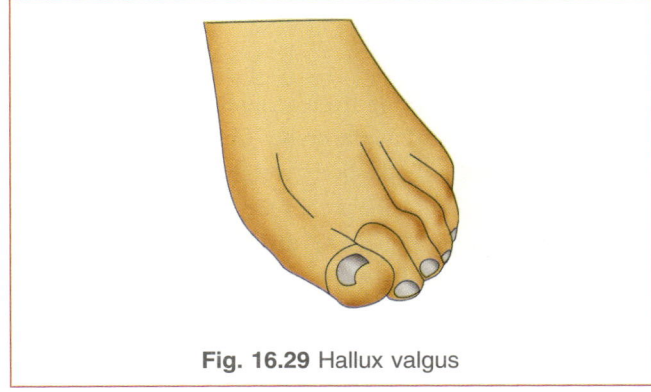

Fig. 16.29 Hallux valgus

SECTION 4

and lumbar plexus; (2) the connection of the afferent on to the efferent neuron in the spinal cord at segments L2, 3, and 4; and (3) the efferent neuron, which extends from the spinal cord to the motor end plates of the quadriceps femoris muscle via the lumbar plexus and femoral nerve. Absence of the knee jerk indicates a lesion in this reflex arc. An exaggerated knee jerk signifies damage to the motor neuron, which normally influences the activity of this reflex arc. The ankle jerk depends on the normal functioning of another simple reflex arc, acting at the level of the fifth lumbar and second sacral segments of the cord. The Babinski test normally results in planter flexion of the big toe. In a positive Babinski test, stimulation of the sole is followed by dorsiflexion of the big toe and indicates damage to the upper motor neuron. (Babies normally have a positive Babinski test.)

Case-2

In laymans language, this girl "sprained" her left ankle. Over inversion causes a strain on the lateral ligaments of the ankle joint. In this case the localized tenderness is found below and in front of the lateral malleolus which would indicate that some of the fibers of anterior talofibular ligament had been torn. The resulting hemorrhage was responsible for the swelling in the area. The movements of eversion and inversion of the foot takes place in the subtalar and transverse tarsal joints.

Case-3

1. The ankle is a very stable joint. The body of the talus is held firmly in position in the mortise formed by the lower end of the tibia and the medial and lateral malleoli. This arrangement is further strengthened by a very strong medial or deltoid ligament and a less strong lateral ligament.

2. Fracture dislocation that involves rotation and over-eversion of the foot, is usually associated with spiral fracture of the lateral malleolus and a transverse fracture across the medial malleolus. The medial ligament is so strong that it pulls off medial malleolus.

Case-4

This patient was suffering from acute foot strain. This new job has put lots of load on the arches of her foot. The arches were carrying not only the body weight, but also weight of loaded trays. Normally, the arches are supported in position by the shape of the bones, by the strong ligaments and-most important of all is tone of muscles in an active foot. Once untrained muscles become fatigued, they stretch. In the case of the medial longitudinal arch, the head of the talus starts to sag down between the calcaneum and the

navicular bone. The calcaneo-navicular ligament and the other plantar ligaments first become over stretched and then may even tear. At this stage there is pain and swelling of the foot. The tendons of the long muscles also stretch, producing pain in the leg. The feet should be rested and elevated to eliminate the swelling. Physiotherapy to the muscles should then be started. When such a patient returns to work, the hours of duty should be gradually increased so that the muscles are trained to carry the work load. A person who continues to walk on a foot with acute foot strain will end up with permanently flat feet.

MCQs

1. The ankle jerk is a reflex twitch of the triceps surae (gastrocnemius and soleus) induced by tapping the tendocalcaneus (Achilles tendon). The reflex center is in
   A. The fifth lumbar segment
   B. The first sacral segment
   C. The fourth lumbar segment
   D. The third lumbar segment

2. Which one of the following statements does NOT apply to the inferior tibiofibular joint?
   A. It is a synovial joint allowing slight gliding movement
   B. It is a fibrous joint
   C. The rough areas at the lower ends of the tibia and fibula are united by interosseous ligament
   D. It is a secondary cartilaginous joint

3. A 51-year-old housewife undergoes successful surgery for excision of a right Baker's cyst. Approximately three months after surgery, the patient is experiencing decreased sensation over the upper one-third of the lateral border of her right leg. She also reports dragging of her right foot during ambulation. Which of the following muscles is most likely involved?
   A. Tibials posterior
   B. Peroneus brevis
   C. Peroneus longus
   D. Tibialis anterior

4. An 18-year-old male patient presents to the hospital with a crushing injury to his right ankle. The attending physician feels for femoral, dorsalis pedis, and posterior tibial pulses and finds that they are intact and symmetric bilaterally. In which of the following locations did the student palpate the posterior tibial pulse?
   A. Deep in the popliteal fossa
   B. Immediately anterior to the medial malleolus

C. Immediately posterior to the lateral malleolus

D. Immediately posterior to the medial malleolus

5. A 16-year-old girl presents with difficulty in walking after injuring her ankle while playing. She is diagnosed with a Pott's fracture. Which of the following types of forceful movement causes this injury?

    A. Avulsion

    B. Dorsiflexion

    C. Eversion

    D. Inversion

6. A patient with a diabetic ulcer in the anterior midline of the ankle region experienced loss of cutaneous sensation on the dorsal surface of the foot. Which nerve was most likely damaged?

    A. Deep peroneal nerve

    B. Saphenous

    C. Superficial peroneal

    D. Sural

7. While playing a 13-year-old girl twists her ankle. Her foot is forcibly everted. Which of the following ligament is most likely to be injured?

    A. Anterior talofibular

    B. Anterior tibiofibular

    C. Calcaneofibular

    D. Deltoid

8. A worker falls from a height and lands on his feet. Radiographs reveal a fracture of the sustentaculum tali. The muscle passing immediately beneath it that would be adversely affected is the:

    A. Flexor digitorum longus

    B. Flexor hallucis longus

    C. Tibialis anterior

    D. Tibialis posterior

9. A deep laceration, 2 cm in length, immediately posterior to the medial malleolus, may injure any of the following *except*:

    A. peroneal artery

    B. tibial nerve

    C. tendon of tibialis posterior

    D. tendon of flexor digitorum longus

10. A long distance runner complains of foot pain. Upon examination, the physician diagnoses tendinitis of the peroneus longus tendon. Because the tenderness is located deep on the sole of the foot, it appears that the irritation occurred where the tendon lies against bone, covered by a structure called

    A. long plantar ligament

    B. plantar aponeurosis

    C. bifurcate ligament

    D. spring ligament

11. Compression of the lateral plantar nerve as it passes between the flexor digitorum brevis and quadratus plantae could result in weakness of any of the following actions *except*:

    A. abduction of the great toe

    B. adduction of the middle toe

    C. abduction of the little toe

    D. adduction of the great toe

12. While walking barefoot on the road, a 24-year-old construction worker steps on a sharp glass piece which punctures the sole of his foot. In the hospital during examination he can no longer spread his toes apart (without using his hands). Which nerve must have been injured?

    A. deep peroneal

    B. lateral plantar

    C. medial plantar

    D. sural

13. A 34-year-old male has difficulty walking after sustaining a traumatic injury to his right leg. Physical examination reveals a right foot that is dorsiflexed and everted. The patient is unable to stand on his tip of the toes. What is the most likely area of sensory loss in this patient?

    A. Medial side of the leg

    B. Medial side of the foot

    C. Dorsum of the foot

    D. Sole of the foot

14. A football player tears his tendocalcaneus. You would expect to find weakness in:

    A. dorsiflexion of the foot

    B. eversion of the foot

    C. extension of the knee

    D. plantar flexion of the foot

15. A patient's ankle joint will have the greatest stability when:

    A. The foot is dorsi flexed

    B. The foot is plantarflexed

    C. The foot is everted

    D. The foot is inverted

16. Your female patient is unable to walk on her toe-tip. You immediately suspect damage to which of the following nerves?

291

A. Sural nerve

B. Tibial nerve

C. Common peroneal nerve

D. Superficial peroneal nerve

17. A barefoot child steps on some glass on the sole of his foot and complains of numbness of the little toe. Which of these nerves is likely to be injured?

A Medial plantar

B Lateral plantar

C Tibial

D Superficial peroneal

18. An important component of pes planus, or flatfoot, is abnormal stretching of the structure that is mainly responsible for supporting the medial longitudinal arch of the foot. Which of the following structures is the main support of this arch?

A. Long plantar ligament

B. Plantar calcaneo cuboid ligament

C. Plantar calcaneo navicular ligament

D. Tibialis anterior tendon

19. Ankle joint ligaments are more easily sprained when the foot is in plantar flexion than in dorsiflexion. Which of the following ligaments of ankle is most likely to be sprained during plantar flexion?

A. Anterior talofibular

B. Calcaneofibular

C. Posterior talofibular

D. Tibiocalcaneal

Answers to MCQs

1. B

2. A

3. A

4. D

5. C

6. C

7. D

8. B

9. A

10. A

11. A

12. B

13. D

14. D

15. A

16. B

17. B

18. C

19. A

SECTION 4

Major questions

1. Describe the common peroneal nerve under-origin and root value, course, branches and distribution and applied anatomy

2. Describe the sciatic nerve under-origin and root value, course, branches and distribution and applied anatomy

3. Describe the boundaries and contents of the femoral triangle. Add a note on femoral sheath, femoral canal and femoral hernia

4. Describe the hip joint under-type, articulating parts of the bones, ligaments stabilizing, movements and muscles producing them and applied anatomy

5. Describe the knee joint under- type, articulating parts of the bones, capsule, extra capsular and intracapsular ligaments. Movements and muscles producing them and applied anatomy.

6. Describe the arches of foot under-types, formation, factor maintaining them (supporting) and applied anatomy

7. Given account of origin, course, branches and applied aspects of femoral artery.

8. Describe the gluteus maximus under- attachments, nerve supply, actions, structure under cover of it.

9. Describe the boundaries and contents of the popliteal fossa

10. Define inversion and eversion, mention the joints involved and describe the invertors.

Short notes

1. Femoral canal
2. Femoral nerve
3. Great saphenous vein
4. Superficial inguinal lymph nodes
5. Adductor canal
6. Obturator nerve
7. Patella
8. Adductor magnus muscle
9. Gluteus medius and minimums muscles
10. Neck of the femur and its blood supply and applied anatomy
11. Piriformis muscle
12. Ilio-femoral ligament
13. Tibial collateral ligament of the knee joint
14. Cruciate ligaments of the knee joint
15. Menisci of the knee joint
16. Popliteus muscle
17. Ilio-tibial tract
18. Bursae related to the knee joint
19. Tendocalcaneus
20. Superficial peroneal nerve
21. Cutaneous innervation of the dorsum of the foot
22. Deltoid ligament of the ankle joint
23. Spring ligament
24. Extensor retinaculae around the ankle joint
25. Flexor retinaculum around the ankle joint
26. Peroneus longus muscle
27. Medial longitudinal arch
28. Subtalar joint
29. Dorsalis pedis artery
30. Profunda femoris artery

SECTION

5

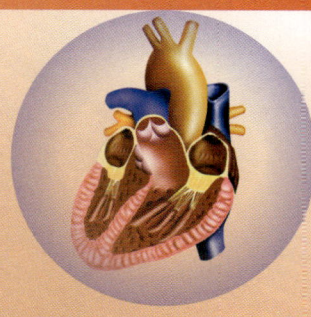

Thorax

Thoracic Wall and Osteology of the Thorax

17

- Thoracic cage
- Sternum
- Ribs
- Thoracic vertebrae
- Joints of the thorax
- Inlet of the thorax
- Muscles of the thoracic wall
- Respiratory movements
- Intercostal nerves
- Arteries of the thoracic wall
- MCQs

Objectives

- To know the bones and cartilages constituting the thoracic cage
- To identify the different types of ribs and parts of the typical rib
- To know the parts and relations of first rib
- To identify the typical and atypical thoracic vertebrae and their parts
- To explain the anatomy of respiratory movements and to know the muscles involved in it
- To explain the attachments and actions of the intercostal muscles
- To explain the structures passing through the thoracic inlet and its clinical significance
- To explain the origin, course, branches, distribution and functional components present in the intercostal nerve
- To understand the anatomy of 'intercostal nerve block' and involvement of intercostal nerve in various referred pain
- To explain the arterial supply and venous drainage of the thoracic wall and their clinical significance

The thorax includes the primary organs of the respiratory and cardiovascular system. It can be studied under thoracic wall and thoracic cavity. The thoracic cavity has a central compartment called mediastinum and pulmonary cavities on either side housing the lungs. Though mammary glands are located in the wall of the thorax, it is discussed in pectoral region of the upper limb.

The thoracic wall includes thoracic cage (thoracic skeleton), muscles between the ribs, skin and fascia. The same structures covering the posterior aspect is discussed in page 306.

THORACIC CAGE

The vital organs of the thorax (heart and lungs) are well protected inside the bony thoracic cage (Fig. 17.1). It is formed anteriorly by the sternum. On either sides, by the ribs and their costal cartilages and posteriorly, by the thoracic vertebral bodies with intervertebral discs.

Though the skeletal framework of the thoracic cage provides rigidity, its joints and flexibility of the ribs can sustain external blows and compressions. It is designed in such a way that it can alter the volume of thoracic cavity for respiration.

STERNUM

Sternum is a flat bone, present in front of the thoracic cage. It presents the following parts: Manubrium, Body and Xiphoid process (Fig. 17. 3).

The **manubrium** is the upper part of the sternum. It articulates with the medial ends of clavicles and first costal cartilages. Its upper end is easily palpable and is called jugular notch (suprasternal notch).

Sternal angle (joint between manubrium and body) is an important landmark for counting the ribs. The 2nd costal cartilage can be felt at the sides of this angle.

The **body** is larger part of the sternum - On each side, it receives ribs through their costal cartilages (3rd to 6th rib).

The **xiphoid process** - It is the most variable part of the sternum. It is a cartilaginous structure in young people but ossified in adults. Its joint with the body of the sternum

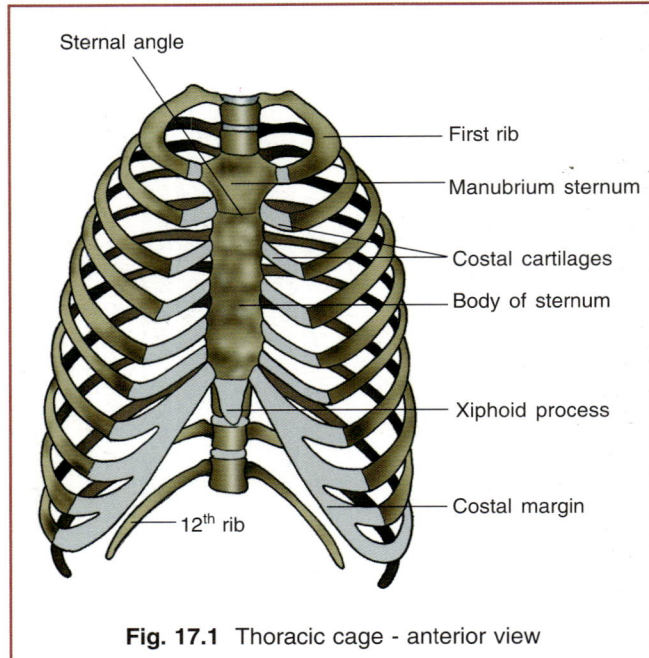

Fig. 17.1 Thoracic cage - anterior view

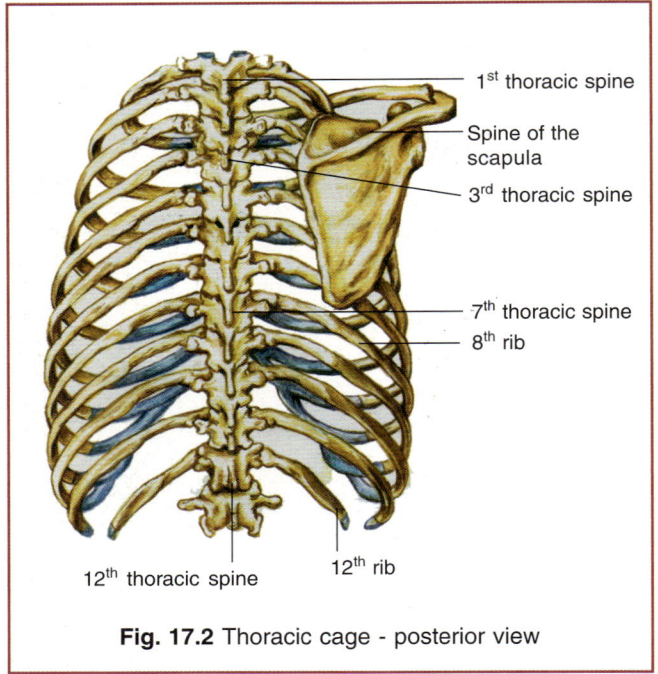

Fig. 17.2 Thoracic cage - posterior view

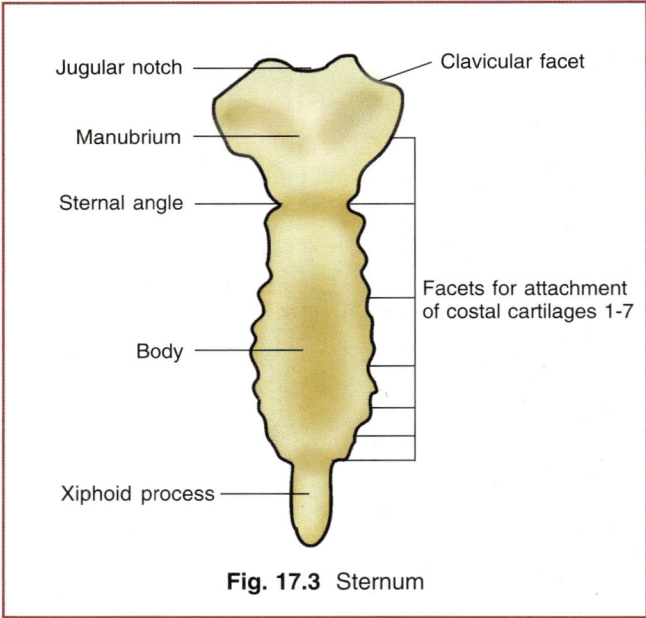

Fig. 17.3 Sternum

(Xiphisternal joint) laterally corresponds to 7th costal cartilage. It is a midline marker for central tendon of diaphragm, inferior border of the heart and upper limit of the liver.

- The fracture of the sternal body is usually comminuted fracture (broken into several pieces), but displacement of the fragments is uncommon because of muscle attachments. Sternal fracture is common in road accidents, with its backward displacement, compressing aorta, heart or liver.

- Sternum may be divided in the median plane (median sternotomy) for the surgeries of heart and its blood vessels. The flexibility of ribs and costal cartilages enables spreading of the halves of the sternum.

- The sternal body is often used for bone marrow aspiration

RIBS (COSTAE)

There are 12 pairs of ribs in the body. Each rib anteriorly articulates with the sternum, through its costal cartilage (1st to 7th). The lower ribs articulate anteriorly with the higher costal cartilages (8th to 10th). The anterior ends of the last two ribs are free and are called floating ribs (Vertebral). Posteriorly each rib articulates with the thoracic vertebrae.

The 3rd to 9th ribs present almost the same features, hence are referred as 'typical ribs'. The 1st, 2nd, 10th, 11th and 12th ribs are atypical.

Typical rib

Each typical rib has an anterior end, shaft and posterior end (Fig. 17.4).

a. Anterior end: It joins the corresponding costal cartilage by primary cartilaginous joint

b. Posterior end presents head, neck and tubercle.

Head: It comprises two facets. The lower facet of the head articulates with body of the corresponding vertebra

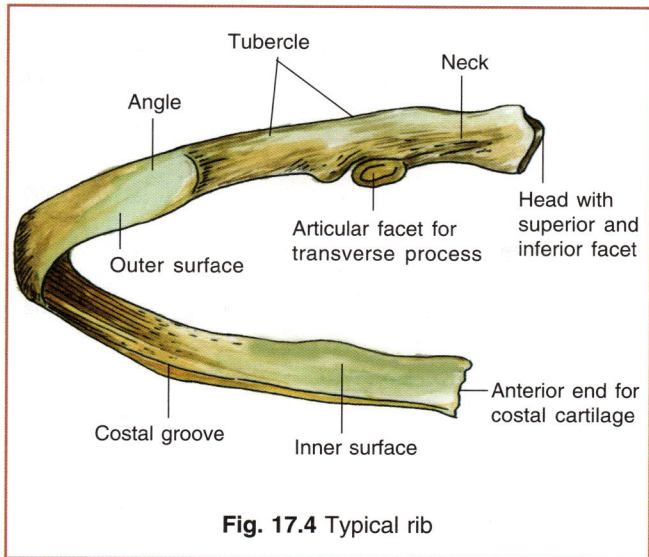

Fig. 17.4 Typical rib

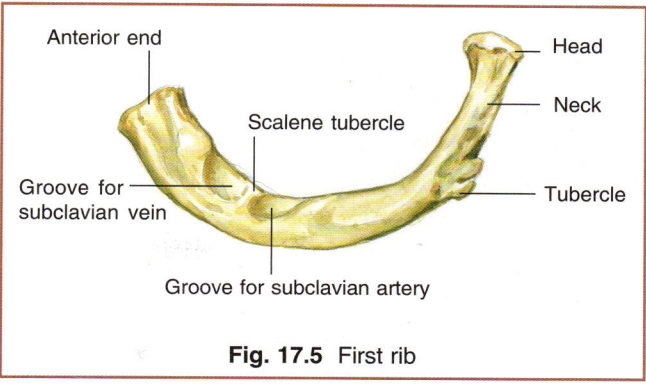

Fig. 17.5 First rib

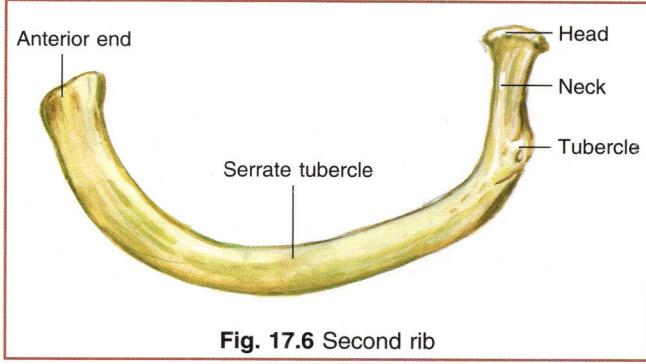

Fig. 17.6 Second rib

(plane synovial joint). The upper facet of the head articulates with body of the vertebra above. The two facets are separated by a crest, which corresponds to the intervertebral disc.

Neck: It is the narrow succeeding part of the head. It lies in front of the transverse process of the corresponding vertebra.

Tubercle: It is the rough portion between neck and shaft. It has medial articular and lateral non-articular parts. The medial articular part articulates with transverse process of corresponding vertebra by a plane synovial joint (costotransverse joint). The lateral part provides attachment to lateral costotransverse ligament.

Shaft: It is the elongated flat part of the rib. It presents angulation about 5 to 6 cm lateral to the tubercle. The shaft is also twisted so that its inner surface faces upwards behind the angle and faces downwards in front of the angle. The shaft presents upper and lower borders, outer and inner surfaces. They provide attachments to mainly intercostal muscles.

Costal groove: The lower part of the inner surface presents costal groove, which is occupied by posterior intercostal vein, artery and intercostal nerve from above downwards.

First rib

- It is the shortest, broadest and most curved among the ribs (Fig.17.5).
- The head presents only one facet for the body of 1st thoracic vertebra.

- The neck of the first rib is related to following structures in front from medial to lateral - sympathetic chain, first posterior intercostal vein, superior intercostal artery and first thoracic nerve. All these structures are related to the apex of the lung. A tumor growing from the apex can (Pancoast tumor) compress all these structures.
- The shaft has no twisting hence presents superior and inferior surfaces, outer and inner borders.
- The inner border presents scalene tubercle for the insertion of scalenus anterior muscle.
- Its superior surface is grooved by subclavian vein in front and subclavian artery behind the scalene tubercle.
- The shaft has no costal groove.

Second rib

- The second rib is also highly curved like the first rib (Fig.17.6).
- Shaft has no twisting and presents outer convex and inner concave surface.
- The head presents two articular facets for the bodies of 1st and 2nd thoracic vertebrae
- It has a rough area on its upper/outer surface called 'serrate tubercle' providing attachment to serratus anterior muscle.
- A short costal groove is present on the posterior part of the inner surface.

Eleventh and Twelfth Ribs

- There is no neck and tubercle.
- The head presents only one facet.
- Their anterior end is pointed.
- Costal groove and angle are absent in twelfth rib, however in eleventh rib it may be ill defined.

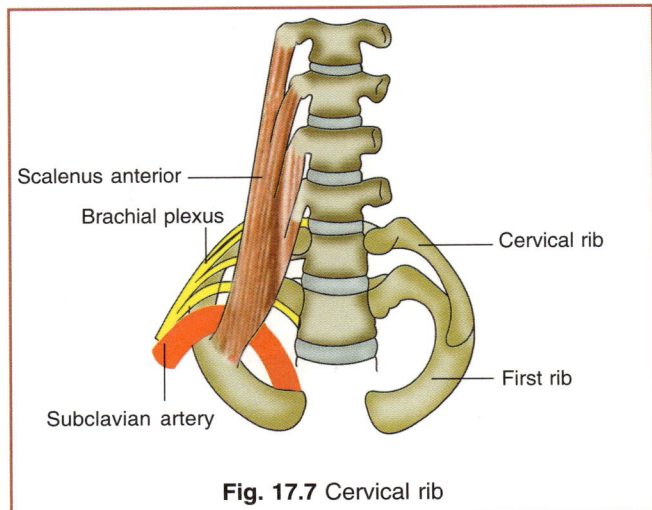

Fig. 17.7 Cervical rib

- The middle ribs are most commonly fractured from blows or from crushing injuries (automobile injuries). The weak point of the rib is near (anterior) its angle, however, direct violence may fracture a rib anywhere. Fracture involving this site can penetrate the lungs, liver or spleen. Fractures of the lower ribs may tear the diaphragm and result in diaphragmatic hernia. Rib fractures are painful.
- Ribs may be fractured occasionally during muscular strains (coughing).
- Rib dislocation can occur where costal cartilage articulates with sternum
- Rib separation is the dislocation at the articulation between costal cartilage and ribs
- In coarctation of aorta, X-rays show notching of the ribs due to pressure by intercostal arteries
- Supernumerary ribs: Presence of cervical or lumbar ribs is also known. Presence of Cervical rib can lead to compression of neurovascular structures. Absence of 12th pair of ribs is also known.

Cervical rib syndrome/Scalenus anterior syndrome/thoracic outlet syndrome:

- Clinically the thoracic inlet is referred as thoracic outlet.
- Presence of cervical rib (Fig. 17.7) or a congenitally hypertrophied scalenus anterior muscle can compress the subclavian artery or lower trunk of the brachial plexus.
- Compression of the subclavian artery causes pallor and coldness of the upper limb, feeble radial pulse.
- Compression of the subclavian vein causes distension of the superficial veins of the upper limb, edema and pain in the upper limb
- Compression of the lower trunk of the brachial plexus causes numbness, tingling and pain along the medial border of the hand (C8 and T1) and little finger, wasting of small muscles of the hand

Costal cartilages

The anterior ends of the ribs continue as costal cartilages, providing elasticity to thoracic wall. The cartilages increase in length through first 7 and then gradually decrease. The first 7 costal cartilages directly articulate with sternum, the 8th, 9th and 10th articulates with costal cartilages superior to them forming '**costal margin'.** The 11th and 12th costal cartilages form caps on the anterior ends of the corresponding ribs.

Costal cartilages provide resilience to the thoracic cage and prevent fractures of ribs and sternum. Because of its elasticity, chest compression may produce injury within the thorax without fractures in children. In elderly people, the costal cartilages become brittle and they may undergo calcification. They become radiopaque in X-rays.

CASE -1

On examining a routine postero-anterior chest radiograph of an 85-year-old woman, it was noticed that many of the costal cartilages showed scattered radiopaque areas. What is the likely explanation for these opacities?

CASE -2

A 60-year-old man and a 10-year-old boy were both involved in a severe automobile accident. In both cases the thorax was badly crushed. On X-ray examination, the man had five fractured ribs, but the boy had no fractures. Comment on these findings.

CASE -3

A 32-year-old patient complains of pain while taking a deep breath. Palpation reveals tenderness over midaxillary region of ribs 5 and 6 on the right side. Radiologic findings confirm fractures of these ribs

a. How did you count the correct rib numbers?
b. Do the ribs move during breathing?

S E C T I O N 5

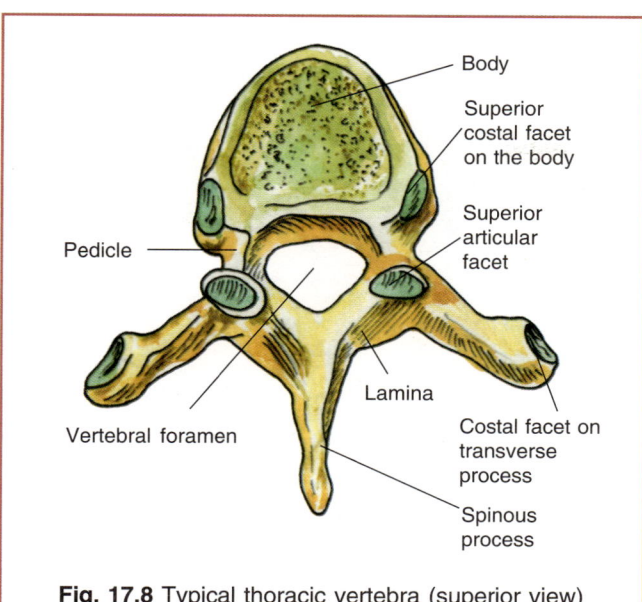

Fig. 17.8 Typical thoracic vertebra (superior view)

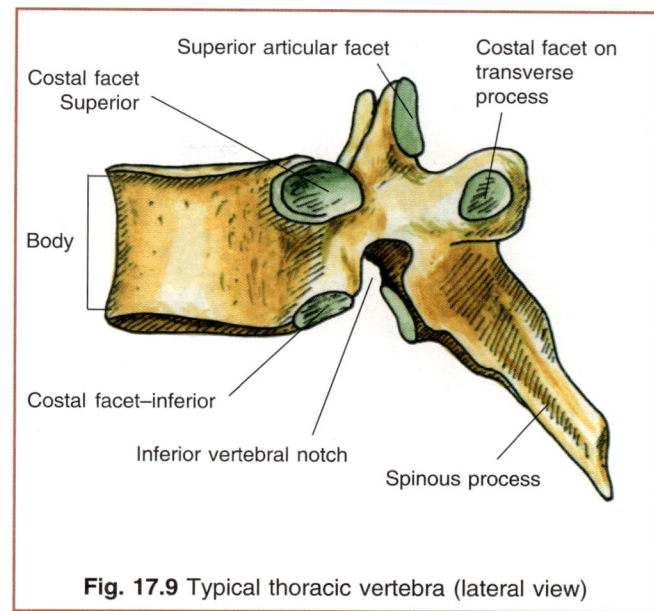

Fig. 17.9 Typical thoracic vertebra (lateral view)

c. How do you explain the pain?

d. What other structures may be at risk?

THORACIC VERTEBRAE

Thoracic vertebrae are 12 in number of which 2nd to 8th thoracic vertebrae are typical, while 1st and 9th to 12th thoracic vertebrae are atypical (Fig. 17.8 superior view and Fig. 17.9 lateral view)

Typical thoracic vertebra

- The body is heart shaped.
- Vertebral foramen is circular.
- The pedicles arise from the lower part of the body and are directed backwards.
- The superior articular facets are directed backwards and laterally and the inferior downwards and medially.
- Transverse process projects backwards and laterally and presents a facet for articulation with the tubercle of the corresponding rib.
- Spinous process is pointed and directed downwards.
- The body presents two superior costal facets close to the upper border and two small inferior costal facets close to the lower border (posterolaterally).

First thoracic vertebra

It is more or less like a typical thorax vertebra. Its body has a complete superior costal facet on each side for the head of the 1st rib, but inferior facet is half (demifacet) for the

head of the 2nd rib. Its spine is nearly horizontal and superior vertebral notch is well marked (unlike typical thoracic vertebra)

Tenth thoracic vertebra

Its body has only one complete costal facet on each side near its upper part.

Eleventh thoracic vertebra

Its body has one complete facet on each side, which are placed near the upper part of the pedicle. Its transverse process does not have any articular facet.

Twelfth thoracic vertebra

Its shape is like a lumbar vertebra. The costal facet on each side is placed near lower part of the body.

JOINTS OF THE THORAX

Manubriosternal joint

Between the body and the manubrium of the sternum. It is a secondary cartilaginous joint.

Costovertebral joint

The head of a typical rib articulates with the numerically corresponding vertebra and the vertebra above. It is a plane synovial joint (Figs 17.10 and 17.11).

Costotransverse joint

The tubercle of a typical rib articulates with the transverse process of the corresponding vertebra. It is a synovial joint (Figs 17.10 and 17.11).

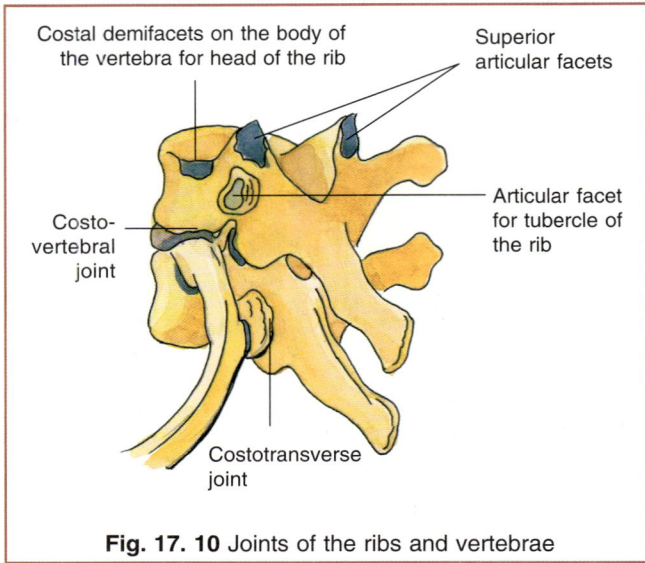

Fig. 17. 10 Joints of the ribs and vertebrae

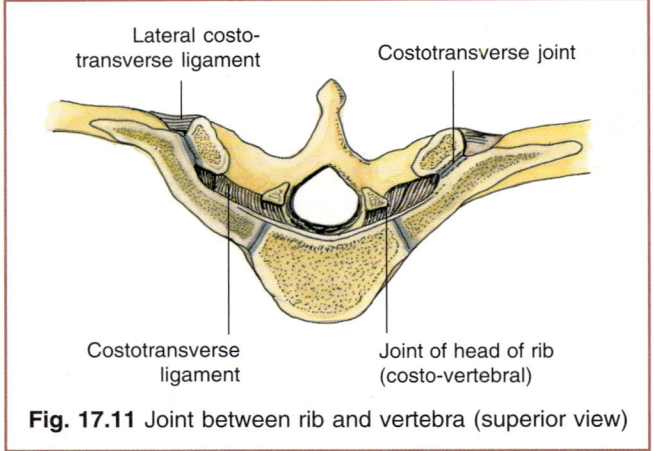

Fig. 17.11 Joint between rib and vertebra (superior view)

Costochondral joint

Each rib continues anteriorly with its cartilage. It is a primary cartilaginous joint.

Chondrosternal joint (between costal cartilages and sternum)

The first chondrosternal joint is primary cartilaginous, and it does not permit any movement. The remaining 2nd to 7th costal cartilages articulate with the sternum by synovial joints.

INLET OF THE THORAX

It is bounded posteriorly by body of 1st thoracic vertebra, on each side by 1st rib and its costal cartilage and anteriorly

by superior border of manubrium sterni. The aperture slopes anteroinferiorly due to obliquity of 1st pair of ribs.

This kidney shaped aperture transmits structures between neck and thorax.

The adult superior thoracic aperture measures about 6.5 cm anteroposteriorly and 11 cm transversely. Following are the important structures passing through it (Fig.17.12)

In the midline:

Sternothyroid and sternohyoid muscles, Inferior thyroid veins, Trachea and oesophagus

On the right side of the midline:
Brachiocephalic artery, Rt.brachiocephalic vein

On the left side of the midline:
Left common carotid artery, left brachiocephalic vein, left recurrent laryngeal nerve and thoracic duct (Fig.17.12)

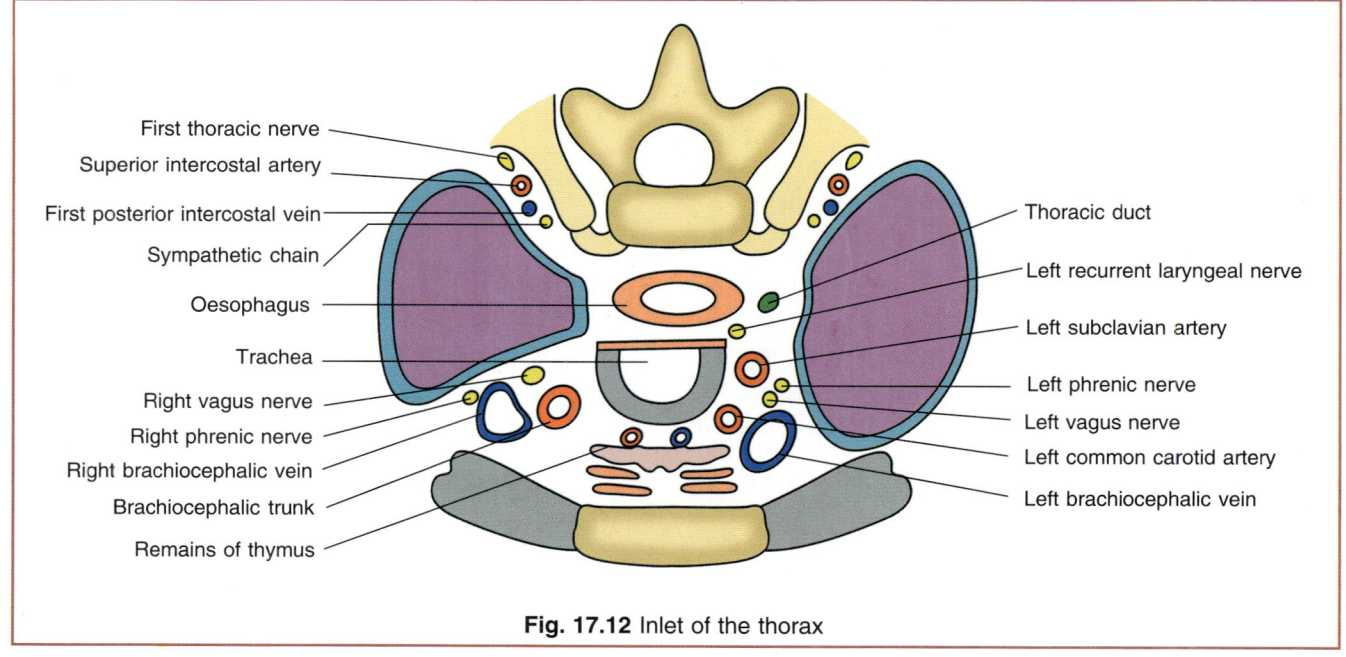

Fig. 17.12 Inlet of the thorax

Outlet of the thorax (Inferior thoracic aperture)

It is irregular in outline and it is closed by the diaphragm. It is also oblique, the posterior thoracic wall is longer than anterior.

MUSCLES OF THE THORACIC WALL

Thoracic wall muscles include intercostal, subcostal, sternocostalis, levator costae and serratus posterior.

The thoracic cage forms the skeletal framework of the walls of the thorax. The gaps between the ribs are called **intercostal spaces**, which are filled up by intercostal muscles (Figs 17.13 to 17.15) They are:

1. External intercostal muscles

- In each intercostal space they extend from the angle of the ribs posteriorly to costochondral junction anteriorly.
- Between the lateral margin of the sternum and costochondral junction it is represented by external intercostal (anterior intercostal) membrane.
- Each muscle arises from inferior border of upper ribs and is attached to superior border of lower ribs.
- The direction of the muscle fibres are downwards and medially.
- They elevate the ribs during forced inspiration.

2. Internal intercostal muscles

- They are present deep to the external intercostal muscle and its fibres are directed right angle to the direction of external intercostal muscles.

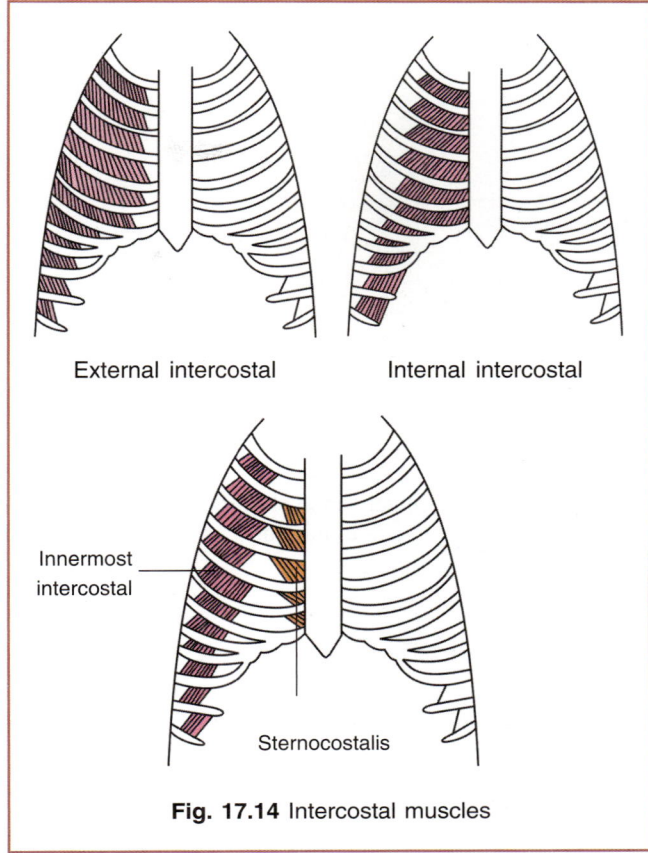

External intercostal　　　　　　　Internal intercostal

Innermost intercostal

Sternocostalis

Fig. 17.14 Intercostal muscles

- In each intercostal space they extend from the angle of the ribs posteriorly to lateral border of the sternum anteriorly.
- In the posterior part of the intercostal space (beyond the angles of the ribs) it is represented by internal intercostal membrane (posterior intercostal).
- Each muscle arises from the floor of the costal grooves and inserted to superior border of the ribs inferior to them.
- Its interchondral part elevates the ribs (inspiration) and interosseous part depresses the ribs (expiration).

3. Innermost intercostal muscles (Intercostalis intimi)

- They are present deep to the internal intercostal muscle in the middle and lateral part of the intercostal spaces, but separated from them by intercostal nerve and vessels.
- The direction of the muscle fibres are same as internal intercostal muscles
- They extend from inner surface of the upper ribs to inner surface of the ribs below (Fig.17.15)

Subcostalis, Sternocostalis and Intercostalis intimi muscles are often grouped as Transversus thoracis.

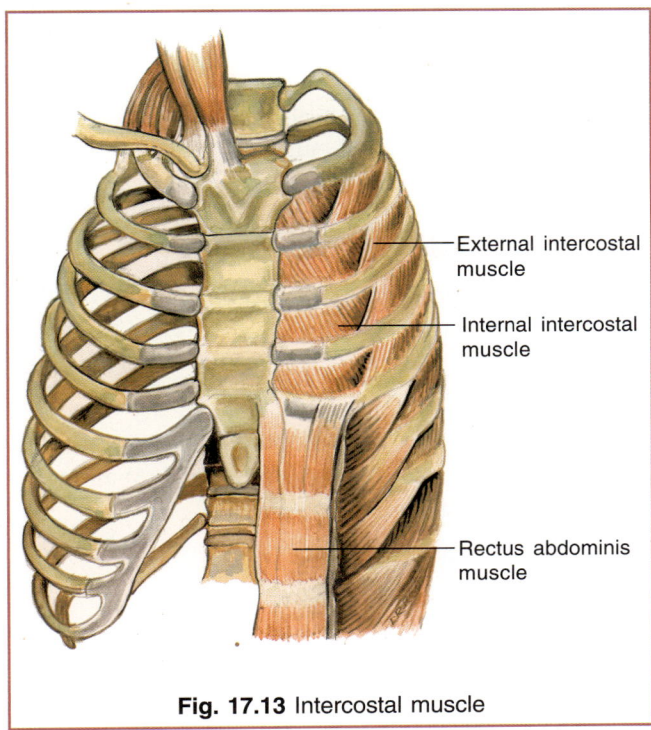

External intercostal muscle

Internal intercostal muscle

Rectus abdominis muscle

Fig. 17.13 Intercostal muscle

S E C T I O N 5

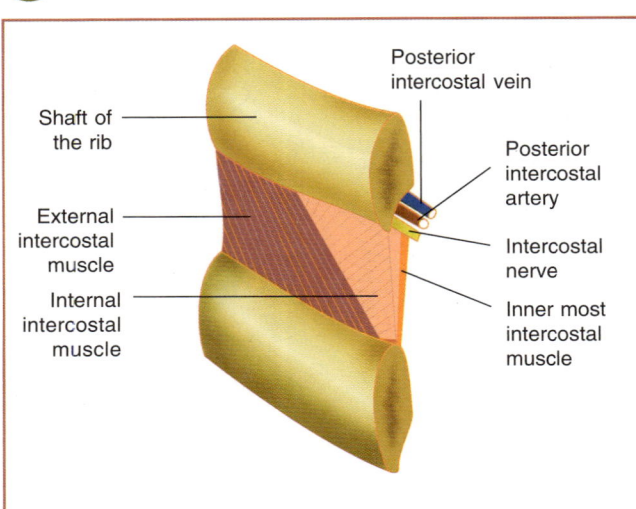

Fig. 17.15 Intercostal space showing arrangement of the muscles

Subcostalis

They arise from inner surface of lower ribs near their angles and extend to superior border of 2 or 3 ribs below. They are better defined in lower intercostal spaces only.

Sternocostalis

It arises from the posterior surface of the lower part of the sternum. It extends to inner surface of 2nd to 6th costal cartilages (Fig.17.15).

All these muscles are supplied by the intercostal nerves (Thoracic spinal nerves).

The main action of the intercostal muscles is to prevent retraction of the intercostal spaces during inspiration, and bulging during expiration.

The role of intercostal muscles in producing the movements of the ribs appear to be related mainly in forced respiration, the diaphragm being primary muscle of inspiration and expiration is passive (due to elastic tissues of the lungs).

Levator costarum, Serratus posterior superior and Serratus posterior inferior muscles also contribute to the thoracic wall.

RESPIRATORY MOVEMENTS

Inspiratory movement

Increase in thoracic volume (decrease in intrapulmonary pressure) is achieved by movement of thoracic wall and diaphragm.

The increase in anteroposterior diameter of the thorax is due to contraction of intercostal muscles. Movement of the ribs (2nd to 6th) at the costo vertebral joints around an axis passing through necks of the ribs causes anterior ends

of the ribs to rise. Since anterior ends of the ribs are directed downwards, their elevation results in anteroposterior movement of the sternum. This is called '**pump handle movement**'.

The increase in transverse diameter of the thorax is also due to contraction of intercostal muscles. Movements of lower ribs elevates the middle part of the ribs, thus increasing transverse diameter. This is called '**bucket handle movement**'

The increase in vertical diameter is due to contraction of the diaphragm. When diaphragm contracts, it descends, which leads to increase in vertical diameter of the thorax.

With increase in the thoracic volume, the pressure inside the lung is reduced. So air is drawn into the lungs through, nose, mouth, larynx and trachea.

Expiratory movement

The air is expelled out from the lung, due to elastic recoiling tendency of the lungs. It is a passive act. The diaphragm and intercostal muscle relax, thus decreasing the thoracic volume and increasing the pressure inside the lungs.

Muscles involved

Chief muscles of Inspiration: Diaphragm, External intercostal and Interchondral portion of the internal intercostal muscle.

Chief muscles of Expiration: Interosseus part of the internal intercostal muscle

---

CASE -4

A mother, on looking at her newborn baby lying on its back in a cradle, was astonished and horrified to see its anterior abdominal wall bulging in and out with each respiration. Can you explain this in anatomical terms?

Typical intercostal space

The spaces between the typical ribs that are traversed by intercostal nerves supplying only thorax are known as 'typical intercostal spaces'. The 3rd, 4th, 5th and 6th intercostal spaces are typical.

Each space is directed downwards and forward. It is narrow at the posterior part (towards vertebra) and wider at the anterior part (towards sternum).

Contents

Intercostal muscles, nerves and vessels.

Endothoracic fascia

The thoracic cage is internally lined by thin fibroareolar membrane called endothoracic fascia. It connects the costal part of the parietal pleura to the inner aspect of the thoracic wall. It is better defined over the apices of the lungs as the suprapleural membrane.

Suprapleural membrane (Sibson's fascia)

It is the thickened part of the endothoracic fascia (or from scalenus minimus/pleuralis muscle) covering the cervical pleura and the apex of the lung which lies deep to it. It is attached to the inner border of the 1st rib and its costal cartilage and tip of the transverse process of 7th cervical vertebra. It prevents puffing off of lung apex during expiratory phase of respiration.

CASE -5

A Carpenter who had received knife wound in the neck two years back noticed that when he blew his nose or sneezed, the skin above the clavicle bulged upward. Explain this upward bulging of the skin in anatomical terms.

INTERCOSTAL NERVES

The 12 pairs of thoracic spinal nerves supply the thoracic wall after dividing into anterior and posterior primary rami. The posterior rami of thoracic spinal nerves pass posteriorly to supply the muscles and skin of the back. The anterior primary rami of 1st to 11th thoracic spinal nerves are called intercostal nerves since they course through intercostal space. The anterior primary ramus of 12th thoracic spinal nerve is called subcostal nerve.

The anterior primary ramus of 1st thoracic spinal nerve divides into 2 branches. The larger branch joins with anterior primary ramus (ventral ramus) of 8th cervical spinal nerve to form lower trunk of the brachial plexus. It means T1 fibres are distributed through upper limb. The smaller branch of anterior primary ramus of 1st thoracic spinal nerve form 1st intercostal nerve, which courses along the under surface of the 1st rib. **It does not give any cutaneous branch**.

The 2nd intercostal nerve gives lateral cutaneous branch and is called 'intercostobrachial nerve', which supplies skin of the floor of the axilla. The 7th to 11th intercostal nerves in addition to intercostal spaces, also supplies anterior abdominal wall.

Typical intercostal nerves

The 3rd to 6th intercostal nerves, which are confined only to thoracic wall, are called 'typical intercostal nerves' (Fig. 17.16).

Course

a. At the posterior ends of the intercostal space (vertebral end), each intercostal nerve travel between parietal pleura and posterior intercostal membrane, crossing behind the sympathetic chain.

b. Each nerve, medial to the angle of the rib enter the costal groove along with intercostal vessels. The arrangement of the structures from above downwards in a costal groove is '**VAN**'-vein, artery and nerve.

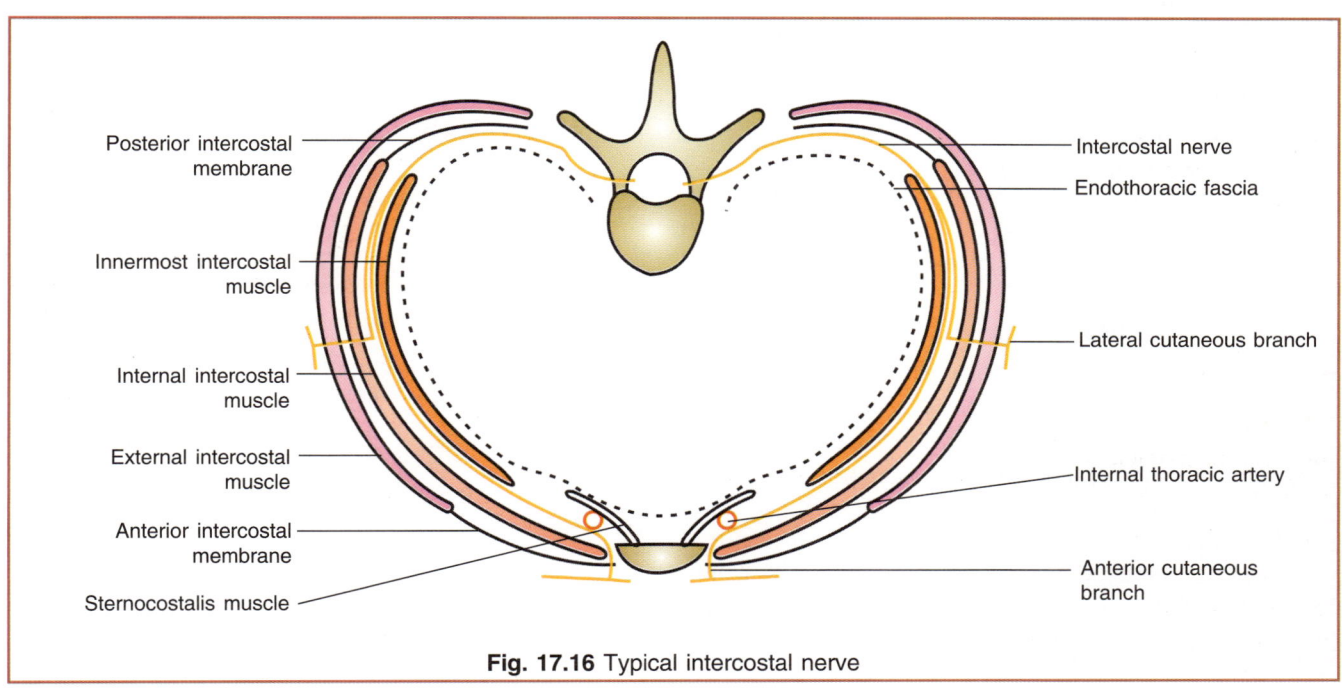

Fig. 17.16 Typical intercostal nerve

c. The nerve proceeds between internal intercostal and innermost intercostal muscles.

d. Near the anterior ends of the intercostal space (sternal end), each nerve crosses in front of the internal thoracic artery, pierces internal intercostal muscle, anterior intercostal membrane, pectoralis major muscle. It terminates as anterior cutaneous nerve

Branches and Distribution

1. **Collateral branch:** It arises near the angle of the rib and proceeds in the lower part of the same intercostal space (upper margin of the lower ribs). It may join the main trunk in the anterior part of the intercostal space. It supplies intercostal muscles and parietal pleura.

2. **Lateral cutaneous branch:** It arises near the angle of the rib, runs with main trunk. At the midaxillary line it pierces the intercostal muscles and becomes superficial. It divides into anterior and posterior branches, which supplies skin of the lateral thoracic wall.

3. **Muscular branches:** It supplies intercostal muscles, subcostal, sternocostalis, and 4th and 5th typical intercostal nerve also supplies serratus posterior superior.

4. **Sensory branches:** The intercostal nerves apart from supplying skin and muscles, they also carry sensory (pain) fibres from parietal pleura. (The atypical, thoracoabdominal intercostal nerves, apart from supplying skin and muscles of the anterior abdominal wall, it also supplies parietal peritoneum.)

5. **Anterior cutaneous branches:** They are the continuation of intercostal nerves, pierces the muscles on either side of the sternum to become superficial). After dividing into medial and lateral branches, it supplies the skin of the anterior aspect of the sternum.

Components of Intercostal nerve

1. Afferent-cutaneous sensation from thoracic and abdominal wall

2. Afferent-sensation from costal and peripheral part of the diaphragmatic pleura

3. Efferent-Motor fibres to intercostal muscles

4. Efferent-Sympathetic fibres present in it is, supplies sweat glands (sudomotor), erector pilorum muscle of the dermis (pilomotor) and the smooth muscles present at the wall of the blood vessels (vasomotor)

- **Intercostal nerve block:** To produce anesthesia in one or two intercostal space, anaesthetic solution is injected around the intercostal nerve. The Intercostal nerve can be blocked anywhere proximal to the mid-axillary line, where the lateral cutaneous branch originates. In children, the block is commonly carried out at the posterior axillary line. In adults, the most popular site for Intercostal nerve block is at the angle of the rib (6–8 cm from the spinous processes of vertebrae). At the angle of the rib, the rib is relatively superficial and easy to palpate and the costal groove is the widest, theoretically reducing the probability of pleural puncture. Blockade medial to the angle of the rib is not recommended because the nerve lies deep to the posterior intercostal membrane with very little tissue between it and the parietal pleura, while the overlying sacrospinalis muscle makes rib palpation difficult. Blockade distal to the anterior axillary line is more difficult because the nerve has left the costal groove and re-entered the intercostal space and lies in the substance of the internal intercostal muscle. Intercostal nerve block is used in a great variety of acute and chronic pain conditions affecting the thorax and upper abdomen. Complete loss of sensation usually does not occur unless 2 or more intercostal nerves are anaesthetized.

- **Herpes Zoster Infection:** Herpes zoster, commonly known as shingles is a viral disease characterized by a painful skin rashes with blisters in a limited area on one side of the body, often in a stripe. Years or decades after a chickenpox infection, the virus may break out of nerve cell bodies (example; dorsal root ganglia) and travel down nerve axons to cause viral infection of the skin in the region, supplied by that particular spinal nerve (dermatome). It can also associate with muscular weakness.

- The diseases of the thoracic vertebrae may irritate the intercostal nerves and pus from the tuberculous thoracic vertebrae may track along the neurovascular plane.

ARTERIES OF THE THORACIC WALL

Internal thoracic artery (Internal mammary artery)

Origin: It arises from the under surface of the 1st part of the subclavian artery.

Course

The artery is crossed by phrenic nerve near its origin. It descends lateral to the sternum, deep to the costal cartilages anterior to sternocostalis muscle. At the 6th intercostal space it ends by dividing into 2 terminal branches; superior epigastric artery and musculophrenic artery. Internal thoracic artery is accompanied by venae commitantes (pair of veins)

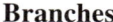

Branches

1. **Anterior intercostal arteries:** In the upper 6 intercostal space, there are 2 anterior intercostal arteries. The upper branch, anastomose with main trunk of the posterior intercostal artery, whereas the lower branch anastomose with collateral branch of the posterior intercostal artery.

2. **Pericardiophrenic artery:** It accompanies the phrenic nerve

3. Pericardial, thymic, sternal and mediastinal branches

4. Perforating branches in 2nd and 3rd intercostal space in females supply mammary gland

5. The superior epigastric artery enters rectus sheath through xiphoid and sternal origins of diaphragm.

6. The musculophrenic artery descends obliquely parallel to costal margin. Apart from supplying diaphragm, it also gives anterior intercostal arteries of 7th to 9th intercostal space.

- The internal thoracic artery is the cardiac surgeon's artery of choice for coronary artery bypass grafting. It has superior long-term patency compared to saphenous vein grafts. Several histological (more elastic tissue), physiological (release more nitric oxide, which inhibits proliferation of smooth muscles in tunica intima) and anatomical (nearer to the coronary artery) advantages of internal thoracic artery is claimed.

Intercostal arteries

In each intercostal space there are 2 anterior intercostal arteries and 1 posterior intercostal artery (with exception of 10th and 11th intercostal spaces).

In the upper 6 intercostal space, anterior intercostal arteries are branches of internal thoracic artery, while in 7th to 9th intercostal space, they are branches of musculophrenic artery.

Posterior intercostal arteries

In the upper 2 intercostal spaces, it arises from superior intercostal artery (a branch of the costocervical trunk of the subclavian artery). In the remaining spaces it arises from descending thoracic aorta (Fig.17.18).

Right posterior intercostal arteries are longer, since thoracic aorta is slightly to the left of the vertebral column and have to cross in front of the vertebral bodies. Each posterior intercostal artery is accompanied by posterior intercostal vein and intercostal nerve in the costal groove.

Anteriorly they end by anastomosing with upper anterior intercostal arteries. The 3rd right posterior intercostal artery can give origin to right bronchial artery.

The anastomoses between anterior and posterior intercostal arteries provide a connection between subclavian artery and thoracic aorta. These anastomoses become important in case of coarctation of aorta providing collateral circulation.

The venous drainage of the thoracic wall is discussed in the chapter–posterior mediastinum

Lymphatic drainage of the thoracic wall

Parasternal nodes

These are placed along the internal thoracic vessels. They drain deeper tissue of the anterior thoracic wall and anterior abdominal wall (up to the level of umbilicus) and also mammary gland. The efferent lymphatic vessels arising from them join broncho mediastinal trunk (refer lymphatic drainage of lungs).

Posterior intercostal nodes

These are located at the posterior ends of the intercostal spaces. They drain part of the mammary gland and posterolateral wall of the thoracic wall. Their efferent vessels drain into thoracic duct.

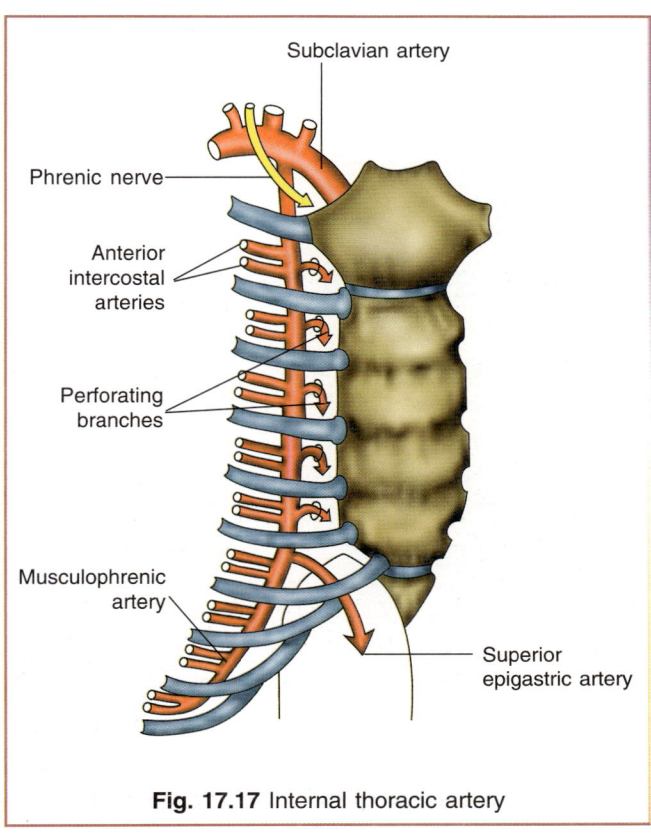

Fig. 17.17 Internal thoracic artery

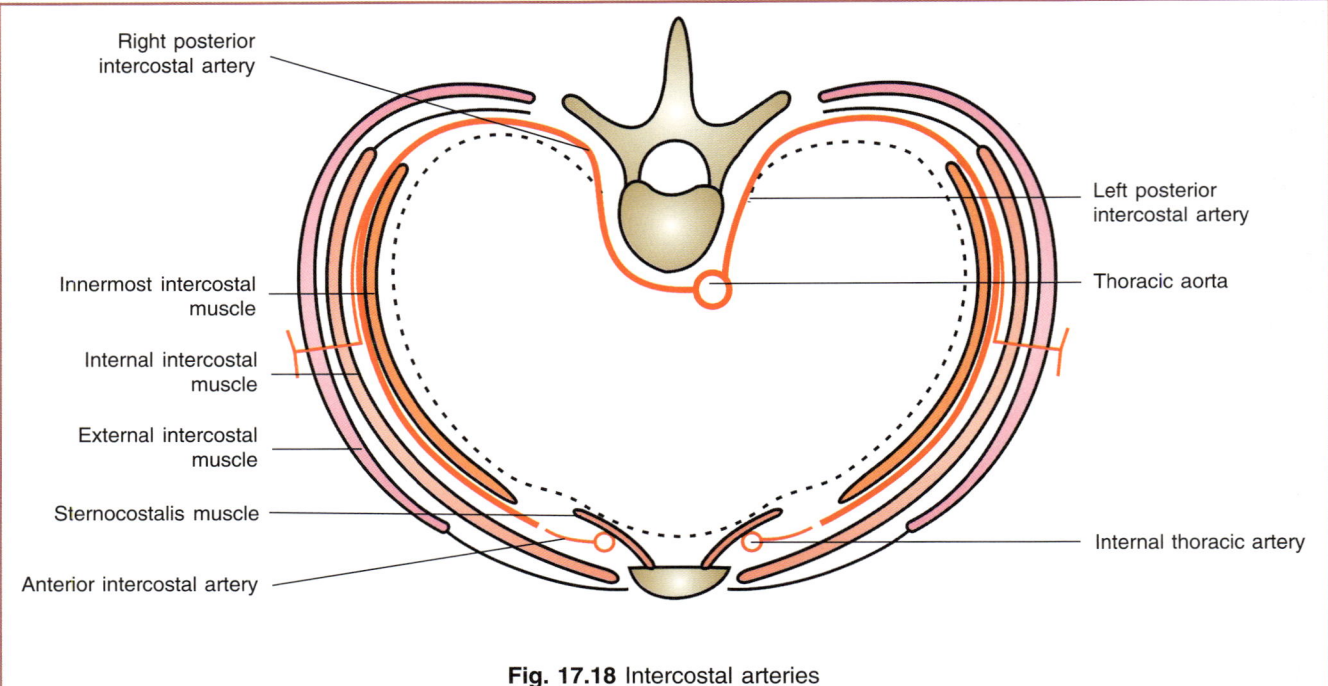

Fig. 17.18 Intercostal arteries

Labels: Right posterior intercostal artery; Innermost intercostal muscle; Internal intercostal muscle; External intercostal muscle; Sternocostalis muscle; Anterior intercostal artery; Left posterior intercostal artery; Thoracic aorta; Internal thoracic artery

Clinical examination of thoracic wall:

1. **Inspection and Palpation:** Usually inspection and palpation are discussed together because there is an intimate relationship between these two procedures in the chest examination. Palpation not only confirms the results of inspection, but also discovers diagnostic signs.

2. **Percussion:** The chest is percussed to confirm the cardiac borders, size, contour and position in the thorax,

3. **Auscultation:** The purpose of auscultation of the heart is to find the normal and abnormal sounds of the heart. It plays a very important role in the diagnosis of heart diseases.

- **Funnel chest (Pectus excavatum):** It is the most common congenital deformity of the anterior wall of the chest, in which several ribs and the sternum grow abnormally. This produces a caved-in or sunken appearance of the chest. It can either be present at birth or not develop until puberty.

- Pectus excavatum is sometimes referred to as cobbler's chest, sunken chest or funnel chest. The hallmark of the condition is a sunken appearance of the sternum. The heart can be displaced and/or rotated.

- **Pigeon test (Pectus carinatum):** It is a deformity of the chest characterized by a protrusion of the sternum and ribs. It is the opposite of pectus excavatum. Pectus carinatum is an overgrowth of cartilage causing the sternum to protrude forward. People with pectus carinatum usually develop normal hearts and lungs. In moderate to severe cases of pectus carinatum, the chest wall is rigidly held in an outward position. Thus, respiration is inefficient and the individual needs to use the diaphragm and accessory muscles for respiration, rather than normal chest muscles, during strenuous exercise. This negatively affects gas exchange and causes a decrease in stamina. Children with pectus deformities often tire sooner than their peers, due to shortness of breath and fatigue.

Surface landmarks

Sternal notch

It is above the manubrium sterni. In normal condition trachea is felt deep to the notch.

Sternal angle (Angle of Louis)

It is also called Louis angle. It is formed by the protrusion of the conjunction composed of sternum and manubrium sterni. It connects bilaterally to each of the right and left second costal cartilage. It acts as an important landmark for counting rib and intercostal spaces, and indicates the bifurcation of the trachea, the upper level of the atria of heart, the demarcation of upper and lower part of mediastinum, and the fifth thoracic vertebra as well.

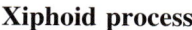
Xiphoid process

It is the protruding triangular part of the lower end of the sternum with its base connected to the sternum. The length of xiphoid process in normal subject varies widely.

Thoracic spines

It marks the posterior midline. The seventh cervical spinous process at the base of the neck is most prominent, usually serves as the hallmark for counting the thoracic vertebrae which start just following it. The spinous process of the scapulae corresponds medially to third thoracic spine and inferior angle of the scapulae to seventh thoracic spine.

> ### CASE -6
>
> A patient with tenderness over the spine of the thoracic vertebra that is on a level with the inferior angle of the scapula. To which thoracic vertebra does the spine belong?

Solutions to the clinical case studies

Case-1

In old age the costal cartilages may undergo ossification. They then become radioopaque and this may give rise to some confusion when examining a chest radiograph of an elderly patient.

Case-2

The thoracic wall of the child is very elastic, and fractures of ribs in children are rare. But in aged people the ribs become brittle and are more prone to be fractured.

Case-3

a. The ribs are usually counted from the level of sternal angle which corresponds to second costal cartilage. There are other bony land marks which also help to determine the correct rib number like, xyphisternal joint corresponds to seventh costal cartilage.

b. Ribs move during respiratory movements (Refer bucket handle and pump handle movement in respiratory movements)

c. Pain is due to fracture of the ribs

d. Lungs

Case-4

Abdominal breathing is normal in infants because the lungs have not expanded enough and so only minimum chest expansion can be noted. As child grows the abdominal breathing gets replaced by chest breathing. A newborn does not breathe evenly like we adults do, in and out. Instead, they breathe in clusters of many breaths followed by long pauses that can be terrifying for new parents.

Case-5

The suprapleural membrane was damaged by knife and was not repaired during surgery. Subsequently, herniation of the cervical pleura and apex of the lung took place, which resulted in the skin above the clavicle bulging upward during forced expiration.

Case-6

Seventh thoracic vertebra

MCQs

1. The second costal cartilage can be located by palpating the:
   A. Costal margin
   B. Sternal angle
   C. Sternal notch
   D. Sternoclavicular joint

2. The tubercle of the 7th rib articulates with which structure?
   A. Body of vertebra T6
   B. Body of vertebra T7
   C. Body of vertebra T8
   D. Transverse process of vertebra T7

3. A physician is demonstrating the correct technique for inserting a subclavian central venous line. He has a medical student palpating the clavicle, then the chest wall below it. The first bony structure that can be palpated below the inferior margin of the medial portion of the clavicle is the
   A. Acromion
   B. Atlas
   C. First rib
   D. Second rib

4. A wrestler's chest is compressed during a match, causing a posterior displacement of the clavicle at the sternoclavicular joint. Which of the following structures would be mostly at risk?
   A. Aorta
   B. Oesophagus
   C. Trachea
   D. Superior vena cava

5. A medical student inserting an intercostal drain for the first time forgets her anatomy and passes it at the lower border of the rib. The structure most likely to be damaged is the
   A. Intercostal artery

B. Intercostal nerve

C. Intercostal vein

D. Internal intercostal muscle

6. A 23-year-old female college student is involved in an automobile accident. She sustains a blunt force injury to the chest, resulting in fracture of the left seventh rib. The patient is experiencing severe pain from this fracture. To relieve this pain, a resident administers a local anesthetic. Which of the following sites would be the most appropriate site for this injection?

   A. Seventh intercostal space immediately below the seventh rib in the midclavicular line

   B. Seventh intercostal space immediately below the seventh rib just lateral to the angle of the rib

   C. Seventh intercostal space immediately below the seventh rib just medial to the angle of the rib

   D. Sixth intercostal space immediately above the seventh   rib in the midclavicular line

7. Which of the following layers provides a natural cleavage plane for surgical separation of the costal pleura from the thoracic wall?

   A. Deep fascia

   B. Endothoracic fascia

   C. Parietal pleura

   D. Visceral pleura

8. A patient runs into the hospital complaining of dyspnea (shortness of breathe). He complains that breathing in air is difficult. Which of the following is a muscle of inspiration?

   A. Rectus abdominus

   B. Internal intercostal

   C. Innermost intercostal

   D. Interchondral part of internal intercostal

9. A doctor informs his colleague to insert a catheter in a patient at the seventh intercostal space. Which of the following is the correct insertion point of catheter

   A. Just above seventh rib

   B. Just below seventh rib

   C. Just above the eighth rib

   D. Just below the eighth rib

Answers to MCQs

1. B

2. D

3. D

4. C

5. B

6. B

7. B

8. D

9. C

- Pleura and its subdivision
- Pleural reflections
- Pleural recesses
- Nerve supply and blood supply to the pleura
- MCQs

Objectives

- To explain the different subdivisions of the pleura, their nerve supply and its clinical relevance
- To explain the anatomy of the pleural recesses and their clinical relevance
- To explain the anatomy of the thoracocentesis

PLEURA AND ITS SUBDIVISION

It is a fibroserous membrane covering the lungs. This membrane is lined by mesothelial cells, which secrete serous fluid into the pleural cavity. Each pleural sac is invaginated by the lung from the medial side; hence it consists of a visceral and a parietal layer with pleural cavity in between them (Figs 18.1 and 18.2).

1. **Visceral (pulmonary) pleura:** It closely invests the lungs, except at the hilum.

2. **Parietal pleura:** It lines inner aspect of the thoracic wall, upper surface of the diaphragm, mediastinum and under surface of the suprapleural membrane. It is named according to the structures it lines. They are

Costal pleura

It lines the inner surface of the sternum, ribs and their costal cartilages and intercostal muscles. All these structures are separated from it by endothoracic fascia. At the first intercostal space, the internal thoracic artery

is directly related to it. Posteriorly it is reflected in front of the sympathetic chain.

Diaphragmatic pleura

It covers the upper surface of the diaphragm.

Cervical pleura

The costal pleura, above the level of 1st rib form cervical pleura. It extends to the root of the neck covering the apex of the lung. Its upper surface is covered by suprapleural membrane.

Mediastinal pleura

It covers the lateral aspect of the mediastinum. The heart with pericardium is separated from medial surface of lung by mediastinal pleura. It is reflected over the root of the lung and extends below the root as double layered fold called **pulmonary ligament**. Through this the parietal pleura continues with visceral pleura. There is a potential space between the two layers of the pulmonary ligament, which provides a dead space for expansion of inferior pulmonary veins during increased

SECTION 5

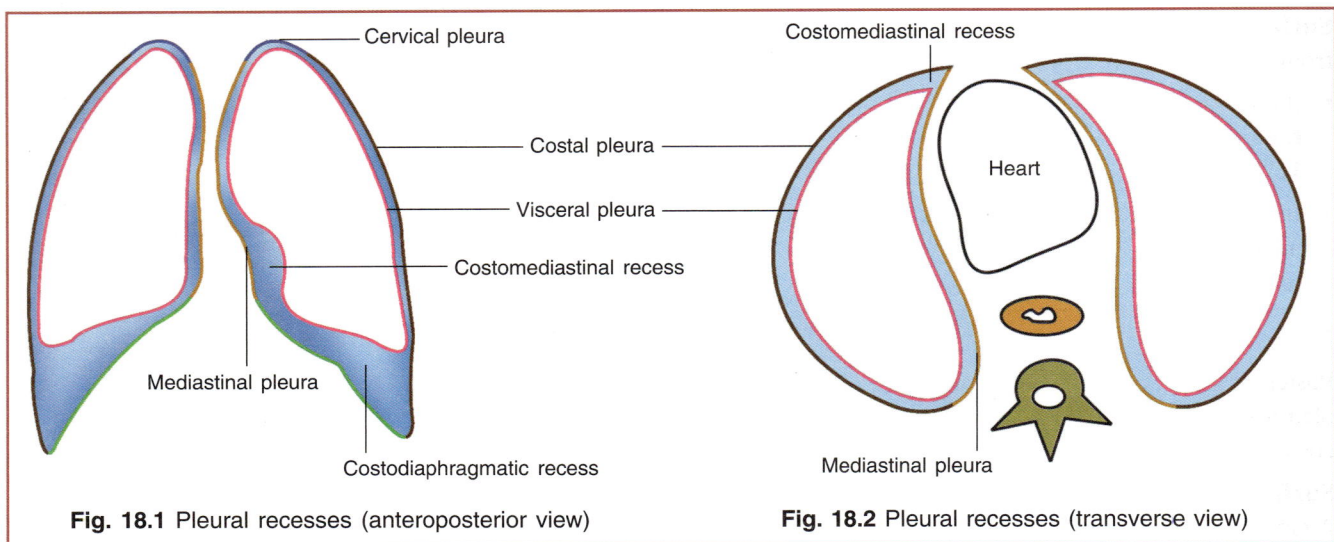

Fig. 18.1 Pleural recesses (anteroposterior view)

Fig. 18.2 Pleural recesses (transverse view)

venous return and also for descent of root of the lung during inspiration.

The space between the visceral and parietal pleura forms the pleural cavity (or pleural space). Normally it contains a small volume of pleural fluid and is a narrow space. The fluid allows the lungs to glide freely without friction over thoracic wall during breathing movements. The lymphatic vessels drain the pleural fluid continuously. The pressure inside the pleural cavity is negative (about −2 mm Hg and during inspiration it drops to about −8 mm Hg), which is necessary to retain the visceral pleura in contact with parietal pleura. When the negative pressure collapse (entry of air or fluid), the lungs will collapse because of its elastic recoiling tendency. It pulls the visceral pleura away from the parietal pleura.

The lungs are comparable to an inflated balloon when they are distended. If the distension is not maintained, their inherent elasticity will cause them to collapse. An inflamed balloon remains (lungs) distended even when the airway passages are open because the outer surface of the lungs (visceral pleura) adhere to the inner surface of the thoracic walls (parietal pleura) as a result of surface tension provided by the pleural fluid.

PLEURAL REFLECTIONS

Costomediastinal line

Anteriorly the costal pleura become continuous with the mediastinal pleura, and is called costomediastinal pleural reflection. It is related to anterior border of the lungs extending from the apex of the lung.

Surface marking: A line connecting the following points will mark the costomediastinal reflection.

- A point behind the sternoclavicular joint, a point near the midpoint of the sternal angle.

- Further the costomediastinal line differs on right and left side. On right side the third point is xiphisternal angle near the midline.

- On left side the third point is at the level of 4th costal cartilage. From this point, draw oblique line descending close to the lateral margin of the sternum up to the left 6th costal cartilage (Fig.18.3).

Costodiaphragmatic line

Inferiorly the costal pleura continue with the diaphragmatic pleura along the costodiaphragmatic pleural reflection.

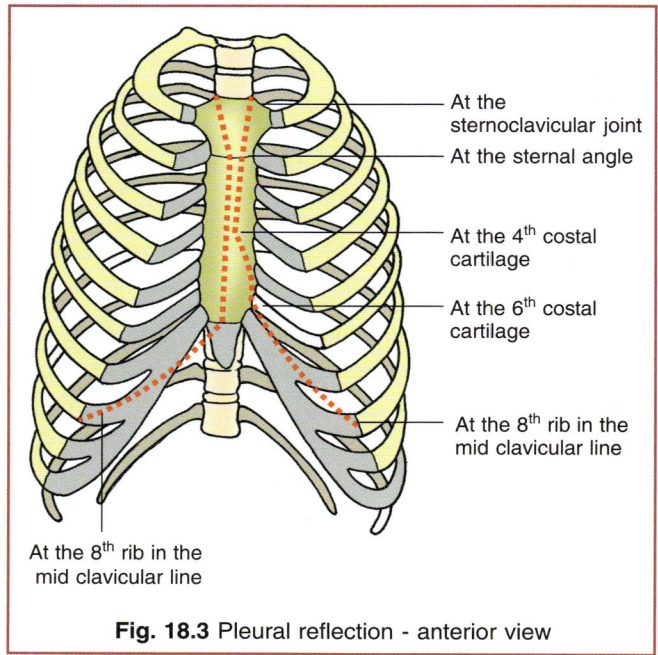

At the sternoclavicular joint

At the sternal angle

At the 4th costal cartilage

At the 6th costal cartilage

At the 8th rib in the mid clavicular line

At the 8th rib in the mid clavicular line

Fig. 18.3 Pleural reflection - anterior view

Surface marking: On the right side, the marking begins from xiphisternal angle.

- It crosses **8th rib in the midclavicular line, 10th rib in the midaxillary line** and ends at a point **2 cm lateral to 12th thoracic spine.**

- It suggests that the lower limit of pleura in the midclavicular line is 8th rib and 10th rib in midaxillary line (Fig.18.3).

Costovertebral line

Posteriorly the costal pleura continues with the mediastinal pleura by the side of the vertebral column and is called costo vertebral pleural reflection.

Surface marking: A vertical line connecting a point 2 cm lateral to the 12th thoracic spine to a point 2 cm lateral to the 7th cervical spine (vertebral prominence) (Fig.18.4).

Cervical pleura

It is marked by a curved line extending posteriorly from a point 2 cm lateral to the 7th cervical spine, a point 2.5 cm above the junction of medial and middle third of the clavicle and finally to a point at the sternoclavicular joint.

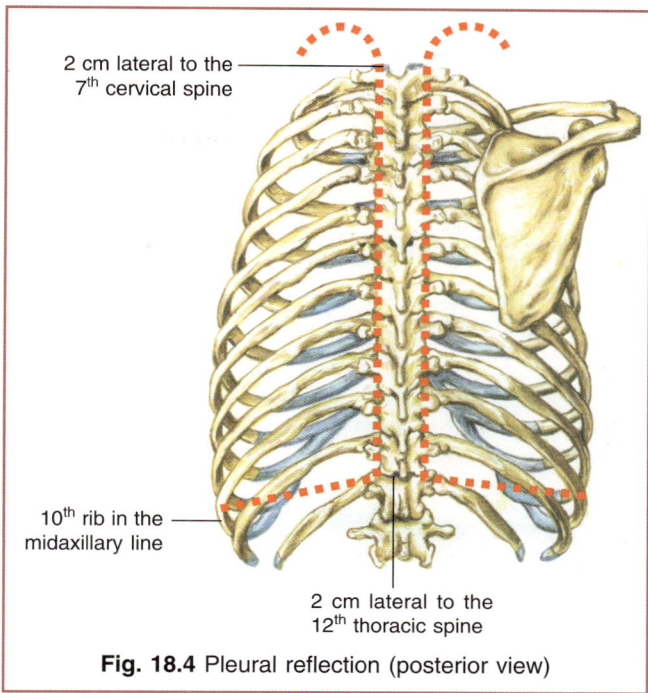

2 cm lateral to the 7th cervical spine

10th rib in the midaxillary line

2 cm lateral to the 12th thoracic spine

Fig. 18.4 Pleural reflection (posterior view)

It is related to anterior borders of the lungs (during deep inspiration). The right costodiaphragmatic recess is narrow and uniform in size. The left costomediastinal recess is well defined between 4th to 6th costal cartilages due to the cardiac notch of the left lung (deviation in the anterior border of the left lung). Because of this cardiac notch, a small portion of the right ventricle is not covered by lung and this area is dull on percussion (area of superficial cardiac dullness) (Fig. 18.5).

PLEURAL RECESSES

The pleural recesses are extended part of the pleural cavity along the lines of pleural reflections. The lungs do not extend into these spaces during quiet breathing. There are two pleural recesses

1. Costomediastinal recess:

This space is present along the costomediastinal pleural reflection (junction of the costal and mediastinal pleura).

2. Costodiaphragmatic recess:

- This space is present along the costodiaphragmatic pleural reflection (between costal and diaphragmatic pleura).

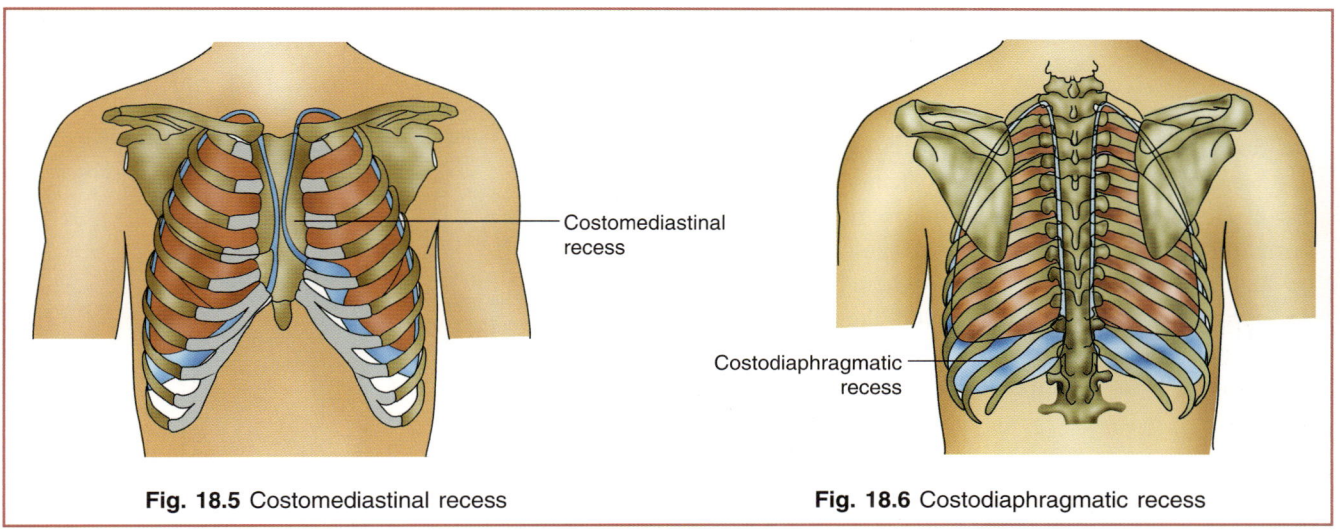

Costomediastinal recess

Fig. 18.5 Costomediastinal recess

Costodiaphragmatic recess

Fig. 18.6 Costodiaphragmatic recess

S E C T I O N 5

- During deep inspiration this space gets obliterated due to downward movement of the lung.
- The recess is deep along the midaxillary line.
- It is the most dependent part of the pleural cavity. If fluid appears in the pleural cavity, it collects first in the costodiaphragmatic recess.
- Excess pleural fluid is drained from costodiaphragmatic recess, hence the relations of this recess is very important.
- On right side it is related to liver and posterior surface of the right kidney and on the left side to spleen, fundus of the stomach and posterior surface of the left kidney (Fig. 18.6).

NERVE AND BLOOD SUPPLY TO THE PLEURA

Nerve supply to Pleura

- The costal pleura and peripheral part of the diaphragmatic pleura are supplied by intercostal nerves.
- The central part of the diaphragmatic pleura and mediastinal pleura are supplied by phrenic nerve (C3, C4, C5).
- These somatic nerves carry pain sensation from the pleura when it is infected. Irritation of the parietal pleura may produce local pain or referred pain projected to dermatomes supplied by the same spinal segment. For example irritation of the mediastinal or central part of the diaphragmatic pleura results in referred pain to the root of the neck and over the shoulder (phrenic nerve C3, C4 and supraclavicular nerve C3, C4).
- The visceral pleura is innervated by autonomic (sympathetic and parasympathetic) nerves supplying the lungs. The visceral pleura is not sensitive to pain or other general sensations.

CASE -1

A 12-year-old boy was rescued from a lake, (who has not learnt to swim). The next day he developed a severe cold, and three days later his general condition deteriorated. He became more febrile and started to cough up blood-stained sputum. At first, he had no chest pain, but later, when he coughed, he experienced severe pain over the right fifth intercostal space in the midclavicular line. The diagnosis of lobar pneumonia was made. Explain the following

a. Why did he not experience chest pain early in the disease?

b. What is the pain due to and why is it worse on coughing?

Blood supply to the pleura

The blood supply to the parietal pleurae is the same vessels supplying thoracic wall (anterior and posterior intercostal vessels) and visceral pleurae is supplied by bronchial vessels.

1. **Pleurisy (pleuritis):**

   It is the inflammation of the pleura. It is characterized with sharp, stabbing pain, which gets aggravated with increased respiratory movements (exertion, such as climbing stairs).

   During normal respiratory movements, the sliding between parietal and visceral pleura is smooth, without any sound during auscultation of the lungs, but in pleurisy, there will be **friction (pleural rub)**, which is detectable with a stethoscope. It sounds like a clump of hair being rolled between the fingers. The inflamed surfaces of the pleura may also cause the parietal and visceral layers of pleura to adhere.

2. **Pneumothorax (air in the pleural space):** The entry of the air into the pleural cavity can result from either penetrating wound of the parietal pleura (bullet entry) or rupture of lung substance into the pleural cavity. Spontaneous pneumothorax is not due to trauma.

   The air in the pleural cavity leads to collapse of the lungs on the affected side. Fractured ribs may also tear the visceral pleura and lung, thus producing the pneumothorax.

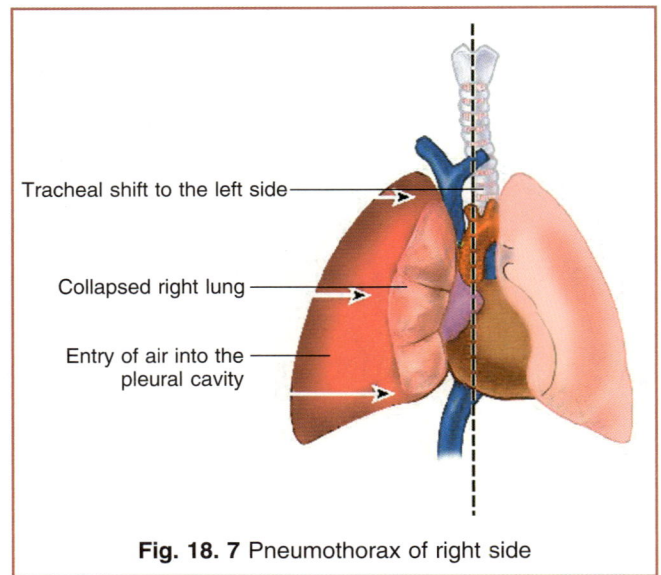

Tracheal shift to the left side

Collapsed right lung

Entry of air into the pleural cavity

Fig. 18. 7 Pneumothorax of right side

SECTION 5

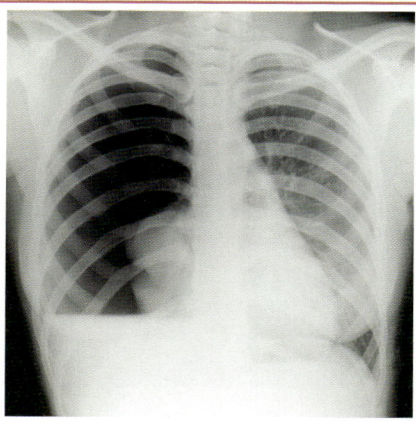

Fig. 18.8 Radiograph showing pneumothorax (Right sided)

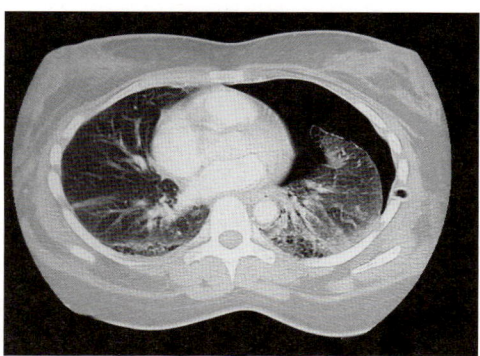

Fig. 18. 9 CT of pneumothorax (Left sided)

The lowering of oxygen tension in blood gives rise to shortness of breath and cyanosis. The mediastinum shifts to the normal side compressing the normal lung also. **The mediastinal shift can be confirmed by palpating the trachea just above the suprasternal notch.** Shift to the same side is also possible due to the absorption while to the opposite side is due to collapse.

When the lungs collapses, it occupies less volume within the pulmonary cavity and the size of the pulmonary cavity is reduced. This can be confirmed with a radiographic picture, with elevation of diaphragm on the affected side, narrowing of the intercostal spaces (ribs closer together) and displacement of the mediastinum (Figs 18.7 to 18.9).

CASE - 2

A 38-year-old patient with a known history of emphysema (dilatation of alveoli and destruction of alveolar walls with tendency to form cystic spaces)

suddenly experiences severe pain in the chest, and he is breathless, and is obviously in a state of shock. On examination, the trachea is found displaced to the right in the suprasternal notch and the apex beat of the heart can be felt in the left 5th intercostal space **just** lateral to the sternum. Assuming the patient has had a spontaneous pneumothorax, explain the following:

a. Why are the trachea and apex beat displaced to the right?

b. Why has the left lung collapsed?

Tension pneumothorax:

It is the presence of air in the pleural space under pressure. The lung collapses, and a mediastinal shift interferes with the expansion of the contralateral lung and compromises venous return to the heart via the IVC. This condition is extremely dangerous and requires urgent intervention. The signs and symptoms of tensionpneumothorax are tachypnea (abnormally rapid respiration rate), contralateral tracheal deviation, distended veins of the neck, dyspnea (difficulty distress in breathing), and hypotension. It is treated with a needle thoracocentesis, followed by chest tube placement (Fig. 18.10).

CASE - 3

A twenty-five-year-old man was brought to the emergency department of the hospital after sustaining a single gunshot wound to the right side of his chest. The paramedics found the patient awake and combative with a palpable pulse, systolic BP of 100 mmHg, and respiratory rate 30/minute. An occlusive dressing was taped over the entry site in the fifth intercostal space, midaxillary line. On arrival, the patient's vital signs were deteriorated.

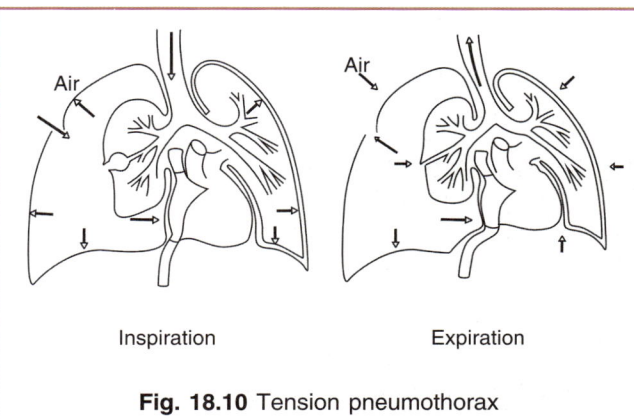

Inspiration   Expiration

Fig. 18.10 Tension pneumothorax

S E C T I O N   5

You note that the patient's trachea is deviated to the left, his jugular veins are distended, he has no breathing sounds on the right side of his chest, he has palpable crepitus (cracking or popping sounds and sensations experienced under skin) and on percussion he has hyper-resonance on the right side of the chest. The physician diagnoses this as tension pneumothorax and inserts a 14 gauge needle in the right midclavicular line at the second intercostal space - air is heard escaping. A chest tube is inserted at the fifth intercostal space in the midaxillary line and connected to a chest drainage device. The patient was stabilized and transferred to the Intensive Care Unit (ICU).

a. What might have created the tension pneumothorax?

b. Why did the resident insert the chest tube into the fifth intercostal space?

c. What structures did the chest tube pass through to enter the pleural cavity?

d. What is tension pneumothorax?

e. What are the signs and symptoms of tension pneumothorax?

3. Pleural effusion (escape of fluid into the pleural cavity):

It is the accumulation of significant amount of fluid in the pleural cavity. It is associated with the **disappearance of friction rub.** The condition gives rise to dullness on percussion and reduction in the intensity of the breath sounds. The lung on the affected side, the mediastinum shifts to the

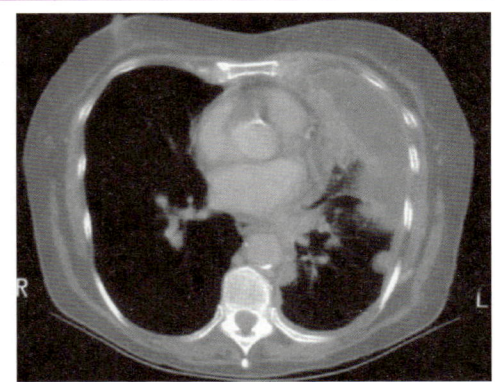

Fig. 18.12 CT showing pleural effusion

normal side, which can be confirmed by shift of the trachea. The fluid level in hydropneumothorax can be confirmed by radiographic examination (instead of horizontal fluid level line, it will be curved).

Accumulation of significant amount of fluid in the pleural cavity is called **hydrothorax** and it may result from pleural effusion. The accumulation of blood in the pleural cavity is called **hemothorax**, which is due to rupture of intercostal or internal thoracic vessels or even from laceration of lungs. The accumulation of pus in the pleural cavity is referred as **pyothorax**. The accumulation of lymph fluid in the pleural cavity is called **chylothorax**, usually due to rupture of the thoracic duct or interference in lymphatic drainage from the pleural cavity (Figs 18.11 and 18.12).

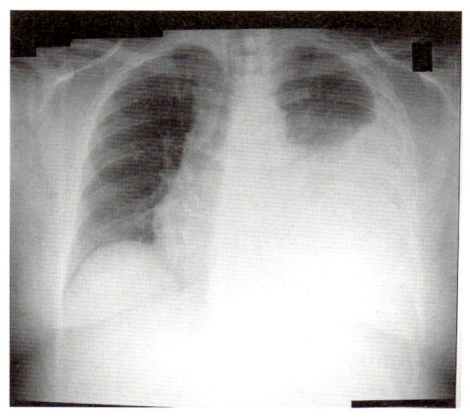

Fig. 18.11 Radiograph of left-sided pleural effusion

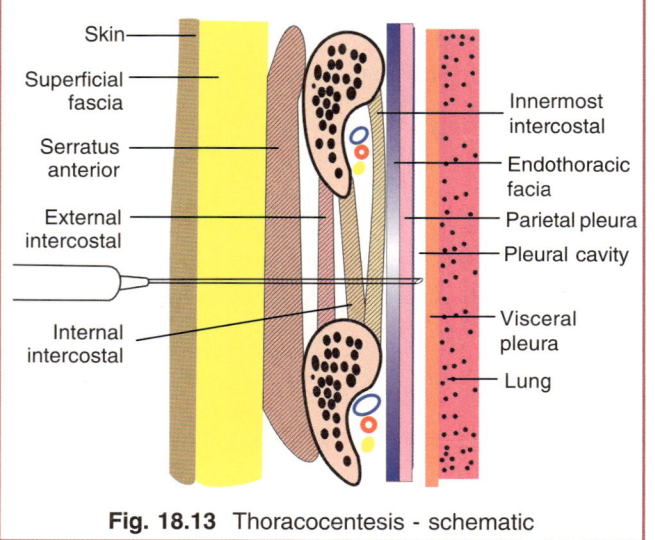

Skin
Superficial fascia
Serratus anterior
External intercostal
Internal intercostal
Innermost intercostal
Endothoracic facia
Parietal pleura
Pleural cavity
Visceral pleura
Lung

Fig. 18.13 Thoracocentesis - schematic

SECTION 5

4. Thoracocentesis or pleural tap: It is a procedure to remove the excess fluid or blood or pus from the pleural cavity. This is performed with the patient in sitting posture. Usually the needle is inserted in the posterior axillary line or the midaxillary line through the lower part of **8th or 9th intercostal space.** The excess fluid accumulates in costodiaphragmatic recess. Performing thoracocentesis in either of these spaces **during expiration** will avoid the injury to the lung. The needle passes in succession through the skin, fasciae, serratus anterior, intercostal muscles, endothoracic fascia and the costal pleura. To avoid damage to the intercostal nerve and vessels, the needle is inserted along the superior border of the lower rib, high enough to avoid the collateral branch - which runs along the upper border of the rib (Fig. 14.10).

CASE 4

A post graduate medical student obtained a sample of pleural fluid from a patient's right pleural cavity. He inserted the needle close to the lower border of the eighth rib in the anterior axillary line. The next morning he was surprised to hear that the patient has complaint of altered skin sensation extending from the point where the needle was inserted downward and forward to the midline of the abdominal wall above the umbilicus.

Can you explain the cause of altered sensation in anatomical terms?

5. **Insertion of a chest tube:** This is a procedure to remove major amount of air, blood, fluid, pus or any combination of these substances from the pleural cavity. A short incision is made in the 5th or 6th intercostal space in the midaxillary line. The tube inserted is directed upwards towards cervical pleura for removal of air or the tube can be directed downwards for fluid drainage. The outer end of the tube is connected to a controlled suction (or under water seal), to prevent air from being sucked back into the pleural cavity. Failure of removal of fluid may cause the lung to develop a resistant fibrous covering that inhibits expansion unless it is peeled.

Solutions to the clinical case studies:

Case-1

a. Diseases of the lung does not cause pain until the parietal pleura is involved. Lung tissue and visceral pleura are not innervated with pain fibres. The costal pleura are innervated by intercostal nerves, which have pain endings in the pleura. The boy had pneumonia of the right middle lobe, which later spread to the pleurae, causing pleurisy. Once the parietal pleura was involved he experienced pain he could localize.

b. Movement of the inflamed pleural surfaces against one another, as in deep inspiration or coughing, accentuated the pain.

Case-2

a. The patient has had a left-sided pneumothorax. The air has entered the left pleural cavity as the result of rupture of one of the emphysematous cysts of the left lung. The air in the left pleural cavity displaced the mobile mediastinum over to the right

b. The left lung collapsed immediately when air entered the left pleural cavity, since the air pressures within the bronchial tree and in the pleural cavity were then equal. The elastic recoil of the lung tissue caused the lung to collapse

Case-3

a. The nature of some injuries to the chest wall may create an opening that acts like a one-way valve. Trauma may create an inward swinging flap in the chest wall. Air is sucked into the pleural cavity during inspiration, but during expiration the chest wall closes on itself, preventing air from escaping.

b. Insertion of the chest tube at the fifth intercostal space allows the release and escape of air from the pleural space into the chest drainage device. In addition, it allows the physician to intervene immediately and prevent a potentially life threatening event by arresting further damage to a potentially injured diaphragm.

c. Skin, fat, external intercostal muscle, internal intercostal muscle, innermost intercostal muscle, endothoracic fascia and parietal pleura.

d. It is the presence of air in the pleural space under pressure. The lung collapses, and a mediastinal shift interferes with the expansion of the contralateral lung and compromises venous return to the heart via the IVC. This condition is extremely dangerous and requires urgent intervention. Other possible injuries leading to tension pneumothorax are explained.

e. Tachypnea, contralateral tracheal deviation, hyper resonance, distended neck veins, dyspnea, and hypotension.

Case-4.

The needle was inserted incorrectly and thereby it damaged the 8th intercostal nerve. This produced altered sensation (paresthesia) in the 8th thoracic dermatome. Needles should always be inserted close to the upper border of a rib, i.e., as far away from the neurovascular bundle as possible.

MCQs

1. You are caring for a 68-year-old male who has copious amounts of fluid in the left pleural cavity due to acute pleurisy. When you examine him as he sits up in bed (trunk upright), where would the fluid tend to accumulate?

   A. Costodiaphragmatic recess
   B. Costomediastinal recess
   C. Cupola
   D. Hilar reflection

2. A needle inserted into the 9th intercostal space along the midaxillary line would enter which space?

   A. Cardiac notch
   B. Costodiaphragmatic recess
   C. Costomediastinal recess
   D. Cupola

3. The pleural cavity near the cardiac notch is known as the:

   A. Costodiaphragmatic recess
   B. Costomediastinal recess
   C. Cupola
   D. Hilum

4. You must remove fluid from the pleural cavity of your patient (thoracocentesis). You decide to insert the aspiration needle over the top of a rib, into an intercostal space inferior to the lower border of the lung in the mid axillary line at the end of normal expiration. The highest level at which this procedure might safely be done without injuring the lung is the

   A. Fourth intercostal space
   B. Fifth intercostal space
   C. Sixth intercostal space
   D. Eighth intercostal space

5. While performing the above procedure, the lower border of the lung will lie at the level of which rib in the midclavicular line?

   A. Fifth
   B. Sixth
   C. Seventh
   D. Eighth

6. A 24-year-old patient suffering from lobar pneumonia complains of severe pain during breathing, suggesting the involvement of the parietal pleura. Which of the following combination of nerves carry pain fibres from parietal pleura?

   A. Phrenic nerves and Intercostal nerves
   B. Vagus and Phrenic nerves
   C. Greater splanchnic and Phrenic nerves
   D. Intercostal and Vagus nerves

Answers to MCQs
1. A
2. B
3. B
4. D
5. B
6. A

SECTION 5

- External features of the lungs
- Medial surface of the lung
- Blood supply to lungs
- Microscopic structure
- MCQs
- Apex of the lungs
- Broncho pulmonary segments
- Nerve supply to lungs
- Lymphatic drainage of the lungs

Objectives

- To explain the external features of right and left lungs
- To mark the position of fissures of the lung on a cadaver or a patient (surface marking) and explain how do you auscultate different lobes of lungs in a patient
- To explain the relations of the apex of the lung and its clinical relevance
- With the help of a diagram, be able to explain the relations of medial surface of right and left lungs
- To define bronchopulmonary segments and be able to explain their clinical relevance
- To explain the source of sympathetic and parasympathetic nerve supply to the lung and list the effect of their stimulation on lung functions
- To explain the lymphatic drainage of lung with their clinical relevance

Lungs are a pair of respiratory organs. Its main function is to oxygenate the blood by bringing the inspired air into close relation with venous blood within the lungs.

The healthy lungs in living are light, soft, porous, highly elastic and spongy in texture. In the newborn, it is rosy pink in colour. In adults, it is dark slaty grey due to the deposition of carbonaceous particles.

Each lung occupies the pulmonary cavities (space on either side of the mediastinum) and is covered by pleura (or invaginates into pleural sac). Because of the negative intrapleural pressure, the parietal and visceral pleurae can slide over each other during respiration.

EXTERNAL FEATURES OF THE LUNGS

Each lung presents an apex, a base, three surfaces (costal, medial and inferior/base) and three borders - anterior, posterior and inferior (Fig.19.1).

The right lung is larger and heavier than the left, but it is shorter and wider because the right dome of the diaphragm is higher.

Anterior border:

The anterior border of the right lung is relatively straight. The anterior border of the left lung has a deep cardiac notch (an indentation consequent to the deviation of the apex of the heart to the left side). The portion of the superior lobe

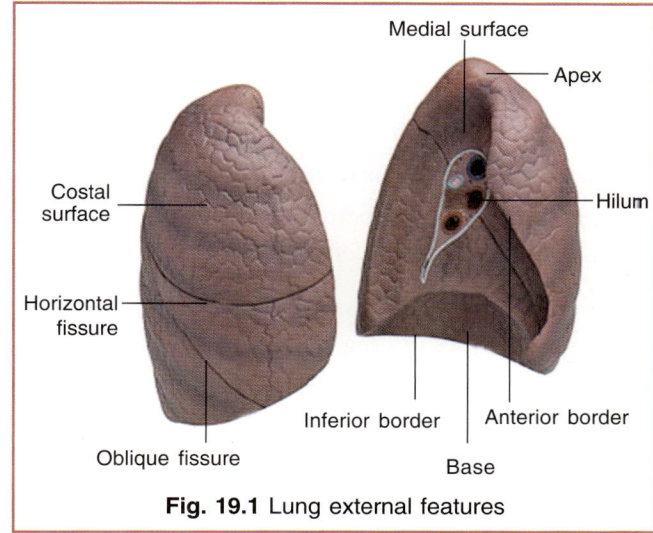

Fig. 19.1 Lung external features

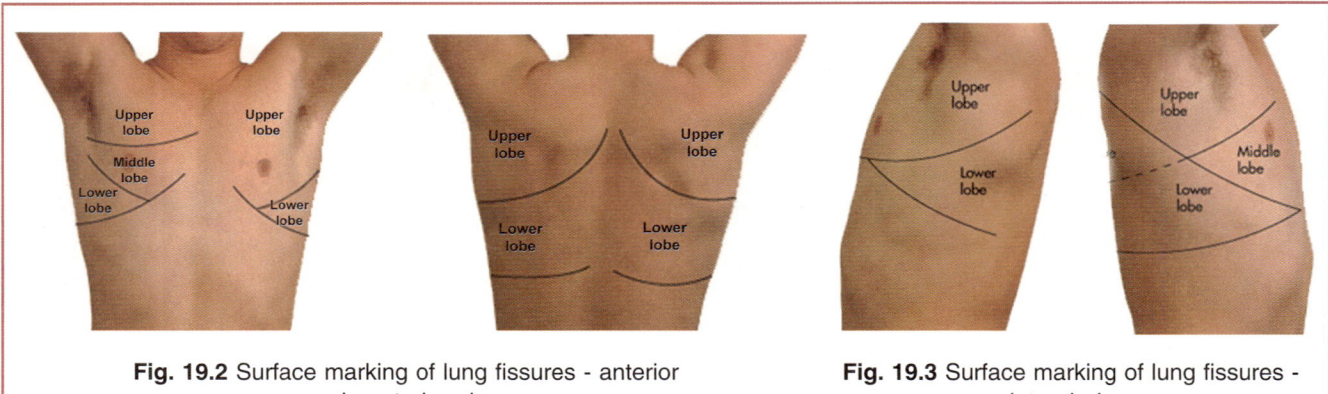

Fig. 19.2 Surface marking of lung fissures - anterior and posterior view

Fig. 19.3 Surface marking of lung fissures - lateral view

below the cardiac notch resembles a tongue and is called **lingula.** It moves across the costomediastinal recess during full inspiration.

Posterior border:

The posterior border is ill defined and separates vertebral part of the medial surface from costal surface.

Inferior border:

The inferior border separates costal surface from the inferior surface or base

Fissures and lobes of the lung

The right lung is divided into 3 lobes by oblique and horizontal fissure, while left lung has only oblique fissure, dividing it into superior and inferior lobes (Figs 19.2 and 19.3).

Surface marking of Oblique fissure:

It roughly corresponds to medial border of the scapula in the fully abducted position of the arm. Connecting the following three points mark the oblique fissure.

- The first point is at 2 cm lateral to the T3 spine.
- The second point is at 5th rib in mid-axillary line
- It reaches 6th costal cartilage 7–8 cm lateral to the midline (6th costochondral junction)

Surface markings of Horizontal fissure:

It begins at the anterior border of right lung at right 4th costal cartilage, then it meet the oblique fissure in midaxillary line

Variations in lobes of lung

The oblique and horizontal fissures may be incomplete or absent in some lungs, with consequent reduction in number of lobes. The left lung sometimes has three lobes and right lung only two. The most common accessory lobe is '**azygos lobe**', which appears in right lung in approximately 1% of

people. It appears above the hilum of right lung, separated by the rest of the lung by a deep groove lodging the arch of the azygos vein.

APEX OF THE LUNG

It is the blunt superior end of the lung above the level of 1st rib. It extends into the root of the neck about 2.5 cm above the medial end of the clavicle. Apex is covered by cervical pleura and externally by suprapleural membrane.

Relations of the apex and its clinical significance

In front: The subclavian artery scalenus anterior muscle and subclavian vein pass in front of the apex.

Medially: The trachea, oesophagus, phrenic and vagus nerve, (left recurrent laryngeal on the left side) are related to its medial surface.

Laterally: Scalenus medius muscle.

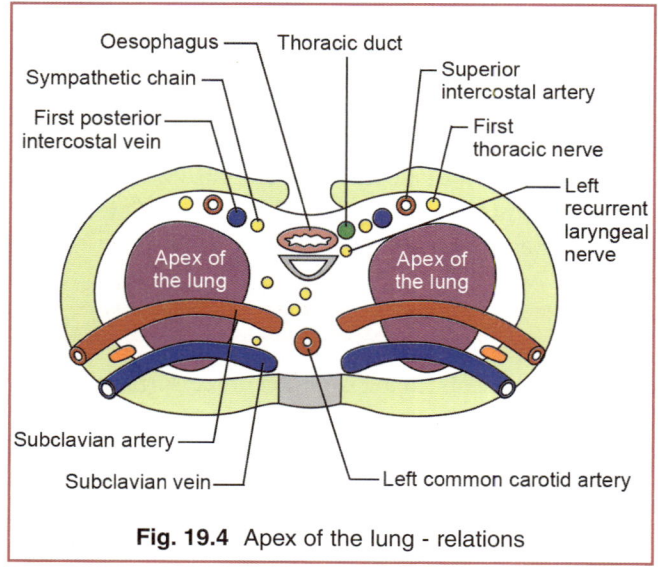

Fig. 19.4 Apex of the lung - relations

SECTION 5

Posteriorly: It is related to structures present in front of the neck of the first rib (from medial to lateral) – sympathetic chain, first posterior intercostal vein, superior intercostal artery, ventral ramus of first thoracic nerve forming lower trunk of the brachial plexus (Fig.19.4).

- The malignancy of the apex of the lung may present as symptoms and signs produced due to spread of cancer to neighboring structures.
- The compression of subclavian vein results in venous engorgement and edema in the arm or neck and face (brachiocephalic vein or SVC).
- The diminished radial pulse is due to the compression of the subclavian artery.
- Infiltration of phrenic nerve cause paralysis of the diaphragm on the affected side (hemidiaphragm)

Pancoast tumor:

Further the erosion of the 1st or 2nd ribs causes pain in the ulnar distribution and wasting of hand muscles (T1 fibres of lower trunk of the brachial plexus). The compression of the sympathetic chain can cause Horner's syndrome.

Base

It is concave inferior surface of the lung and rests on upper surface of the diaphragm. The diaphragmatic pleura and diaphragm separates the base of the right lung from right lobe of the liver, and left lung from left lobe of the liver, fundus of stomach and spleen.

Costal surface is related to thoracic wall (ribs, costal cartilages and intercostal spaces) and presents impressions of ribs and costal cartilages. It is covered by costal pleura and endothoracic fascia.

MEDIAL SURFACE OF THE LUNG

It is further divided into an anterior mediastinal part and posterior vertebral part.

The posterior vertebral part is related to bodies of the thoracic vertebrae and intervertebral discs between them.

The **mediastinal part** is related to mediastinum. It presents hilum of the lung, cardiac impression. There are many structures related to mediastinal surface and some of them leave impressions on the cadaveric lungs (except the

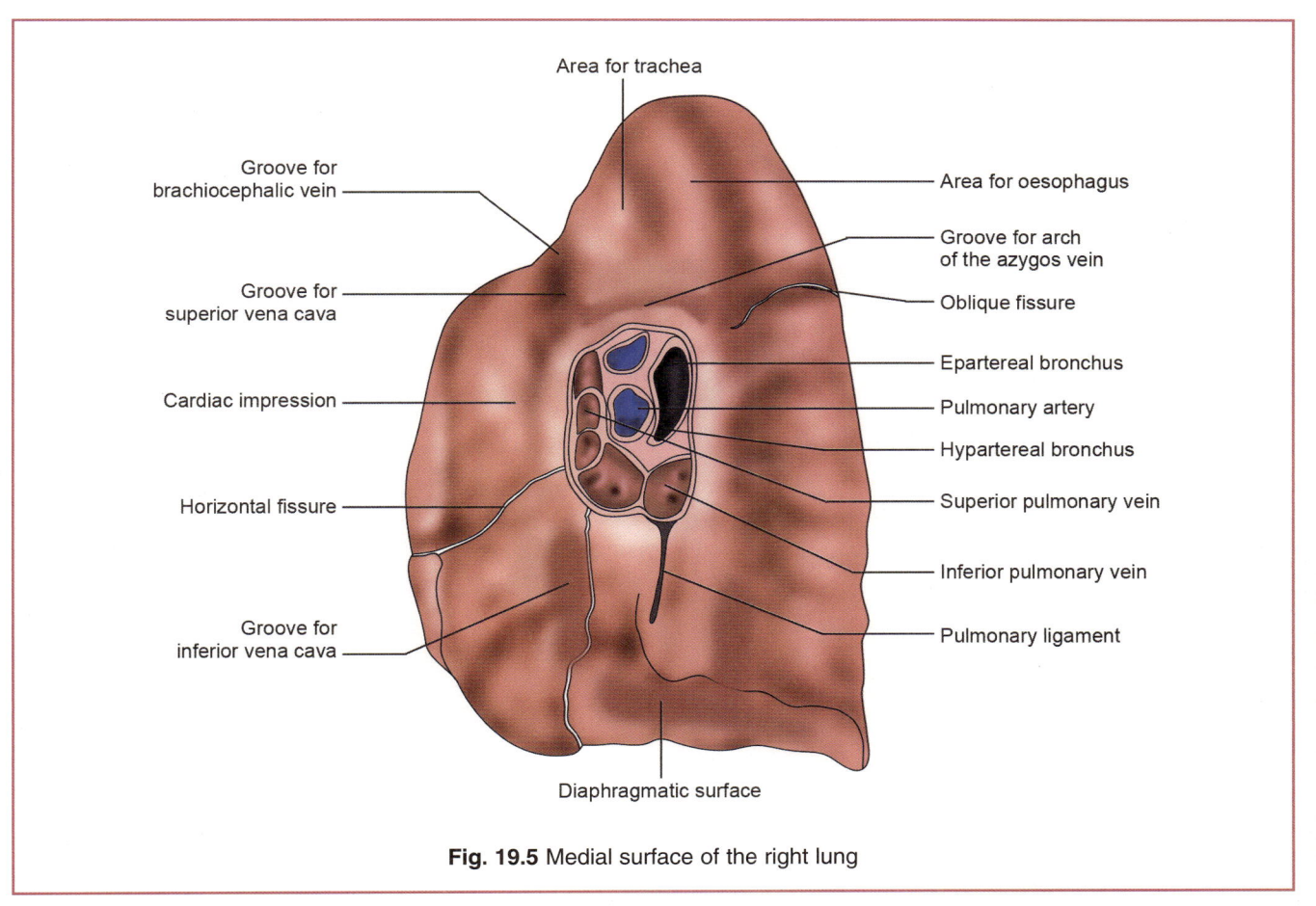

Fig. **19.5** Medial surface of the right lung

SECTION 5

heart, which is evident during surgery or fresh cadaveric or postmortem specimens) and are shown in Figs. 19.5 and 19.6

Mediastinal surface of the Right lung

1. Cardiac impression – in front and below the hilum, related to right atrium and anterior part of the right ventricle (Figs 19.5 and 19.7)
2. Arch of the azygos vein – Above the hilum, a prominent arched groove
3. Groove for superior vena cava—The upper part of the cardiac impression continuous with groove for superior vena cava
4. Groove for the inferior vena cava—It is placed postero-inferior to the cardiac impression
5. Trachea—related posterior to the groove for superior vena cava
6. Oesophagus—it makes a shallow groove behind the trachea, hilum and pulmonary ligament, but this shallow groove does not extend up to the inferior margin of the lung
7. Phrenic nerve descends **in front of the hilum**, along the right margin of the superior and inferior vena cava.

8. Vagus nerve descends along the trachea, then descends behind the hilum.
9. The right subclavian artery may produce a notch just below the apex and the right 1st rib produces a notch just below the pulmonary artery at the anterior border.

Mediastinal surface of the Left lung

1. Cardiac impression—A large cardiac impression is present in front and below the hilum related to left ventricle (Figs 19.6 and 19.8).
2. Pulmonary trunk—is related just in front of the hilum (between cardiac impression and hilum)
3. Arch of aorta—is related to a deep groove immediately above the hilum
4. Descending thoracic aorta—the groove for arch of aorta continues behind the hilum and pulmonary ligament for descending thoracic aorta, up to the inferior border of the lung.
5. Left subclavian artery—the groove for the left subclavian artery begins from groove for arch of aorta and extends upwards just in front of the apex

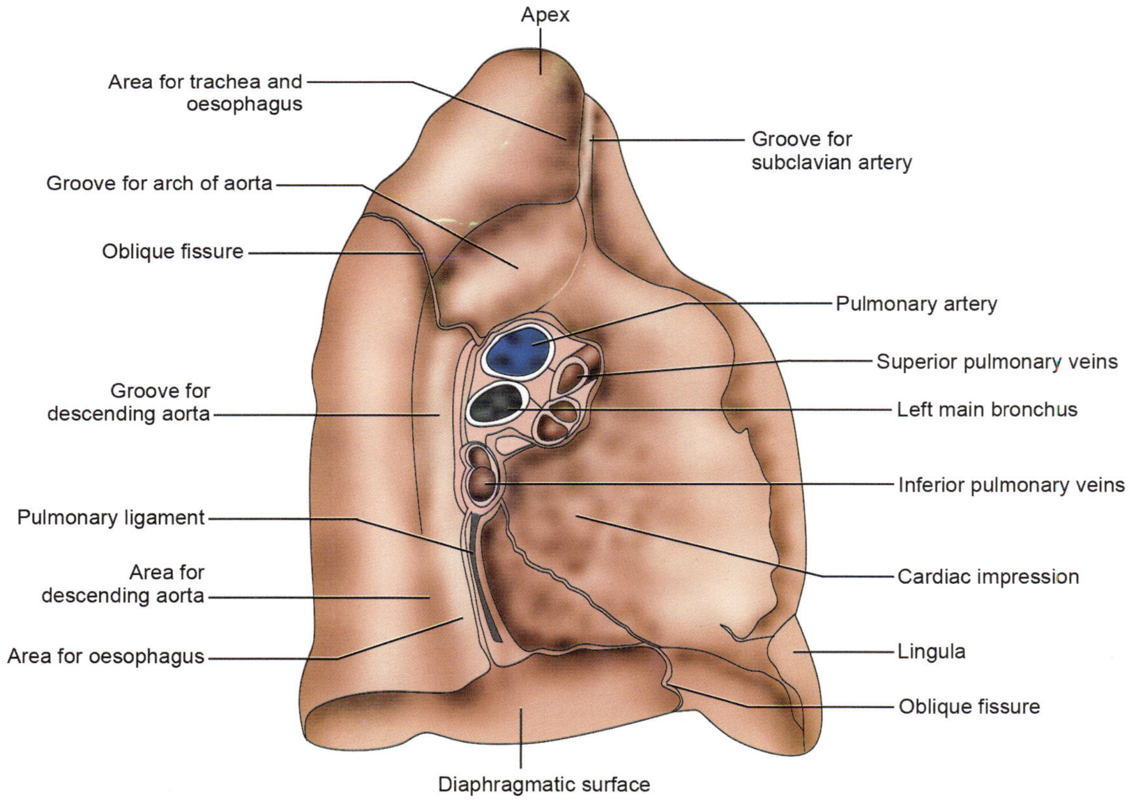

Fig. 19.6 Medial surface of the left lung

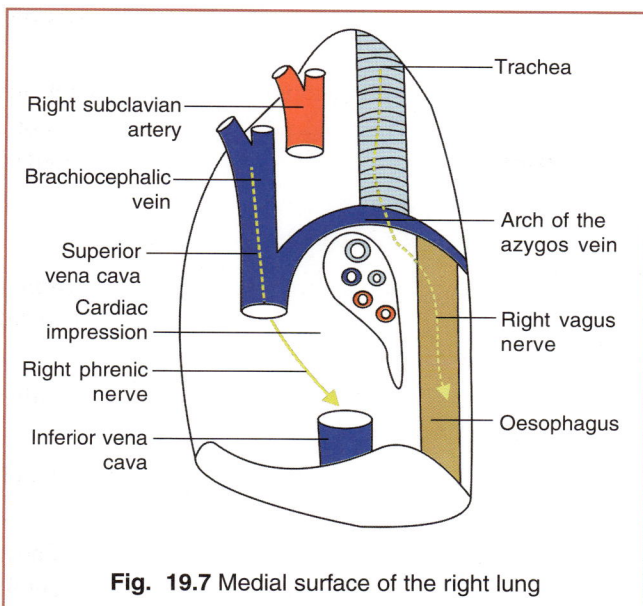

Fig. 19.7 Medial surface of the right lung

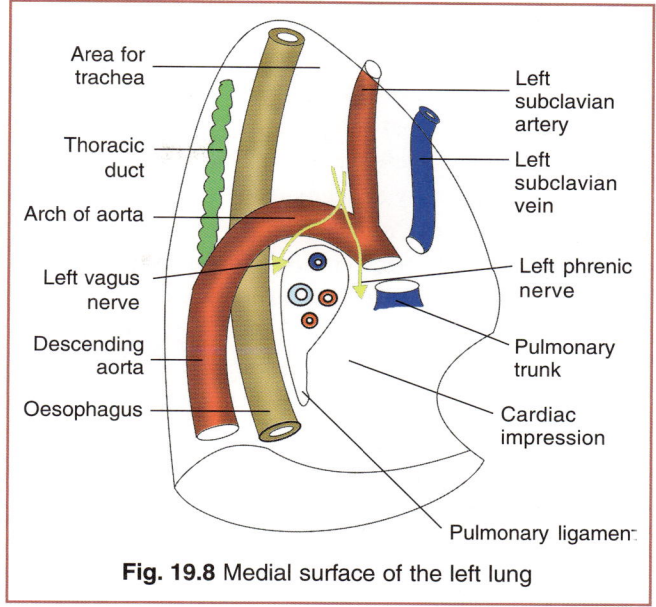

Fig. 19.8 Medial surface of the left lung

6. Oesophagus—is related just behind the groove for left subclavian artery along with the thoracic duct. The oesophagus is related again, in front of the descending thoracic aorta, behind and below the lower end of the pulmonary ligament

7. Nerves—The left vagus and left phrenic nerve cross each other above the hilum, deep to the groove for the arch of aorta. Then the vagus descends behind the hilum along with the oesophagus and phrenic descends in front of the hilum. The left recurrent laryngeal nerve winds around the arch of aorta, is also related to medial surface of the left lung.

Root of the lung

It connects the hilum of the lung to the mediastinum. The root contains the principal bronchus on the left side, eparterial and hyparterial bronchus on right side pulmonary vessels, bronchial vessels, lymphatics and nerves.

It extends from T5 to T7 vertebra.

Relations:

Hilum of the lung

Hilum is an area through which the structures enter or emerge out from the lung. It consists of a pair of pulmonary veins, one pulmonary artery, two bronchi on the right side and one bronchus on the left side, bronchial vessels, lymphatics, lymph nodes and nerve fibres.

The arrangement of the structures at the hilum from above downwards is as follows:

Right lung

• Eparterial bronchus (Fig.19.9)

• Pulmonary artery

• Hyparterial bronchus

• Inferior pulmonary vein

Left lung

• Pulmonary artery (Fig.19.9)

• Left principal bronchus

• Inferior pulmonary vein

How to identify these structures in a cadaveric specimen?

The bronchus is identified by the presence of rigid cartilage in its wall. The anterior most structure is superior pulmonary vein and the inferior most is the inferior pulmonary vein.

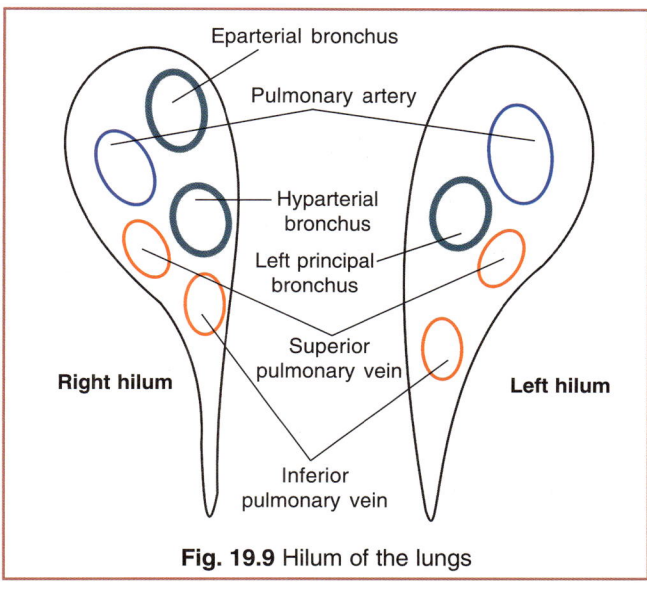

Fig. 19.9 Hilum of the lungs

S E C T I O N   5

Bronchial tree

Trachea divides into right and left principal bronchi at the root of the lung. Each principal bronchus again divides into secondary (or lobar) bronchi, one for each lung (3 on right lung and 2 on left lung). Each secondary bronchus subdivides into tertiary or segmental bronchi. There are 10 such tertiary bronchi in each lung. The tertiary bronchi divide repeatedly to form 'terminal' and further 'respiratory bronchioles'. **The wall of the bronchus is made up of cartilages while they are absent in bronchioles.** The respiratory bronchiole terminates in alveoli where oxygenation of blood takes place (Fig. 19.10).

The right principal bronchus is shorter, wider and more vertical than the left principal bronchus. Therefore an, aspirated foreign body is more likely to enter the right lung than left. The right principal bronchus is 2.5 cm long, soon divides into two, the upper lobar bronchus (eparterial) passes above the pulmonary artery), and the lower (hyparterial) bronchus enter the lung below the pulmonary artery at the level of T5 vertebra.

BRONCHOPULMONARY SEGMENTS

Definition:

These are well-defined pyramidal shaped independent units of the lung aerated by tertiary (segmental) bronchi with separate branch of pulmonary artery accompanying it (Fig. 19.11).

- The apex of each segment is directed towards the hilum and base towards lung surface.
- Each segment is separated from the other by connective tissue septa.

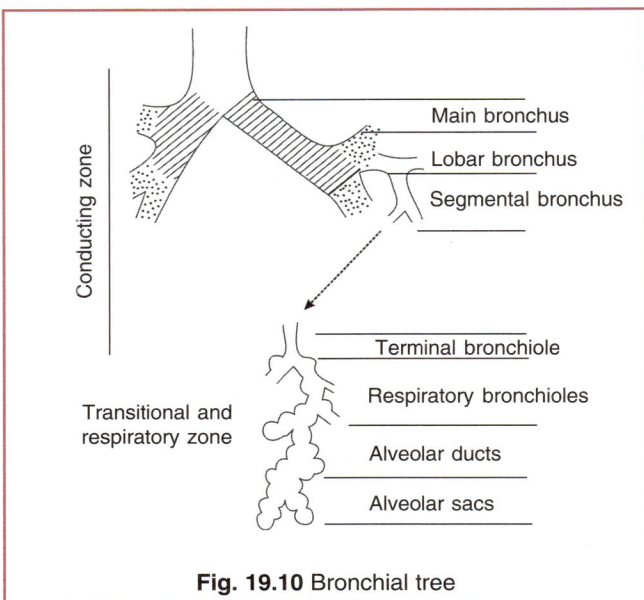

Fig. 19.10 Bronchial tree

Labels in figure: Conducting zone; Main bronchus; Lobar bronchus; Segmental bronchus; Terminal bronchiole; Respiratory bronchioles; Transitional and respiratory zone; Alveolar ducts; Alveolar sacs

- The tributaries of the pulmonary veins carrying oxygenated blood traverse the connective tissue septa placed between the bronchopulmonary segments.
- However the branches of the bronchial artery follow the segmental bronchus.
- There are 10 bronchopulmonary segments in each lung, which are (Figs 19.12 and 19.13)

1. Though the spreading of infection from one segment to the other is prevented to some extent by this

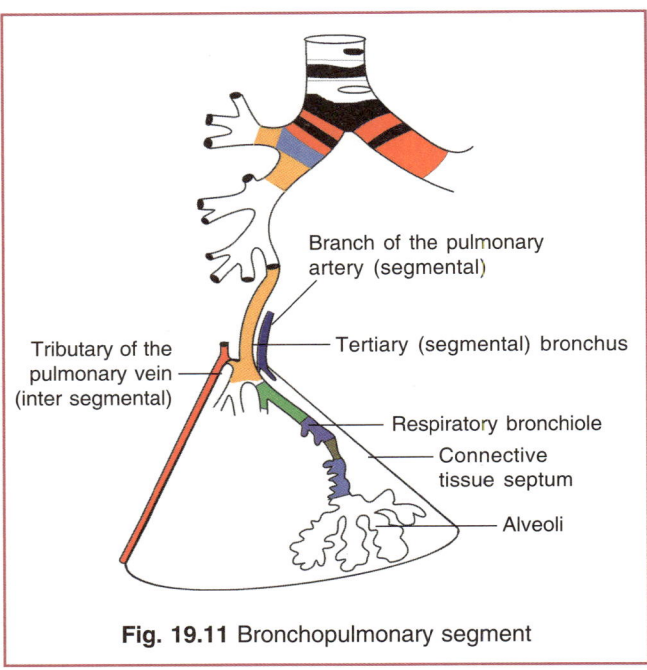

Fig. 19.11 Bronchopulmonary segment

Labels in figure: Branch of the pulmonary artery (segmental); Tributary of the pulmonary vein (inter segmental); Tertiary (segmental) bronchus; Respiratory bronchiole; Connective tissue septum; Alveoli

RIGHT LUNG	LEFT LUNG
Upper lobe	**Upper lobe**
1. Apical	1. Apico-posterior
2. Posterior	2. Anterior
3. Anterior	3. Posterior (may be separate)
Middle lobe	
4. Lateral	4. Superior lingular
5. Medial	5. Inferior lingular
Lower lobe	**Lower lobe**
6. Superior (apical basal)	6. Apical basal
7. Medial basal	7. Anterior basal
8. Anterior basal	8. Lateral basal
9. Lateral basal	9. Posterior basal
10. Posterior basal	10. Medial basal (may be suppressed)

SECTION 5

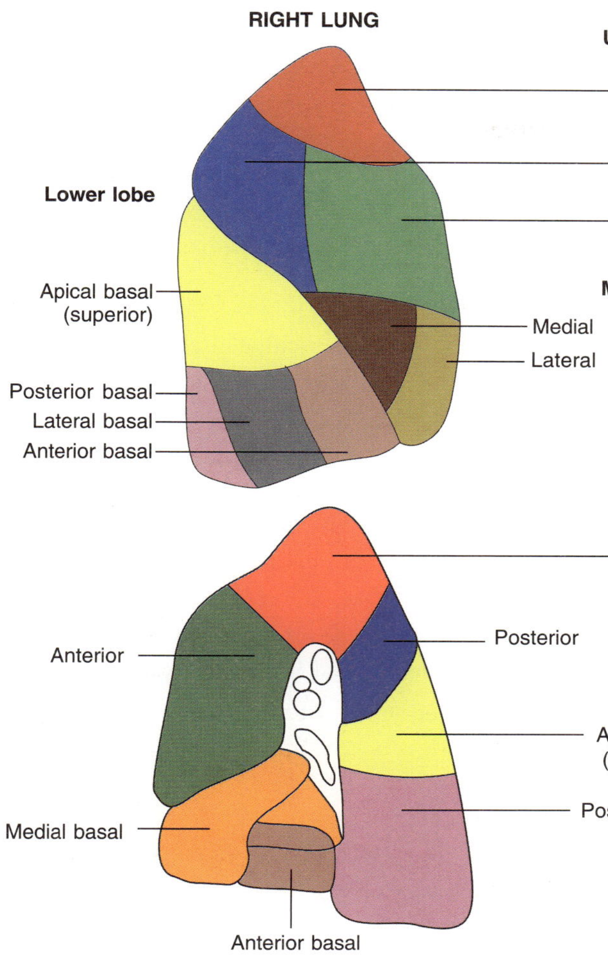

RIGHT LUNG

Upper lobe

Apical

Posterior

Anterior

Lower lobe

Apical basal
(superior)

Posterior basal
Lateral basal
Anterior basal

Middle lobe

Medial
Lateral

Apical

Posterior

Anterior

Apical basal
(superior)

Posterior basal

Medial basal

Anterior basal

Fig. 19.12 Bronchopulmonary segments of the right lung

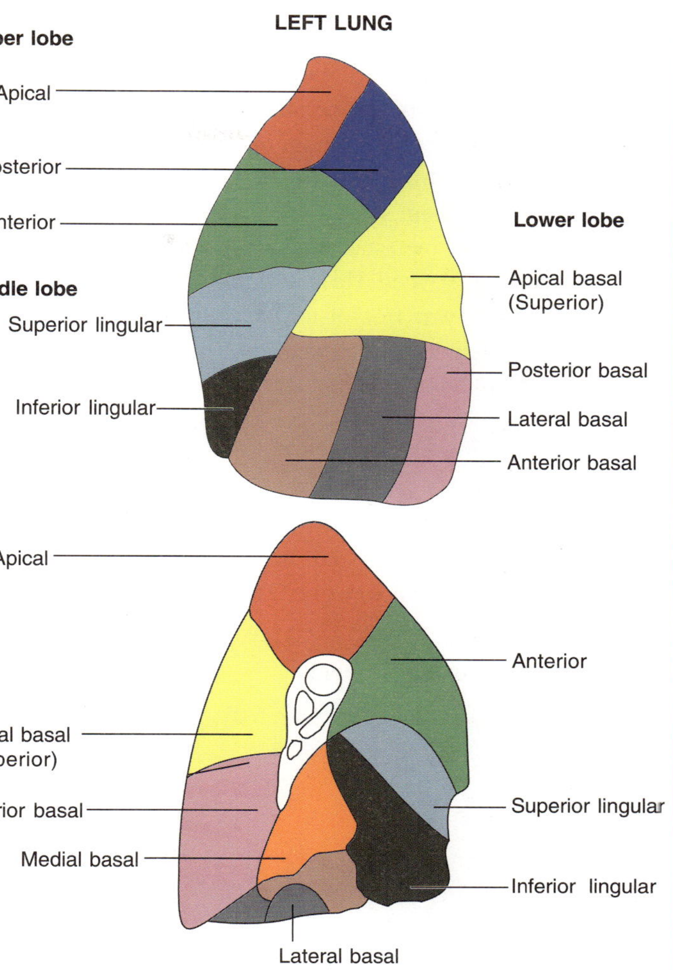

LEFT LUNG

Apical

Posterior

Anterior

Lower lobe

Apical basal
(Superior)

Posterior basal

Lateral basal

Anterior basal

Superior lingular

Inferior lingular

Apical

Anterior

Apical basal
(superior)

Medial basal

Superior lingular

Inferior lingular

Lateral basal

Fig. 19.13 Bronchopulmonary segments of the left lung

connective tissue septum, the tuberculosis or carcinoma of the lung can break this barrier.

2. The apical (superior) segment of the lower lobe and posterior segment of the upper lobe are common sites (more commonly on right side) for lung abscess due to aspiration of infected material. These are the most dependent segments in supine position.

3. Being independent units of the lung, the diseased bronchopulmonary segments can be surgically removed. During surgical resection of certain bronchopulmonary segments the diseased segmental bronchus is identified by dissection and it is clamped along with the blood vessels. This helps to identify the segment, as the surface of the segment will darken due to loss of blood supply and air.

4. It is important to note that the apical (superior) segmental bronchus is directed backwards. In supine

position of the body, this segmental bronchus is directed posteriorly (most dependent) and foreign bodies entered into the right lung is most likely to enter through this segmental bronchus into **superior (apical) bronchopulmonary segment of the lower lobe** (Fig. 19.14).

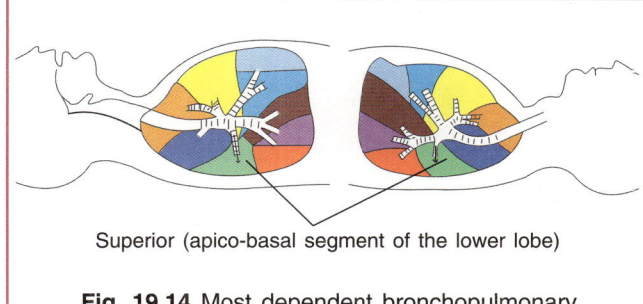

Superior (apico-basal segment of the lower lobe)

Fig. 19.14 Most dependent bronchopulmonary segments in supine position

CASE - 1

A 67-year-old male who had been a heavy cigarette smoker for nearly 50 years was diagnosed with lung cancer. Radiologic and bronchoscopic examinations revealed a relatively small tumour in one of the tertiary bronchi of the middle lobe of the right lung. This segment of the patient's lung was removed. As there was no evidence of metastasis of the tumour, no further treatment was prescribed. He quit smoking and 5 years after the surgery was free of any detectable cancer. Why was it possible to remove only a portion of the diseased lung rather than a lobe or the entire structure?

Auscultation of lungs and percussion of the thorax:

These are important techniques used during physical examinations. The auscultation is listening to the sounds with the help of a stethoscope. It assesses the airflow through the tracheobronchial tree. The percussion refers

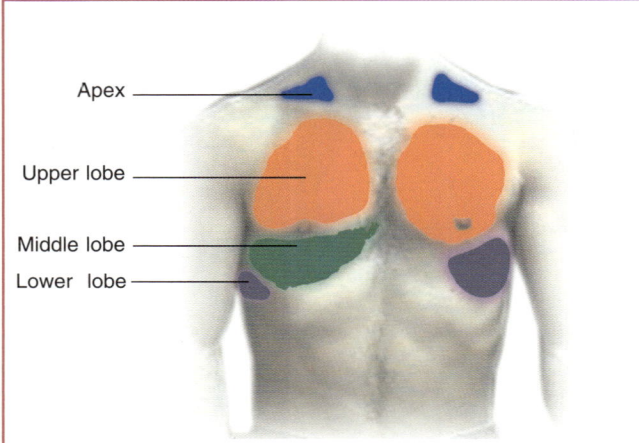

Fig. 19.15 Surface projection of lobes of lungs - anterior view

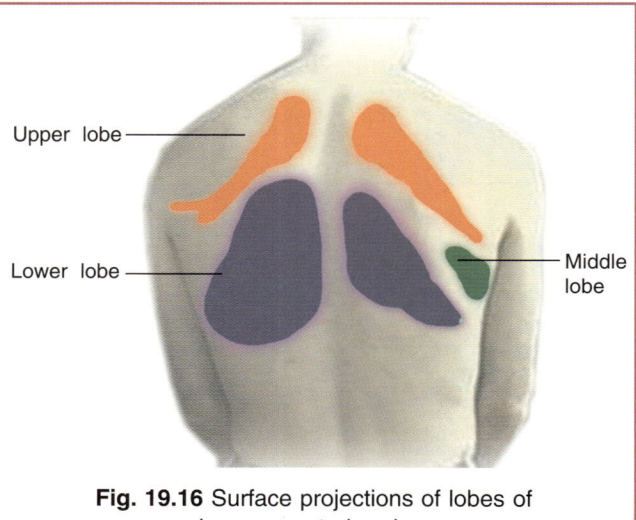

Fig. 19.16 Surface projections of lobes of lungs - posterior view

to tapping the thorax over the chest wall with the fingers to detect the resonance sounds of the lungs. It helps to know whether the underlying tissue is air filled (resonant sound), fluid filled (dull sound), or solid (flat sound). The knowledge of normal anatomy of the lung and its projections, portions covered by the bones (example scapula), muscles is important to know where flat and resonant sounds should be expected.

Auscultation sites (Figs 19.15 and 19.16)

- Apex of the lung is auscultated above the medial third of the clavicle anteriorly and upper part of suprascapular region posteriorly

- The upper lobe of the right lung is best heard anteriorly in the area extending from the clavicle to the level of 4th costal cartilage, while that of the left lung is best heard in the area up to the level of 6th costal cartilage

- The middle lobe is heard anteriorly between right 4th and 6th ribs in front of the midaxillary line

- The apical or superior segment of the lower lobe (on both sides) is heard posteriorly in the interval between the medial border of the scapula and the vertebral spines

- The basal segment of the lower lobe (on both sides) are heard posteriorly in the infrascapular region up to the level of 10th rib

  When clinicians refer to 'auscultating the base of the lung', they are not usually referring to diaphragmatic surface of lungs, instead postero-inferior part of the lower lobe (i.e. basal segments).

BLOOD SUPPLY TO THE LUNG

Pulmonary vessels

Each pulmonary artery arises from pulmonary trunk at the level of sternal angle carrying deoxygenated blood to the lungs for oxygenation. The branches of the pulmonary arteries and bronchi are paired in the lung, running in parallel course.

The branches of pulmonary arteries accompanying the bronchiole are thin walled without any muscles in its wall. These arteries end up in forming capillaries, which are placed close to the alveoli of the lung. The venous ends of the capillaries join to form intersegmental veins running in between the bronchopulmonary segment. Finally two pulmonary veins carrying oxygenated blood emerge from the hilum of the lungs drains into the left atrium. The right pair of pulmonary veins cross posterior to the base of the heart.

Pulmonary embolism:

- An obstruction of a pulmonary artery by a blood clot (embolus) can cause death. The embolus in the pulmonary artery forms when blood clot or fat globule or air bubble travels through veins and reach the lung after traversing the right atrium and right ventricle.

- For example, a blood clot arising from a fracture site can dislodge and travels through a person's body to his or her lungs obstructing the pulmonary artery or its branch. The blockage results in a lung or a portion of the lung that is ventilated with air but not perfused with blood. The patient suffers acute respiratory distress because of decrease in oxygenation of the blood. The right side of the heart may become acutely dilated and this results in death within few minutes. A small embolus can block the artery supplying the bronchopulmonary segment causing a pulmonary infarct, an area of necrotic (dead) lung tissue.

Bronchial vessels

The bronchial arteries supply intrapulmonary bronchial tree and connective tissue of lung parenchyma.

On right side there is one bronchial artery arising from left bronchial or 3rd right posterior intercostal artery or descending aorta.

On the left side there are two bronchial arteries (upper and lower) arising from descending aorta at level of tracheal bifurcation. The right bronchial vein drains into azygos vein while left bronchial vein opens into either the left superior intercostals vein or the accessory hemiazygos vein.

NERVE SUPPLY TO LUNGS

The sympathetic and parasympathetic nerves supplying the lungs are derived from anterior and posterior pulmonary plexus placed in front and behind the root of the lung. These are extensions from cardiac plexus (Table 19.1).

LYMPHATIC DRAINAGE

The lymphatic vessels of the lungs can be classified into superficial and deep lymphatic plexus (Fig. 19.17)

- The superficial lymphatic plexus lies deep to the visceral pleura and drains the lung parenchyma and visceral pleura. Lymphatic vessels arising from them drains into **bronchopulmonary lymph nodes** (hilar lymph nodes) at the hilum of the lung.

- The deep lymphatic plexus is located in the submucosa of the bronchi and in the peribronchial connective tissue along the bronchial tree. A lymph vessel from these deep plexus drains initially into **pulmonary lymph nodes**, located along the lobar bronchi.

- Lymphatic vessels from these nodes continue to follow the bronchi to the hilum of the lung where they also drain into the bronchopulmonary lymph nodes, hence lymph from both superficial and deep plexus are drained into bronchopulmonary lymph nodes.

- Lymph vessels arising from them drain into superior and inferior **tracheobronchial lymph nodes** (placed superior and inferior to the bifurcation of the trachea and main bronchus respectively). These lymph nodes enlarge in carcinoma of the lungs and also in pulmonary tuberculosis.

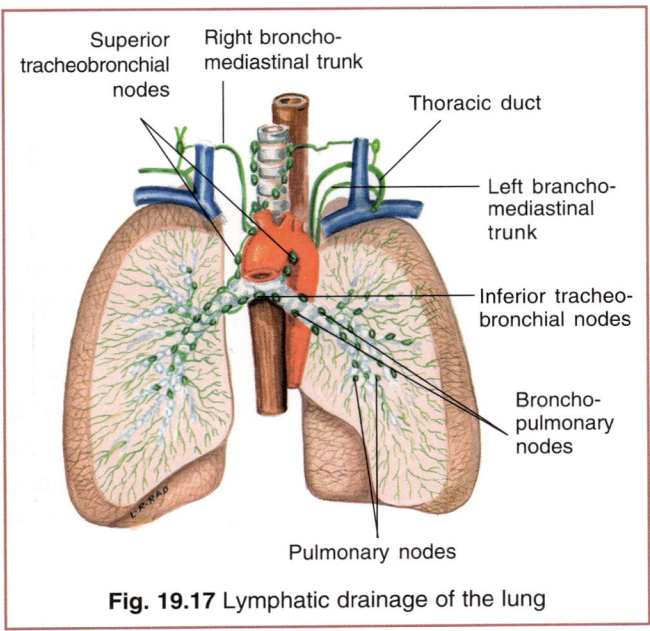

Superior tracheobronchial nodes

Right broncho-mediastinal trunk

Thoracic duct

Left broncho-mediastinal trunk

Inferior tracheo-bronchial nodes

Broncho-pulmonary nodes

Pulmonary nodes

Fig. 19.17 Lymphatic drainage of the lung

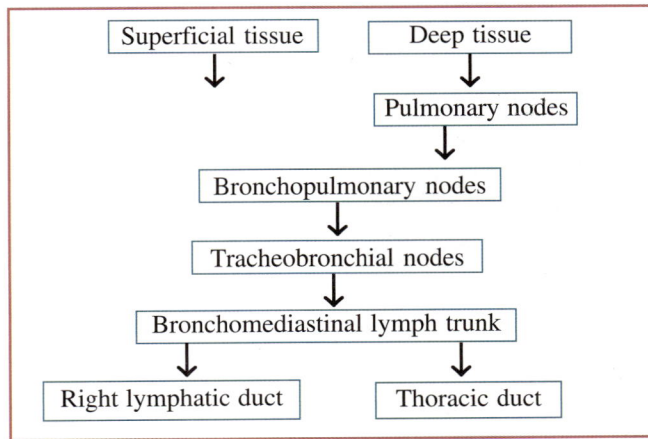

Superficial tissue	Deep tissue
↓	↓
	Pulmonary nodes
	↓
Bronchopulmonary nodes	
↓	
Tracheobronchial nodes	
↓	
Bronchomediastinal lymph trunk	
↓	↓
Right lymphatic duct	Thoracic duct

Table 19.1 Nerve supply to the lungs	
Parasympathetic	**Sympathetic**
• Vagus	• Upper thoracic segments of spinal cord
• Bronchoconstrictors (Motor to smooth muscles in the wall of the bronchial tree, the attack of bronchial asthma is due to spasm of smooth muscles of bronchioles) This may be precipitated by (excessive vagal stimulation) exposure to cold air, dust, smoke	• Bronchodilators (Inhibitor to smooth muscles in the wall of the bronchial tree)
• Secretomotor to the glands in the mucous membrane of the respiratory tract	• Inhibitor to the glands in the mucous membrane of the respiratory tract
• Vasodilator (inhibitory to the pulmonary vessels)	• Vasoconstrictor (motor to the pulmonary vessels)
• Concerned with reflex control of respiratory activity	• Convey painful stimuli such as chemical irritants, ischemia or excessive stretch
• Parasympathetic fibres are cholinergic	• Sympathetic fibres are adrenergic (Sympathetic drugs like adrenaline cause bronchodilation

- The right lung drains primarily through the consecutive sets of nodes on right side, and the superior lobe of the left lung drains primarily through the corresponding side of the left side. Many, but not all, of the lymphatics from the lower lobe of the left lung, however drain into the right superior tracheobronchial lymph nodes; the lymph then continues to follow the right side pathway.

- The lymph from the tracheobronchial lymph nodes passes to right and left bronchomediastinal lymph trunks. These lymph trunks may end at the junction of internal jugular and subclavian vein of the respective sides or right bronchomediastinal lymph trunk may join right lymphatic duct and left bronchomediastinal lymph trunk into thoracic duct.

CASE-2

A 55-year-old man states that his wife had recently noticed an alteration in his voice. He has lost 18 kgs, in weight and has persistent cough with blood-stained sputum. He smokes fifteen cigarettes a day. On examination, the left vocal cord is immobile and lies in the adducted position. A postero-anterior chest radiograph reveals a large mass in the upper lobe of the left lung with an increase in width of the mediastinal shadow on the left side.

a. Explain in anatomical basis for the alteration in the voice

b. Relate the voice change to the other findings.

c. Trace the lymphatic drainage from the lung to the systemic circulation.

Radiographic anatomy of the lungs

The most common radiographic study of the thorax is the posteroanterior (PA) X-ray. The anterior aspect of the patients' thorax is placed against the X-ray detector and the shoulders move anteriorly to move the scapula away to expose the superior parts of the lungs (Figs 19.18 and 19.19).

The patient is asked to take a deep breath and hold it. The deep inspiration causes the diaphragmatic dome to descend, moving the inferior margin of lungs into costomediastinal recesses. The inferior margins should appear as sharp, acute angles. Pleural effusions if any do not allow the inferior margin to descend into the recess and the usual radiolucent air density here is replaced with a hazy radiopacity.

The PA radiograph of the chest is viewed as if you were facing the patient (an anteroposterior [AP] view). The bony structures like clavicles, ribs, lower cervical and upper thoracic vertebrae are identified and also uncommon cervical ribs, missing ribs, forked ribs and fused ribs should be detected.

Among the soft tissue structures, the trachea is identified in the midline in the superior mediastinum as a translucent air column. The lung fields are translucent (because of low density), but bronchovascular markings are seen as opacities throughout the lungs. In case of pneumonia the affected area appears to be radiodense instead of radiolucent. The hilum is recognized as an opaque area because it contains large blood vessels and lymph nodes. The right

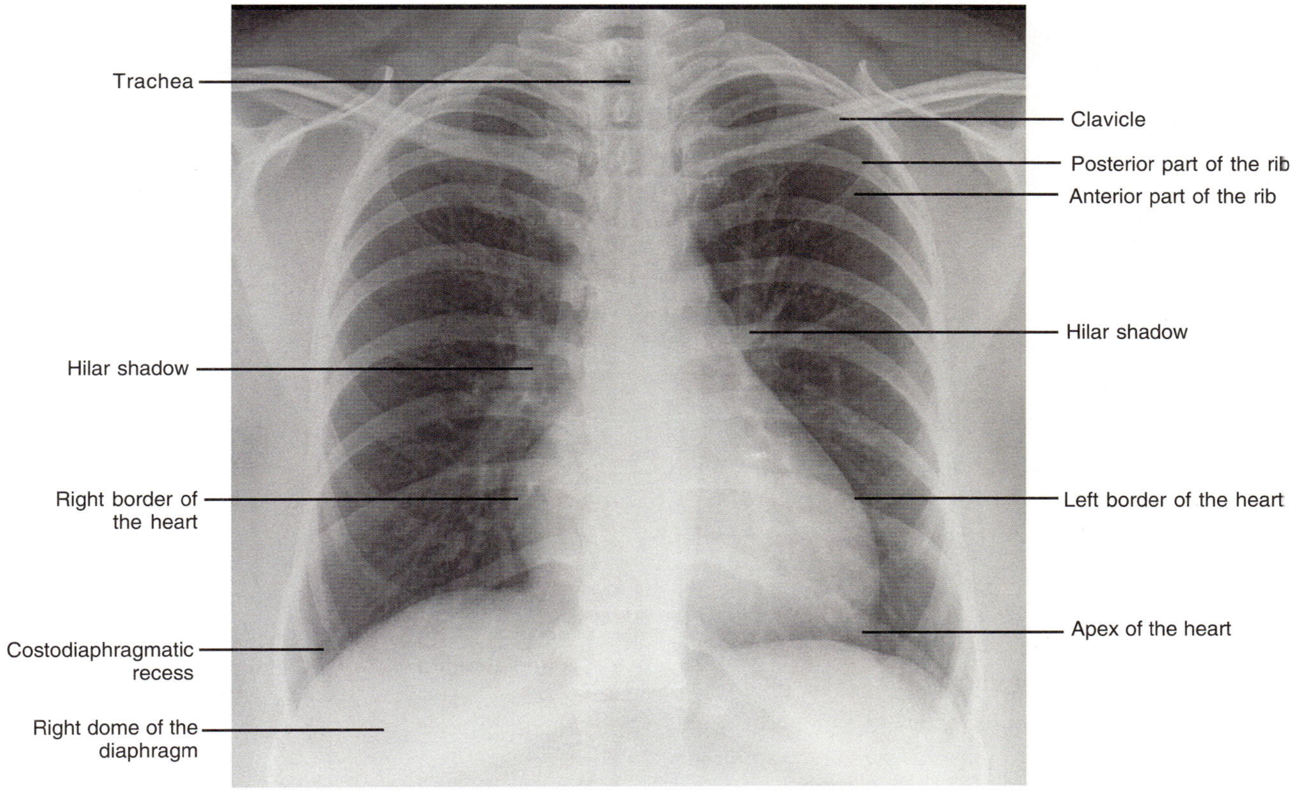

Trachea

Clavicle

Posterior part of the rib

Anterior part of the rib

Hilar shadow

Hilar shadow

Right border of
the heart

Left border of the heart

Costodiaphragmatic
recess

Apex of the heart

Right dome of the
diaphragm

Fig. 19.18 Chest radiograph—PA view

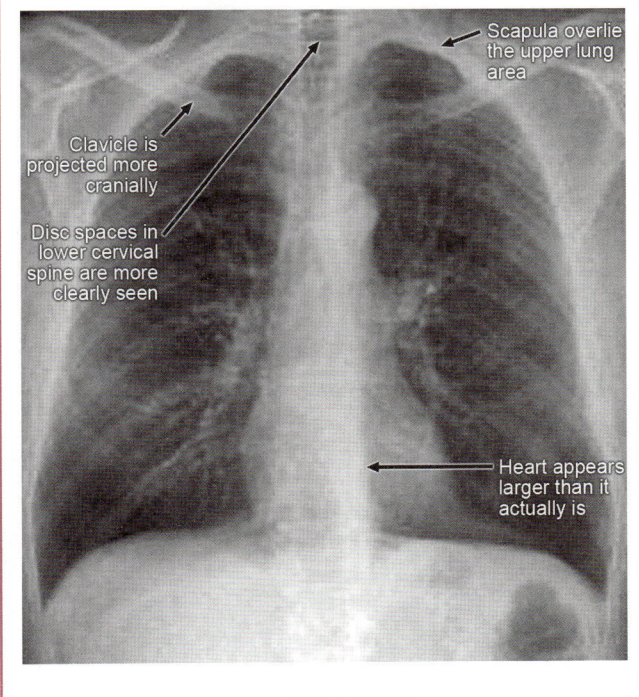

Scapula overlie
the upper lung
area

Clavicle is
projected more
cranially

Disc spaces in
lower cervical
spine are more
clearly seen

Heart appears
larger than it
actually is

Fig. 19.19 Chest X-ray—AP view

and left domes of the diaphragms are visible with a translucent area beneath the left dome of the diaphragm which is due to the gas in the fundus of the stomach.

MICROSCOPIC STRUCTURE

The alveoli of the lung are lined by simple squamous cells. The alveoli are set close to the capillaries derived from the pulmonary artery (carrying deoxygenated blood). The structures intervening between air of lung alveoli and blood of pulmonary capillaries constitute air-blood barrier. The structures include (Fig. 19.21):

a. Flattened epithelium of the alveoli

b. Its basement membrane

c. Basement membrane of the capillary

d. Endothelial cells lining the capillaries

The average thickness of this barrier is about 0.2 µm. The total surface area of alveoli is about 70–100 sq. meters (both lungs).

SECTION 5

329

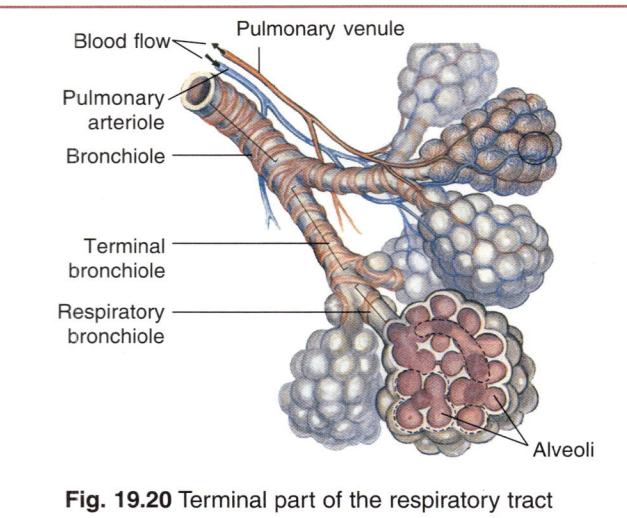

Fig. 19.20 Terminal part of the respiratory tract

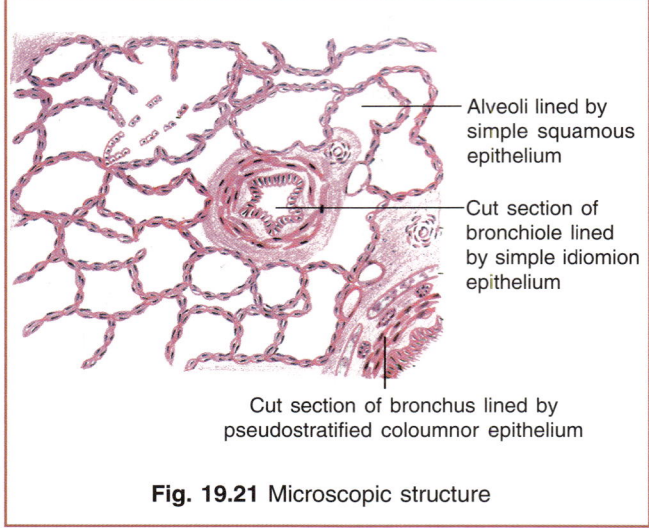

Fig. 19.21 Microscopic structure

The alveoli also present some specialized cells, which secrete fluid which acts as 'surfactant' by reducing the surface tension and thereby preventing the collapse of alveoli during expiration.

- Pulmonary surfactant is not produced until the end of foetal life. In premature infants, the alveoli collapse during exhalation and must be completely reinflated during each inspiration, an effort that requires tremendous expenditure of energy. This can lead to exhaustion and respiratory failure. The condition is called **infant respiratory distress syndrome** (IRDS).

Bronchoscopy:

- A bronchoscope is introduced through respiratory passage to examine the internal surface of the main bronchi in the lung. The tube is inserted through the nose or mouth and guided inferiorly through the larynx and trachea. At the bifurcation of the trachea, the **'carina'** is identified. It is the cartilaginous projection. In case of carcinoma, if the tracheobronchial lymph node that are placed between the two main bronchi is enlarged, it can distort the carina. The mucous membrane covering the carina is highly sensitive and is associated with cough reflex. For example, when a foreign body is aspirated, the people choke and cough. In such case, the person is inverted to make use of the gravity to expel the foreign body. Forceps may be attached to the tip of the tube to remove trapped objects, take biopsy samples or retrieve samples of mucous for examination.

Aspiration of foreign body:

- The right principal bronchus is wider, shorter and more vertical and hence the aspirated foreign bodies

or food is more likely to enter it. Infections are more common on the right lung for the same reason. The apical segment of the lower lobe and posterior segment of the upper lobe are common sites of lung abscess caused by aspiration because these segments are most dependent parts of the lung.

Pneumonia:

- Infection and inflammation of the lungs in which fluid accumulates in the alveoli (Fig. 19.22).

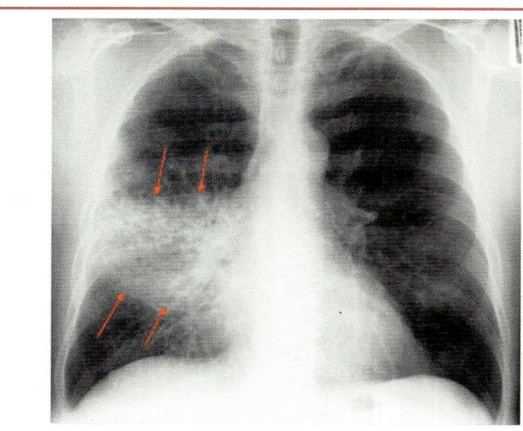

Fig. 19.22 Pneumonia

Tuberculosis (TB):

- It is caused by bacterium Mycobacterium tuberculosis, which primarily enters the body in inhaled air. The TB typically affects the lungs but can spread through lymph vessels to the other organs. The symptoms of TB are coughing, fever and chest pain. The **posterior segment of the right upper lobe** is frequently the site of tuberculosis

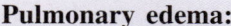

Pulmonary edema:

- It is the accumulation of the fluid in the lung alveoli. It occurs in inflammation of the lung tissue. It mainly occurs in pneumonia or left ventricular failure due to myocardial infarction, mitral stenosis, mitral regurgitation or systemic hypertension. It is characterized by dyspnea, sweating and cyanosis.

Bronchogenic carcinoma

- It is the most common cancer in men. Cancer cells spread mostly by the lymphatics. Over 90% of the lung cancer patients are smokers. The three most common types of lung cancer are
- Squamous cell carcinoma (20 to 40% cases)
- Adenocarcinoma (25 to 30%)
- Small cell carcinoma (20%)

    The anterior segment of the upper lobe is frequently the site for carcinoma. The lung cancer involving a phrenic nerve may result in paralysis of one half of the diaphragm (hemidiaphragm). Since left recurrent laryngeal nerve is related to medial surface of left lung near its apex, may cause hoarseness due to paralysis of vocal cord.

Lung resection:

For surgical resection of diseased bronchopulmonary segment, a sound knowledge of bronchopulmonary segments and their interpretation in radiographs and other medical images are essential. Tumours or abscesses are often confined to a bronchopulmonary segments, may be surgically resected. In case of carcinoma of the lung, whole lung (pneumonectomy), a lobe (lobectomy), or a bronchopulmonary segment (segmentectomy) may be removed.

Asthma

Asthma is a common chronic inflammatory disease of the respiratory tract characterized by variable and recurring symptoms, airflow obstruction, and bronchospasm. It is characterized by wheezing, cough, chest tightness, and shortness of breath.

CASE - 3

A patient presents with a cold which she has been suffering from the past 48 hours. This morning she experienced blood in her sputum (hemoptysis) when she coughs. When she coughs you notice that she bends her chest to the right and has a pained expression (it is a really sharp pain). She also tells you that it hurts when

take a deep breath and is harder to even to do so (Dyspnea). Upon asking the patient to locate the pain, she points to the right side of her chest (The patient abducts the right arm and places the palm of the left hand over the lateral aspect of the right breast and fingers over the medial wall of the right axilla). With the patient seated upright, auscultation reveals the following findings at the 2nd and 3rd intercostal spaces along the right midaxillary line: 1. Fine rales (crepitation or clicking) at the end of deep inspiration. 2. Percussion dullness is found at the same site

a. Which lobe of the lung is affected?

b. Explain the basis for dyspnea in this patient?

c. Use your knowledge of the nerve supply of the thorax to explain the sharp pain experienced when coughing

d. Examine the chest radiograph and identify all lobes and the structures defining the borders of the cardiovascular shadow.

CASE - 4

A 65-year-old obese lady with the past history of thrombophlebitis in the leg was admitted to the hospital, for a surgery of hip replacement after traumatic neck fracture of the femur. Her cardiac functions were normal. During postoperative period she was reluctant to undergo routine physical therapy and always preferred to be on the bed. She suddenly developed dyspnea, anginal pain, hemoptysis, cyanosis and also deterioration of mental function. A CT angiogram revealed a 'pulmonary embolism' in the left pulmonary artery bifurcation. A catheter introduced into the pulmonary artery has shattered the clot and the patient was discharged from the hospital after couple of weeks.

a. What is 'pulmonary embolism'?

b. How do you correlate this patients reluctance to do exercise during postoperative period and development of pulmonary embolism?

c. Trace the venous pathway by which a 'thrombus' travel from calf vein to pulmonary artery.

Answers to the case studies:

Case – 1.

The Bronchopulmonary segments are independent units of the lungs, hence removal of one or other segment may not affect oxygenation process. The spreading of infection/tumor from one segment to the other is prevented to some extent by this connective tissue septum.

Case-2

This patient, a smoker, has an advanced carcinoma of the bronchus in the upper lobe of the left lung that has metastasized (spread) to the tracheobronchial lymph nodes. Enlargement of these nodes has resulted in pressure on the left recurrent laryngeal nerve as it passes under the arch of the aorta. Partial injury of the recurrent laryngeal nerve results in paralysis of the abductor muscles of the vocal cords, leaving the adductor muscles unopposed. The left vocal cord was therefore adducted and immobile.

Case-3

a. Consolidation of the upper lobe of the right lung

b. The patient's dyspnea indicates inadequate ventilation or perfusion of the lungs.

c. The patient's chest pain appears to be somatic pain originating from the parietal pleura of the right pleural space. The movements of the chest wall and diaphragm during inspiration stretch the parietal pleura of the pleural spaces. The increased tension in the parietal pleura elicits a sharp, knife-like pain if the parietal pleura is inflamed. Sharp chest pain produced by the stretching of inflamed parietal pleura is called pleuritic pain.

d. Refer Figs 19.18 and 19.19.

Case-4

a. An obstruction or a sudden blockage of a pulmonary artery by a blood clot (embolus) or fat globule, blood clot or air bubble is called pulmonary embolism (a clot that forms in one part of the body and travels in the bloodstream to another part of the body is called an embolus).

b. Immobilization of legs after surgery is a predisposing factor, which can cause deep vein thrombosis (DVT). During postoperative period, there is minimum activity of the legs, which can cause venous stasis and thrombosis. The emboli enter venous circulation to reach the right side of the heart and may cause life threatening pulmonary embolism.

Rarely, pulmonary embolism leads to localized destruction of lung tissue called pulmonary infarction by blocking the arterial blood supply. Infarction is more likely to happen in people with chronic heart or lung disease. Although pulmonary infarction may be so mild as to cause no symptoms, massive embolism (more than 50% blockage of the pulmonary arterial circulation) and infarction can be fatal.

Usually, the first symptom is labored breathing, which may be accompanied by chest pain. Other symptoms include a rapid pulse, a productive cough (sputum may be blood-tinged), slight fever, and fluid build up in the lungs.

c. The embolus from deep veins of the leg enters popliteal vein and then successively through femoral, external iliac, common iliac, inferior vena cava, right atrium, right ventricle, pulmonary trunk and pulmonary artery.

MCQs

1. During routine cadaveric dissection, a medical student attempted to pass his index finger posterio-inferior to the root of the lung, but he found that the passage was blocked. Which structure would most likely be responsible for this?
   A. Costodiaphragmatic recess
   B. Inferior vena cava
   C. Left pulmonary vein
   D. Pulmonary ligament

2. A 50-year-old patient attends the clinic with the complaints of cough with blood, fever 39°C for 7 days. On auscultation of the chest posteriorly the physician could not hear the normal breathe sounds above the fifth rib. Which of the following lobe was the physician auscultating?
   A. Inferior lobe
   B. Superior lobe
   C. Lingula
   D. Middle lobe

3. During a pneumectomy the surgeon started operating anterior to the right hilum of the lung. Which of the following structures will be incised (cut) first?
   A. Thoracic duct
   B. Pulmonary artery
   C. Right bronchus
   D. Pulmonary vein

4. A 50-year-old male with a chronic history of smoking presented with a hoarse voice and inability to abduct his left vocal cords. The patient also had a mass in the upper lobe of his left lung. Which of the following structures of the lung could have involved the left recurrent laryngeal nerve?
   A. Tracheobranchial nodes
   B. Thoracic duct
   C. Parasternal nodes
   D. Bronchopulmonary nodes

SECTION 5

5. While examining the chest of a patient, you attempt to identify the oblique fissure. The oblique fissure lies parallel to a line interconnecting the _____ spinous process posteriorly, _____ rib in the midaxillary line, _____ costal cartilage anteriorly. Select the correct sequence

    A. T3, 5th, 6th
    B. T3, 6th, 7th
    C. T4, 5th, 6th
    D. T5, 6th, 7th

6. The enlargement of which of the following group of lymph nodes is most likely to compress left recurrent laryngeal nerve?

    A. Bronchopulmonary nodes
    B. Tracheobronchial nodes
    C. Pulmonary nodes
    D. Thoracic duct

7. A chest radiograph shows a tumor at the cardiac notch on the upper lobe of the left lung in a 45-year-old woman. The tumor is located in which of the following bronchopulmonary segments?

    A. Apical
    B. Medial
    C. Posterior
    D. Superior lingular

8. During dental procedure, it is possible that small fragments may be aspirated into the trachea and can cause aspiration pneumonia. If the patient is sitting upright during the procedure, which of the following is the most common site of aspiration pneumonia?

    A. Left lower lobe
    B. Left upper lobe
    C. Right upper lobe
    D. Right lower lobe

9. A 16-year old boy while lying supine in bed and eating, aspirates a peanut. Which of the following bronchopulmonary segments would this foreign object is most likely enter?

    A. Apical segment of the left upper lobe
    B. Apical segment of the right upper lobe
    C. Medial segment of the right middle lobe
    D. Superior segment of the right lower lobe

10. Which part of the left lung might partially fill the costomediastinal recess in full inspiration?

    A. Apex
    B. Cupola

C. Hilum
D. Lingula

11. The oblique fissure of the right lung separates which structures?

    A. Upper from middle
    B. Lower lobe from upper lobe only
    C. Lower lobe from both upper and middle lobes
    D. Lower lobe from middle lobe only

12. A 35-year-old man was stabbed at the back with a knife that just nicked his left lung halfway between its apex and diaphragmatic surface. Which part of the lung was most likely injured?

    A. Hilum
    B. Inferior lobe
    C. Lingula
    D. Middle lobe

13. A 4-year-old girl is brought in with coughing, and you are told by her mother that she had been playing with some beads and had apparently aspirated one (gotten it into her airway). Where would you expect it to most likely be?

    A. Left main bronchus
    B. Lingular segment of left lung
    C. Right main bronchus
    D. Terminal bronchiole of right lung, lower lobe

14. A sick person, lying supine in bed, aspirates (breathes in) some fluid into her lungs while swallowing. It would most likely end up in which of the following bronchopulmonary segments?

    A. Anterior segmental bronchus of right superior lobe
    B. medial segmental bronchus of right middle lobe
    C. superior segmental bronchus of right inferior lobe
    D. medial basal segmental bronchus of left inferior lobe

15. A 10-year-old boy underwent tonsillectomy under general anesthesia. At home he laid supine in bed for two weeks and developed fever and chest pain with cough. He returned to the hospital and was diagnosed as having right lung pneumonia due to aspiration of infectious material during the tonsillectomy. In which bronchopulmonary segment of the lung is fluid (pus) most likely have been accumulated by the simple force of gravity?

    A. Anterior basal segment—inferior lobe
    B. Anterior segment—superior lobe
    C. Lateral segment—middle lobe
    D. Superior segment—inferior lobe

SECTION 5

333

16. A 24-year-old man involved in street fight was brought to the hospital with a deep laceration in the right fourth intercostal space around the midclavicular line. Which lobe is most likely to be damaged?

   A. Upper lobe
   B. Middle lobe
   C. Lower lobe
   D. Lingula

17. A patient was brought to the emergency department with a knife wound at the right fifth intercostal space in the midaxillary line. Which of the following structures is likely to have been damaged?

   A. Middle lobe of the right lung
   B. Right atrium
   C. Right pulmonary artery
   D. Upper lobe of right lung

18. A 93-year-old lady, who is on a liquid diet was fed in bed. She refuses to sit up, so the nurse had to feed her while she is lying on her back. Halfway through the feeding, the patient aspirates the liquid and subsequently develops pneumonia. Which of the following is the most likely site affected by pneumonia?

   A. Anterior segment of the right upper lobe
   B. Apical segment of the right lower lobe
   C. Inferior lingular segment of the left upper lobe
   D. Lateral segment of the right middle lobe

19. A thoracic CT scan of a patient reveals that a neoplasm of the right lung has expanded medially into the wall of the pericardium, and has compressed nerve fibers that coursed on the surface of the pericardium anterior to the root of the lung. Which of the following signs or symptoms might you expect in this individual?

   A. Decreased heart rate and cardiac output
   B. Hoarseness
   C. Right hemidiaphragm
   D. Slow gastric emptying

20. A 55-year-old woman is undergoing radiographic evaluation for bronchogenic carcinoma that is discovered incidentally in the lateral segmental bronchus. The tumor is most likely located in which of the following lobes of the lung?

   A. Lower lobe of left lung
   B. Lower lobe of right lung
   C. Middle lobe of right lung
   D. Upper lobe of left lung

Answers to the MCQs

1. D
2. B
3. D
4. A
5. A
6. B
7. D
8. D
9. D
10. D
11. C
12. B
13. C
14. C
15. D
16. B
17. D
18. B
19. C
20. C

SECTION 5

Pericardium and Heart 20

- Pericardium
- Heart - External features
- Chambers of the heart-Right atrium
- Right ventricle
- Left atrium
- Left ventricle
- MCQs

Objectives

- To list different subdivisions of the pericardium, their nerve supply and its clinical relevance
- To explain the anatomy of the pericardial sinuses and their clinical relevance
- To understand the anatomy of the pericardiocentesis
- To explain the external features of the heart
- To mark the borders of the heart on a cadaver or a patient
- To explain the internal features of each chambers of the heart including the features of the valves
- To locate the auscultation areas of the cardiac valves in a cadaver or in a patient
- To identify the normal features observed in a PA-view of chest X-ray

PERICARDIUM

Heart is covered by a fibro-serous membrane called 'pericardium'. Pericardium consists of outer fibrous layer and inner serous layer. The pericardium keeps the heart in position and prevents its over-distention. The pericardium has the following parts.

The inner serous pericardium has an outer parietal layer, which blends with fibrous pericardium. The visceral layer (epicardium) of the serous pericardium is closely applied

to the heart. The space between the two layers of serous pericardium is called 'pericardial cavity', which contains thin layer of fluid, (which allows the free movement of the heart within the fibrous pericardium).

Fibrous pericardium

- It is a tough non-elastic external layer of the pericardium.
- Superiorly it continues with the tunica adventitia of great vessels entering or emerging from the heart and also with pretracheal layer of the deep cervical fascia.
- Anteriorly it is attached to the posterior surface of the body of the sternum by superior and inferior sterno pericardial ligaments.
- Posteriorly it is separated from the posterior mediastinum by loose connective tissue.
- Inferiorly it is attached to the central tendon of the diaphragm by pericardiophrenic ligament.
- The central tendon of the diaphragm and the fibrous pericardium is developmentally from the same source, the septum transversum.

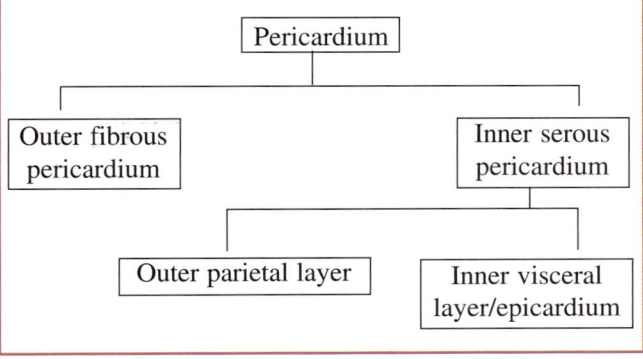

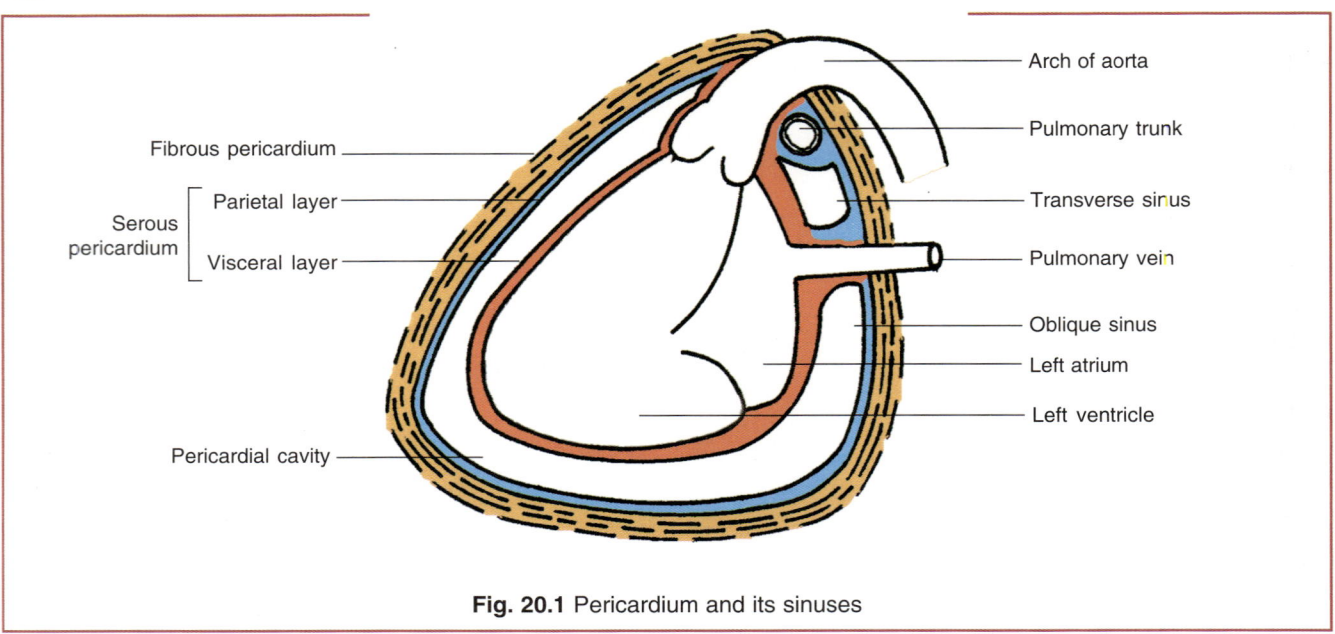

Fig. 20.1 Pericardium and its sinuses

- The fibrous pericardium protects the heart against sudden overfilling because it is so unyielding.

- The ascending aorta carries the pericardium superiorly beyond the heart to the level of sternal angle (Fig. 20.1).

Serous pericardium

- It is thin glistening membrane having an outer parietal layer and inner visceral layer. It is made up of single layer of mesothelial cells resting on the basement membrane.

- It's parietal layer lines the inner surface of the fibrous pericardium and inner visceral layer (epicardium) covers the external surface of the heart.

- The visceral layer becomes continuous with parietal layer where aorta and pulmonary trunk leave the heart and SVC, IVC and pulmonary veins enter the heart.

Pericardial sinuses

These are parts of the pericardial cavity formed around the sites of reflection between serous and visceral pericardium. The pericardial sinuses are formed during the development of the heart, as a consequence of the folding of the developing heart tube (Figs 20.1 and 20.2)

1. **Transverse sinus:** It is a transverse gap behind the pulmonary trunk and ascending aorta and in front of the superior vena cava.

   Boundaries:

   Anteriorly: Visceral pericardium covering ascending aorta and pulmonary trunk

Posteriorly: Visceral pericardium covering anterior surface of the left atrium.

On each side it opens into pericardial cavity.

2. **Oblique sinus:** It is part of the pericardial cavity behind the left atrium.

   Boundaries:

   Anteriorly: Visceral pericardium covering posterior surface of the left atrium

   Posteriorly: Parietal pericardium and fibrous pericardium further outside.

   On right side it is bound by pericardial reflection from inferior vena cava to right pulmonary veins and left side by pericardial reflection from left pulmonary veins.

   The oblique sinus opens inferiorly into the pericardial cavity. Fingers can be passed just behind the apex of the heart and traced upwards through this inferior opening of the oblique sinus.

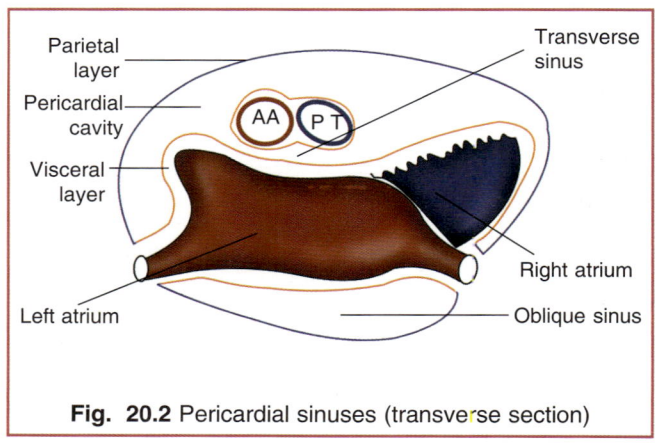

Fig. 20.2 Pericardial sinuses (transverse section)

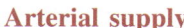

Arterial supply

- The fibrous and parietal layer are supplied by branches of internal thoracic artery and descending thoracic aorta. It is also supplied by pericardiophrenic artery.
- The visceral layer is supplied by coronary arteries.

Nerve supply

- The fibrous and parietal layers are supplied by phrenic nerve (C3–5).
- The visceral layer is supplied by vagus and sympathetic nerves.
- The pain sensation from the fibrous pericardium is carried by phrenic nerve and is referred to the skin above the clavicle (which is supplied by supraclavicular nerves sharing root value C3,4)

1. **Surgical significance of Transverse Pericardial sinus:** During cardiac surgeries, after opening of the pericardial cavity, a finger can be passed through the transverse pericardial sinus that lie posterior to the ascending aorta and pulmonary trunk. By passing a surgical clamp or a ligature around these large vessels, inserting the tubes of the coronary bypass machine, the surgeons can stop or divert the circulation of blood in these arteries while performing cardiac surgery.

2. **Pericarditis, Pericardial Rub and Pericardial Effusion:** The inflammation of pericardium in several diseases is called pericarditis. It causes chest pain. The serous pericardium becomes rough. The smooth opposing layers of serous pericardium, normally makes no detectable sound during auscultation. In case of pericarditis, friction between the two layers of the serous pericardium sounds like the **rustle of silk** when listening with a stethoscope. This is called **pericardial friction rub**. A chronic inflammation of the pericardium adversely affects the functioning of the heart. The accumulation of the fluid in the pericardial cavity is called **pericardial effusion**, which occurs in certain inflammatory diseases. In pericardial effusion, the heart will not be able to expand fully.

3. **Cardiac Tamponade:** The compression of the heart due to excessive pericardial effusion is called cardiac tamponade. If extensive pericardial effusion exists, the pericardial sac does not allow full expansion of the heart due to tough, inelastic nature of the fibrous pericardium. It causes a decrease in the cardiac output. The accumulation of the blood in the pericardial cavity is called **hemopericardium**, it can

also produce cardiac tamponade. In chest radiograph it appears as a globular shadow.

4. **Pericardiocentesis:** In case of cardiac tamponade, it is necessary to drain excess fluid from the pericardial cavity. The procedure by which the excessive fluid of the pericardial cavity is removed is called Pericardiocentesis. There are two approaches for this procedure

a. Parasternal route: A needle may be inserted through the left 5th or 6th intercostal space near the lateral border of the sternum. This approach is possible through the cardiac notch in the left lung and shallower notch in the left pleural cavity. This is the area, where heart and the pericardium is not overlapped by lung and pleura (area of superficial cardiac dullness).

b. Subcostal route: The needle is introduced at the left costoxiphoid angle in an upward, backward direction to enter the pericardial cavity (through the rectus sheath and central tendon of the diaphragm). The needle is inserted at an angle of 45° towards the left scapula.

In this approach, the needle will not enter into pleural cavity, because both anterior border of left lung (cardiac notch) and costomediastinal reflection of pleura deviates laterally below the level of left 4th costal cartilage. However care must be taken not to puncture the internal thoracic artery or its terminal branches (Fig. 20.3). In acute cardiac tamponade an emergency thoracotomy may be performed.

CASE -1

A 26-year-old male is brought into the emergency room after having been kicked on the chest by his opponent team mate while playing foot-ball. After examination,

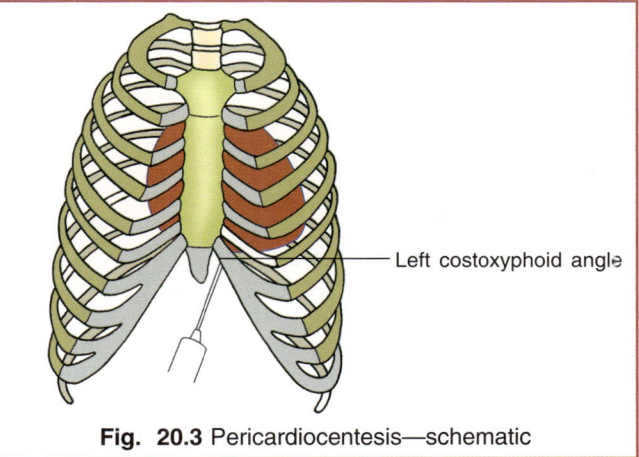

Fig. 20.3 Pericardiocentesis—schematic

SECTION 5

it is concluded that the most likely immediate complication of this condition is cardiac tamponade (bleeding into the pericardial cavity). The physician decide to draw off some amount of the blood from the cavity to relieve the pressure on the heart.

a. What is cardiac tamponade?

b. How does the pericardial tamponade appear in a chest radiograph?

c. What are the two approaches for pericardiocentesis?

HEART—EXTERNAL FEATURES

Human heart is a hollow muscular organ, which pumps blood to various parts of the body to meet the nutritive requirement. It is slightly larger than one own clenched fist.

Situation

The heart is placed obliquely in the thoracic cavity (middle mediastinum) between the two lungs and behind the sternum (Fig. 20.4).

The measurement

The normal adult heart measures about 12 cm vertically and about 6 cm antero-posteriorly. The average weight of the male heart is 300 g and female heart is 250 g.
The heart consists of four chambers.

The right and left atria, right and left ventricles. The auricles are the extensions (appendages) of atria.

Circulation of blood

The right atrium receives deoxygenated blood from the whole body through the superior and inferior vena cavae and coronary sinus. When it contracts, the blood passes to the right ventricle through the right atrioventricular orifice. When the right ventricle contracts, blood passes to the lungs through the pulmonary trunk and pulmonary arteries. In the lungs it gets oxygenated, returns to the left atrium through the pulmonary veins and reaches the left ventricle through the left atrioventricular orifice. When the left ventricle contracts, the blood passes to the aorta and through its branches to the different parts of the body.

External features

Heart consists of an apex, a base, three surfaces and three borders (Figs 20.5 to 20.7).

Apex of the heart:

- It is conical and is formed by the left ventricle.
- It is situated in the left 5th intercostal space, about 9 cm from the median plane. It remains motionless throughout the cardiac cycle. The sounds of mitral valve closure is best heard during auscultation at this place (apex beat)

Base or posterior surface:

- It is the fixed part of the heart during cardiac motion
- It is formed by two atria (2/3rd by posterior surface of left atrium and 1/3rd by right atrium).

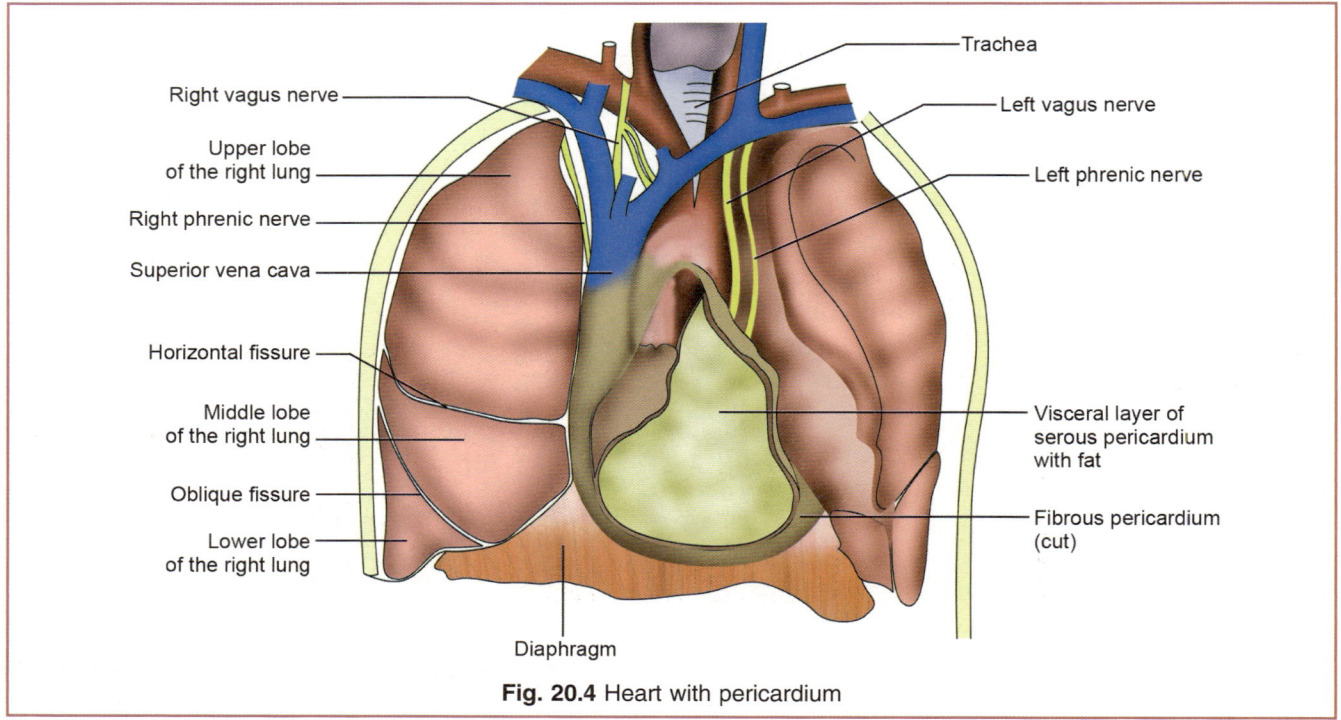

Fig. 20.4 Heart with pericardium

Labels: Right vagus nerve, Upper lobe of the right lung, Right phrenic nerve, Superior vena cava, Horizontal fissure, Middle lobe of the right lung, Oblique fissure, Lower lobe of the right lung, Diaphragm, Trachea, Left vagus nerve, Left phrenic nerve, Visceral layer of serous pericardium with fat, Fibrous pericardium (cut)

- Posteriorly it is related to the bodies of the vertebrae T6-T9 and is separated from them by **right pair** of pulmonary veins, **oesophagus**, descending thoracic aorta (Fig. 20.5).
- Enlargement of left atrium in mitral stenosis **may compress oesophagus** and produce difficulty in swallowing.

Sternocostal surface:

- It is formed mainly by right ventricle and also right atrium with its auricle, and part of the left ventricle.
- This surface is related to posterior aspect of the sternum and adjoining costal cartilages (3rd to 6th costal cartilage) but separated by pericardium, anterior margins of lung with pleura.
- Due to the cardiac notch of left lung, lungs do not cover a portion of right ventricle on this surface. This area is called **area of superficial cardiac dullness**.
- The sternocostal surface presents anterior part of the coronary sulcus and anterior interventricular sulcus (Figs 20.5 and 20.6).

Diaphragmatic (inferior) surface:

- It rests on the central portion of the diaphragm and separates the heart from liver and fundus of stomach.
- The diaphragmatic surface is formed by two ventricles, 2/3rd by left ventricle and 1/3rd by right ventricle.
- This surface is traversed by posterior interventricular sulcus (Figs 20.5 and 20.7).

Left surface:

- It is formed by left ventricle and partly by left atrium and its auricle.
- The major part of this surface is related to medial surface of the left lung.

Right border:

- It is vertical and formed by right atrium only.
- It extends from the right side of the superior vena caval orifice to inferior vena caval orifice.
- A shallow sulcus 'sulcus terminalis' runs along the right border.
- The right border separates sternocostal surface from the base of the heart. This border is closely related to right pericardiophrenic vessels.

Inferior border

- It is horizontal formed mainly by right ventricle and partly by left ventricle.
- This border extends from inferior vena caval orifice to apex of the heart.

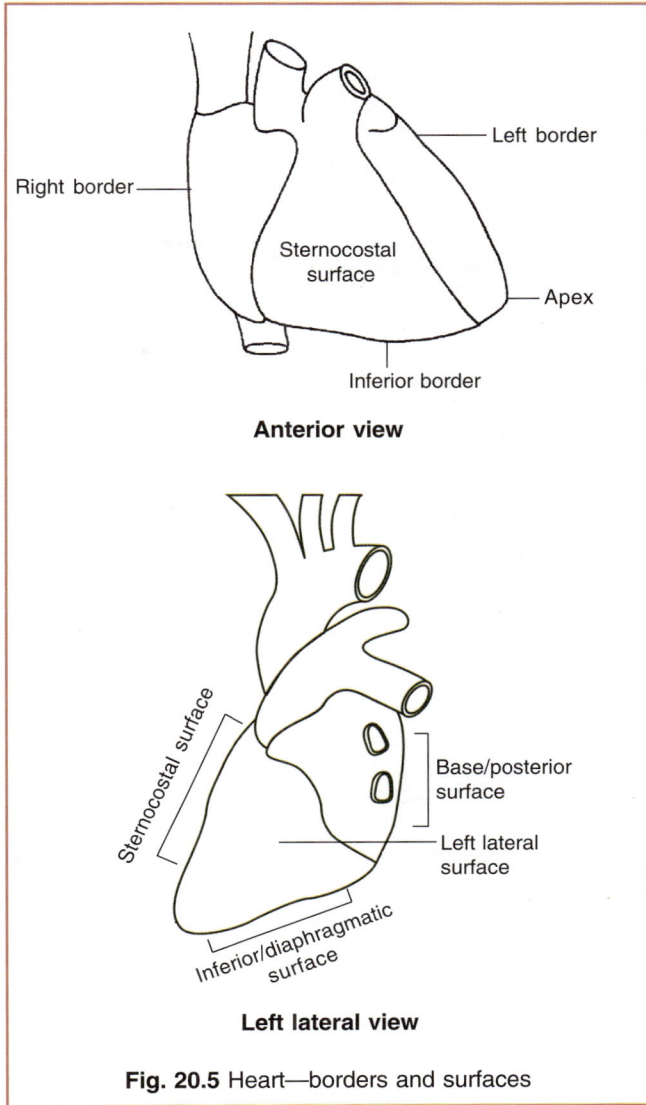

Anterior view

Left lateral view

Fig. 20.5 Heart—borders and surfaces

- Inferior border separates diaphragmatic surface from the sternocostal surface.

Left border:

- It is ill defined and extends from apex of the heart to the left auricle.
- It is formed by left ventricle and partly by left auricle.
- Left border separates sternocostal surface from left surface.

Coronary sulcus

- The atria are separated from ventricles externally by atrioventricular groove or **coronary sulcus.**
- The right anterior coronary sulcus extend downwards and is occupied by right coronary artery
- The left anterior coronary sulcus intervenes between left auricle and left ventricle and is occupied by

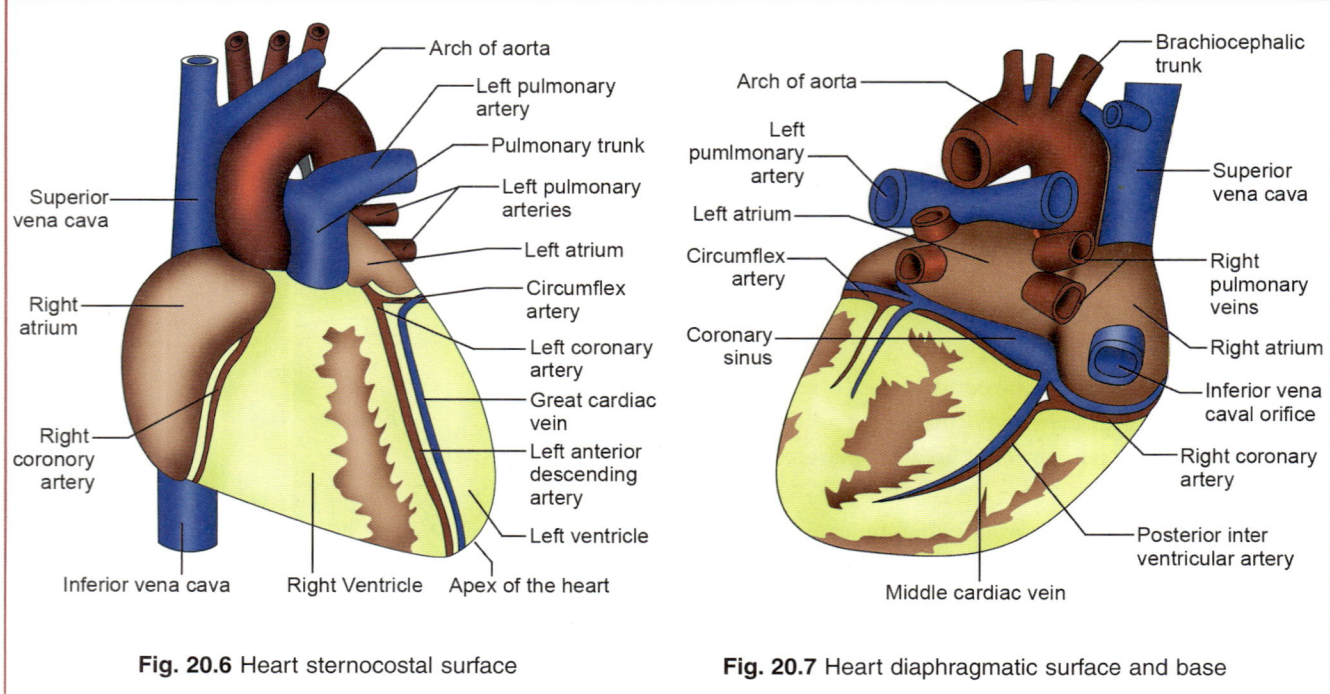

Fig. 20.6 Heart sternocostal surface

Fig. 20.7 Heart diaphragmatic surface and base

circumflex branch of left coronary artery and great cardiac vein

- The posterior part of the coronary sulcus intervenes between base of the heart and its diaphragmatic surface. On the left side, it is occupied by coronary sinus and circumflex artery and on right side by right coronary artery and small cardiac vein.

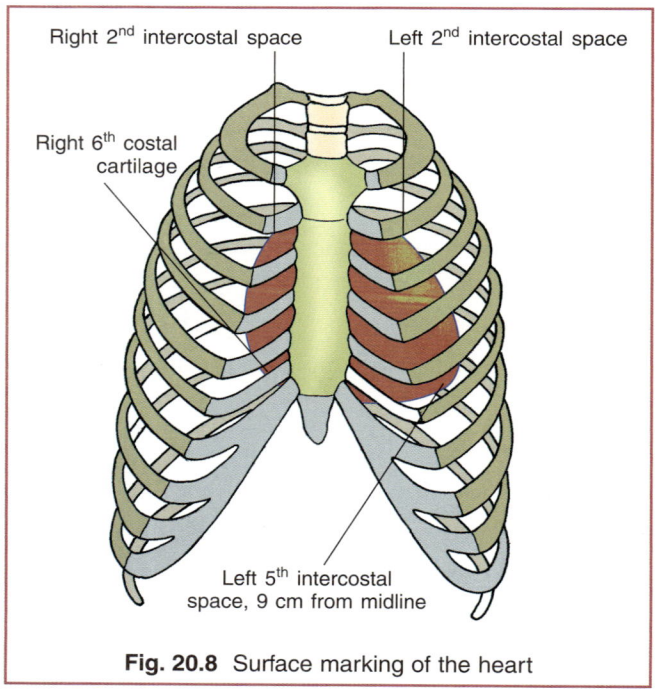

Fig. 20.8 Surface marking of the heart

- The right and left ventricles are separated externally by anterior interventricular sulcus (on sternocostal surface) and posterior interventricular sulcus (on diaphragmatic surface). They are occupied by anterior and posterior inteventricular arteries respectively.

Crux of the heart:

It is the meeting point of posterior interventricular, atrioventricular and interatrial grooves.

Surface marking of the heart

The outline of the heart can be marked by connecting the following points (Fig. 20.8).

Apex: A point 9 cm away from midline in the left 5th intercostal space

Right margin: A point at the lower part of right 2nd intercostal space close to sternum to a point at right 6th costal cartilage, 1–2 cm from sternal margin.

Inferior margin: A point from right 6th costal cartilage to apex of the heart.

Left margin: A point from the apex of the heart to a point on the left 2nd intercostal space 1–2 cm lateral to the sternal margin

Superior margin: It is marked by connecting the upper part of right and left margins.

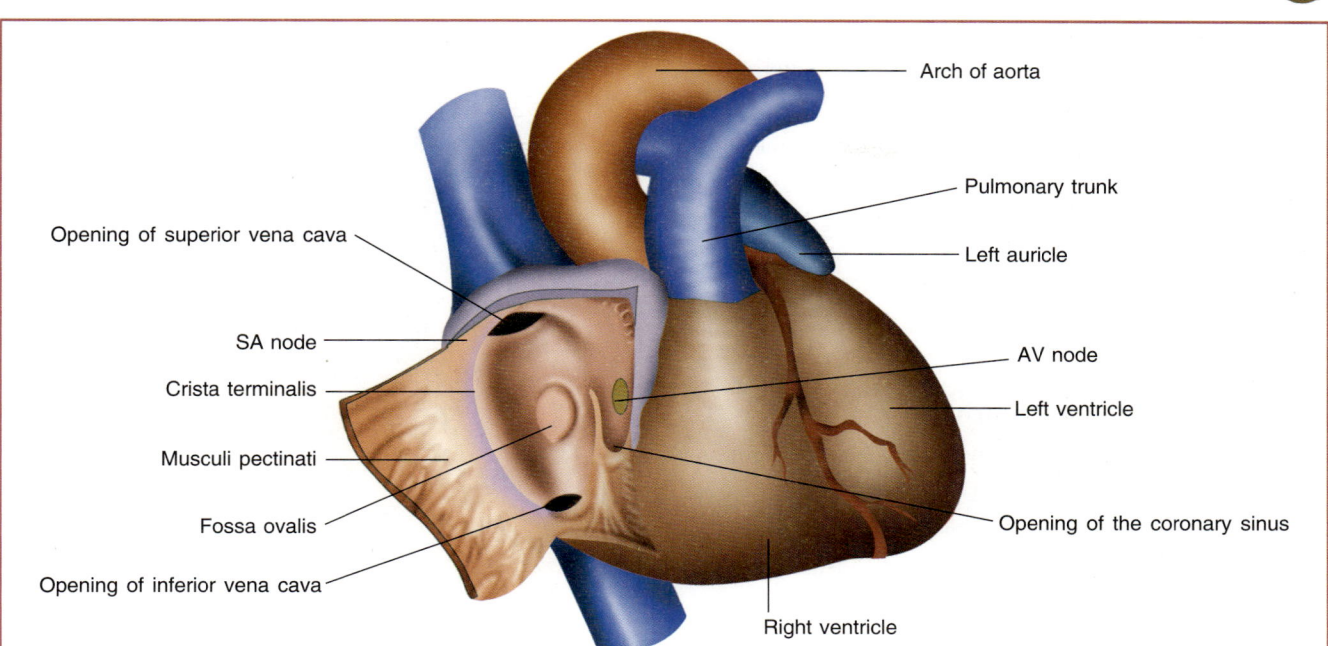

Fig. 20.9 Interior of the right atrium

CHAMBERS OF THE HEART—RIGHT ATRIUM

Right atrium

External features

- It forms the part of the sternocostal surface, entire right border and right 1/3rd of the base.
- Right auricle is the conical projection of right atrium towards ascending aorta.
- Sulcus terminalis is a shallow groove, which extends from superior vena caval orifice to inferior vena caval orifice. It corresponds to a ridge inside the right atrium called 'crista terminalis'.

Interior of the right atrium

The cavity of the right atrium presents three walls (anterior, posterior and septal).

1. Anterior rough wall

- **Crista terminalis** is a smooth muscular ridge, which extends from the upper part of the inter-atrial septum. It passes in front of the superior vena caval orifice and then descends along the right border of the heart. Below it ends by joining with right horn of Eustachian valve (valve guarding IVC orifice)
- Crista terminalis separates anterior rough wall from the posterior smooth wall. Upper part of the crista terminalis lodges sinuatrial node (SA node).

- **Musculi pectinati (Pectinate muscles)** are parallelly placed muscular ridges extending from crista terminalis and are directed towards the right atrioventricular orifice (Fig. 20.9).

2. Posterior smooth wall

- It is also called sinus venarum. It presents the following openings for major veins, which bring deoxygenated blood from the body and the heart itself.
- Opening of the superior vena cava – in the upper part
- Opening of the inferior vena cava – in the lower part. This opening is guarded by a semilunar valve called 'Eustachian valve' which presents right and left horns (Fig. 20.9).
- Opening of coronary sinus: The venous blood from musculature of the heart is drained into coronary sinus which opens into the right atrium between inferior vena caval orifice and right atrioventricular orifice.

3. Septal wall

- It separates the right atrium from left atrium, which is placed posteriorly and to the left. It presents the following features (Fig. 20.9).
- **Fossa ovalis** is an oval depression. In the foetal life the right and left atria are communicated through a foramen called 'foramen ovale'. This opening is closed immediately after the birth. The depression below this opening forms fossa ovalis.

- **Limbus fossa ovalis** – It is the sharp margin surrounding the fossa ovalis in its upper, anterior and posterior margins

- **Triangle of Koch** is a triangular area behind the septal leaflet of the tricuspid valve and the opening of coronary sinus. The atrioventricular node (AV node) is lodged in this area.

- **Torus aorticus** is a bulging produced by the right posterior aortic sinus of the ascending aorta in the septal wall.

Development of the right atrium

1. The anterior rough wall is developed from the right half of the primitive atrium

2. The posterior smooth wall is developed from absorption of body and right horn of the sinus venosus

3. The fossa ovalis of the septal wall is developed from septum primum and remaining part of the septal wall (including limbus fossa ovalis) is developed from septum secundum.

4. The crista terminalis, valve of IVC and valve of coronary sinus are developed from right venous valve.

Right atrioventricular orifice

It is an oval opening communicating right atrium with right ventricle. The blood flows in postero-anterior direction since the plane of the orifice is vertical. This orifice is guarded by tricuspid valve.

Right atrioventricular/Tricuspid valve

- It guards the right atrio-ventricular orifice (Figs 20.13 and 20.14).

- It consists of three cusps or leaflets. They are named anterior, posterior and septal. They are attached to the corresponding sides of the orifice. The other end (free margin) of each cusp extends into the cavity of right ventricle.

- This free margin provides attachments to the 'chordae tendineae' (tendinous cords).

- The chordae tendineae arise from the apical part of the papillary muscles present in the rough part of the right ventricle.

The papillary muscles contract when rest of the ventricle contracts (during ventricular systole), and they pull on the chordae tendineae to prevent the AV valve from everting. The regurgitation of blood from the right ventricle back into the right atrium is blocked during ventricular systole by the valve cusps.

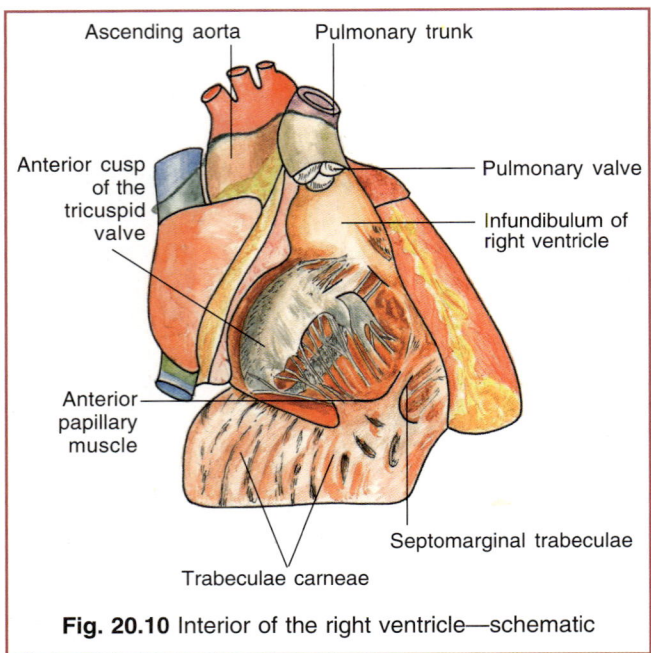

Fig. 20.10 Interior of the right ventricle—schematic

RIGHT VENTRICLE

Right ventricle forms sternocostal surface, diaphragmatic surface and inferior border of the heart.

Internal features

The interior of the right ventricle is semilunar on cross section due to bulging of interventricular septum towards the right ventricular cavity. The interior of the right ventricle consists of two parts:

- Rough inflowing part (ventricle proper)
- Smooth out flowing part (infundibulum)

Rough inflowing part

It receives blood from the right atrium. Roughness of this part is due to the presence of muscular ridges called 'trabeculae carneae'. Trabeculae carneae are of three types (Figs 20.10 and 20.11).

1. **Ridges:** These are muscular elevations, e.g. supraventricular crest which separates the smooth part from the rough part of the right ventricle.

2. **Bridges:** The two ends are connected to the wall of the ventricle with central free portion, e.g. **septo-marginal trabecula (moderator band)** which extends from the interventricular septum to the base of the anterior papillary muscle. It conveys right branch of the atrioventricular (AV) bundle.

3. **Papillary muscles:** These are conical muscular projections usually three in number (anterior, posterior and septal). The **anterior papillary muscle** is the largest

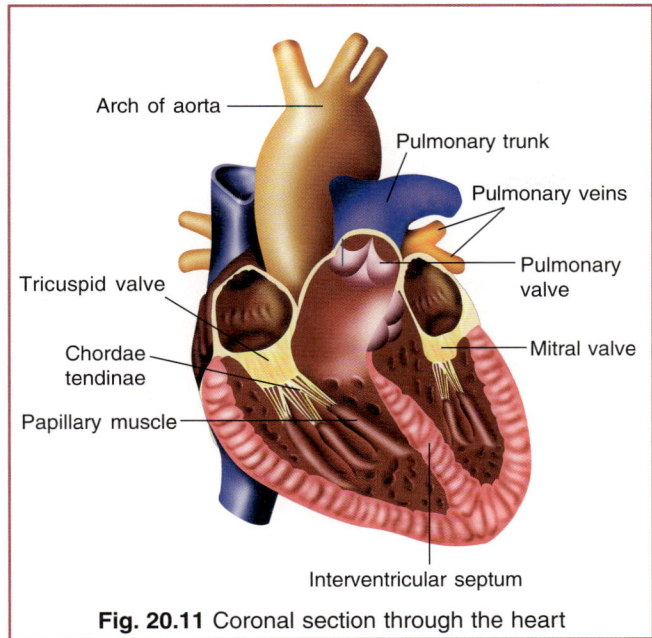

Fig. 20.11 Coronal section through the heart

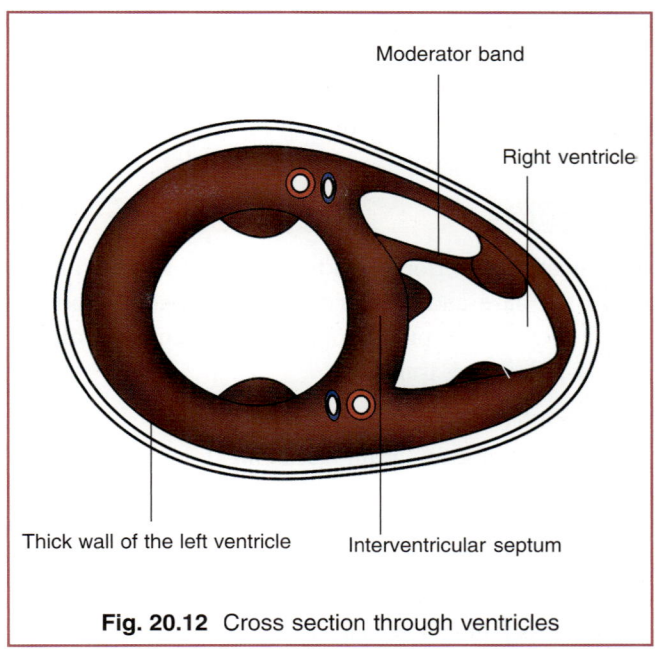

Fig. 20.12 Cross section through ventricles

and most prominent. It arises from the anterior wall of the right ventricle and its chordae tendineae are attached to anterior and posterior cusps of the tricuspid valve. The **posterior papillary muscle** arises from the inferior wall of the right ventricle and its chordae tendineae are attached to posterior and septal cusps. The **septal papillary muscle** arises from interventricular septum and their chordae tendineae are attached to the anterior and septal cusps. The septal papillary muscles are usually divided into a number of small ridges.

Smooth out flowing part (infundibulum)

The apex of the infundibulum presents pulmonary orifice, which is guarded by three semilunar cusps. The free margins of the cusps are directed into the pulmonary trunk.

The right atrium contracts when the right ventricle is empty and relaxed; The blood that enters the right ventricle takes a 'U' shaped path to enter the pulmonary trunk. This change in direction is due to the presence of supraventricular crest (which separates smooth and rough part of the right ventricle).

Development

1. The rough inflowing part is developed from right half of the primitive ventricle
2. The smooth outflowing part is developed from absorption of bulbus cordis (bulboventricular cavity)

Pulmonary valve

It is the most superficial (anterior) and upper most valve. It has 3 semilunar cusps (leaflets) which are right anterior,

left anterior and posterior. There is a thickening in the middle part of the free margins of each cusp called 'nodule'. The margin on either side of the nodule is called 'lunule'. The pulmonary trunk shows little dilatation above the valve called pulmonary sinus.

Interventricular septum

- It is a strong obliquely placed partition between right and left ventricles (Figs 20.11 and 20.12).

- It has muscular (rough) and membranous (smooth) parts. The muscular part is rough due to trabeculae carneae.

- Posterosuperiorly the partition between the two ventricles is formed by a thin membrane called '**pars membranacia septi**' (membranous part).

- The septal leaflet of the tricuspid valve is attached to the middle of the membranous part on its right surface dividing them into superior and inferior parts.

- The inferior part is 'interventricular' separating right and left ventricles.

- The superior part is 'atrioventricular' separating right atrium from the left ventricle.

- The anterior 2/3rd of the septum is supplied by anterior interventricular artery (branch of left coronary artery) and posterior 1/3rd by posterior interventricular artery (branch of right coronary artery)

- The membranous part presents AV bundle and the muscular part has right and left terminal branch of the AV bundle.

- The muscular part is developed from primitive inter-ventricular septum. The membranous part is developed from proliferation of AV cushion (posterior atrio-ventricular part) and proximal bulbar septum (anterior interventricular part).

LEFT ATRIUM

It is situated posteriorly and to the left of right atrium. It forms the base and part of left surface and left border. Left auricle is the projection of left atrium towards the root of pulmonary trunk.

Interior of the left atrium

- The wall of the left atrium is slightly thicker than that of the right atrium.
- A major part of the interior is smooth except at the auricle, which presents musculi pectinati. The posterior wall of the left atrium receives the openings of four valveless pulmonary veins (Fig. 20.11).
- Anteriorly, it communicates with left ventricle through left atrioventricular orifice, which is guarded by 'mitral valve'.
- The septal wall separating it from the right atrium presents a 'lunate fossa' corresponding to the fossa ovalis.

LEFT VENTRICLE

It forms the sternocostal, diaphragmatic and left surfaces and left border of the heart. The apex of the heart is formed by left ventricle. The wall of the left ventricle is three times thicker than that of right ventricle to pump the oxygenated blood to all parts of the body.

Interior of the left ventricle

- The interior is circular in cross section due to bulging of the interventricular septum towards the cavity of right ventricle (Fig. 20.12).
- The interior of the left ventricle also presents an inflowing rough part and a smooth out flowing part (Fig. 20.11).
- The rough inflowing part presents left atrioventricular orifice with mitral valve and trabeculae carneae.
- The trabeculae carneae are finer and more numerous than those of the right ventricle. It presents anterior and posterior papillary muscles.
- The out-flowing part of the left ventricle is called 'aortic vestibule', leading to aortic orifice.

The summit of the vestibule presents three semilunar cusps (aortic valve). Above the cusps the wall of the ascending aorta presents three dilatations called 'aortic sinuses'.

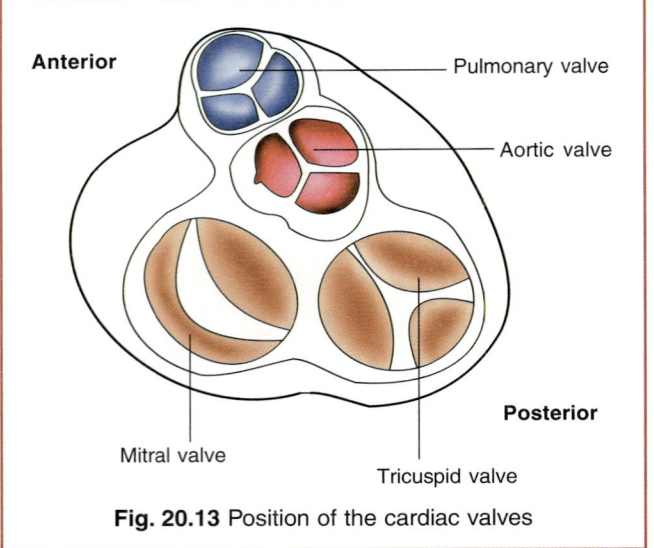

Fig. 20.13 Position of the cardiac valves

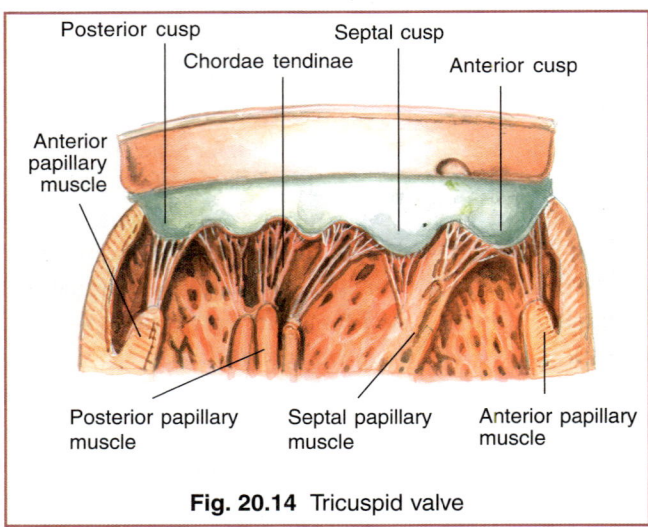

Fig. 20.14 Tricuspid valve

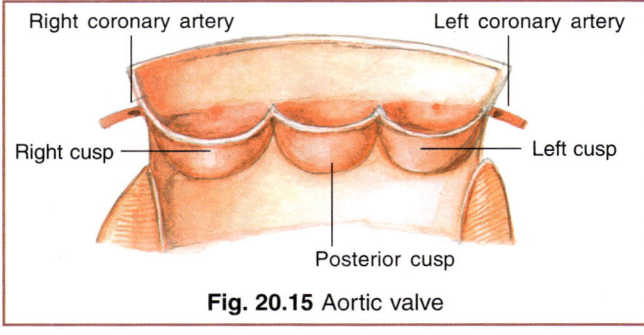

Fig. 20.15 Aortic valve

Left atrioventricular/bicuspid/mitral valve

- It consists of two cusps anterior and posterior (Figs 20.11 and 20.13).
- These cusps are attached to the margin of left atrio-ventricular orifice. Their free ends provide attachment to the chordae tendineae. These chordae tendineae arise from papillary muscles present in the left ventricle.

- The cords become taut just before and during systole, preventing the cusps from being forced into the left atrium

- The mitral valve is most strained because it must resist the powerful contraction of left ventricle. Therefore it is often involved in valve disorders.

Aortic valve

The aortic valve also presents three semilunar cusps (leaflets) which are named as anterior, right posterior and left posterior. The aortic valve is stronger than pulmonary valve. It also presents 'nodule' and 'lunule'. At the level of the cusps, the aorta shows dilatation called aortic sinuses and they are also named according to their position, anterior, right posterior and left posterior. The anterior aortic sinus gives origin to right coronary artery and left posterior aortic sinus gives origin to left coronary artery. The right posterior aortic sinus will not give origin to any coronary artery and is called 'non coronary' which produces a bulge in the right atrium called 'torus aorticus' (Figs 20.13 and 20.15).

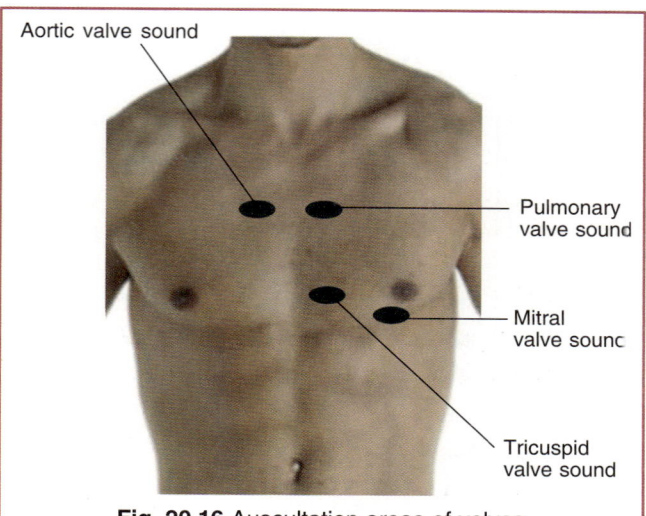

Fig. 20.16 Auscultation areas of valves

Surface markings of the valves/orifice

Pulmonary orifice: Draw 2.5 cm transverse line partly behind the left 3rd costal cartilage and partly behind the adjacent left half of sternum

Aortic orifice: Draw oblique line, 2.5 cm long behind the left half of the body of sternum at the level of 3rd intercostal space

---

Mitral orifice: Draw 3 cm long oblique line behind the left half of the sternum opposite the left 4th costal margin

Tricuspid orifice: Draw 4 cm long line vertically behind the right half of the sternum opposite the 4th intercostal space .

Areas of auscultation of Cardiac valves

Pulmonary valve: Second intercostal space to the left of the sternum (pulmonary valve murmurs, ventricular septal defect murmurs, continuous murmurs of patent ductus arteriosus)

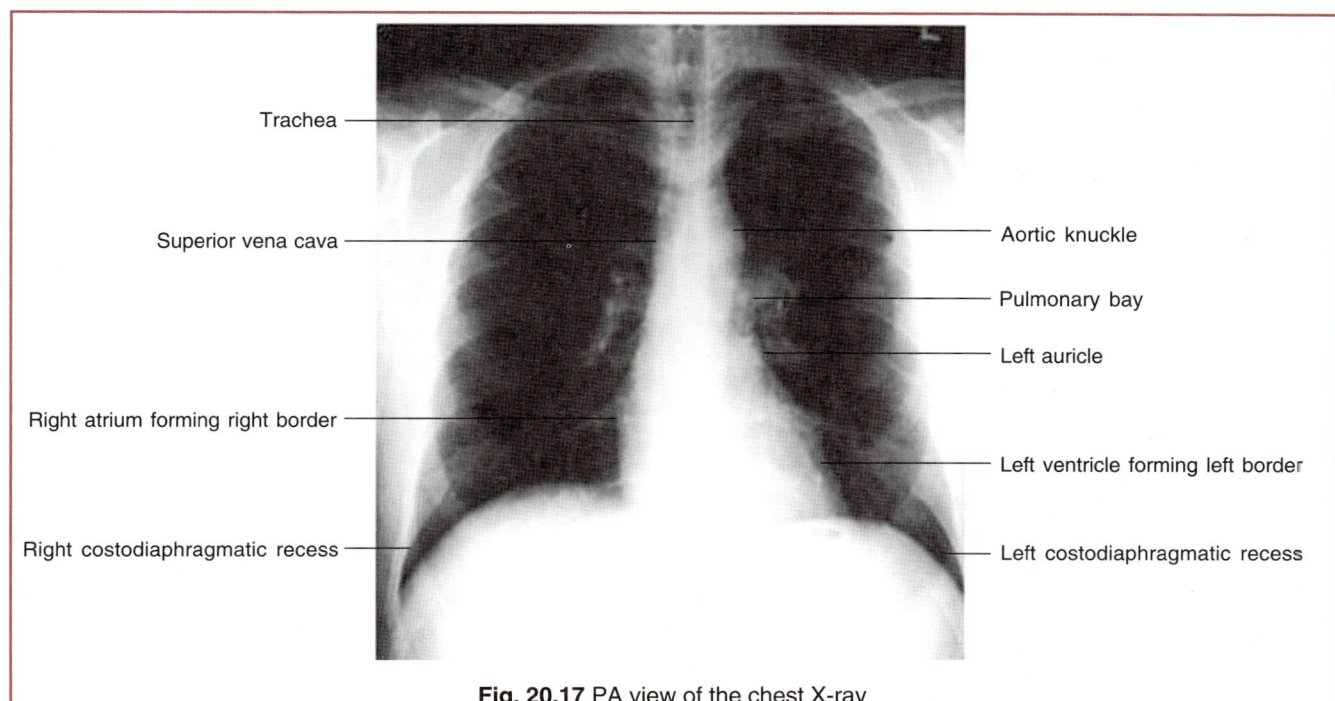

Fig. 20.17 PA view of the chest X-ray

Aortic valve: Second intercostal space to the right of the sternum

Tricuspid valve: Left 4th intercostal space (tricuspid and aortic regurgitation)

Mitral valve: Left 5th intercostal space 9 cm away from midline (apex of the heart) (Fig. 20.16).

Radiological Anatomy of the Heart (PA View)

In a PA chest X-ray, following features of the heart needs to be identified (Fig. 20.17)

- Cardiac shadow of normal sized heart is equal to **half the diameter of the chest**. When it exceeds this ratio (1 : 2), it is suggestive of cardiac enlargement

- Right margin of cardiac shadow is formed by SVC, Right atrium and, IVC

- Left margin of cardiac shadow is formed by Aortic knuckle (produced by arch of aorta), pulmonary bay, left auricle and left ventricle

- **Aortic knuckle:** Aortic knuckle or knob is formed by the posterior part of the arch of the aorta protruding from the mediastinum in radiograph of the chest. It may be indistinct in young people and very prominent in older people. Below the aortic knuckle is the air space called aortopulmonary window. Failure to identify this clear space indicates the pathology.

- The aortic window is a normally radiolucent region below the aortic arch. It is formed by the bifurcation of the trachea and traversed by the left pulmonary artery. It is visible in the left anterior oblique radiograph of the heart and great vessels.

Echocardiography (ECHO) is a method by which the position and motion of the heart is recorded. Pericardial effusion can be detected by this technique. Doppler echocardiography is a technique that demonstrates and records the flow of blood through the heart. This is very useful in diagnosis and analysis of problems with blood flow through the heart, such as septal defects, valvular stenosis and regurgitation. However it is not possible to properly visualise the structures at the base of the heart in ECHO, this drawback is overcome by the transoesophageal echography

Valvular heart diseases: The defect and dysfunctions of the valves will interfere with pumping efficiency of the heart. The valvular heart disease produces either stenosis (narrowing) or insufficiency.

a) Stenosis is a failure of a valve to **open fully**, slowing the blood flow from a chamber

b) Insufficiency (or regurgitation) is failure of valve to **close completely**. It occurs due to structural changes in the valve (nodule formation on the edges of the cusps). It leads to regurgitation of the blood back into the chambers from which it was just ejected.

Both stenosis and regurgitation results in increased work load for the heart and produces turbulence in blood flow. This turbulence results in vibrations which are audible as 'murmurs'.

Clinically the valvular dysfunction may be insignificant in some cases, but in others it may be severe and fatal. The valvular diseases may be congenital or acquired. The diseases of the valves of the heart usually arise from the history of rheumatic fever in childhood. Damaged or defective cardiac valves can be repaired or replaced by artificial valves (made up of synthetic material).

Mitral valve insufficiency (regurgitation/ incompetence):

The mitral valve fails to close during systole and the blood regurgitates into the left atrium. So during diastole there is overfilling left ventricle. Eventually it leads to enlargement of the left ventricle and left ventricular failure.

It is caused by various mechanisms related to structural or functional abnormalities of the mitral valve, adjacent myocardium, or both. Significant mitral valve regurgitation occurs in about 2% of the population with a similar prevalence in males and females.

Patients with chronic, severe mitral regurgitation may remain asymptomatic for years because the regurgitant volume load is well tolerated as a result of compensatory ventricular and atrial dilation. When symptoms do develop, the most common are dyspnea, fatigue, paroxysmal nocturnal dyspnea, and palpitations caused by atrial fibrillation. The chest radiograph demonstrates left atrial enlargement and cardiomegaly.

Mitral valve stenosis: Mitral valve stenosis refers to narrowing of the mitral valve orifice, resulting in impedance of filling of the left ventricle in diastole. It is usually caused by rheumatic heart disease during childhood.

Patients with mitral valve stenosis typically presents it more than 20 years after an episode of rheumatic fever.

Patients with mitral stenosis may present with exertional dyspnea, fatigue, atrial arrhythmias, angina-like chest pain, hemoptysis, or even right-sided heart failure.

On chest radiography, the characteristic findings of mitral stenosis are pulmonary congestion, enlargement of the main pulmonary arteries, and enlargement of the left atrium without cardiomegaly.

An electrocardiogram (ECG) may reveal evidence of left atrial enlargement, atrial fibrillation or, in advanced disease, right ventricular hypertrophy consistent with pulmonary hypertension.

The enlarged left atrium, may compress oesophagus causing dysphagia and on left recurrent laryngeal nerve (hoarseness of voice).

The embolic event of mitral stenosis: The stasis of the blood in the left auricle encourages clot formation. The detached clots form emboli, enter the left ventricle, ascending aorta then into circulation and cause various types of problems depending on sites blocked. It can causes gangrene of lower limb (due to occlusion of femoral artery) or myocardial infarction (due to occlusion of coronary artery) or stroke (occlusion of cerebral artery) or renal infarct (due to occlusion of segmental branch of renal artery).

Aortic valve insufficiency (regurgitation/ incompetence: Aortic regurgitation is incompetence or insufficiency of aortic valve that allow the blood to flow back into the left ventricle. The cusps are unable to close properly due to structural changes. The left ventricle has to repump the blood with every heart beat, leading to an increased work load and **enlargement of left ventricle.**

Aortic valve stenosis: The aortic stenosis is abnormal narrowing of the aortic valve. It is the most common valve abnormalities. It is usually arises from the history of rheumatic fever in the childhood. Aortic stenosis cause extra work for the heart and cause **enlargement of the left ventricle**. The signs and symptoms include angina (chest pain), fainting (syncope) and shortness of breath (associated with exertion or excitement).

Pulmonary valve insufficiency (regurgitation/ incompetence): The structural changes in the pulmonary valves (becoming thick) or damage by disease, cause incomplete closure of this valve. It results in backward flow of blood into the right ventricle **during diastole.** Mild cases usually do not cause any symptoms, but severe regurgitation may contribute to

right ventricular hypertrophy, and in later stages, right heart failure.

Pulmonary valve stenosis: Pulmonary stenosis is narrowing of the pulmonary outflow tract causing obstruction of blood flow from the right ventricle to the pulmonary artery **during systole.** Most cases are congenital; many remain asymptomatic until adulthood. When symptoms develop, they resemble those of aortic stenosis (syncope, angina, dyspnea) and can cause variable degree of right **ventricular hypertrophy.**

Structure of the heart

Heart consists of three coats from outside to inside – epicardium, myocardium and endocardium.

1. **Epicardium:** It is a thin outer covering (mesothelium) derived from the visceral layer of serous pericardium.

2. **Myocardium:** It is made up of cardiac muscles, which present striations with centrally placed nucleus. The muscle fibres branch and anastamose with adjacent fibres. Intercalated discs connect the adjacent muscle cells (myocytes). Some of the cardiac muscle fibres are specialized to form 'Purkinje fibres', which constitute the conducting system of the heart.

   The wall of the ventricle is thicker than that of the atria. The cardiac muscle fibres are anchored to the **fibrous skeleton of the heart**

3. **Endocardium:** It is the lining endothelial cells of the chambers.

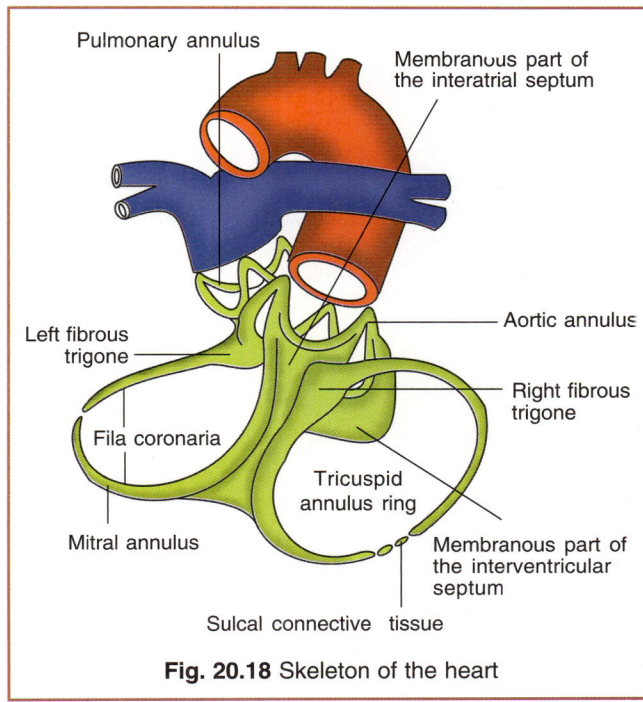

Fig. 20.18 Skeleton of the heart

Fibrous skeleton of the heart

The fibrous skeleton of the heart provides attachment of atrial and ventricular musculature and supports the valves of the heart (keep them competent). The continuity between atrial and ventricular musculature is disturbed by the fibrous skeleton, hence propogation of impulses from atria to ventricle (SA node to AV node) is by specialized conducting system of the heart (Fig. 20.18).

The skeleton consists of four fibrous rings (or annulus) at right and left atrioventricular orifices, pulmonary and aortic orifices.

- The pulmonary annulus are the anterior most, while aortic annulus is placed behind and little to the right of the pulmonary annulus.

- These two annulus is connected by a fibrous structure called **tendon of infundibulum**.

- The right (tricuspid) and left (mitral) atrioventricular annulus are placed further behind the aortic annulus. The right and left atrioventricular annulus are connected by a fibrous structure called **trigonum fibrosum dextrum**. The left margin of the trigonum connects mitral annulus with aortic annulus called trigonum fibrosum sinistrum.

- The left bottom of the aortic annulus forms left fibrous trigone, which gives attachment to the anterior filum coronarium of the mitral annulus. The right bottom of the aortic annulus forms right fibrous trigone, which provides attachment to posterior filum coronarium of the mitral annulus. Thus the mitral annulus is formed by anterior and posterior fila coronaria and the gap between their ends is connected by sulcal connective tissue

- The tricuspid annulus is also made up of anterior and posterior fila coronaria and sulcal connective tissue. These fila coronaria are connected to right fibrous trigone (central fibrous body).

CASE - 2

A 40-year-old woman comes to your clinic tired and complaining of shortness of breath and fatigue. Her history is unremarkable except for a vague history of fever and joint pain as a child. She recently fatigue and difficulty sleeping that she attributes to job stress. On examination, her heart rate is 120 beats/min, and the rhythm has no discernible pattern (irregularly irregular). Auscultation of the heart indicates a systolic murmur (during left ventricular ejection of blood) that is harsh in character. It is diagnosed as atrial fibrillation due to

---

left atrial enlargement. It was due to mitral stenosis due to rheumatic heart disease.

a. Name the cardiac valves and give their surface markings

b. Give the surface markings of auscultation area of each cardiac valve

c. Give an account of structure and functions of valves of the heart

---

Answers to the clinical case studies

Case-1

a) Refer the clinical anatomy section

b) Globular shadow

c) The safest site at which to insert the needle of the syringe in order to miss the pleura would be just to the left of the xiphisternal junction.

Case-2

a), b) and c) Refer the text

MCQs

1. You are examining the heart of a victim of fatal trauma and note a tear at the junction of the SVC and the right atrium. This tear would likely damage the

   A. SA node
   B. AV node
   C. AV bundle
   D. Right bundle branch

2. You are examining the AV bundle histologically. In which of the following tissue samples will you find the AV bundle?

   A. Right atrium
   B. Left atrium
   C. Interatrial septum
   D. Membranous interventricular septum

3. The sternocostal surface of the heart is formed primarily by the anterior wall of which heart chamber?

   A. Left atrium
   B. Left ventricle
   C. Right atrium
   D. Right ventricle

4. A patient involved in an automobile accident presents with a sharp object puncture in the middle of the sternum at about the level of the 4th or 5th costal cartilage. If the object also penetrated pericardium and heart wall, which heart chamber would most likely be damaged?

A. Left atrium

B. Left ventricle

C. Right ventricle

D. Right atrium

5. A 23-year-old male injured in an industrial explosion was found to have multiple small metal fragments in his thoracic cavity. Since the pericardium was torn inferiorly, the surgeon began to explore for fragments in the pericardial sac. Slipping his hand under the apex of the heart, he slid his fingers upward and to the right within the sac until they were stopped by the cul-de-sac formed by the pericardial reflection near the base of the heart. Her finger tips were then in the:

A. Coronary sinus

B. Oblique sinus

C. Coronary sulcus

D. Costomediastinal recess

6. In cardiac surgery it is sometimes necessary to clamp off all arterial flow out of the heart. This could be done within the pericardial sac by inserting the index finger immediately behind the two great arteries and compressing them with the thumb of the same hand. The index finger would have to be inserted into which space?

A. Cardiac notch

B. Coronary sinus

C. Oblique pericardial sinus

D. Transverse pericardial sinus

7. During a heart transplant procedure, the surgeon inserted his left index finger through the transverse pericardial sinus, and then pulled forward on the two large vessels lying ventral to his finger. Which vessels were these?

A. Pulmonary trunk and brachiocephalic trunk

B. Pulmonary trunk and ascending aorta

C. Pulmonary trunk and superior vena cava

D. Superior vena cava and aorta

8. A stethoscope placed over the left second intercostal space just lateral to the sternum would be best positioned to detect sounds associated with which heart valve?

A. Aortic

B. Pulmonary

C. Mitral

D. Tricuspid

9. A 3rd-year medical student was doing her first physical exam. In order to properly place her stethoscope to listen to heart sounds, she palpated bony landmarks. She began at the jugular notch, then slid her fingers down to the sternal angle. At which rib (costal cartilage) level were her fingers?

A. 1

B. 3

C. 2

D. 4

10. The heart sound associated with the mitral valve is best heard:

A. In the jugular notch

B. In the second left intercostal space

C. In the second right intercostal space

D. In the left fifth intercostal space

11. Which heart valve has leaflets described as "anterior, left and right"?

A. Aortic

B. Pulmonary

C. Left atrioventricular

D. Right atrioventricular

12. In preparation for thoracic surgery, a median sternal splitting procedure was carried out. But an improper depth setting on the saw blade resulted in a slight nick on the underlying sternocostal surface of the heart. Which heart chamber would most likely have been opened had the blade completely penetrated this wall?

A. Left atrium

B. Left ventricle

C. Right atrium

D. Right ventricle

13. The sound associated with tricuspid stenosis (narrowing) in a 40-year-old male would be best heard at which location on the anterior chest wall?

A. Below the left nipple

B. In the right 2nd intercostal space near the sternum

C. Over the apex of the heart

D. Left 4th intercostal space

14. Traumatic, acceleration/deceleration injuries to the aorta usually occur where its mobile and fixed portions meet. This would be at the:

A. Ligamentum arteriosum

B. Junction of aortic arch with the descending portion

C. Junction of the ascending aorta with the heart

D. Origin of the brachiocephalic artery on the arch

15. Which of the following structures does NOT lie in the coronary sulcus?

 A. circumflex artery

 B. coronary sinus

 C. right coronary artery

 D. right marginal artery

16. Which of the following posterior mediastinal structures is most closely applied to the posterior surface of the pericardial sac?

 A. Aorta

 B. Azygos vein

 C. Oesophagus

 D. Thoracic duct

17. A 22-year-old male involved in an automobile accident presents with symptoms suggestive of myocardial contusion due to blunt trauma, specifically compression of the sternocostal surface of the heart by the sternum when his chest hit the steering wheel. Which heart chamber was most likely damaged?

 A. Left atrium

 B. Left ventricle

 C. Right atrium

 D. Right ventricle

18. While listening to a patient's heart sounds with a stethoscope, you identify a high-pitched sound in the second right intercostal space, just lateral to the edge of the sternum. Your correct conclusion is that you have detected stenosis of which heart valve?

 A. Aortic

 B. Mitral

 C. Pulmonary

 D. Tricuspid

19. The following anatomic structures are penetrated by a needle while performing a pericardiocentesis *except*

 A. Skin and subcutaneous tissue

 B. The aponeuroses of the external and internal oblique muscles

 C. The left parietal and visceral layers of pleura

 D. The rectus abdominis muscle

20. A patient arrives in the emergency room after having been stabbed. He has suffered a penetrating wound in the left fourth intercostal space immediately lateral to the sternal border. Which of the following thoracic structures is most likely to have been injured?

 A. Left atrium

B. Left ventricle

C. Right atrium

D. Right ventricle

21. A 35-year-old woman suffers severe chest trauma. She is unconscious and her blood pressure is substantially decreased. She has sustained a tear in one of the pulmonary veins at the point at which the vein enters the heart. Into which of the following spaces is the patient bleeding?

 A. Between the epicardium and the parietal pericardium

 B. Between the fibrous pericardium and the parietal pleura

 C. Between the myocardium and the epicardium

 D. Between the parietal pericardium and the fibrous pericardium

22. In reviewing a lateral projection of a barium swallow of a patient, a physician notes that the anterior wall of the oesophagus is compressed by an enlarged structure immediately anterior to it. The most likely structure compressing the oesophagus is the

 A. Right ventricle

 B. Left ventricle

 C. Right auricular appendage

 D. Left atrium

23. A patient has been admitted to the hospital after suffering from a knife wound of the chest just to the left of the sternum. He is slightly cyanotic, and there is a distension of veins of the neck during inspiration. You suspect that the patient has a cardiac tamponade and order a pericardiocentesis. What is the last tissue layer that the needle must traverse in order to reach the accumulating blood?

 A. Epicardium

 B. Fibrous pericardium

 C. Mediastinal pleura

 D. Parietal layer of serous pericardium

24. A cardiac surgeon is performing a median sternotomy to gain access to the heart for a coronary artery bypass. While cutting through the sternum, a large quantity of blood suddenly erupts from the chest. The cardiac surgeon immediately suspects that the saw has lacerated a structure in the mediastinum posterior to the body of the sternum.

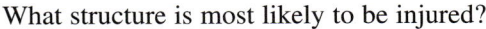

What structure is most likely to be injured?

A. The azygos vein

B. The arch of the aorta

C. The left atrium

D. The right ventricle

25. If the oesophageal mass expands anteriorly into the middle mediastinum, what structure might initially become compressed?

A. Left ventricle

B. Right ventricle

C. Right atrium

D. Left atrium

26. Cardiac tamponade is a life-threatening situation characterized by blood or fluid collecting around the heart, restricting its contractions until a patient experiences hypotension and shock. One of the etiology of cardiac tamponade is a collection of transudative fluid in a patient with renal failure. In which of the following locations would this fluid be found?

A. Between the fibrous pericardium and the visceral pleura

B. Between the myocardium and the endocardium

C. Between the parietal serous pericardium and the fibrous pericardium

D. Between the visceral and parietal serous pericardium

Answers to MCQs

1. A
2. D
3. D
4. C
5. B
6. D
7. B
8. B
9. C
10. D
11. A
12. D
13. D
14. A
15. D
16. C
17. D
18. A
19. C
20. D
21. A
22. D
23. D
24. D
25. D
26. D

SECTION 5

Blood Supply and Nerve Supply to the Heart

21

- Blood supply to the heart
- Nerve supply to the heart
- Conducting system of the heart
- MCQs

Objectives

- To explain the origin, course, branches and distribution of right and left coronary arteries
- To explain the arterial supply to the different parts of the conducting system of the heart and its clinical relevance
- To explain the venous drainage of the heart
- To explain the source of sympathetic and parasympathetic nerve supply to the heart and to list the effect of their stimulation on heart function
- To trace the pain pathway from the heart to the spinal cord and to explain the anatomical basis of referred pain
- To know the clinical methods employed in identifying the coronary obstruction and methods to restore the coronary circulation

BLOOD SUPPLY TO THE HEART

Arterial supply

The blood within the chambers of the heart will only supply the endocardium and subendocardial tissue. The thick musculature of the heart needs additional source of arterial supply. Heart is supplied by right and left coronary arteries (Figs 21.1 and 21. 2).

1. Right coronary artery

Origin:

It arises from anterior aortic sinus of the ascending aorta.

Course:

a. The artery appears between right auricle and pulmonary trunk and passes into right anterior coronary sulcus.

b. It descends obliquely downwards towards lower part of the right border and curves around this border to enter the right posterior coronary sulcus. The course of the artery up to this point is referred as 1st segment.

c. It reaches the crux and ends a little to the left of the crux by anostomosing with circumflex branch of the left

coronary artery. This part of the artery (in the right posterior coronary sulcus) is referred as 2nd segment

Branches

1. Right conus artery:

It forms an arterial circle around the pulmonary trunk by anastomosing with similar branch from the left coronary artery. This arterial circle is called 'annulus of Vieussens'.

2. Atrial branches:

- They are classified into anterior, lateral and posterior groups.
- One of the anterior atrial branches is called '**artery to the sinuatrial node**'. This nodal branch forms a loop at the base of the superior vena cava and gives a prominent branch called 'ramus cristae terminalis', which traverses the SA node.

3. Ventricular branches:

These arteries are classified into anterior and posterior groups. The anterior group traverses the sternocostal surface and posterior group diaphragmatic surface.

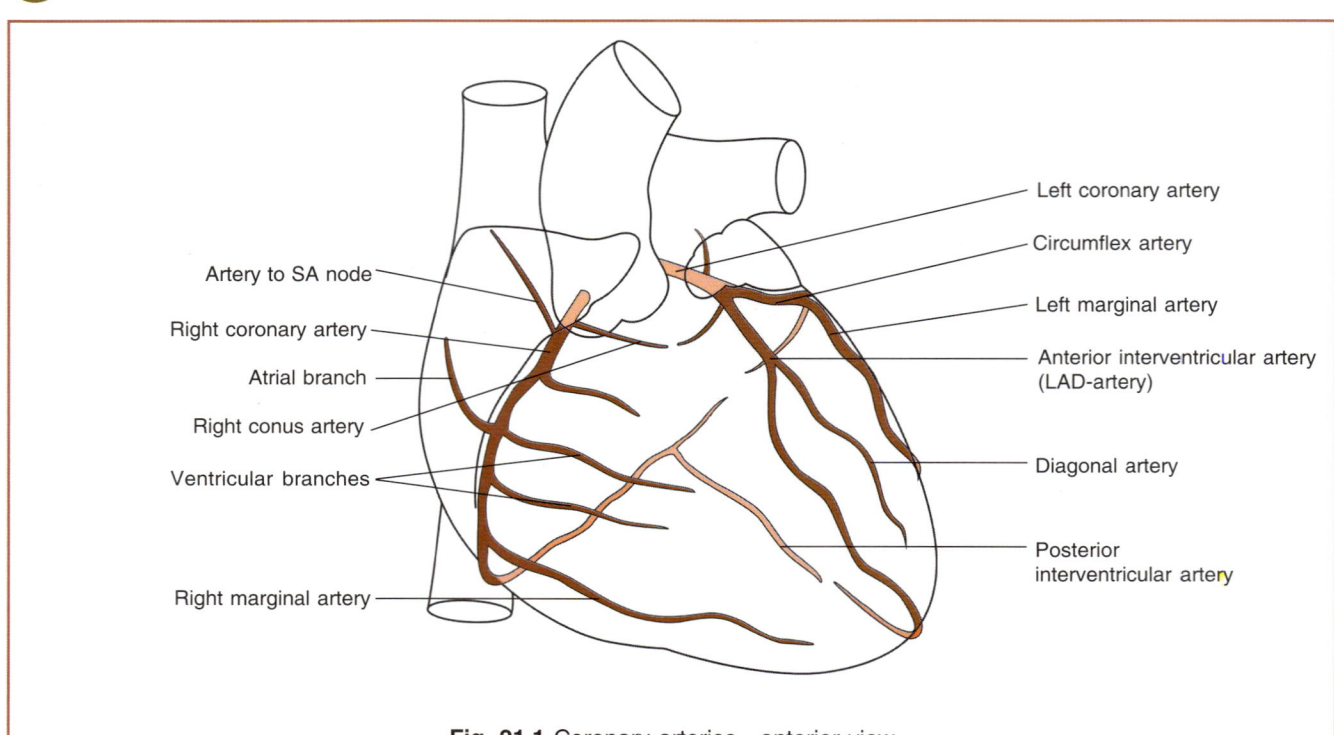

Fig. 21.1 Coronary arteries—anterior view

4. Right marginal artery:

This branch arises when right coronary artery crosses the right border of the heart. This marginal branch passes along the inferior border of the heart up to the apex.

5. Posterior interventricular artery (Clinically referred as Posterior descending artery/PDA):

This branch arises close to the crux and proceeds in posterior interventricular groove. This artery is accompanied by middle cardiac vein. The posterior interventricular artery gives many septal branches and one of the upper septal branch supplies AV node.

Areas of distribution of right coronary artery

a. Right atrium.

b. Greater part of the right ventricle except a part at the anterior interventricular groove.

c. Small portion of left ventricle adjoining posterior interventricular groove.

d. The entire conducting system of the heart except the left branch of the AV bundle. (AV bundle can be supplied by left coronary artery)

e. Posterior 1/3rd of the interventricular septum.

2. Left coronary artery

Origin

It arises from the left posterior aortic sinus of the ascending aorta.

Course

a. The artery passes between pulmonary trunk and left auricle and enters left anterior coronary sulcus. Soon it divides into two (or three) branches.

Branches

1. The anterior interventricular artery (Clinically referred as Left anterior descending/LAD):

It descends in the anterior interventricular groove. It is accompanied by 'great cardiac vein'. The anterior interventricular artery gives following branches:

a. Right anterior ventricular branches

b. Left anterior ventricular branches: One of these branches is large and is called '**left diagonal artery**'.

c. Left conus artery: It forms an arterial ring around the pulmonary trunk along with right conus artery

d. Septal branches: Supply anterior 2/3rd of the interventricular septum.

2. Circumflex artery:

This artery traverses the left anterior coronary sulcus and then curves around the left border of the heart. It partly runs in the left posterior coronary sulcus. It terminates (little to the left of the crux) with terminal branches of the right coronary artery. Circumflex artery gives following branches.

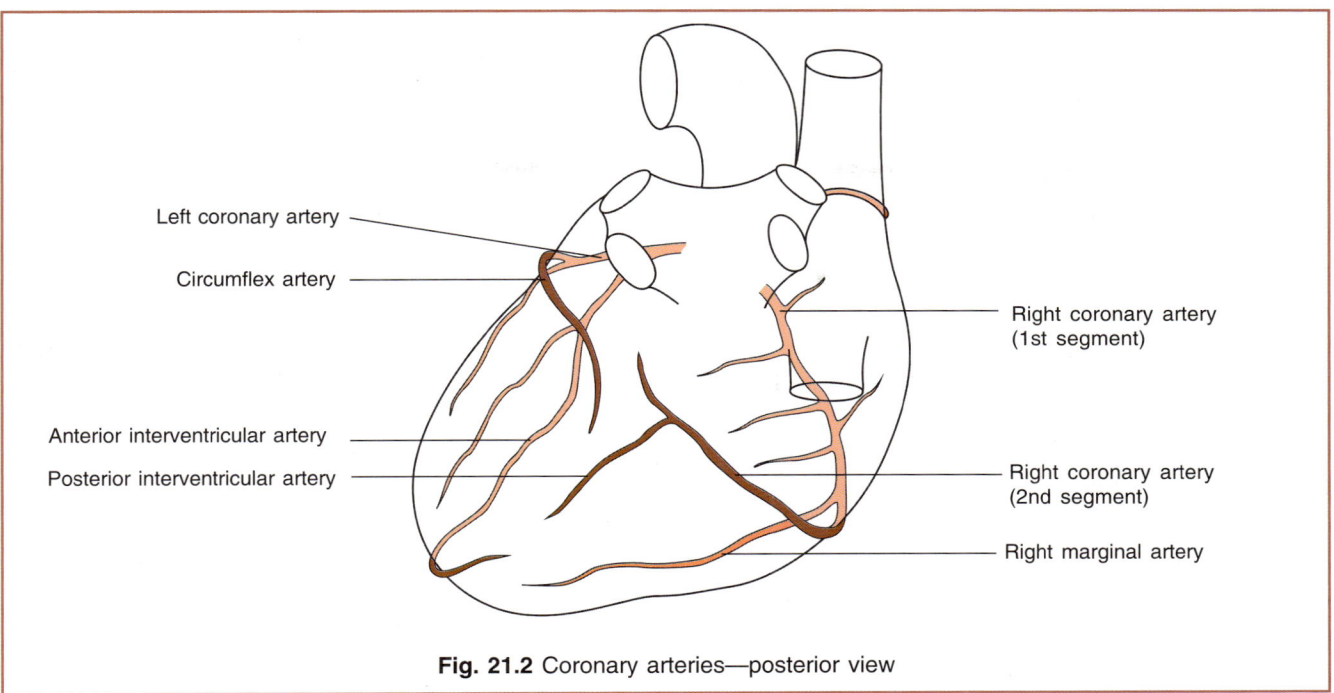

Fig. 21.2 Coronary arteries—posterior view

a. **Left marginal artery:** It descends along the left border up to the apex of the heart.

b. Anterior and posterior ventricular branches

c. Atrial branches are classified into anterior, posterior and lateral groups

d. Kugel's anastomotic artery traverses the anterior interatrial sulcus to establish direct or indirect anastomosis with right coronary artery.

Areas of distribution of Left coronary artery

a. Left atrium.

b. Greater part of the left ventricle except at the posterior interventricular groove.

c. Small part of the right ventricle at the anterior interventricular groove.

d. A part of the left branch of the AV bundle.

Dominant Coronary circulation

About 70% of individuals have a 'right dominant' coronary circulation. This means the right coronary artery gives rise to the posterior interventricular artery. When this branch arises from the left coronary's circumflex branch, then the heart is considered 'left dominant'. If both right and left coronary arteries contribute to this branch, then the circulation is considered 'balanced'.

In case of left dominance, the AV node and AV bundle are supplied by left coronary artery (Figs 21.3 and 21.4).

Special features of the coronary arteries

• The diameter of the coronary artery varies from 1.5 to 5.5 mm

• Left coronary artery is larger in caliber, supplying greater volume of the myocardium

• Coronary arteries are the only vessels where blood flows in diastole

• Posterior interventricular artery normally arises from right coronary artery and is referred as 'right dominance'.

• The branches of the coronary arteries are generally considered as functional end arteries.

• Sympathetic stimulation constricts the epicardial arteries and dilates the intra-muscular arteries.

Venous drainage of the heart

The venous blood from the musculature of the heart is drained into the right atrium through

A. Coronary sinus

B. Anterior cardiac veins

C. Venae cordis minimae (Thebesian veins)

Coronary sinus

It is a venous sac about 2 to 3 cm long, situated in the left posterior coronary sulcus. It opens into the right atrium by an orifice, which is guarded by a valve. Following are the tributaries of the coronary sinus (Figs 21.5 and 21.6)

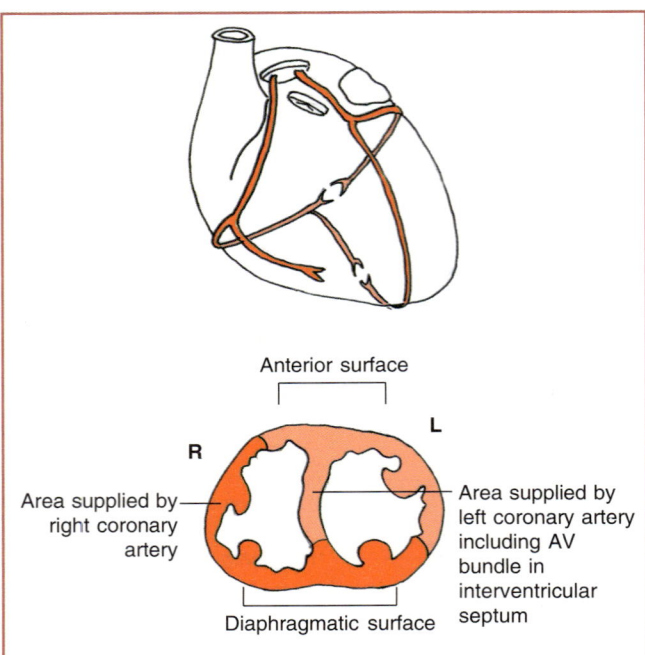

Fig. 21.3 Arterial supply to the interventricular septum

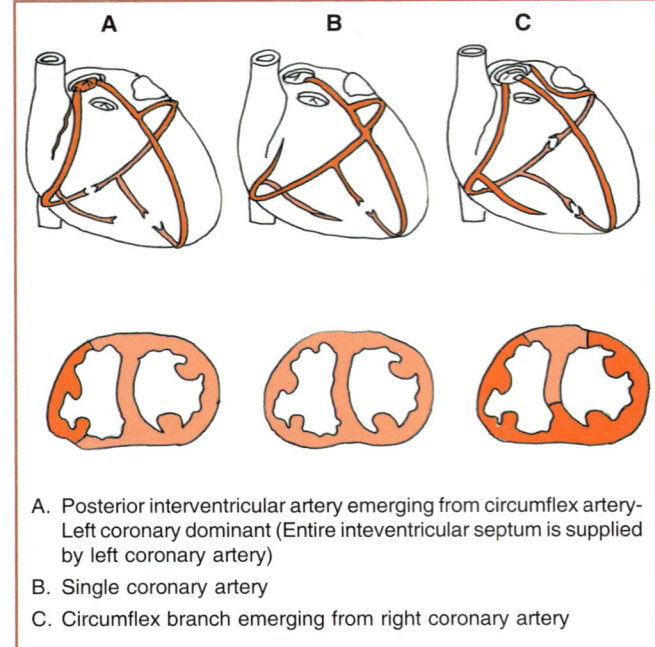

A. Posterior interventricular artery emerging from circumflex artery-Left coronary dominant (Entire inteventricular septum is supplied by left coronary artery)
B. Single coronary artery
C. Circumflex branch emerging from right coronary artery

Fig. 21.4 Major variations in arterial supply

1. Great cardiac vein:

It begins near the apex, ascends in the anterior interventricular groove and then traverses the coronary sulcus. It receives left marginal vein.

2. Small cardiac vein:

It passes along the right posterior coronary sulcus.

3. Middle cardiac vein:

It begins near the apex and traverses the posterior interventricular groove.

4. Posterior vein of the left ventricle:

It is present on the diaphragmatic surface of the left ventricle.

5. Oblique vein of the left atrium (of Marshall):

It descends obliquely on the back of the left atrium to join the coronary sinus.

Anterior cardiac veins

They drain anterior part of the right ventricle and are usually two or three in number. They ascend to open directly into right atrium, crossing first segments of right coronary artery.

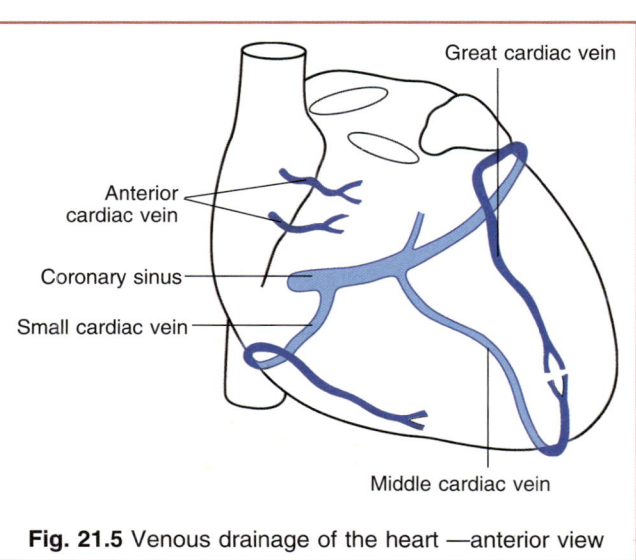

Fig. 21.5 Venous drainage of the heart —anterior view

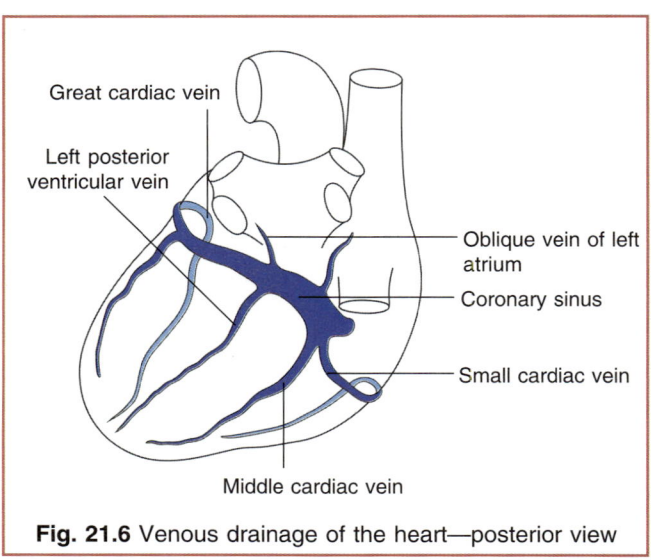

Fig. 21.6 Venous drainage of the heart—posterior view

Venae cordis minimae

They are numerous in the right atrium and ventricle. They open into all the chambers.

NERVE SUPPLY TO THE HEART

Though the cardiac muscle contracts rhythmically and automatically, the nerves supplying the heart alter the cardiac rate.

The sympathetic and parasympathetic fibres supplying the heart form two cardiac plexuses-superficial and deep. The fibres arising from these plexus follow the coronary arteries and to the components of conducting system, particularly the SA node.

Sympathetic source

The preganglionic fibres arise from upper 5 or 6 thoracic segment (T1-T6) of the spinal cord (lateral horn/ intermediate horn) to reach sympathetic ganglion where the fibres synapse. The post ganglionic fibres from all the three cervical sympathetic ganglion and upper 5 or 6 thoracic sympathetic ganglion reach cardiac plexus.

Parasympathetic source

It is derived from right and left **vagus nerves**. The vagus nerve gives cardiac branches in the neck (cervical cardiac branch) and also few in the thorax.

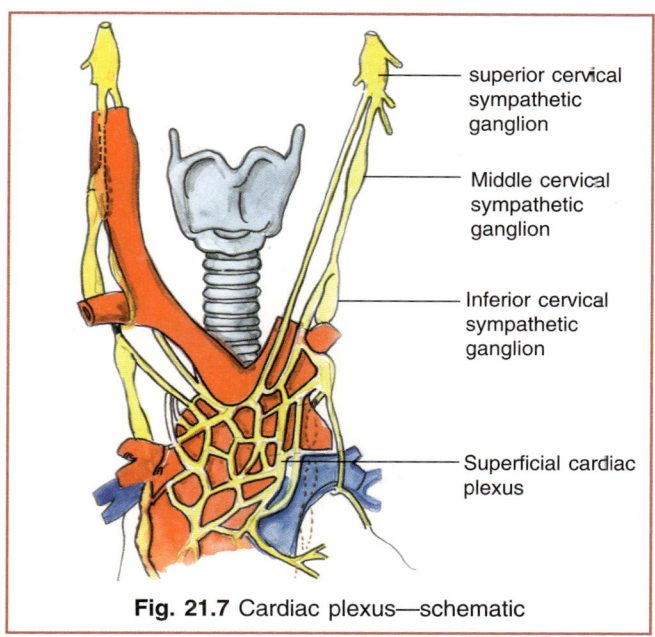

Fig. 21.7 Cardiac plexus—schematic

These are preganglionic (or presynaptic) fibres, which make synapses with small ganglia close to the myocardium.

a. Superficial cardiac plexus

It is situated below the arch of aorta and in front of the right pulmonary artery. Fibres from the superficial cardiac plexus pass into deep cardiac plexus and pulmonary plexus (Figs 21.7 and 21.8).

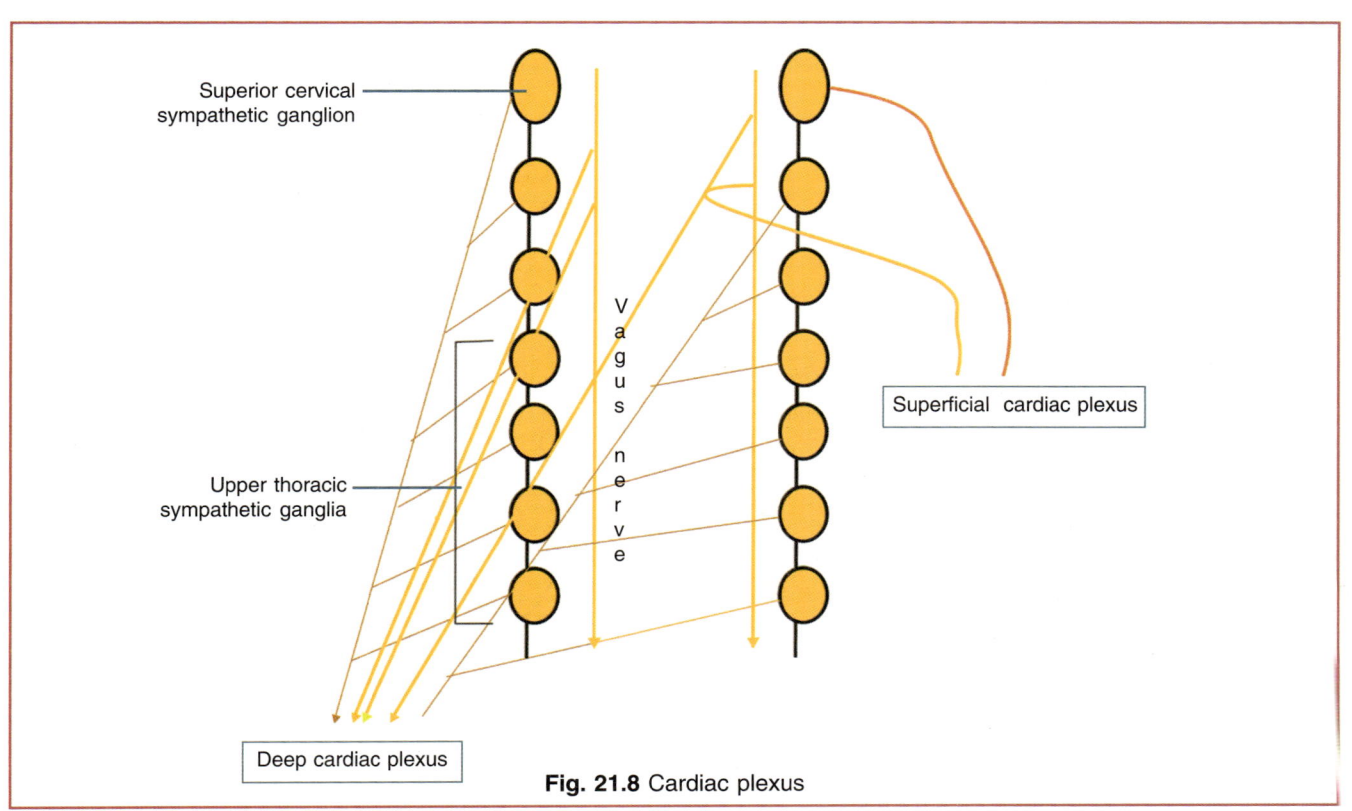

Fig. 21.8 Cardiac plexus

SECTION 5

Formation

1. A branch from the left superior cervical sympathetic ganglion.

2. Lower cervical cardiac branch of the left vagus nerve.

b. Deep cardiac plexus

It is situated in front of the bifurcation of the trachea.

Formation

1. Cardiac branches of both (right and left) cervical sympathetic ganglia (except from left superior)

2. Cardiac branches from the upper four or five thoracic sympathetic ganglia

3. Cardiac branches of the both vagus (except lower cervical cardiac branch of left vagus)

Functions

- Sympathetic fibres increase the heart rate, impulse conduction, force of contraction (increases cardiac output) and increased blood flow through coronary vessels to support the increased activity (Most adrenergic receptors/b_2 on coronary blood vessels, when activated cause relaxation of smooth muscles in the wall of the coronary arteries, therefore dilation of the arteries occur, this supplies more oxygen and nutrients to the myocardium.)

- Sympathetic fibres also carry pain sensation (due to ischemia of the heart) from the heart. These afferent fibres reach the sympathetic ganglia and then through

white ramus communicans joins the spinal nerve. Then through the dorsal root of the spinal nerve it enters the spinal cord (Fig. 21.9)

- Parasympathetic stimulation slows the heart rate, reduces the force of contraction and constricts the coronary arteries (Post synaptic parasympathetic fibres release acetyl choline).

CONDUCTING SYSTEM OF THE HEART

The conducting system consists of specialized cardiac muscle fibres. It includes pacemaker and Purkinje muscle fibres. These structures are capable of initiating and conducting the cardiac impulses, which produces the coordinated contraction of atrium and ventricles (Fig. 21.10)

1. Sinuatrial node (SA node)

It is known as the 'pace maker' of the heart. It is situated in the **upper part of the crista terminalis**. The SA node initiates and regulates the impulses for the contraction of the heart. The sympathetic fibres stimulate the SA node while parasympathetic inhibit it. The impulses from the SA node reach atrioventricular node through the walls of the right atrium (in the interatrial septum and crista terminalis).

2. Atrioventricular node (AV node)

It is located in the **triangle of Koch,** which is placed in the lower part of the inter-atrial septum. The impulses are then conveyed to the ventricle through AV bundle.

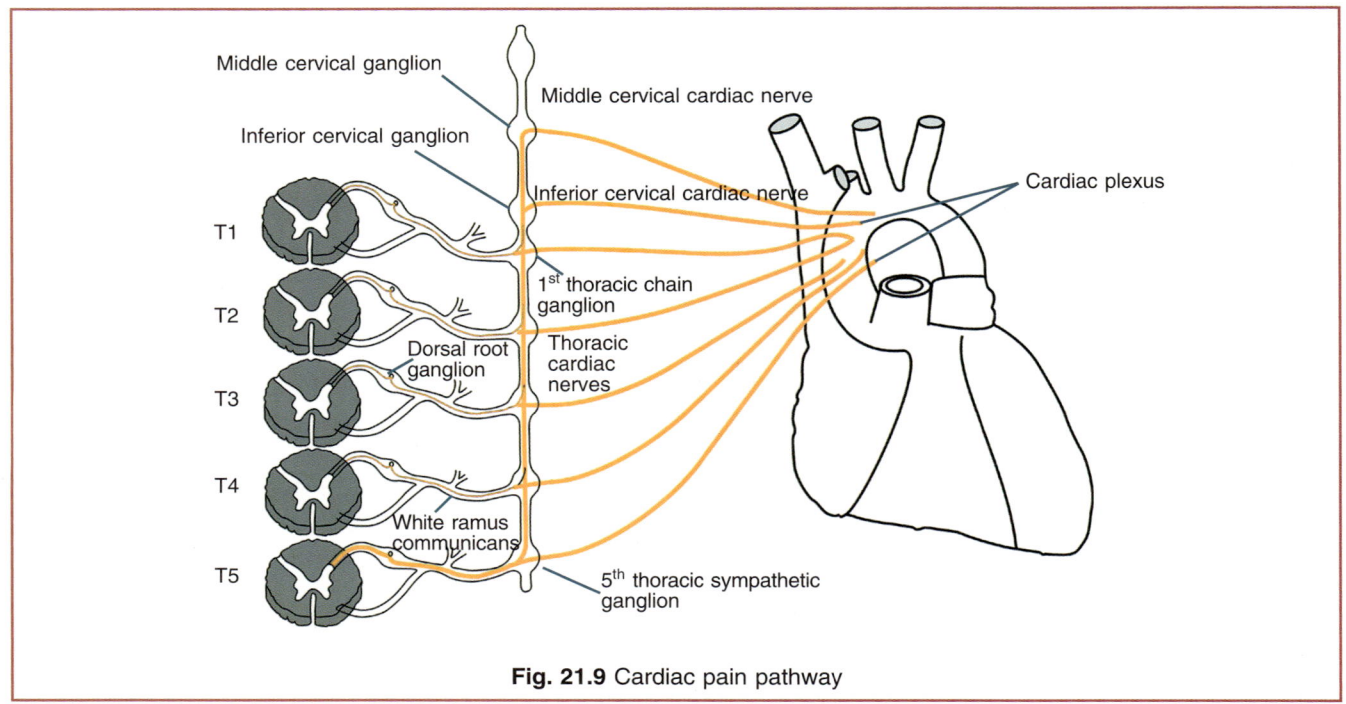

Fig. 21.9 Cardiac pain pathway

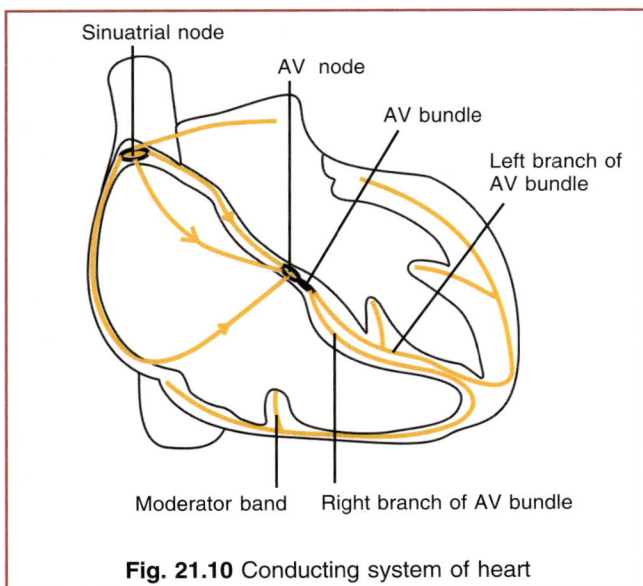

Fig. 21.10 Conducting system of heart

(Diagram labels: Sinuatrial node, AV node, AV bundle, Left branch of AV bundle, Moderator band, Right branch of AV bundle)

3. Atrioventricular bundle (AV bundle or bundle of His)

It begins from the AV node, traverses the **membranus part of the interventricular septum**. The AV bundle is the only bridge between the atrial and ventricular myocardium. At the junction of membranous and muscular part of the interventricular septum, the AV bundle divides into right and left branches.

a. The right branch passes to the right side of the interventricular septum. Majority of the fibres enters septo-marginal trabecula (moderator band) to reach the base of the anterior papillary muscle. The remaining fibres ramify on the musculature of the right ventricle forming subendocardial plexus.

b. The left branch is distributed in the wall of the left ventricle and also anterior and posterior papillary muscles of the mitral valve.

4. Purkinje fibers (Subendocardial branches)

They are located just beneath the endocardium of the ventricles. These fibers are specialized myocardial fibres. The Purkinje fibers are specialized to rapidly conduct impulses (numerous sodium ion channels and mitochondria, fewer myofibrils than the surrounding muscle tissue). Purkinje fibers take up stain differently than the surrounding muscle cells, and, on a slide, they often appear lighter and larger than their neighbours. They are binucleated.

Blood supply to conducting system

- Usually SA node is supplied by right coronary artery, but in 35% individuals, can be supplied by branch of left coronary artery.

- Usually AV node and AV bundle are supplied by right coronary artery, but in 20% the circumflex branch of left coronary artery supplies it. The AV bundle may be supplied by LAD artery.

- The right bundle branch receives blood from both right and left coronary arteries

- The left bundle branch from the left coronary artery

- In left coronary dominance, entire interventricular septum receives branches from left coronary artery

Lymphatic drainage of the heart

Lymphatic vessels arising from the musculature of the heart forms subepicardial lymphatic plexus. Lymphatic vessels arising from these plexus follow the coronary artery and finally a single lymphatic vessel is formed which ascends between pulmonary trunk and left atrium to end in inferior tracheobronchial lymph node, usually on the right side.

Angina pectoris: Angina pectoris is the term referring to pain originating from heart. It is a severe constricting pain as tightness in the thorax, deep to the sternum. The pain is the result of **ischemia of the myocardium.** This ischemia cause cellular necrosis (infarction) in myocardium, because of which the myocardium will not able to pump the blood.

The common cause for angina is narrowing of the coronary artery. This results in reduced blood flow, reduced oxygen supply to the cardiac muscle cells. This limited anaerobic metabolism of the myocytes, causes **lactic acid** accumulation and reduced pH. The pain receptors are stimulated by lactic acid.

Strenuous exercise, sudden exposure to cold and stress are the added factors in a patient with narrowed coronary vessels that cause angina, because all these require increased activity of the heart. After a heavy meal more blood flow into the digestive tract, for which some blood may be diverted from heart also. This can also cause angina in patients with narrowed coronary vessels followed by a heavy meal.

The angina is relieved by rest which reduces the work load on the heart. **Sublingual nitroglycerin** is placed under the tongue for rapid absorption, which dilates the coronary arteries. Such angina warns the patient about occlusion or narrowed coronary arteries indicating health care intervention.

The pain resulting from myocardial infarction is more severe than angina pectoris and the pain does not subside after 1–2 minute of rest. **The stable angina is**

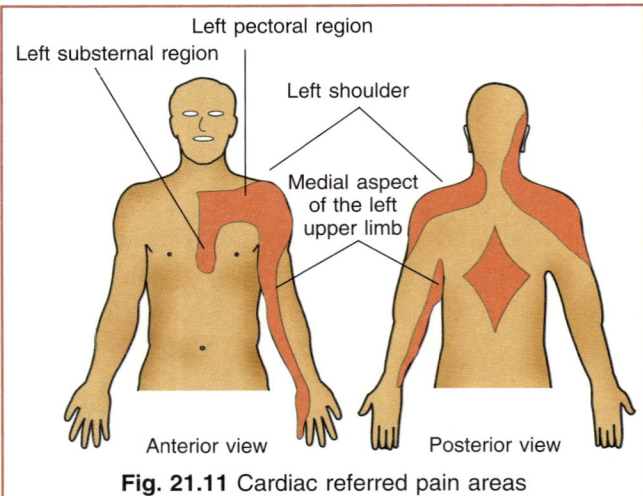

Fig. 21.11 Cardiac referred pain areas

characterized by chest discomfort and pain precipitated by some activity (running, walking, etc.) with minimal or non-existent symptoms at rest. In **unstable angina**, the chest discomfort and pain occurs even at rest and it is severe and of new onset (i.e., within 4–6 weeks). The pathophysiology of unstable angina is the reduction of coronary flow due to transient **platelet aggregation** on apparently normal endothelium, coronary artery spasms or coronary thrombosis.

Cardiac referred pain: The pain sensation from the heart is derived from ischemia of the myocardium. The ischemia causes accumulation of certain metabolic products which are stimulus to pain receptors. (Heart is insensitive to touch, cold, heat or cutting). The sympathetic fibres carry pain sensation from the heart. These afferent fibres reach the sympathetic ganglia (thoracic, middle and inferior cervical) and then through white ramus communicants joins the spinal nerve. Then through the dorsal root of the spinal nerve (especially on the left side, hence pain is referred in left arm) it enters the spinal cord at the level of T1 to T5 segment.

The cardiac referred pain (angina pectoris) is felt as radiates from the substernal and left pectoral regions to the left shoulder and the medial aspect of the left upper limb (Fig. 21.11).

The referred pain at the substernal area and pectoral region is due to common innervation (T2-T5) to that part of the body wall (somatic nerve/intercostal) and heart (visceral) by T2 to T5 segment of the spinal cord.

The referred pain at the shoulder and medial aspect of the upper limb is because T1 and T2 segment of the spinal cord also supply upper limb through brachial plexus. Skin of the floor of the axilla or medial side of the arm is supplied by T2 (Intercostobrachial nerve).

The cardiac pain is usually referred to the left side because cardiac lesions mostly occur in the left half of the heart, but if the lesion is in right half of the heart, the pain will be referred to the right side.

Coronary angiography: This is a radiographic technique in which the coronary arteries are visualized. A catheter is introduced into the femoral artery or radial artery then guided into ascending aorta with the help of a monitor. Under the fluoroscopic control, the tip of the catheter is placed just inside the coronary artery. A radiopaque contrast material is injected and radiographs are taken. The radiograph shows the lumen of the

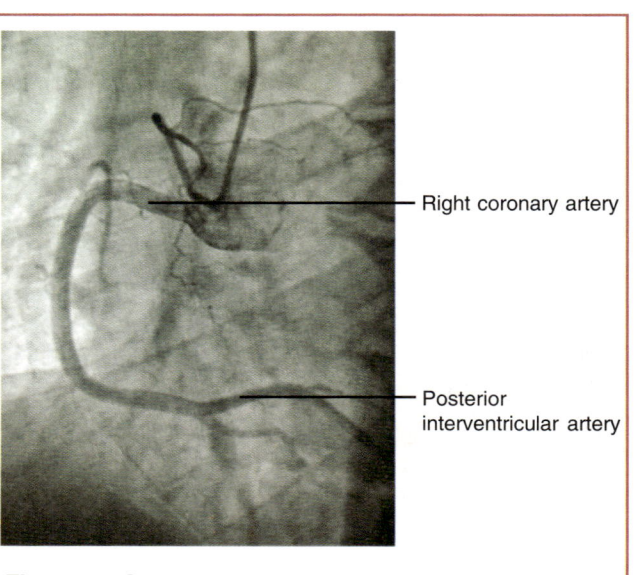

Right coronary artery

Posterior interventricular artery

Fig. 21.12 Coronary angiography of right coronary artery

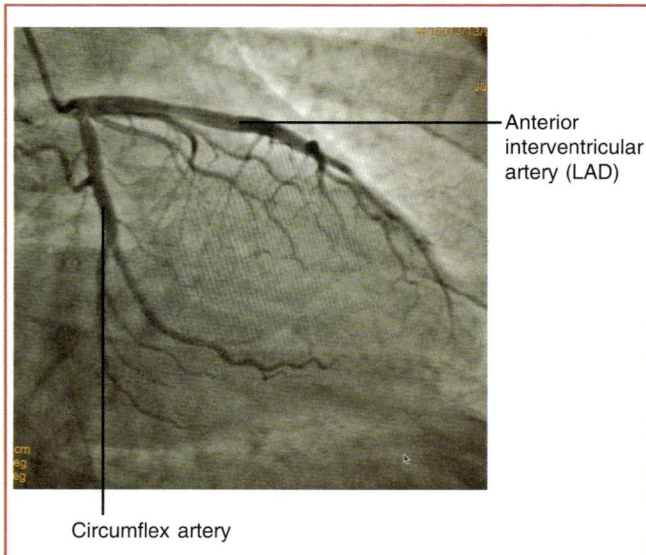

Anterior interventricular artery (LAD)

Circumflex artery

Fig. 21.13 Coronary angiography of left coronary artery

coronary arteries and its branches and also stenotic area if any (Figs 21.12 and 21.13).

Myocardial infarction (Heart attack): A sudden occlusion of the coronary artery or its major branch by an embolus causes infarction of the myocardium (and followed by its necrosis) in the area of the heart supplied by it. This is called 'myocardial infarction'. An area of the myocardium that has undergone necrosis constitutes a myocardial infarction.

The most common cause for such sudden occlusion of the coronary artery is due to atherosclerotic changes in the coronary artery. Apart from severe chest pain (tightness in the chest), the victims of heart attack may also have dyspnea, nausea, vomiting, sweating, pain in the left arm pit and medial side of the arm. Abnormalities in the electrical activity usually occur with heart attacks and ECG can identify the areas of heart muscle that are deprived of oxygen and/or areas of muscle that have died. Apart from ECG, estimation of cardiac enzymes will also help in diagnosing the myocardial infarction. Cardiac enzymes are proteins that are released into the blood by dying heart muscles.

These cardiac enzymes are **creatine phosphokinase (CPK)**, special sub-fractions of CPK, and **troponin**, and their levels can be measured in blood. These cardiac enzymes typically are elevated in the blood several hours after the onset of a heart attack.

The three most common sites of coronary artery occlusion are

1. Left anterior descending (LAD)/Anterior interventricular artery branch of left coronary artery (40–50%)

2. Right coronary artery (30–40%)

3. Circumflex branch of the left coronary artery (15–20%)

Coronary atherosclerosis: It is characterized by deposition of cholesterol, calcium and cellular waste. As these atherosclerotic plaque build up in the tunica intima of the coronary arteries, a stenosis (narrowing) of the lumen develops slowly. As coronary atherosclerosis progress, the collateral channels are established which may initially permit adequate perfusion of the heart. But when heart needs to perform increased amounts of work (for example strenuous exercise), these collateral channels are not sufficient and which results in angina or myocardial infarction if there is total obstruction (Fig. 21.14).

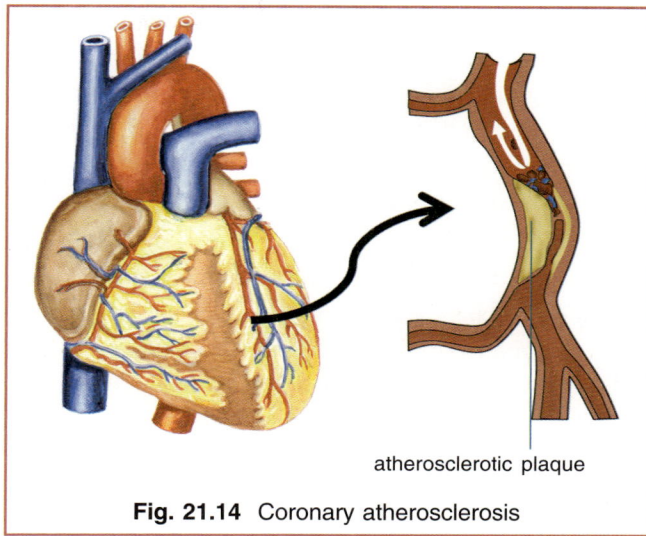

atherosclerotic plaque

Fig. 21.14 Coronary atherosclerosis

Coronary angioplasty: In certain people with coronary obstruction, the cardiologists use percutaneous transluminal coronary angioplasty. A catheter with inflatable balloon attached to its tip is introduced to the lumen of coronary artery at the site of obstruction. Then the balloon is inflated, flattening the atherosclerotic plaque against the arterial wall. The artery is stretched to increase the size of the lumen, thus improving the blood flow. Sometime '**thrombokinase/streptokinase**' an enzyme dissolves the blood clot is injected through the catheter. It is also possible to introduce 'intravascular stent' to maintain the dilation. These intravascular stents are rigid or semi rigid tubular meshes (Fig. 21.15).

Coronary bypass Graft (CABG): It is also called "the cabbage procedure", which is indicated in patients with

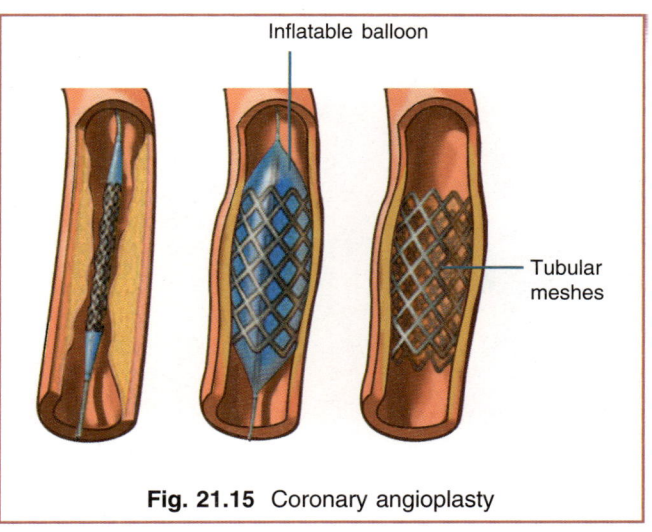

Inflatable balloon

Tubular meshes

Fig. 21.15 Coronary angioplasty

SECTION 5

coronary obstruction and severe angina. A segment of the vein or an artery from elsewhere in the patient's body is grafted into the coronary artery to improve the circulation. The one end of the arterial graft is connected to aorta or coronary artery proximal to the block and another end to the coronary artery distal to the site of the block.

A portion of the great saphenous vein is commonly used for coronary graft because its diameter is equal or greater than coronary arteries and can be easily dissected from the lower limb. The portion of the great saphenous vein is grafted in reverse direction due to the presence of valves. Other alternatives include usage of radial artery and internal thoracic artery (Fig. 21.16).

Electrocardiography (ECG or EKG): It is a noninvasive recording procedure for interpretation of the electrical activity of the heart. The ECG works mostly by detecting and amplifying the tiny electrical changes (depolarisation) that is triggered by the cells in the sinuatrial node, spreads out through the atrium, passes through "intrinsic conduction pathways" and then spreads all over the ventricles. This is detected as tiny rises and falls in the voltage between two electrodes placed on either side of the heart which is displayed as a wavy line either on a screen or on paper. This display indicates the overall rhythm of the heart and weaknesses in different parts of the heart muscle.

The heart function is also tested by exercise tolerance test (treadmill stress test).

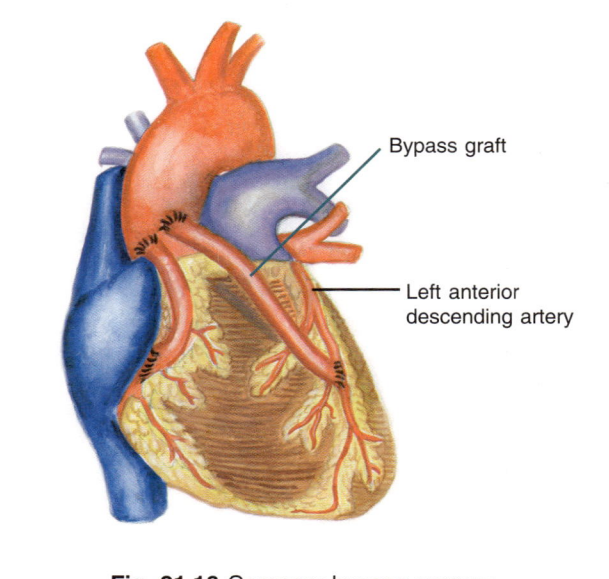

Fig. 21.16 Coronary bypass surgery

- Bypass graft
- Left anterior descending artery

Artificial cardiac pacemaker: The AV node is damaged by various forms of heart diseases. The only route for impulse transmission from the atria to the ventricles is through the AV node. Therefore, damage to this node is called **'heart block'**. It interferes with the ability of the ventricles to receive the impulses. Without these signals, the ventricles beat at an intrinsic rate that is slower than that of the atria and too slow to maintain adequate circulation. In such cases an **artificial pacemaker** set to discharge impulses at the appropriate rate is usually implanted.

The pacemaker consists of a battery pack, a wire and an electrode. An electrode connected to a catheter is inserted to a vein and then guided towards superior vena cava, right atrium, right ventricle with a fluoroscope. Here the electrode is firmly fixed to the trabeculae carneae of the ventricle. The opposite end of the electrode lead is connected to the pacemaker generator. The pacemaker produces electrical impulses that are spread into the musculature of the ventricles for its contraction at predetermined rate. Modern pacemakers are externally programmable and allow the cardiologist to select the optimum pacing models for individual patients.

Fibrillation and defibrillation of Heart:

Atrial fibrillation: It is the most common cardiac arrhythmia (abnormal heart rhythm) and involves the two atria of the heart. Instead of a coordinated contraction, the atria present rapid, irregular and uncoordinated contraction of atrial wall. It can often be identified by taking a pulse and observing that the heartbeats don't occur at regular intervals. However, a stronger indicator of atrial fibrillation is the absence of P waves on an electrocardiogram (ECG or EKG). Atrial fibrillation is often asymptomatic and is not in itself generally life-threatening, but it may result in palpitations, fainting, chest pain or congestive heart failure. People with AF usually have a significantly increased risk of stroke.

Ventricular fibrillation: It is a condition in which there is uncoordinated contraction of the ventricles of the heart. Ventricular fibrillation is a medical emergency. Ventricular fibrillation is a cause of cardiac arrest and sudden death.

Defibrillation of Heart: An electric shock may be given to the heart through the thoracic wall via large electrodes. This shock causes cessation of all cardiac movements and few seconds later the heart may begin to beat more normally.

Restarting Heart (Cardiopulmonary resuscitation/ CPR): is an emergency procedure for people with cardiac arrest or, in some circumstances like respiratory arrest. CPR is performed both in hospitals and in pre-hospital settings (by first-aid workers). CPR involves physical intervention to create artificial circulation through rhythmic pressing on the patient's chest to manually pump blood through the heart, called chest compressions, and usually involves the rescuer exhaling into the patient (or using a device to simulate this) to ventilate the lungs and pass oxygen into the blood, called artificial respiration. Some protocols now downplay the importance of the artificial respirations, and focus on the chest compressions only. Despite its name, CPR is unlikely to restart the heart; its main purpose is to maintain a flow of oxygenated blood to the brain and the heart, which are both the most essential organs to human life and are most vulnerable to damage from lack of oxygen (hypoxia).

CASE - 1

A 48-year-old male software engineer while doing his regular exercise, when he first noticed a diffuse substernal pain that radiated across his chest to the left shoulder and medial side of the left arm. Having been a sports person almost all his life; however he continued his regular exercise as well as swimming. The bouts of pain became recurrent with strenuous exercise and subsided during rest. Thinking the pain would go away, he did not seek medical assistance. During one particularly long and strenuous session of swimming, he experienced a crushing pain in the chest, and was slumped to the floor. He was rushed to the nearest hospital and placed immediately in the intensive care unit. Tests revealed, among other things, an elevated serum cholesterol level and an abnormal ECG. The patient was placed on anticoagulant and vasodilatory drug therapy and prescribed total bed rest for 10 days, followed by a long period of convalescence that included modified diet, rest, moderate exercise, and reduction of stress. His condition improved steadily and he has suffered no recurrences of this disorder.

The underlying cause usually is a narrowing of the diameter of one or more of the major arteries of the heart as a result of atherosclerotic plaque formation on the internal walls of these vessels. The patient's elevated cholesterol level combined with the pain upon exertion would tend to support a diagnosis of reduced coronary artery capacity. When the patient was at rest, the arteries

apparently were capable of carrying an adequate blood supply, but with increased demand, as occurs in exercise, the heart became deprived of its required oxygen level, resulting in ischemia and pain.

a. What is the term for the recurring pain experienced by the patient upon exertion?

b. Describe the sensory nerve supply to the heart

c. Explain the referred pain experienced with this condition

d. Trace the pain pathway from the heart to spinal cord

CASE - 2

A 65-year-old man complains of tight chest pressure and shortness of breath after lifting several boxes in his garage approximately 2 hours earlier. He says he believes his heart is skipping beats. His medical history is significant for hypertension and cigarette smoking. On examination, his heart rate was 55 beats/min and regular, and his lungs are clear on auscultation. An electrocardiogram shows bradycardia with an increased PR interval and ST-segment elevation in multiple leads including the anterior leads, V1 and V2. Further estimation of cardiac enzymes after several hours, showed an increase in cardiac enzyme levels. The cardiologist decided to perform a coronary bypass surgery. After the surgery the patient recovered well and got discharged from the hospital.

a. What anatomical structures are most likely to be affected?

b. Describe the course and areas of the heart supplied by the right and left coronary arteries, respectively.

c. Describe the venous drainage of the heart

d. Name three blood vessels of the body that can be used for coronary artery graft

e. To perform coronary angiography the cardiologist chooses the right femoral artery. Trace the path of catheter from the femoral artery to the coronary ostia.

CASE - 3

A 58-year-old man presented to the emergency room with pain in his left shoulder that radiated to the scapula. While taking the patient's history it was noted that the patient had many episodes of such attacks in the past two years, with lengthy intervals between them. The patient also said that, such attacks of pain was always

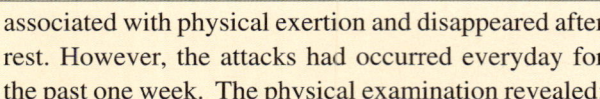
associated with physical exertion and disappeared after rest. However, the attacks had occurred everyday for the past one week. The physical examination revealed:

- shoulder joint within normal limits, range of motion free
- heart slightly enlarged, otherwise within normal limits
- no elevation of cardiac enzymes

Administration of sublingual nitroglycerin resulted in pain relief. He was diagnosed with angina pectoris and discharged until further tests could be performed.

a. What is the anatomical basis of angina pectoris?

b. Describe the blood supply to the heart, listing the major arteries and branches.

c. Why is pain related to myocardial ischemia often "referred"?

d. What is the difference between angina pectoris and myocardial infarction

CASE - 4

A 17-year-old male athlete visited the hospital with complaints of breathlessness, dizziness, weakness, fainting and fatigue. A detailed medical history of the patient was taken and followed by series of tests, which include portable ECG, which recorded heart's electric activity for 48 hours. The ECG is characterized by intermittently nonconducted P waves, not preceded by PR prolongation and not followed by PR shortening. The patient was diagnosed to have Mobitz type II heart block. The cardiologist decided to place an artificial pacemaker to maintain the heart rate.

a. Name the anatomical components of conducting system of heart and their specific locations in the heart

b. What is 'Heart block' and how does it interfere with heart's function?

c. How is the electrical activity of the heart recorded?

d. Describe the arterial supply to the different parts of the conducting system of the heart.

e. How does an artificial 'pacemaker' help in case of heart block?

Solutions to the Clinical case studies:
Case-1

a. This patient was suffering from angina pectoris

b. The heart is supplied by the autonomic nervous system through parasympathetic (vagus nerve) and sympathetic (upper 4 segments of the thoracic portion of the spinal

cord/T1–T4). The two autonomic subdivisions are antagonistic in their action on the heart, the sympathetic causing the heart rate to increase, whereas the parasympathetic is responsible for reducing the rate. The fibres from both subdivisions intermingle and ramify around the aorta as the cardiac plexuses of nerves. In addition, sensory fibres travel from the heart and enter the dorsal roots of the upper four or five thoracic spinal nerves.

c. These same nerves receive afferent fibres from the shoulder and arm (mainly T1 and T2) and from the thoracic wall. Although the mechanism of referred pain is still poorly understood, somehow pain impulses from the heart become intermingled with afferent fibres from the periphery of the body in such a way that somatic pain is also felt (in this case from the left shoulder and arm)

d. Refer text

Case-2

a. Right coronary artery and left anterior descending artery

b. Refer text

c. Refer text

d. Internal thoracic artery, radial artery and tributary or a segment of great saphenous vein

e. Right femoral artery, right external iliac artery, right common iliac artery, abdominal aorta, thoracic aorta, arch of the aorta and ascending aorta.

Case-3

a. Angina pectoris, "chest pain," is due to myocardial ischemia. The pain is frequently precipitated by exercise, stress, or eating. During periods of increased oxygen demand, narrowed arteries may not be able to deliver adequate blood supply. By definition, angina is coupled with exertion, and relieved by 1–2 minutes of rest.

b. Refer text.

c. Cardiac pain is often referred to areas of the body surface which send sensory impulses to the same levels of the spinal cord that receive cardiac sensation. This is true especially on the left side. The sensory nerve fibers from the heart and blood vessel walls travel through the cardiac plexus, sympathetic chain, and up to the dorsal roots and ganglia of spinal nerves T1–T4. Make sure you look up the dermatomes of T1–T4 to see the cutaneous distribution of this part of the spinal cord, as this is the common site of referred pain. The common sites of referred pain include the neck, jaws, shoulders, arms, and epigastric area.

d. Angina pectoris is the chest pain located in the retrosternal area, that may or maynot be caused by exercise, and can or cannot subside with rest (that depends if the angina is stable or unstable). The angina can be a caused by myocardial infarction, or just by ischemia of the muscle. The myocardial infartion is the death of the heart cells by necrosis, and the pain will not be relieved by rest and immediate medical intervention is a must.

Case-4

a. SA node- in the upper part of the crista terminalis, AV node – in the interatrial septum (triangle of Koch), AV bundle – in the membranous part of the interventricular septum, right branch of AV bundle – in rough part of interventricular septum and septomarginal trabaculae, left branch of AV bundle – in rough part of inter-ventricular septum

b. Refer text

c. Refer text

d. Refer text.

e. The pacemaker produces electrical impulses that spread into the musculature of the ventricles for its contraction at predetermined rate. Modern pacemakers are externally programmable and allow the cardiologist to select the optimum pacing modes for individual patients.

MCQs

1. A 55-year-old man is awakened from sleep by crushing substernal chest pain that radiates to his jaw. Upon arrival at the emergency department he is hypotensive and bradycardic. The electrocardiogram demonstrates third degree heart block. The blood supply to the atrioventricular node is usually from a branch of
   A. Circumflex artery
   B. Left coronary artery
   C. Left marginal artery
   D. Right coronary artery

2. A 67-year-old man is brought to the emergency department by ambulance after a cardiac arrest. After defibrillation, an electrocardiogram demonstrates ST segment elevation in leads V2, V3, V4, V5 and V6 consistent with an anterior wall myocardial infarction. The blood supply to the anterior wall of the left ventricle is derived from the following branches *except*
   A. Right coronary artery
   B. Left marginal artery
   C. Diagonal branch of the left anterior descending artery
   D. Circumflex artery

3. A 60-year-old man develops a myocardial infarction and is noted to have a heart rate of 40 beats/min. The cardiologist diagnoses an occlusion of the right coronary artery. Which of the following structures is most likely to be affected?
   A. AV node
   B. AV bundle
   C. Left branch of the AV bundle
   D. Mitral valve

4. As cardiologist, you are concerned about blockage of the artery to the SA node in a patient. The artery typically arises from the
   A. Right coronary artery
   B. Right marginal artery
   C. Posterior interventricular artery
   D. Anterior interventricular artery

5. In a normal coronary artery pattern, the blood supply to majority of the interventricular septum is derived from
   A. Right coronary artery
   B. Posterior interventricular artery
   C. Anterior interventricular artery
   D. Circumflex artery

6. As a cardiologist, you are concerned about blockage of the artery to the AV node in a patient. This artery typically arises from the
   A. Right coronary artery –first segment
   B. Right marginal artery
   C. Posterior interventricular artery
   D. Anterior interventricular artery

7. An elderly lady suffers a coronary occlusion and subsequently it is noted that there is a complete heart block (that is, the right and left bundles of the conduction system have been damaged). The artery most likely involved is the:
   A. Circumflex branch
   B. Anterior interventricular (Left anterior descending)
   C. Posterior interventricular (posterior descending)
   D. Right marginal

8. Blockage of blood flow in the proximal part of the anterior interventricular artery could deprive a large area of heart tissue of blood supply, unless a substantial

retrograde flow into this artery develops via an important anastomosis with which other artery?

A. Circumflex
B. Left marginal
C. Posterior interventricular
D. Right coronary

9. While attempting to suture the distal end of a coronary bypass onto the anterior interventricular artery, the surgeon accidentally passed the needle through the adjacent vein. Which vein was damaged?

A. Anterior cardiac vein
B. Coronary sinus
C. Great cardiac vein
D. Middle cardiac vein

10. Normal cardiac conduction depends upon electrical communication between cardiac muscle cells occurring at gap junctions found in which of the following regions?

A. Atrioventricular bundle (of His)
B. Atrioventricular node
C. Cardiac skeleton
D. Intercalated disks

11. Pain from the heart typically is conducted by fibers of which of the following nerves?

A. Cervical cardiac branches of sympathetic trunk
B. Cervical cardiac branches of vagus nerves
C. Thoracic splanchnic nerves
D. Ventral rami of spinal nerves T1 – T4

12. A 66-year-old man presents to the emergency department with diaphoresis and crushing chest pain that radiates down his left arm. An ECG is performed and shows ST elevation and inverted T waves. His troponin level is high. He is taken to the cardiac catheterization unit, where he is diagnosed with an obstructive myocardial infarction due to a blockage in his left anterior descending artery (LAD). Which of the following best describes the area of myocardium supplied by the LAD?

A. Anterior wall and interventricular septum
B. Atrioventricular node and posterior septum
C. Left atrium and left ventricle
D. Right atrium and posterior wall

13. A 48-year-old man with a history of stable angina presents to the emergency department with an episode of chest pain that is not relieved by rest or nitroglycerin.

After stabilization in the telemetry unit for 2 days, he undergoes a thallium stress test. The results showed reduced perfusion of the lateral wall of the left ventricle. Which artery is most likely to be occluded?

A. Left anterior descending
B. Circumflex
C. Left main coronary
D. Right coronary

14. A 55-year-old male lawyer is brought to the emergency room by his wife. The wife states that her husband complained of a sharp, squeezing chest pain behind the sternum after a meal and has had repeated episodes of chest pain after exertion over the past several months. A diagnosis is made of an acute myocardial infarction (MI) of the AV bundle. What was the most likely site of an occlusion?

A. Posterior interventricular artery
B. Circumflex artery
C. Marginal artery
D. Left marginal artery

15. What part of the cardiac conduction system might have been affected in this patient in Question 14 if the right coronary artery is the site of an occlusion?

A. Stellate ganglion
B. Cardiac plexus
C. Sinoatrial node
D. Atrioventricular bundle

16. Which of the following is a neural structure that carries visceral pain fibers from the heart that results in referred pain over the Tl–5 dermatomes?

A. Ventral roots of the Tl–5 spinal nerves
B. Dorsal roots of the Tl–5 spinal nerves
C. Greater splanchnic nerves
D. Gray rami communicantes of the Tl–5 spinal nerves

17. A 43-year-old woman is diagnosed with a heart block in which contraction of the ventricles is dissociated from that of the atria. The suspected cause is ischemia of the atrioventricular node resulting from coronary artery blockage. In most individuals, the atrioventricular nodal artery is the branch from which of the following vessels?

A. Anterior interventricular artery
B. Circumflex branch of left coronary artery
C. Left marginal artery
D. Posterior interventricular artery

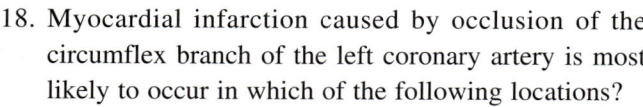

18. Myocardial infarction caused by occlusion of the circumflex branch of the left coronary artery is most likely to occur in which of the following locations?

    A. Apex

    B. Left atrium and left ventricle

    C. Right and left ventricles

    D. Right atrium and right ventricle

19. A 72-year-old woman arrives at the emergency department and states that her left arm is numb and she is diaphoretic. Laboratory studies show an elevated troponin I level. An echocardiogram indicates an abnormality of the anterior interventricular septum. Stenosis of which of the following arteries would most likely cause this condition?

    A. Acute marginal artery

    B. Circumfiex artery

    C. Left anterior descending artery

    D. Posterior descending artery

Answers to MCQs

1. D
2. A
3. A
4. A
5. C
6. C
7. B
8. C
9. C
10. D
11. A
12. A
13. B
14. A
15. C
16. B
17. D
18. B
19. C

SECTION 5

- Mediastinum
- Arch of the aorta
- Vessels of the superior mediastinum
- Nerves of the superior mediastinum

- Trachea
- Thymus
- Phrenic nerve
- MCQs

Objectives

- To know the subdivision of the mediastinum and to list the major structures present in each of them
- To explain the location, extent, relations and branches of the arch of aorta
- To list the major vessels and nerves of the superior mediastinum
- To explain the extent, relations and microscopic structure of the trachea
- To explain the position, structure and functions of thymus
- To explain the origin, course and distributions of phrenic nerve and their clinical relevance
- To draw neat labeled diagrams of the cross section of the thorax at sternal angle, at T3 vertebral level and the junction between T4 and T5 vertebrae.
- To identify the structures in cross section of thorax in CT pictures at same levels.

MEDIASTINUM

The mediastinum is the midline structures between the right and left pleural cavities of thorax. It is bounded in front by sternum, behind by thoracic vertebral bodies and on each side by mediastinal pleura.

It is divided into superior and inferior parts by an imaginary line passing through sternal angle (manubrio-sternal joint) to the disc between T4 and T5 vertebrae. The inferior mediastinum is further divided into anterior, middle and posterior parts by the heart with pericardium (Fig. 22.1).

Superior mediastinum

It is placed behind the manubrium sterni and in front of the upper four thoracic vertebral bodies. Its upper limit is the inlet of thorax, which is obliquely placed between sternal notch in front and disc between C7 and T1 vertebrae.

Contents:

The arch of the aorta is the main content of the superior mediastinum. The sternohyoid and sternothyroid muscles

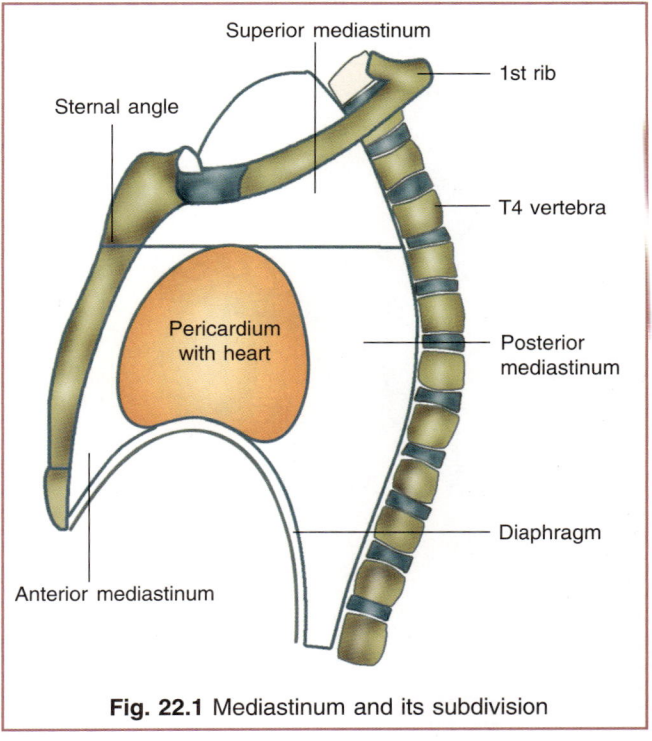

Fig. 22.1 Mediastinum and its subdivision

are also the contents. The remnant of the thymus may be present at the superior mediastinum.

The other contents include

- Branches of arch of aorta,
- Superior vena cava, right and left brachiocephalic veins,
- Right and left vagus and phrenic nerves, left recurrent laryngeal nerves,
- Oesophagus, trachea and thoracic duct.

    The study of the relations of the arch of aorta explains all the structures in the superior mediastinum.

Anterior mediastinum

It is the space behind the body of the sternum and in front of pericardium and heart. The pericardium is connected to inner surface of the body of sternum by sternopericardial ligaments.

Middle mediastinum

It is the space between anterior and posterior mediastinum and is occupied by heart with pericardium.

Posterior mediastinum

It is bound in front by pericardium with heart, bifurcation of trachea and pulmonary vessels in the upper part. Posteriorly it is related to lower eight thoracic vertebral bodies.

Its contents include descending thoracic aorta, oesophagus, azygos and hemiazygos veins, thoracic duct, vagus nerves, thoracic part of the sympathetic chain with their splanchnic nerves.

ARCH OF AORTA (AORTIC ARCH)

It is the continuation of the ascending aorta at the level of sternal angle and continues as descending thoracic aorta at the level of lower border of body of T4 vertebra. It arches behind the manubrium sterni. It passes upwards, backwards and to the left forming an arch. This arch produces a deep groove on the medial surface of the left lung above the hilum.

It gives three **branches** (Fig. 22.2)

1. Brachiocephalic trunk (Innominate artery) - which further divides into right common carotid and right subclavian arteries.
2. Left common carotid artery.
3. Left subclavian artery.

    A fourth branch called 'arteria thyroidea ima' may arise from arch of aorta. At times, the left vertebral artery can also arise from arch of aorta

Relations

Anteriorly and to the left (from anterior to posterior): (Figs 22.3 to 22.6)

- Medial surface of the left lung with pleura
- Left phrenic nerve
- Left superior intercostals vein
- Left vagus nerve
- Inferior cervical cardiac branch of the left vagus nerve (to superficial cardiac plexus)

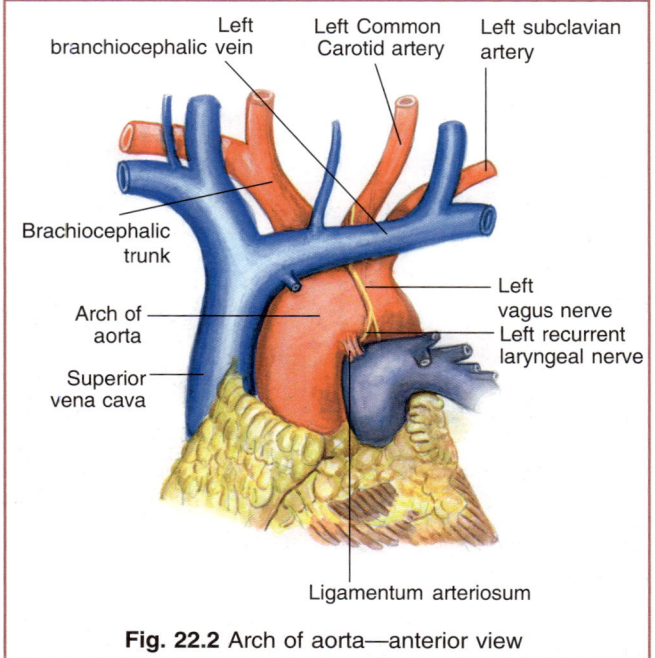

Fig. 22.2 Arch of aorta—anterior view

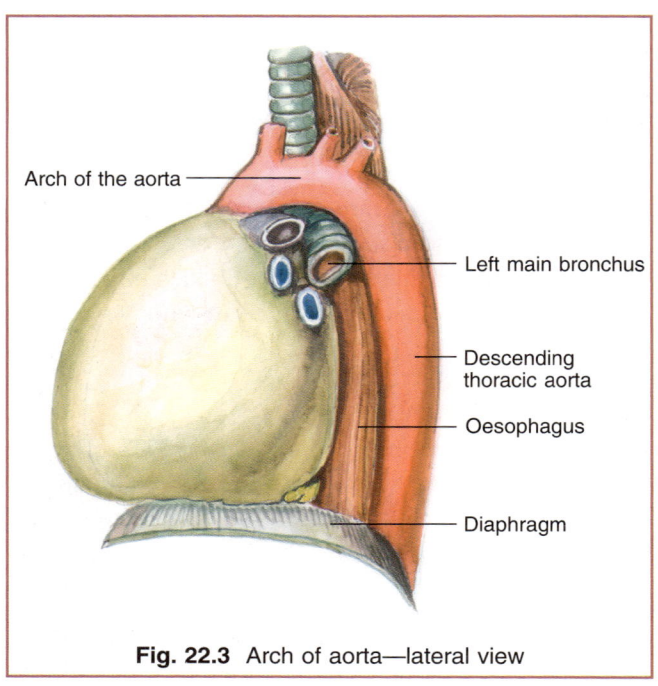

Fig. 22.3 Arch of aorta—lateral view

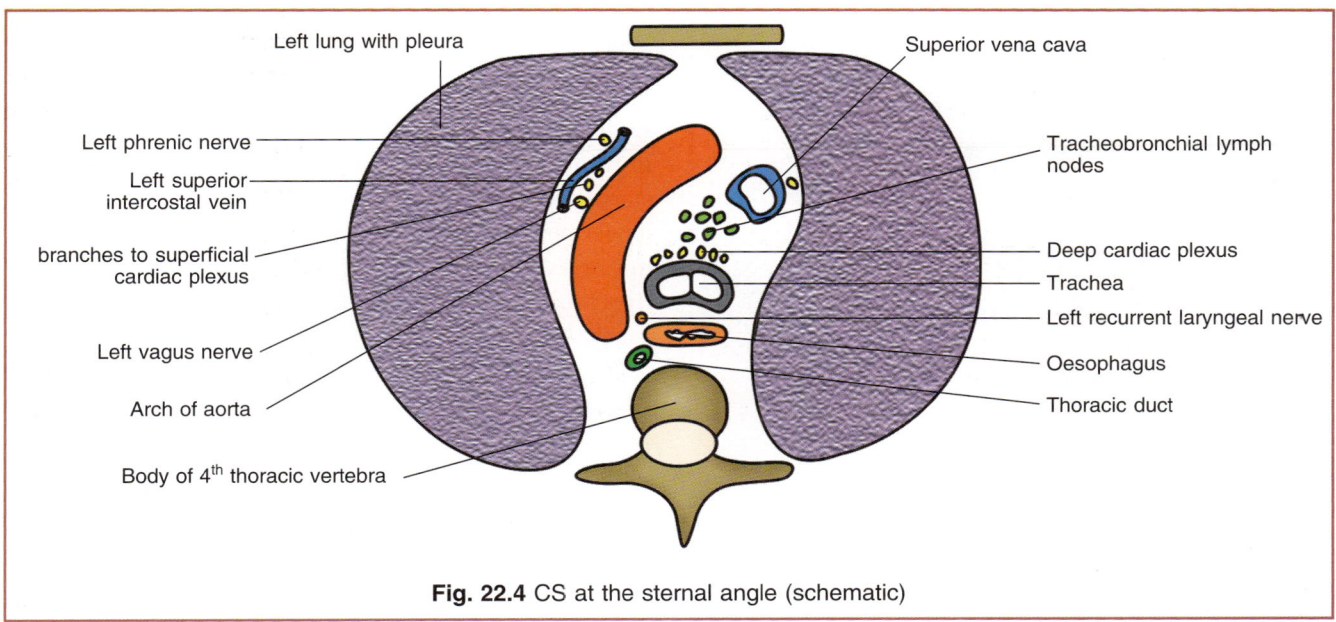

Fig. 22.4 CS at the sternal angle (schematic)

- A branch from left superior cervical sympathetic ganglion (to superficial cardiac plexus)

Posteriorly and to the right (from anterior to posterior):
- Lower end of the trachea with deep cardiac plexus and tracheobronchial lymph nodes in front of it
- Left recurrent laryngeal nerve
- Oesophagus
- Thoracic duct
- Body of the T4 vertebra

Inferiorly:
- Bifurcation of pulmonary trunk,
- left pulmonary artery,
- left main bronchus.
- **The ligamentum arteriosum** is connected to under surface of arch of aorta (distal to the origin of the left subclavian artery) to the left pulmonary artery. The left recurrent laryngeal nerve winds around the ligament

(Note: The right recurrent laryngeal nerve winds around the right subclavian artery in the neck) with superficial cardiac plexus present in front of it. The ligament represents embryological ductus arteriosus (Refer Chapter 24, Development of the Heart, Major Blood Vessels and Respiratory System).

Superiorly:

The three branches of the arch of aorta arise from its upper convex arch. The left brachiocephalic vein cross in front of these branches

1. **Aortic aneurysm:** It is a localized dilatation of the aorta. It occurs due to weakness in the wall of the arch of aorta. The dilated artery may occasionally cause discomfort, a greater concern is the risk of rupture, which causes severe pain, massive internal bleeding that can results in a death if untreated (Fig. 22.7).

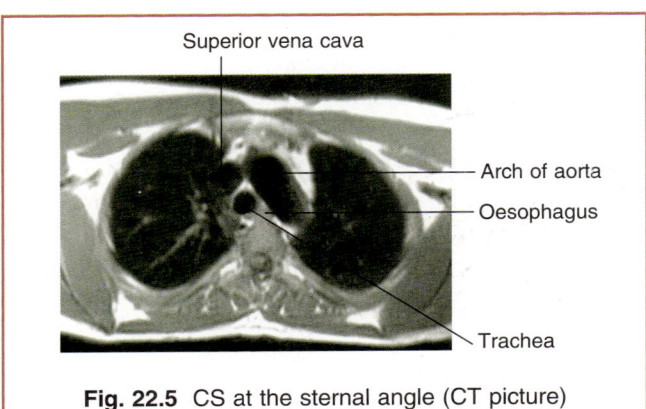

Fig. 22.5 CS at the sternal angle (CT picture)

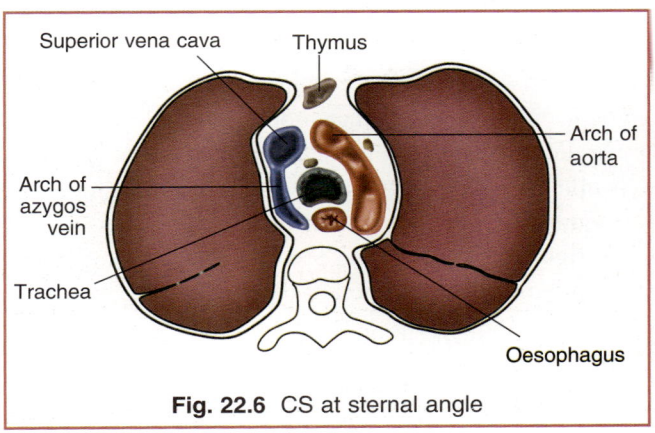

Fig. 22.6 CS at sternal angle

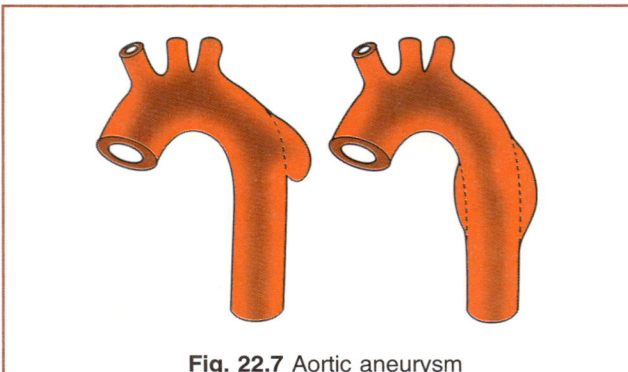

Fig. 22.7 Aortic aneurysm

The change in the structure of the wall of the aorta can occur secondary to trauma, infection, an intrinsic defect in the protein construction of the aortic wall, or due to progressive destruction of aortic wall proteins by enzymes.

The aneurysm usually causes compression of neighboring structures in the superior mediastinum. The signs and symptoms depend on what structures(s) it compresses.

A common symptom is a hoarse voice as the left recurrent laryngeal nerve (a branch of the vagus nerve) is stretched. This is due to the recurrent laryngeal nerve winding around the arch of the aorta.

The pressure on oesophagus can cause dysphagia, pressure on trachea causes stridor and dry cough, pressure on sympathetic chain can cause Horner's syndrome, pressure on veins can cause venous congestion in the neck and upper limb.

It can also cause tracheal tug, which can be felt at suprasternal notch in the extended position of the neck. The treatment of aortic aneurysm involves the placement of an endo-vascular stent via a percutaneous route (usually through the femoral artery) into the diseased portion of the aorta.

CASE -1

A 52-year-old patient (with a history of syphilis in her youth) has a swelling that protrudes from the upper margin of the sternum in the midline of the neck. The swelling expands with each systole of the heart. On examination, the trachea is found to be displaced to the right in the neck, and there is a distinct tugging sensation felt on palpation of the trachea.

What anatomical structure lying within the superior mediastinum is likely to have an expansile swelling that tugs at the trachea?

VESSELS OF THE SUPERIOR MEDIASTINUM

Brachiocephalic veins

Each brachiocephalic vein is formed by the union of internal jugular and subclavian veins posterior to the sternoclavicular joint. The left brachiocephalic vein is longer and crosses from left to right anterior to the three major arteries originating from arch of aorta (brachiocephalic trunk, left common carotid artery and left subclavian artery).

At the level of the inferior border of the 1st right costal cartilage, the right and left brachiocephalic vein joins to form superior vena cava.

The right brachiocephalic vein receives vertebral vein, the first right posterior intercostal vein, the right internal mammary vein.

The left brachiocephalic vein receives left superior intercostals vein, left internal mammary vein, left vertebral vein, inferior thyroid veins and left first posterior intercostal vein (Fig. 22.8).

Superior vena cava

It brings the venous blood from the parts of the body above the diaphragm except for heart and lungs. It extends from the lower border of the 1st right costal cartilage, vertically downwards to the level of right 3rd costal cartilage where it opens into right atrium. The right phrenic nerve descends on the right side of the superior vena cava. The lower end of the superior vena cava is covered by pericardium with ascending aorta on its left side. It forms the posterior boundary of the transverse sinus of the pericardium.

The **azygos vein** after arching over the hilum of the right lung opens into superior vena cava before it pierces the pericardium. The arch of the azygos vein receives right superior intercostal vein just before it pierces the pericardium.

Ascending aorta

It begins from aortic vestibule of the left ventricle and is covered by pericardium with inferior vena cava on its right side. It has an anterior mild bulging called anterior aortic sinus which gives origin to right coronary artery. It has two posterior bulging called right and left posterior aortic sinuses. The left posterior aortic sinus gives origin to left coronary artery. The right posterior aortic sinus is referred as non-coronary which produces a bulge in the cavity of the right atrium called torus aorticus.

Brachiocephalic trunk (Innominate artery)

It is the first branch of the arch of the aorta, ascends behind the manubrium sterni and in front of the trachea. At the right sternoclavicular joint it divides into right common carotid and right subclavian artery.

The **left common carotid artery** ascends in front and to little left of the trachea. The **left subclavian artery** ascends lateral to the trachea.

NERVES OF THE SUPERIOR MEDIASTINUM

Each **vagus nerve** descends in the neck within the carotid sheath.

The **right vagus nerve** enters the thorax anterior to the right subclavian artery, then descends on the right side of the trachea posterior to inferior vena cava and the root of the right lung. The nerve then descends on the right side of the oesophagus.

Near the lower end of the oesophagus the right vagus passes posterior to the vagus and is called posterior gastric nerve. In the thorax it gives branches to cardiac plexus, pulmonary plexus and oesophageal plexus.

The **right recurrent laryngeal nerve** arises from vagus just above the superior mediastinum (in the neck) and winds around the right subclavian artery (the right subclavian artery develops from the right 4th arch artery). It ascends between the trachea and oesophagus (trachea-oesophageal groove) on its way to larynx (Fig. 22.8).

The **left vagus nerve** descends in front of the left common carotid artery and then anterolateral to the arch of aorta. Here the left vagus nerve is separated from left phrenic nerve by left superior intercostal vein. Further the left vagus descends posterior to the root of the left lung along the left side of the oesophagus.

Near the lower end of the oesophagus the left vagus passes in front of the oesophagus as anterior gastric nerve. The left vagus gives branches to pulmonary plexus, cardiac plexus, oesophageal plexus and left recurrent laryngeal nerve.

The **left recurrent laryngeal nerve** arises from left vagus close to the arch of aorta. The left recurrent laryngeal nerve winds around the ligamentum arteriosum and arch of aorta (arch of aorta is partly developed from left 4th arch artery), and then ascends between trachea and oesophagus on its way to larynx (Fig. 22.8).

The vagus nerve also carry sensory fibres (visceral afferent) from heart and lungs which are concerned with reflex activity of these organs

TRACHEA

- Trachea is a part of the respiratory tract.
- It extends from the lower border of the cricoid cartilage (opposite to C6 vertebra) to the lower border of T6 vertebra in the living, and in the standing position.
- The length of the trachea is about 10 cm to 11 cm.
- The trachea bifurcates at the level of sternal angle into right and left principal bronchi, and enters the hilum of the corresponding lungs. The bronchus divides successively to give secondary bronchi, tertiary bronchi and bronchioles. Bronchioles also divide successively, to end in alveoli, where gaseous exchange takes place (Fig. 22.9).

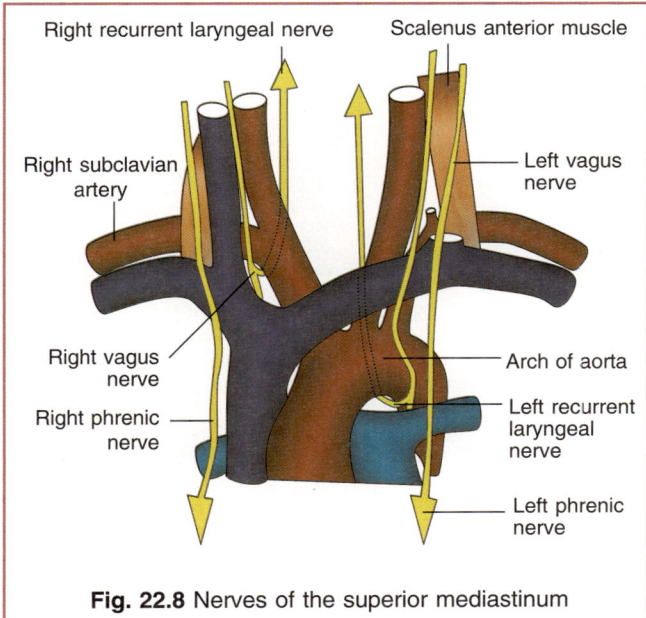

Fig. 22.8 Nerves of the superior mediastinum

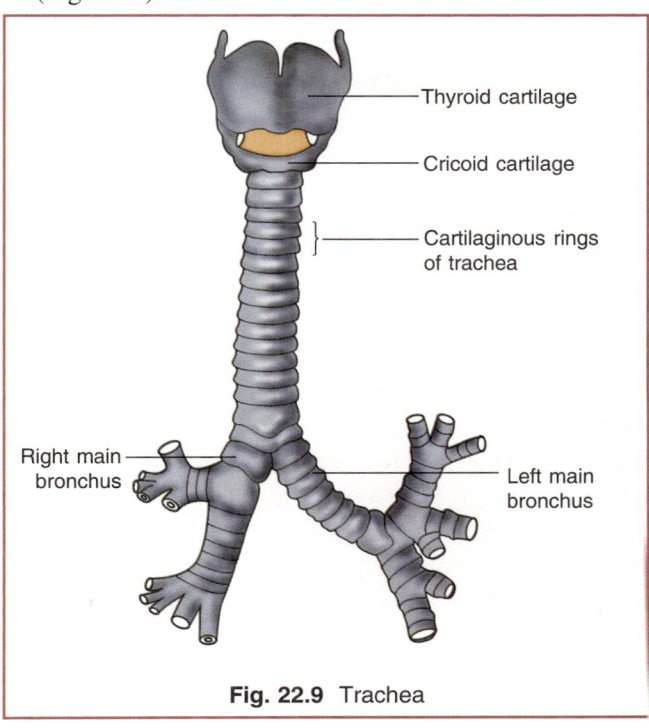

Fig. 22.9 Trachea

SECTION 5

- The diameter of the trachea is 12 mm in adults, but in children it is in millimeters (corresponding almost to their age)

Relations of the cervical part of the trachea and its significance

In case of an upper respiratory obstruction, an emergency tracheostomy is performed in the neck region above the sternal notch. The following structures are related anterior to the upper part (cervical) of the trachea.

Skin, superficial fascia, deep fascia (investing layer), sternohyoid, sternothyroid, isthumus of the thyroid gland, inferior thyroid vein emerging from the lower border of the isthmus, jugular venous arch in the suprasternal space, arteria thyroidea ima (if present), pretracheal lymph nodes.

Oesophagus descends posterior to the trachea. Laterally the trachea is related to thyroid lobes (hence enlarged thyroid lobes can compress trachea) and carotid sheath.

Relations of the thoracic part of the trachea

The anterior relations of trachea in the superior mediastinum include brachiocephalic trunk, left common carotid artery and more importantly the arch of aorta (anteriorly and to the left). An aneurysm of the arch of the aorta can compress this part of the trachea. The other anterior relations include deep cardiac plexus of nerves, tracheobronchial nodes and some time remains of thymus (Figs 22.15 to 22.18).

The recurrent laryngeal nerve ascends in the tracheo-oesophageal groove on either side.

Arterial supply

Trachea is supplied by branches of inferior thyroid and bronchial arteries.

Lymphatic drainage

It drains into lymph nodes present in front (pretracheal) and sides of the trachea (paratracheal).

Nerve supply

It includes both sympathetic and parasympathetic. The parasympathetic vagus is secretomotor to tracheal glands and also motor to trachialis muscle

Carina

It is a hook like ridge inside the trachea at the level of its bifurcation. It is formed by the lowest cartilaginous ring of the trachea. It is about 30 cm from nostrils and 25 cm from incisor teeth. The tracheobronchial lymph node placed just below the bifurcation, if enlarged (in case of carcionoma of the lung) can compress the carina and it becomes flattened and distorted. During bronchoscopy, the carina is examined for such changes (Fig. 22.10).

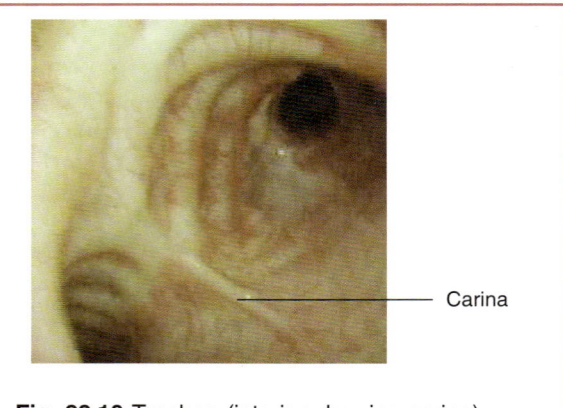

Fig. 22.10 Trachea (interior showing carina)

Structure of the trachea

- Trachea is lined by ciliated pseudo-stratified columnar epithelium with numerous goblet cells
- The submucous coat contains many mucous and serous glands
- The anterior part of the trachea is composed of C-shaped cartilaginous rings (16 to 20 in number). Posteriorly, it is replaced by a fibrous membrane containing smooth muscle fibres (trachealis) which allows the expansion of oesophagus during the passage of food substances (Fig. 22.11).

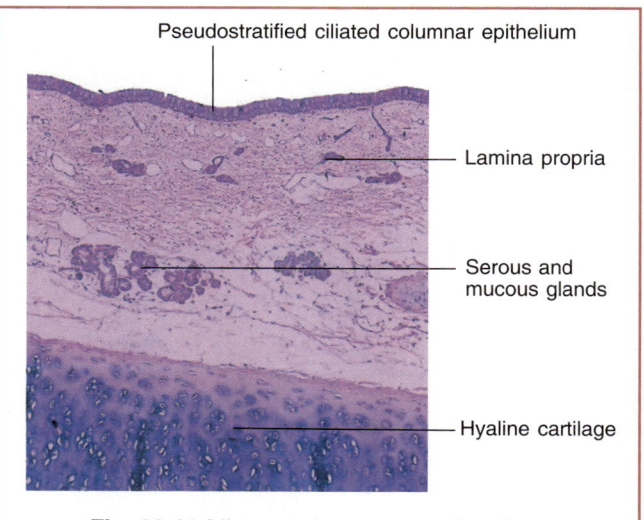

Fig. 22.11 Microscopic structure of trachea

1. Tracheal compressions cause difficulty in breathing (dyspnea). Tracheal compression can arise from enlarged thyroid gland, enlarged lymph nodes or from aneurysm of arch of aorta

2. Tracheostomy is a procedure to make an artificial opening just above the sternal notch in case of obstruction in upper airway.

3. A bronchoscope introduced into trachea can also take biopsies from tracheobronchial lymph nodes at the tracheal bifurcation apart from internal visualisation.

4. The trachea can be felt just above the sterna notch. The deviation of trachea in case of pneumothorax can be felt at this site. The aneurysm of the arch of the aorta can cause tracheal tug.

THYMUS

Thymus is a central lymphatic organ placed in the superior and anterior mediastinum. It is placed in front of the arch of aorta and its branches, left brachiocephalic vein, trachea and upper part of the pericardium. It is irregular in shape, usually having two lobes.

The size of the thymus progressively increases up to puberty (when it weighs about 20 to 30 g). After puberty it undergo involution and converted into fibro-fatty mass.

Thymus is developed from the endoderm of the third pharyngeal pouch and it migrates down along with the inferior parathyroid (Fig. 22.12).

Structure

The substance of the thymus is divided into irregular lobes by connective tissue septa, which also forms a capsule. Each lobule consists of an outer cortex and inner medulla. Because of irregular lobulation medulla may be common for adjacent lobules

The cellular population of thymus consists of mainly reticular epithelial cells (endodermal in origin) and lymphocytes (from bone marrow). The other variety of cells includes macrophages, plasma cells and mast cells. The antigens of the circulating blood are prevented from

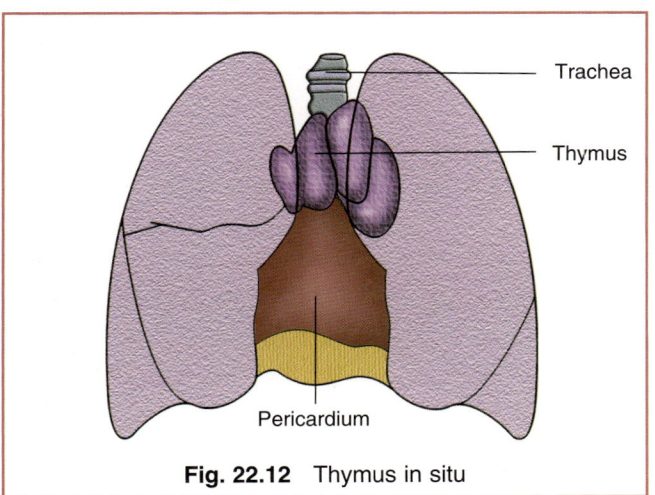

Fig. 22.12   Thymus in situ

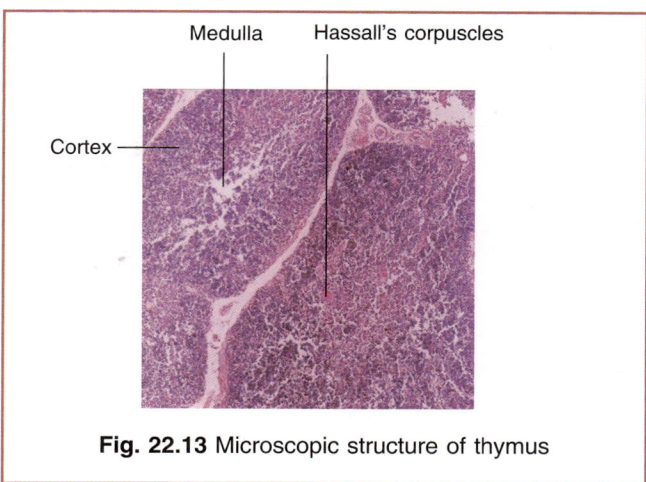

Fig. 22.13 Microscopic structure of thymus

coming in contact with lymphocytes of the thymus by a haemo-thymic barrier. The lymphocytes undergo multiplication, but they have a very short life span for about 3 to 5 days (about 90% of the lymphocytes). These lymphocytes are phagocytosed by macrophages. The remaining lymphocytes enter circulation and appear in secondary lymphatic organs (spleen, lymph nodes etc). About 75% of the circulating lymphocytes are derived from T-lymphocytes.

The degenerating epitheliocytes form 'Hassall's corpuscles' in the centre of the medulla (Fig. 22.13). The lymphocyte phagocytosed by macrophages are also incorporated within the Hassall's corpuscles.

Functions

1. Thymus provide uncommitted immunologically competent T-lymphocytes to the circulation and also to peripheral lymphatic organs

2. During postnatal development thymus influences the growth of the peripheral lymphatic organs. The steroid hormone from the suprarenal cortex and gonads cause involution of thymus after puberty. Hence administration of cortisone to newborn could hinder the immunological activity of the child.

Myasthenia gravis

It is an autoimmune neuromuscular disease (muscle develops early fatigue after few initial contractions) is caused by circulating antibodies that block acetylcholine receptors at the post-synaptic neuromuscular junction (inhibiting the stimulative effect of the neurotransmitter acetylcholine). Up to 75% of patients have an abnormality of the thymus; 25% have thymoma, a tumor (either benign or malignant) of the thymus, and other abnormalities are frequently found. The disease process generally remains stationary after thymectomy (removal of the thymus). Myasthenia is treated medically with cholinesterase inhibitors or immunosuppressant, and, in selected cases by thymectomy.

PHRENIC NERVE

Origin

The phrenic nerve arises from ventral rami of C3, C4 and C5 with main contribution from C4 (Fig. 22.14).

Course

1. In the neck the phrenic nerve descends in front of the scalenus anterior muscle but deep to the prevertebral fascia. The main anterior relations of the nerve in the neck include internal jugular vein and sterno-cleidomastoid muscle.

2. The right and left phrenic nerve enters the superior mediastinum crossing the internal mammary artery on its anterior aspect.

3. Each phrenic nerve descends in front of the hilum along with pericardiophrenic vessels.

4. The right phrenic nerve descends on the right side of the superior vena cava, close to the right border of the

heart. It leaves the thorax along the inferior vena cava through the opening present in the central tendon of the diaphragm (some time it pierces the diaphragm)

5. The left phrenic nerve descends in front and left of the arch of the aorta. Further its course is closely related to left surface of the heart. It pierces the diaphragm to the left of the central tendon.

Distribution

1. Motor fibres to diaphragm

2. Sensory (proprioceptive) fibres from diaphragm

3. Sensory fibres from mediastinal pleura and central part of the diaphragmatic pleura (in case of pleuritis referred pain is felt above the clavicle due to supraclavicular nerve sharing same root value) and also from parietal and fibrous pericardium

4. Sensory fibres from parietal peritoneum lining the under surface of the diaphragm Hence peritonitis involving under surface of diaphragm and adjacent area (ruptured cholecystitis, abscess around the kidney, sub-diaphragmatic abscesses) can cause referred pain above the clavicle.

1. Injury to phrenic nerve results in paralysis of the corresponding half of the diaphragm (hemidia-phragm).

2. **Phrenic nerve block**: Phrenic nerve can be blocked by anesthetic injection. Under ultrasound control, the medication is injected at a point 1 inch above the clavicle, at the groove between the posterior border of the sternocleidomastoid muscle and the scalenus anterior muscle, with a slightly anterior trajectory. After inserting the needle to a depth of approximately 1 inch, aspiration is carried out to identify blood or elicitation of brachial plexus paresthesia; if negative, the solution was slowly injected. This procedure may be helpful in intractable hiccups (spasmodic contraction of the diaphragm due to irritation to phrenic nerve) in cancer patients or during lung surgeries.

3. **Phrenic nerve crush**: It is compressing the nerve injuriously with the forceps. It produces a longer period of paralysis of diaphragm (as it is required in surgical repair of diaphragmatic hernia)

4. **Accessory phrenic nerve** (a branch from nerve to subclavius/upper trunk of the brachial plexus having root value mainly C5) if present, it must also be crushed to produce complete paralysis of the hemidiaphragm

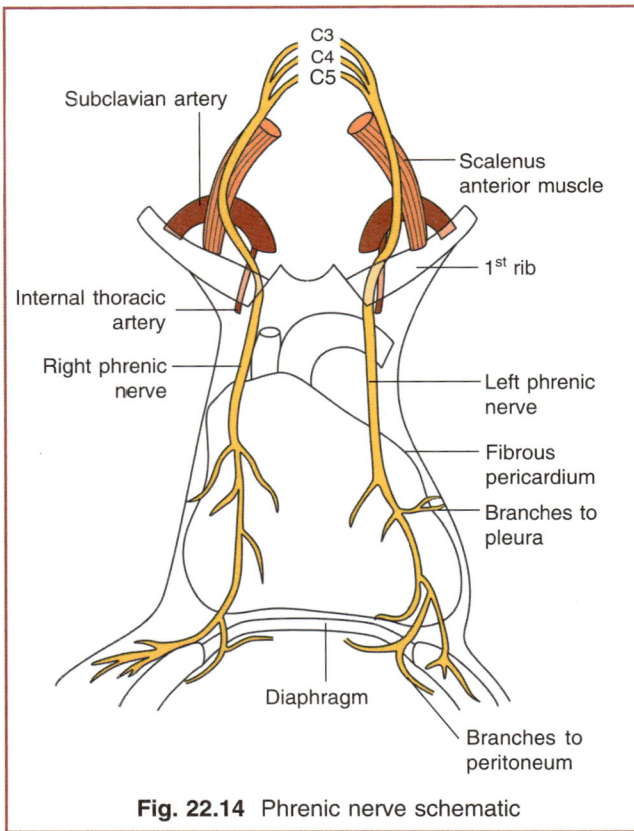
Fig. 22.14 Phrenic nerve schematic

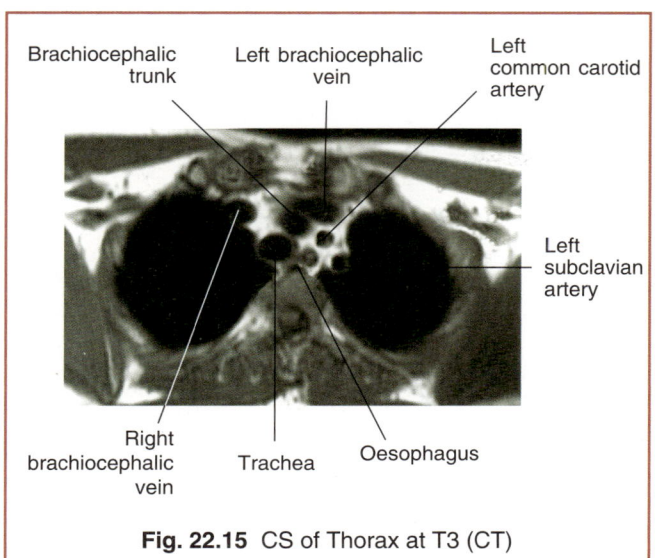

Fig. 22.15 CS of Thorax at T3 (CT)

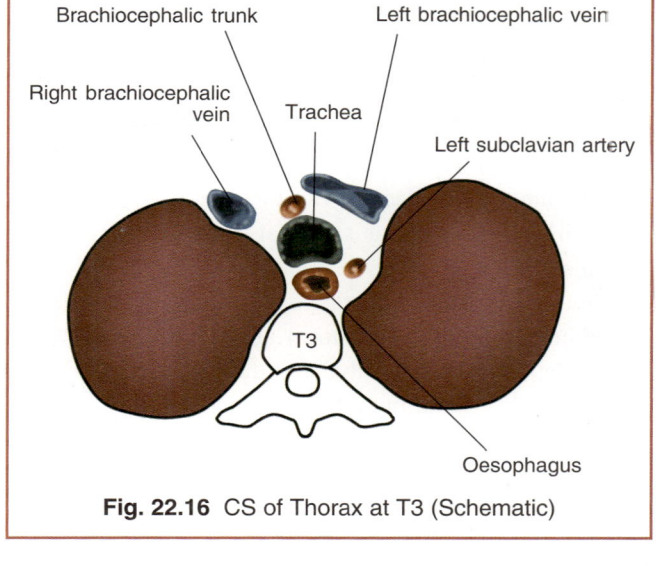

Fig. 22.16 CS of Thorax at T3 (Schematic)

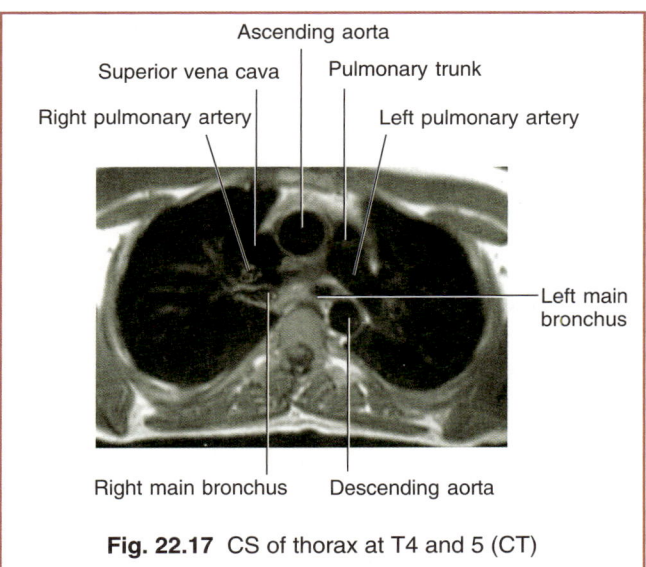

Fig. 22.17 CS of thorax at T4 and 5 (CT)

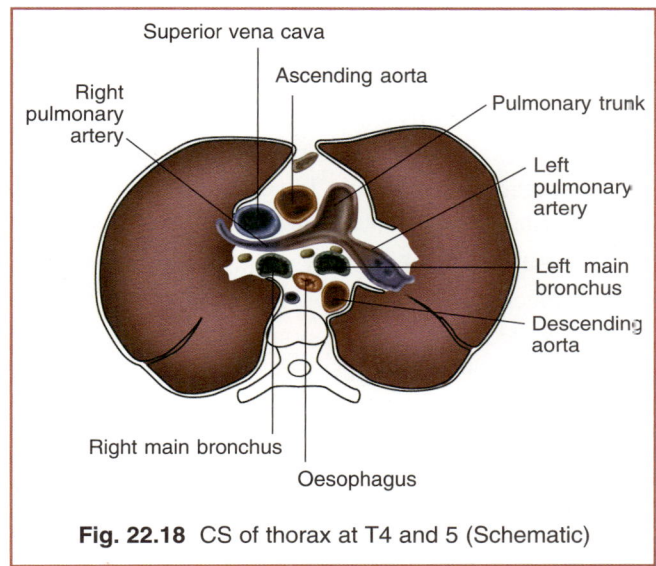

Fig. 22.18 CS of thorax at T4 and 5 (Schematic)

5. **Referred pain**: Pain resulting from irritation of diaphragmatic and mediastinal pleura (in pleurisy) or from the parietal peritoneum lining under surface of the diaphragm (in ruptured gall bladder or abscess around the kidney) carried by phrenic nerve having root value C3,4,5 is referred to shoulder region. This is because skin over the shoulder is supplied by C3 to C5 segment of the spinal cord through supraclavicular nerve.

Solutions to the Clinical case studies:
Case-1

The patient has an aneurysm of the arch of the aorta. With each systole the aneurysm swells and recoils thus pushing down on the bifurcation of the trachea and left primary bronchus. That's a tracheal tug.

MCQs

1. The ductus arteriosus sometimes remains open after birth, requiring a surgical closure. When placing a clamp on the ductus, care must be taken to avoid injury to what important structure immediately dorsal to it?

   A. Left internal thoracic artery

   B. Left phrenic nerve

   C. Left recurrent laryngeal nerve

   D. Thoracic duct

2. An 7-year-old boy is found to have a mid-line tumour of the thymus gland that is impinging posteriorly on a blood vessel. The vessel that is most likely to be affected

A. Left brachiocephalic vein

B. Left pulmonary vein

C. Left bronchial vein

D. Right pulmonary artery

3. A 32-year-old woman presents to her physician with complains of headaches. Her blood pressure is 220/100 mmHg. Her heart rate is 58 beats per minute. Her radial pulses are intact but her femoral pulses are reduced. She undergoes diagnostic angiography. The catheter is advanced from the femoral artery retrograde to the region of the aortic valve and then pulled distally into the first branch of the arch of the aorta. This structure is the

A. Brachiocephalic trunk

B. Left common carotid artery

C. Left subclavian artery

D. Right common carotid artery

4. Upon radiograph examination of the thorax, the doctor noticed that the patients ribs were unusually thin (rib notching). He also had strong radial pulses but a diminished pulse in the lower limbs Which of the following was most likely responsible for this condition

A. Obstruction of arch of aorta proximal to major branches

B. Obstruction of arch of aorta distal to major branches

C. Subclavian artery obstruction

D. Common carotid artery obstruction

5. A surgical procedure is performed in a patient to remove a thymic tumor. Which of the following structures must be avoided during the surgery that is directly posterior to the thymus in the superior mediastinum?

A. Arch of the aorta

B. Esophagus

C. Trachea

D. Left brachiocephalic vein

6. A 64-year-old woman is admitted to the hospital complaining of shortness of breath and difficulty swallowing. The patient coughs up blood during the examination and speaks with a hoarse voice. Diagnosis is made of an oesophageal carcinoma that commonly occurs at a site of constriction of the oesophagus where it is indented by the left main bronchus. What other anatomic structure indents the oesophagus and causes a constriction?

A. Arch of the aorta

B. Inferior vena cava

C. Azygos vein

D. Superior vena cava

7. In the above question, the patient's hoarse voice may have been caused by the compression of the growth on:

A. The left phrenic nerve

B. The left recurrent laryngeal nerve

C. The left vagus nerve

D. The sympathetic trunk on the left

8. A 21-year-old man is diagnosed to have high blood pressure. The blood pressure is significantly higher in both upper limbs than in both lower limbs. Imaging reveals bilateral erosion of the anterior and lateral parts of his ribs. The angiography reveals a narrowing of the aorta. Where is the most likely site of the aortic constriction?

A. Between the brachiocephalic trunk and the left common carotid artery

B. Just distal to the ligamentum arteriosum

C. Between the origin of the subclavian artery and the ligamentum arteriosum

D. In the middle mediastinum

9. In this patient in Question 8, which of the following vessels is there a retrograde flow of blood?

A. Anterior intercostal arteries

B. Posterior intercostal arteries

C. Internal thoracic arteries

D. Right subclavian artery

10. A 57-year-old man, who has smoked cigarettes for 40 years, has a lung cancer that invades his left third intercostal space at the midaxillary line. If cancer cells were carried in the venous drainage of that intercostal space, they would travel first to which of the following intrathoracic veins?

A. Accessory hemiazygos vein

B. Azygos vein

C. Hemiazygos vein

D. Left brachiocephalic vein

11. A patient with intractable hiccups is treated by crushing of the right phrenic nerve in the neck to paralyze the right hemidiaphragm. After this procedure, however, the physician finds that the right half of the patient's diaphragm is not completely paralyzed. The diaphragmatic function is probably being maintained by an accessory phrenic nerve. From which of the following nerves is an accessory phrenic nerve most likely to arise?

SECTION 5

A. Fourth intercostal nerve

B. Left phrenic nerve in thorax

C. Nerve to subclavius

D. Right phrenic nerve in thorax

12. Pain from the diaphragmatic pleura or peritoneum may be referred to the ipsilateral shoulder via the phrenic nerve and a cutaneous nerve that is derived from the same spinal cord segments as the phrenic nerve. Which cutaneous branch of the cervical plexus is involved in this referred pain?

A. Greater occipital nerve

B. Lesser occipital nerve

C. Supraclavicular nerve

D. Suprascapular nerve

Answers to MCQs

1. C
2. A
3. A
4. B
5. C
6. A
7. B
8. B
9. B
10. D
11. C
12. C

SECTION 5

- Oesophagus
- Descending thoracic aorta
- Azygos system of veins
- Thoracic duct
- Autonomic nerves of the thorax
- MCQs

Objectives
- To explain the parts and major relations of the oesophagus
- To know the normal constrictions of the oesophagus
- To explain the microscopic structure of the oesophagus
- To explain the blood supply and lymphatic drainage of the oesophagus and its clinical relevance
- To locate the descending thoracic aorta and to mention their branches
- To explain the formation, course, tributaries of azygos system of veins
- To explain the formation, course and termination of thoracic duct

OESOPHAGUS

- It is a muscular tube of about 25 cm in length.
- It extends from the laryngopharynx (at the level of C6 vertebra/ lower border of cricoid cartilage) to the cardiac end of the stomach (at the level of T11 vertebra)
- The oesophagus has three parts
  Cervical (4 cm)
  Thoracic (20 cm)
  Abdominal (1.25 cm).

Relations of the cervical part of the oesophagus

Anteriorly: Trachea

Posteriorly: Prevertebral fascia and retropharyngeal space (in front of the prevertebral fascia and posterior to the pharynx and upper part of the oesophagus)

Laterally: The recurrent laryngeal nerve ascends in the tracheoesophageal groove. The common carotid artery and lateral lobes of thyroid are related to oesophagus on either side (Fig. 23.1).

Relations of the thoracic part of the oesophagus

Anteriorly (from above downwards): Trachea, arch of aorta, left main bronchus, oblique sinus of the pericardium (separating it from the left atrium)

Posteriorly: Thoracic part of the vertebral column, right posterior intercostal arteries, thoracic duct and azygos vein. The descending thoracic aorta is related to the left in the upper part of the posterior mediastinum and posterior to it in the lower part (Fig. 23.1)

To the left (In the superior mediastinum): Thoracic duct, left recurrent laryngeal nerve, left subclavian artery, upper lobe of the left lung. In the posterior mediastinum, oesophagus is related to left lung where it makes an impression

To the right: Medial surface of the right lung behind the hilum

- Oesophagus passes through the oesophageal orifice of the diaphragm (at the level of 10th thoracic vertebra) and enters the abdominal cavity along with the right and left vagus nerves (posterior and anterior gastric nerves)

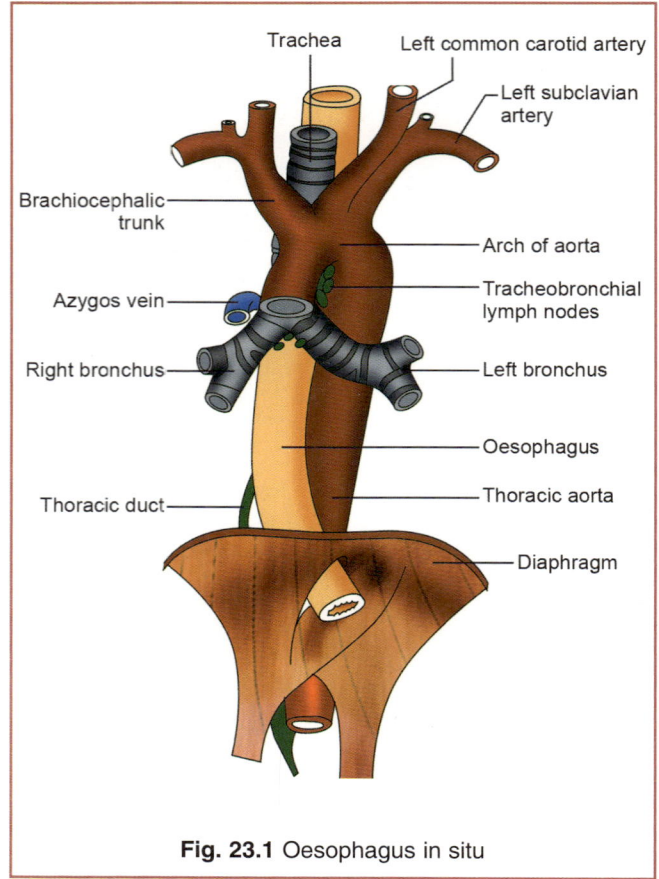

Fig. 23.1 Oesophagus in situ

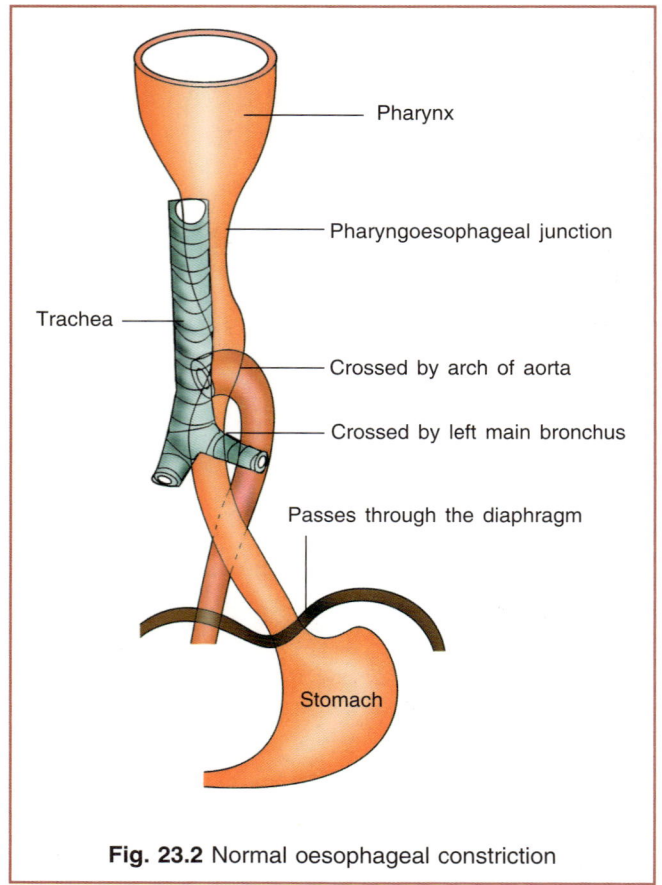

Fig. 23.2 Normal oesophageal constriction

- Though there is no anatomical sphincter at the lower end, the opening of the diaphragm acts as a sphincter. This opening is formed by right crus of the diaphragm. The fascia covering the under surface of the diaphragm is attached to the margins of the oesophagus by **phreno-oesophageal ligament**. Food passes through oesophagus by peristaltic action of its musculature and not by the gravity (one can still swallow if inverted). The lumen of the oesophagus is normally collapsed and prevents reflux of the stomach contents into the oesophagus.

- Oesophagus presents **four normal constrictions**, which are important during instrumentation through it (Fig. 23.2).

1. **First constriction**: at the pharyngoesophageal junction (At the level of C6 vertebra) It is about 6 inches from the incisor teeth.

2. **Second constriction** is where it is crossed by arch of aorta (At the level of T4 vertebra) It is about 9 inches from the incisor teeth.

3. **Third constriction** is where it is crossed by left bronchus (At the level of T6 vertebra) It is about 11 inches from incisor teeth.

4. **Fourth constriction** is where the oesophagus passes through the diaphragm (At the level of T 10 vertebra). It is about 15 or 16 inches from the incisor teeth.

Arterial supply

The oesophagus is supplied by the branches of the following arteries - Inferior thyroid artery, descending thoracic aorta, bronchial arteries and left gastric artery.

The cervical part of the oesophagus drains into inferior thyroid vein, thoracic part into azygos and hemiazygos veins and abdominal part into left gastric vein (one of the sites of portocaval anastomosis).

Lymphatic drainage

The cervical part drains into deep cervical lymph nodes, the thoracic part into posterior mediastinal nodes. The abdominal part drains into left gastric and then into coeliac group of lymph nodes.

Nerve supply

The striated muscles of the upper part of the oesophagus are supplied by vagus nerve. The remaining part by oesophageal plexus which consists of sympathetic and parasympathetic nerve fibres. The sympathetic fibres are derived from T4 and T5 segments of the spinal cord and reach the oesophagus through greater splanchnic nerves. It carries pain sensation (especially from the lower part, which is vulnerable to acid peptic oesophagitis). The referred pain from such oesophagitis is felt at the lower thoracic and epigastric region. This is often referred as heart burn, sometime mistaken for angina.

The parasympathetic nerves are derived from vagus and are motor to musculature of the oesophagus and secretomotor to oesophageal glands.

Microscopic structure of the oesophagus

The wall of the oesophagus is made up of four layers from inside to outside (Fig. 23.3).

1. Mucosa (mucous membrane): It has three parts.

   a. Lining epithelium – stratified squamous non-keratinized epithelium.

   b. Lamina propria – made up of connective tissue fibres.

   c. Muscularis mucosa – layer of smooth muscle fibres.

2. Submucosa – It presents plenty of mucous secreting oesophageal glands.

3. Muscularis externa (muscle coat): It consists of outer longitudinal and inner circular layers. The upper part of oesophagus presents striated, middle part mixed variety and lower part smooth muscle fibres.

4. Outer fibrous coat is made up of areolar tissue.

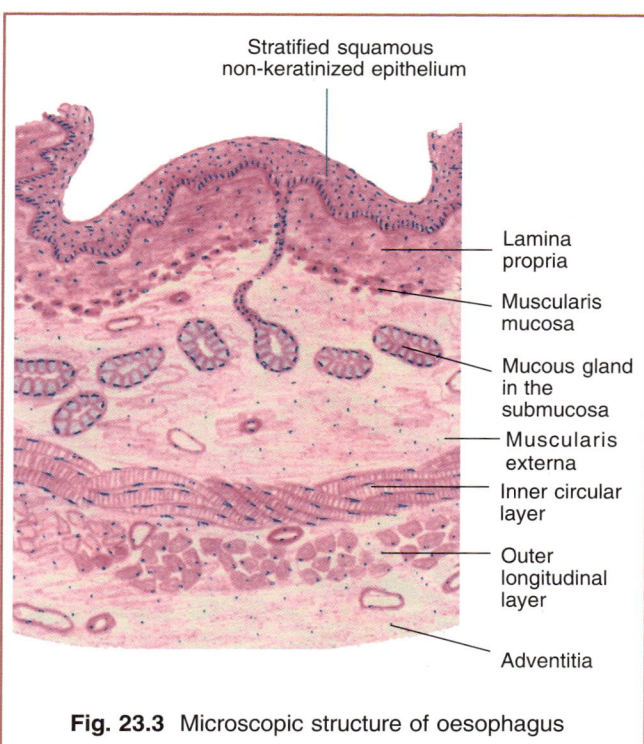

Fig. 23.3 Microscopic structure of oesophagus

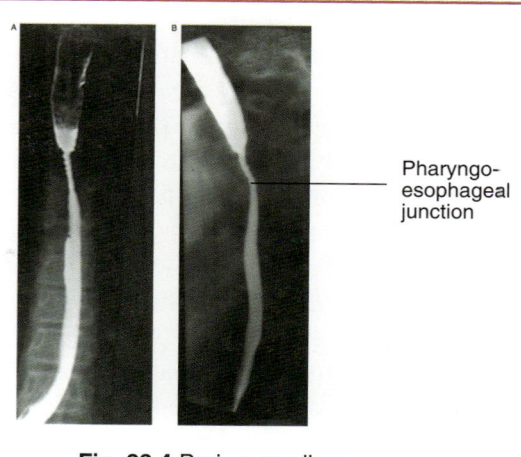

Fig. 23.4 Barium swallow

Pharyngo-esophageal junction

1. **Carcinoma of the oesophagus:** The squamous cell carcinoma arises from the epithelium lining the oesophagus (association with tobacco and alcohol consumption) and the adenocarcinoma arises from glandular cells that are present at the junction of the esophagus and stomach (associated with a history of gastroesophageal reflux). The oesophageal tumors usually lead to dysphagia (difficulty swallowing), pain and other symptoms, and are diagnosed with biopsy. The carcinoma spreads by lymphatics and involves posterior mediastinal lymph nodes, gastric and coeliac nodes. The direct infiltration can involve the lungs.

2. **The gastroesophageal reflux:** The lower end of the oesophagus is guarded by a physiological sphincter which prevents gastroesophageal reflux. However it can become compromised, usually by a loss of muscle tone or sliding hiatal hernia (explained in the chapter-35 diaphragm). The acidic chyme burns and inflames the oesophageal mucosa (oesophagitis). It causes uncomfortable sensation or heart burn, and dysphagia.

3. **Oesophageal varices:** It occurs in portal hypertension. The anastomoses between the tributaries of systemic and portal vessels at the lower end of the oesophagus dilate. The varices (dilated veins) lie immediately beneath the mucosa, where they are subjected to mechanical trauma during deglutition, or by the passage of diagnostic instruments. They produce no symptoms until they rupture, causing massive haematemesis (vomiting of blood). The oesophageal varices can be visualized radiographically by barium swallow.

4. **The oesophagoscopy:** The interior of the oesophagus is examined directly through an

SECTION 5

instrument. Oesophagoscopy is a very useful tool in the diagnosis and treatment of oesophageal diseases. It is a highly reliable diagnostic method for evaluating oesophageal disorders that affect the mucosa or alter the lumen of the organ. The oesophagoscopy allows the procurement of cytology and histology samples. The most common mucosal and luminal abnormalities diagnosed by oesophagoscopy are foreign bodies, oesophagitis, strictures, oesophageal ulcers, fistula and neoplasia.

5. **Achalasia cardia:** In achalasia, the oesophageal sphincter remains contracted, the normal peristalsis is interrupted and food cannot enter the stomach. It is due to congenital absence of the nerve cells of oesophagus. The most common symptom of the achalasia is dysphagia.

6. **Dysphagia:** It means difficulty in swallowing. Any structure related to oesophagus can compress it, causing dysphagia. Such compression can be due to aneurysm of the arch of aorta, enlarged lymph nodes, enlarged left atrium (mitral stenosis), retrosternal goiter, aberrant right subclavian artery. The oesophageal strictures and carcinoma can also cause dysphagia.

7. **Radiological examination:** The interior of the oesophagus can also be examined by a barium swallow radiological method (Fig. 23.4).

CASE - 1

A 55-year-old carpenter is admitted to the hospital as an emergency. He has severe shortness of breath (dyspnea) and great difficulty in swallowing (dysphagia). The patient states that for the past six months he had suffered increasing difficulty and pain in swallowing. He has to restrict himself with a liquid diet and has lost weight. His shortness of breath has been present for the past few weeks. From time to time, he has severe coughing spells, his sputum is blood-tinged, and occasionally he brings up as much as a cupful of blood. He states that for the last few weeks he has become quite hoarse. Fluoroscopic examination of the oesophagus with radiopaque barium demonstrates an obstruction at the level of the bifurcation of the trachea. It was diagnosed as oesophageal cancer that has obstructed the oesophagus at one of its most common site-the level of the tracheal bifurcation. The common sites of esophageal cancer correspond to the physiologic constrictions of the oesophagus.

a. Where are the oesophageal constrictions located?

b. What is the anatomical basis for dyspnea?

c. Why did the patient become hoarse?

d. What lymph nodes are likely to be involved?

DESCENDING THORACIC AORTA

- It descends in the posterior mediastinum of the thorax.

- It enters the abdominal cavity by passing through the diaphragm (aortic opening) at the level of T12 vertebra, where it is accompanied by thoracic duct and azygos vein.

- In the abdomen it continues as abdominal aorta (Fig. 23.5).

Relations

- Anteriorly – root of the left lung, pericardium and heart and oesophagus in the lower part

- Posteriorly – Thoracic part of the vertebral column

- On right side – thoracic duct and azygos vein

- On left side – it forms an impression on the medial surface of the left lung

Branches

- They include third to eleventh posterior intercostal arteries on each side. These arteries supply the thoracic wall.

- The other branches from the thoracic aorta are oesophageal and mediastinal arteries, upper and lower left bronchial arteries and inferior phrenic arteries (Fig. 23.5).

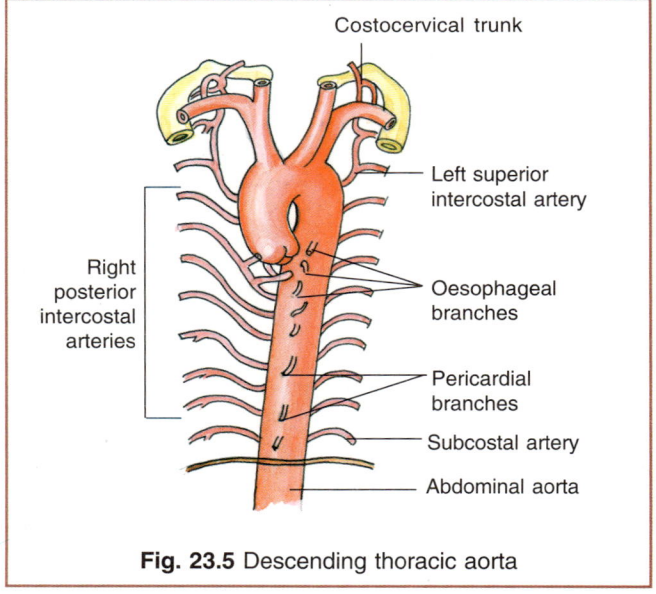

Fig. 23.5 Descending thoracic aorta

S E C T I O N 5

AZYGOS SYSTEM OF VEINS

The intercostal spaces of thorax are drained by anterior and posterior intercostal veins. The anterior intercostal veins terminate in internal thoracic vein. However the mode of termination of posterior intercostal veins differs on two sides. They drain into azygos (azygos = unpaired) system of veins (Fig. 23.6).

Azygos vein

It is an important vein draining the venous blood from the posterior abdominal wall and major portion of the thoracic wall.

Formation

It is formed within the abdominal cavity by many combinations.

- Usually it is formed by the union of right ascending lumbar vein (which is formed by the union of four lumbar veins) and right subcostal vein.

- Sometimes a lumbar azygos vein (a vein arising from the inferior vena cava) can also contribute to the formation of azygos vein.

It ascends through aortic opening of the diaphragm. It ascends in the posterior mediastinum on the right side.

Termination

It arches over the root of right lung and opens into the superior vena cava.

Tributaries

i. The right posterior intercostal veins (4th to 11th)

ii. The right subcostal vein

iii. The right superior intercostal vein formed by the union of right 2nd, 3rd and 4th posterior intercostal vein

iv. **Accessory hemiazygos vein** – which is formed by the union of 5th to 8th left posterior intercostals veins. At the level of T7 vertebra it crosses to the right side posterior to thoracic duct and descending thoracic aorta to join azygos vein

v. **Hemiazygos vein** - which is formed by the union of left ascending lumbar vein and left subcostal vein. It enters the thorax by piercing the left crus of the diaphragm. It ascends in front of the thoracic vertebral bodies and crosses to the right side at the level of T8 vertebra to join azygos vein.

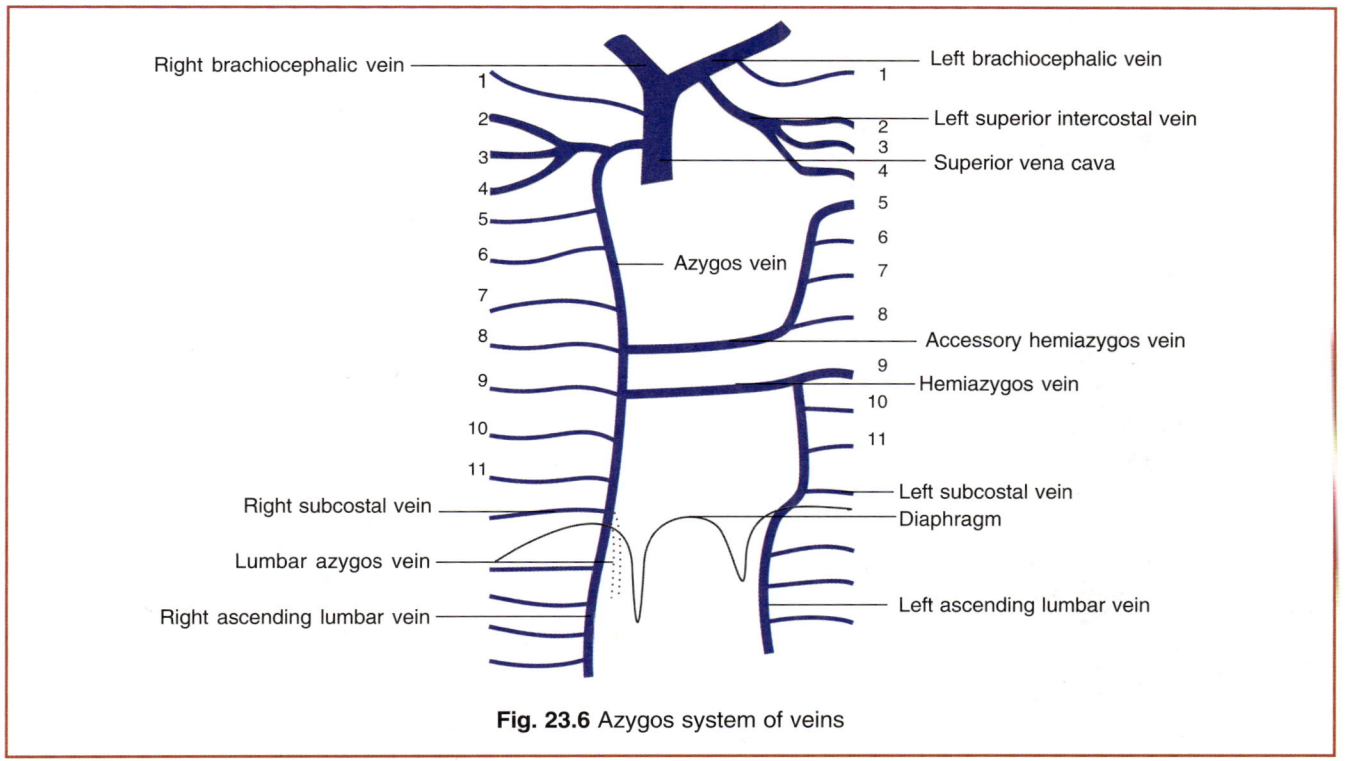

Fig. 23.6 Azygos system of veins

SECTION 5

vi. Right bronchial vein and also some oesophageal, pericardial and mediastinal veins

> The internal thoracic vein would provide a collateral route for drainage if the azygos vein is obstructed. In case of an obstruction, blood could flow from the posterior intercostal veins (which usually drain into the azygos) into the anterior intercostal veins, enter the internal thoracic vein, and drain into the right brachiocephalic vein. This would allow the blood to bypass the blockage.

THORACIC DUCT

It is a major lymphatic vessel draining lymph from the whole body except the right upper limb, right side of the head and neck and right half of the thorax.

It is about 45 cm in length and has beaded appearance with many valves inside

It begins from the cistern chyli (at the level of T12 vertebra) in the abdominal cavity and enters thorax by passing through aortic orifice where it is related to aorta and azygos vein (Figs 23.7 to 23.9).

Course and relations:

• It ascends in the posterior mediastinum in front of the thoracic vertebral bodies and behind the oesophagus.

• At the level of T5 vertebra it inclines to the left and then ascend upwards in the superior mediastinum along the left edge of the oesophagus

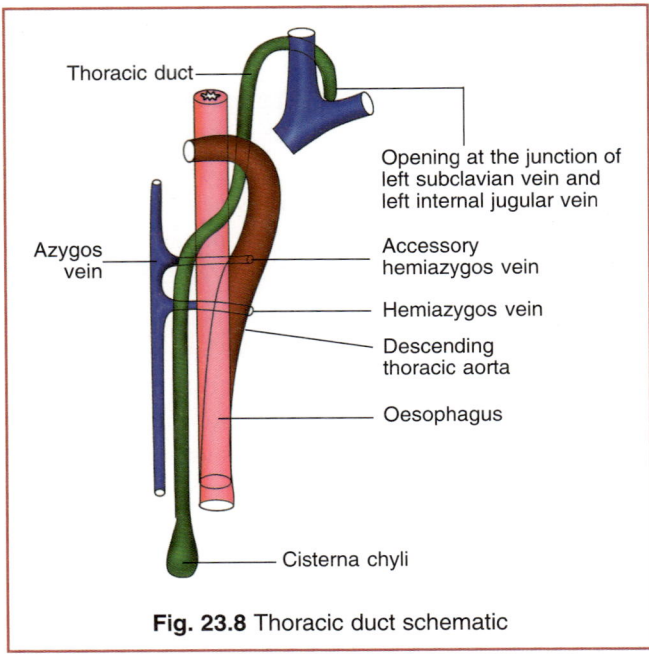

Fig. 23.8 Thoracic duct schematic

• At the root of the neck (at the level of transverse process of C7 vertebra), it arches laterally behind the lower end of the carotid sheath and in front of the vertebral artery and turns downwards.

• It terminates at the junction of left subclavian vein and left internal jugular vein and at this site it is guarded by a valve.

Tributaries:

1. Left jugular lymph trunk bringing lymph from left half of the head and neck area
2. Left subclavian lymph trunk bringing lymph from left upper limb including left mammary gland
3. Left bronchomediastinal lymph trunk bringing lymph from left lung and left half of the mediastinum

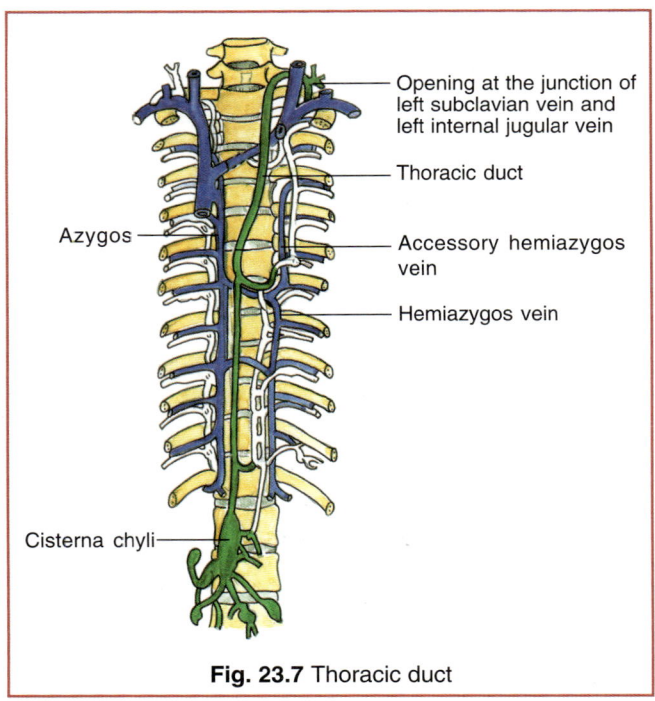

Fig. 23.7 Thoracic duct

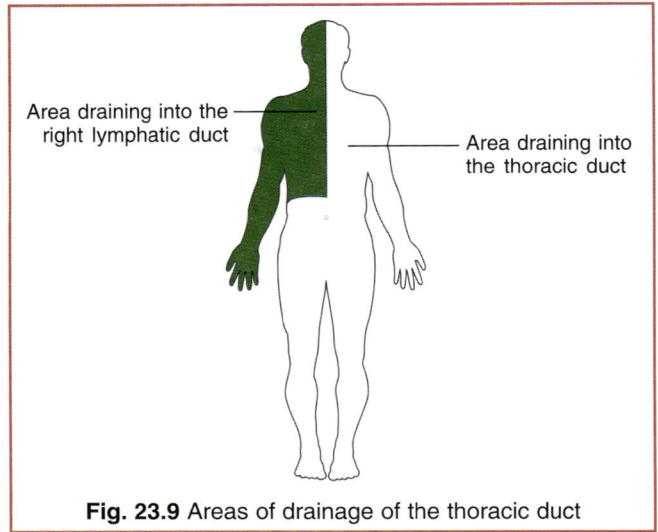

Fig. 23.9 Areas of drainage of the thoracic duct

SECTION 5

4. Lymph vessels draining from left posterior intercostals nodes of the upper six spaces of the left side

5. Descending thoracic lymph trunks (right and left) draining from lower six spaces

6. Ascending lymph trunks (right and left) draining from upper lumbar lymph nodes

> 1. Filarial parasites may obstruct the thoracic duct and sometimes cause rupture of the duct. The chyle (lymph from intestine) may fill pleural (chylothorax) or peritoneal cavity (chyloperitoneum) and sometimes in cavity of the tunica vaginalis.
>
> 2. The terminal part of the thoracic duct may be injured during removal of supraclavicular lymph nodes

CASE-2

A 48-year-old patient is currently recovering from a modified radical neck procedure for squamous cell carcinoma of the tongue. The patient presents tachycardia and was hypotensive with decreasing urinary output and poor skin turgor. He is intermittently combative and semi-conscious. On physical exam, you note the incision line on the left side of his neck to be intact with a bulb suction device protruding through the incision. The surrounding region of the neck is edematous, and a palpable mass roughly 8 cm in diameter is felt. You connect the bulb suction to the wall suction apparatus and approximately 600 ml of milky white fluid is immediately aspirated from the wound with a subsequent diminution in the size of the mass. Over the next few hours, you notice that the patient continues to have worsening hypotension, and the wound has now drained over 1 liter of milky white fluid in the period of six hours. The physician diagnosed a chylothorax.

a. What is chylothorax?

b. How would you explain the milky white fluid following this kind of operation?

c. Which lymphatic channel/duct would be involved?

d. What is the course of the thoracic duct?

e. What structures drain into the thoracic duct?

f. Which lymph nodes are found in the posterior mediastinum?

AUTONOMIC NERVES OF THE THORAX

Thoracic part of the sympathetic chain

- The right and left sympathetic chain is placed on either side of the thoracic vertebral bodies (para-vertebral) close to the heads of the ribs (Fig. 23.10).

- Each chain continues as lumbar part of the sympathetic chain after descending deep to the medial arcuate ligament

- The thoracic part of the sympathetic chain consists of 11 ganglia

- The first thoracic ganglion is often fused with inferior cervical ganglion, which is star shaped (stellate ganglion) placed in front of the neck of the 1st rib

- The thoracic sympathetic ganglia are placed close to the heads of the succeeding ribs.

- Each thoracic sympathetic ganglion is connected with corresponding thoracic spinal nerves by two communications, the pre (white ramus) and post (grey ramus) ganglionic communicants. The white rami communicants bring preganglionic sympathetic fibres from the spinal cord (lateral horn), while grey rami communicants give postganglionic sympathetic fibres to thoracic spinal nerves (to sweat glands, erector pylorum muscle and blood vessels)

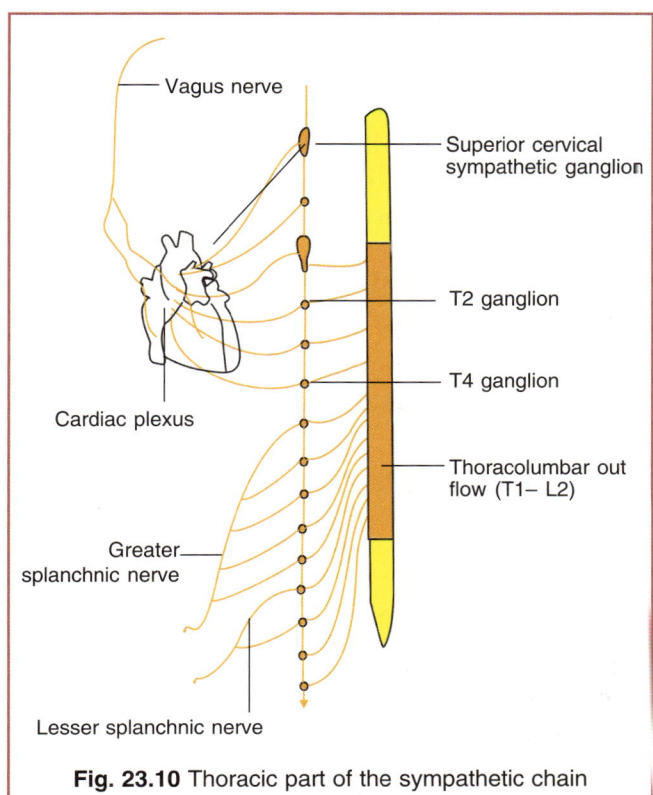

Fig. 23.10 Thoracic part of the sympathetic chain

SECTION 5

- The post-ganglionic sympathetic fibres also passes out as splanchnic nerves

- The greater splanchnic nerve is derived from 5th to 8th thoracic sympathetic ganglia on each side. It descends into the abdomen by piercing the crura of the diaphragm to terminate in celiac ganglion (providing sympathetic fibres to abdominal organs)

- The lesser splanchnic nerve is derived from 9th to 10th thoracic sympathetic ganglia. It ends in aorticorenal ganglion after piercing the crura of the diaphragm.

- The least splanchnic nerve from the 11th thoracic sympathetic ganglion ends in renal ganglion

- The thoracic splanchnic nerves lie on the anterior surfaces of the vertebral bodies.

- The splanchnic nerves lie medial to the sympathetic trunk, which is lying on the heads of the ribs.

- The upper 5 thoracic sympathetic ganglion give cardiac branches to cardiac plexus (for heart) from which the pulmonary plexus supply the lung

- The pain fibres from the viscera (visceral afferent) is also conveyed through these sympathetic nerves and ganglion (without relaying there), but reach spinal cord through dorsal root (neurons are located in the dorsal root ganglion).

Vagus nerve

The parasympathetic fibres to the thoracic and majority of the abdominal organ are derived from vagus nerve. The preganglionic parasympathetic fibres are derived from dorsal nucleus of vagus present in the medulla oblongata.

The course and branches of vagus in the thorax is discussed in page 386, superior mediastinum.

Solutions to the clinical case studies

Case-1

a. Refer text

b. Dyspnea is due to compression of trachea at its bifurcation

c. As a result of the tumor affecting the recurrent laryngeal nerve.

d. Posterior mediastinal lymph nodes, gastric and coeliac nodes

Case-2

a. A pleural effusion composed of lymphatic fluid due to disruption of the thoracic duct.

b. The fluid is lymph, which contains lipids and hence presents as milky white drainage. Given the location of

the surgical procedure - dissection of the left neck - there is a danger of injuring the thoracic duct or its major tributaries, particularly the jugular trunk found within the neck.

c. The thoracic duct begins at the cisterna chyli in the abdomen and extends cranially on the anterior surface of the vertebral bodies. It passes through the diaphragm along with the aorta at the T12 level. It then shifts to the left at T5 to T7 and then empties into the left subclavian vein.

d. The thoracic duct receives branches from the intercostal spaces, and the jugular, subclavian, and broncho-mediastinal trunks of the lymphatic system.

e. The posterior mediastinal lymph nodes lie posterior to the pericardium. These lymph nodes receive lymph from the esophagus, the posterior aspect of the pericardium, and the middle posterior intercostal spaces.

MCQs

1. The sympathetic fibers in the greater thoracic splanchnic nerve terminates in
   A. Brainstem
   B. Coeliac ganglion
   C. Sympathetic chain ganglion
   D. Spinal cord

2. Which nerve fiber would have its cell body in the lateral horn of the spinal cord at segmental level T1?
   A. Afferent fiber from skin around the nipple
   B. Efferent fibers to sweat glands in the lumbar region
   C. Efferent fibers to skin of the forehead
   D. Parasympathetic fibers to the heart

3. The grey rami communicant contain postganglionic sympathetic fibers that innervate which of the following structures in the thoracic region?
   A. Aorta
   B. Heart
   C. Lung
   D. Sweat glands

4. In the midregion of the thorax the thoracic duct lies immediately posterior to the:
   A. Azygos vein
   B. Oesophagus
   C. Superior vena cava
   D. Trachea

5. Lymph nodes can be found in which mediastinal compartment(s)?
   A. Anterior

B. Middle
C. Posterior
D. All of the above

6. Which posterior mediastinal structure is most closely applied to the posterior surface of the pericardial sac?
A. Aorta
B. Azygos vein
C. Oesophagus
D. Thoracic duct

7. A tumor of the posterior mediastinum is most likely to compress which of the following structures?
A. Arch of the aorta
B. Oesophagus
C. Inferior vena cava
D. Pulmonary trunk

8. While performing transesophageal echocardiography on a patient, the posterior wall of the oesophagus, immediately behind the left atrium, was punctured from within. The patient subsequently developed an infection in the space around the oesophagus at this point, namely the:
A. Anterior mediastinum
B. Middle mediastinum
C. Posterior mediastinum
D. Superior mediastinum

9. Since the puncture in the previous question was through the posterior wall of the oesophagus, the doctors were also very concerned about possible damage to a thin-walled vessel just behind the oesophagus, i.e. the:
A. Hemiazygos vein
B. Left bronchial vein
C. Left pulmonary vein
D. Thoracic duct

10. During a surgical procedure, a patient's right sympathetic trunk was accidentally severed just cranial to the level of spinal nerve T1. Which function would be left intact in the affected region?
A. Arrector pili muscle activity
B. Dilation/constriction of blood vessels
C. Sweat production
D. Voluntary muscle activity

11. Most of the drainage of the thoracic body wall reaches the superior vena cava via the azygos vein. A notable exception is the left superior intercostal vein, which normally drains into the:
A. Left brachiocephalic vein

B. Left bronchial vein
C. Left pulmonary vein
D. Left subclavian vein

12. An enlarging lymph node gradually constricts the flow of blood in the azygos venous arch. Which vessel would enlarge as a result of collateral drainage?
A. Superior vena cava
B. Inferior vena cava
C. Internal thoracic vein
D. Right brachiocephalic vein

13. During a procedure to harvest lymph nodes in the posterior mediastinum, the thoracic duct is accidentally cut. The resulting accumulation of lymph in the pleural cavity is referred to as:
A. Pleurisy
B. Chylothorax
C. Pyothorax
D. Hemothorax

14. A cancerous growth from the body of the 9th thoracic vertebra exerts pressure anterolaterally. Which structure lies in direct contact with this growth?
A. Right phrenic nerve
B. Right vagus nerve
C. Right sympathetic trunk
D. Right greater thoracic splanchnic nerve

15. A 48-year-old female patient complains of excessive sweating on the right side of the face and neck and in the right armpit region, which leaves her clothing constantly stained with moisture. It is such a terrible social embarrassment that she has become withdrawn and self-conscious. Since no medical treatment has proven effective, she is considering surgical denervation of the sweat glands in the affected areas. Which structure(s) might be removed or cut in order to alleviate her condition?
A. Cervico-thoracic (stellate) ganglion
B. Dorsal roots of cervical nerves
C. Greater thoracic splanchnic nerve
D. Lumbar sympathetic trunk

16. While viewing an exploratory surgery on a patient injured in an automobile accident, you see the surgeon elevate the oesophagus off the vertebral bodies and look in the area between the azygos vein and descending aorta. What structure was she most likely looking for?
A. Left recurrent laryngeal nerve
B. Right pulmonary artery
C. Sympathetic trunk
D. Thoracic duct

17. The ductus arteriosus sometimes remains open after birth, requiring surgical closure. When placing a clamp on the ductus, care must be taken to avoid injury to what important structure immediately dorsal to it?
    A. Accessory hemiazygos vein
    B. Left internal thoracic artery
    C. Left phrenic nerve
    D. Left recurrent laryngeal nerve

18. A 62-year-old man, suspected of having widespread cancer of the lungs and bronchi, is brought in for bronchoscopic examination. The instrument is inserted into the airway, where it accidentally punctures the thin, brittle posterior wall of the diseased right main bronchus. A sudden gush of blood immediately indicates that the instrument has also torn the wall of the blood vessel immediately behind the right main bronchus, i.e. the:
    A. Azygos vein
    B. Left brachiocephalic artery
    C. Pericardiacophrenic artery
    D. Right pulmonary vein

19. In obstruction of the superior or inferior vena cava, venous blood is returned to the heart by an alternate route via the azygos vein, which becomes dilated in the process. Which of the following structures might it compress as a result?
    A. Trachea
    B. Root of the left lung
    C. Arch of the aorta
    D. Thoracic duct

20. A 58-year-old man undergoes upper gastrointestinal endoscopy to investigate the source of his acute gastrointestinal bleeding. After completion of the procedure, the patient complains of pain and the feeling of a foreign body lodged in his throat. A chest radiograph shows mediastinal air and a widening of the mediastinum. A barium swallow confirms esophageal perforation. Iatrogenic perforation of the esophagus occurs most commonly at which of the following levels?

A. Pharyngoesophageal junction
B. Oesophageal opening of the diaphragm
C. Gastroesophageal junction
D. Site of compression by left primary bronchus and aortic arch

21. A pleural effusion caused by leakage of lymph from thoracic duct lymph into the pleural space (chylothorax) is usually associated with lymphoma or lung cancer. Which of the following best describes the area drained by the thoracic duct?
    A. All of the body above the diaphragm
    B. All of the body except the head and neck
    C. Most of the body below the diaphragm
    D. Thorax and abdomen only
    E. Thorax only

Answers to MCQs

1. B
2. C
3. D
4. B
5. D
6. C
7. B
8. C
9. D
10. D
11. A
12. C
13. B
14. D
15. A
16. D
17. D
18. A
19. D
20. A
21. C

Development of the Heart, Major Blood Vessels and Respiratory System

24

- Development of the Heart
- Development of aortic arch arteries
- Development of major veins
- Circulation before and after birth
- Development of respiratory system
- MCQs

Objectives

- To explain the fate of five dilatations of the primitive heart tube, to explain the formation of inter-atrial and inter-ventricular septum and to discuss the anomalies related to them
- To summarize the development of right and left atria and right and left ventricles
- List the cyanotic and acyanotic congenital cardiac anomalies of the heart and to explain the Fallot's teralogy
- List the cardiac anomalies with left to right shunt and right to left shunt
- To explain the fate of aortic arch arteries on each side and the embryology of patent ductus arteriosus (PDA)
- To know the pre and post-ductal types of coarctation of aorta and to understand the collateral circulation established in post-ductal type
- To explain the foetal circulation and series of events taking after birth in this circulation
- To know the normal state of differentiation of the lung parenchyma and pulmonary vasculature at the sixth month of gestation, and at birth, and changes that occurs postnatally
- To explain the state of surfactant production in the premature neonate with the full term neonate, and state of foetal age at which alveolar type II cells begin to produce surfactants.
- To explain the embryology of 'tracheoesophageal fistula'

DEVELOPMENT OF THE HEART

The cardiovascular system is the first organ system of an embryo to reach functional state

Nutrition at the early stage of development

In early stages of development, the morula is nourished by deutoplasm (cytoplasm of the ovum) and the blastocyst by the secretion from the uterine glands.

In the first two weeks of development, the maternal blood present in the lacunar spaces of the syncytiotrophoblast reach embryo by diffusion. As embryo grows, this diffusion cannot meet the requirement and this induces the formation of vascular system in the embryo.

- Vascular system of the human embryo appears in the middle of the 3rd week
- The human embryonic heart begins beating around 21 days after conception and blood begins to circulate during 24th day.
- The first heart beat can be felt at 5–6 weeks of pregnancy on a sonogram.

What is cardiogenic area?

The splanchnopleuric layer of lateral plate mesoderm in the midline cranial to the prochordal plate is called cardiogenic area (Fig. 24.1). Two blood vessels appear in the cardiogenic area, below the floor of the pericardial sac and are called 'primitive endothelial heart tubes'.

Development of the intraembryonic blood vessels

- Two longitudinal vessels are formed on either side of the notochord on dorsal wall of the yolk sac. These are called 'Dorsal aortae'
- The cranial end of the dorsal aortae continues with primitive endothelial heart tube.
- Caudally dorsal aortae continues with umbilical arteries (which are developed within the connecting stalk) and then breaks up into the capillary plexus in placenta.
- Capillary plexus in placenta forms venules which traverse the connecting stalk as umbilical veins
- The umbilical veins continue with cranial end of the primitive heart tube.

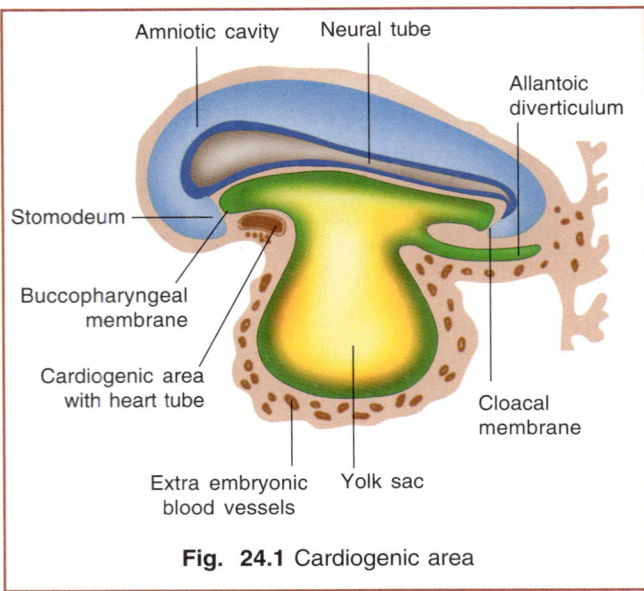

Fig. 24.1 Cardiogenic area

- Thus the caudal end of the primitive endothelial heart tube continues with dorsal aortae and cranial end with umbilical veins.

- The vitelline veins from the yolk sac and cardinal veins from the body wall also end at the cranial end of the primitive endothelial heart tubes (Fig. 24.2). These arrangements are seen before the head fold formation.

Effect of head fold formation on cardiogenic area

With the formation of head fold, there will be changes in the cardiogenic area (Fig. 24.3).

- The heart tubes lies dorsal to the pericardial cavity and the septum transversum lies still caudal to the cardiogenic area.

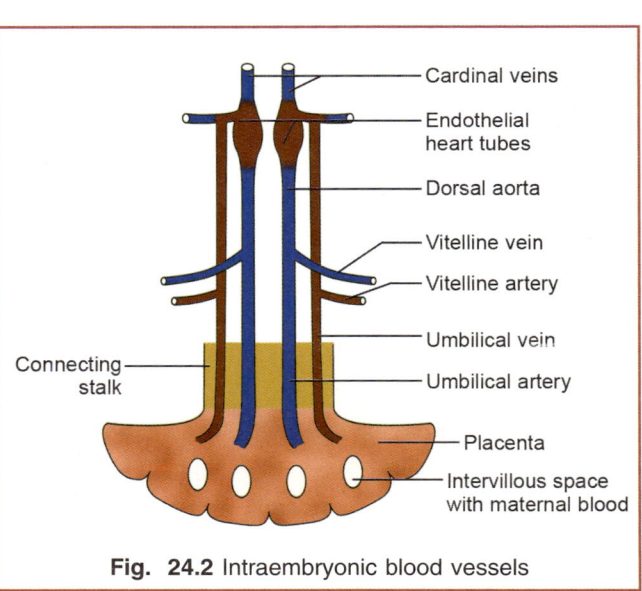

Fig. 24.2 Intraembryonic blood vessels

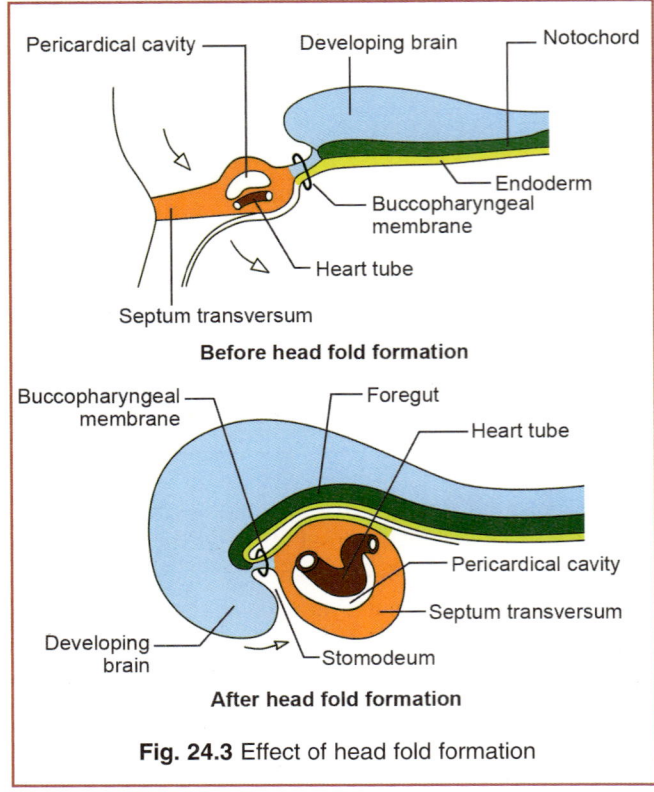

Before head fold formation

After head fold formation

Fig. 24.3 Effect of head fold formation

- Now cranial end of the heart tube continues with dorsal aortae and the caudal end of the heart tube receives-vitelline veins, umbilical veins and common cardinal veins

Definitive heart tube

- The two heart tubes fuse to form a single heart tube (primitive heart)

- The cranial end is arterial (with dorsal aortae) and caudal end is venous (where umbilical, vitelline and cardinal veins open)

  The primitive heart tube shows five dilatations with four constrictions. From cranial to caudal the dilatations are called (Fig. 24.4)

- Truncus arteriosus

- Bulbus cordis

- Primitive ventricle

- Primitive atrium

- Sinus venosus

  The heart tube grows faster than the pericardial cavity. As venous and arterial ends are fixed by pericardium, the heart tube necessarily becomes bent (in order to accommodate itself within the pericardial cavity). Thus a 'Bulboventricular loop' is formed between bulbus cordis and primitive ventricle. Internally these dilatations are separated by a 'Bulboventricular ridge' (Fig. 24.5).

SECTION 5

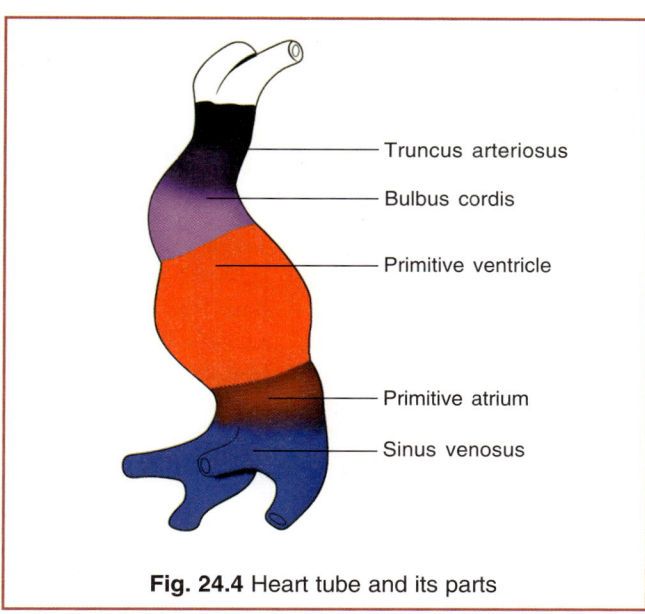

Fig. 24.4 Heart tube and its parts

The ventricle is projected ventrally and to the right side. At the caudal end of the heart tube, the primitive atrium undergoes transverse dilatation. The atrium and sinus venosus are gradually freed from septum transversum. Now the sinus venosus lies dorsal to the primitive atrium and the communication is called 'sinuatrial orifice'. The caudal end of the heart tube remains separate by means of right and left horns of sinus venosus. Each horn receives 3 sets of veins.

The cranial end of the heart tube is connected on either side with corresponding dorsal aorta by 'first arch artery'. The aortic sac is the cranial end of the truncus arteriosus which divides into right and left horns.

The atrium is sandwiched between foregut posteriorly and bulbus cordis anteriorly. The caudal part of the bulbus cordis is absorbed into the ventricle. The atrioventricular groove becomes narrow and its lumen is called 'atrioventricular canal'

Sinus venosus and its fate

The groove separating the sinus venosus and atrium deepens on the left side and is called Sinu atrial fold. Due to thickening of the sinu-atrial fold, the sinuatrial orifice is shifted to the right side. The vertically placed sinuatrial orifice is guarded by two valves projecting towards the atrium. Both these venous valves fuse above the orifice and form 'septum spurium' and below as sinus septum. The right horn of the sinus venosus enlarge and left horn remains small due to major changes in the veins opening into the sinus venosus (Figs 24.6A to C).

* The left horn of the sinus venosus forms the coronary sinus.

* The right horn and body of the sinus venosus is absorbed into the primitive atrium (smooth part of the right atrium)

Septal formation in atrioventricular canal

From the ventral and dorsal wall of the atrioventricular canal, proliferation of mesenchymal tissue forms ventral and dorsal endocardial cushions. At the end of 5th week of intra uterine life, these endocardial cushions fuse to form fused endocardial cushion (atrioventricular cushion or septum intermedium). Thus it divides the atrioventricular canal into right and left portions, so that the right half of the primitive atrium continues with right half of the ventricle and left half of the primitive atrium with left half of the ventricle (Fig. 24.7).

Common atrioventricular canal

This is due to failure in the formation of atrioventricular cushion. It is associated with patent foramen primum and also interventricular foramen. The septal cusp of

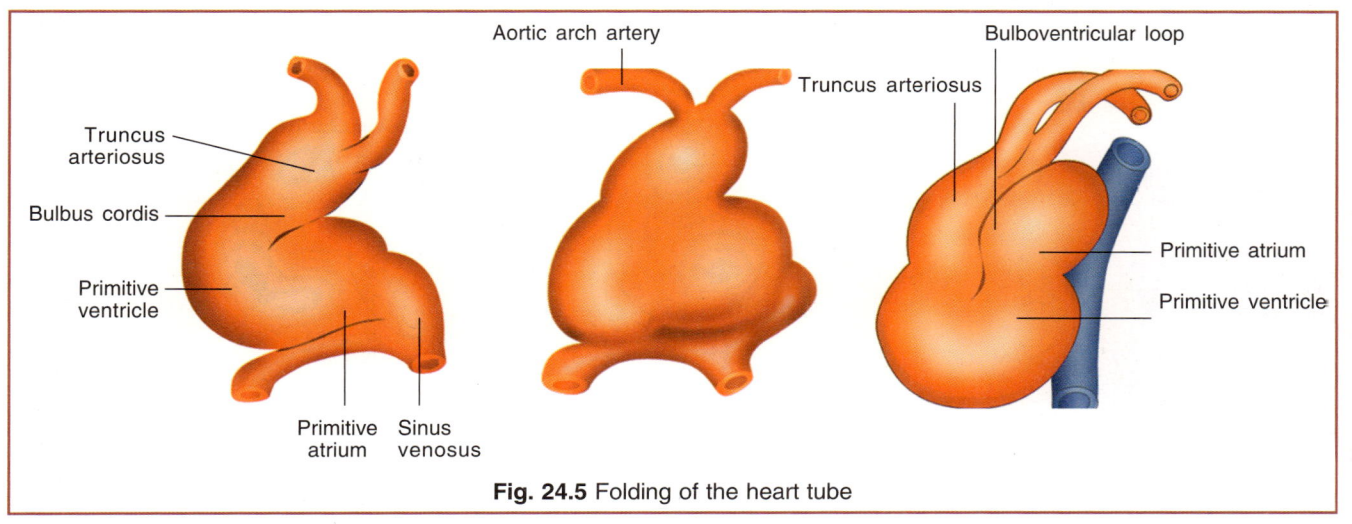

Fig. 24.5 Folding of the heart tube

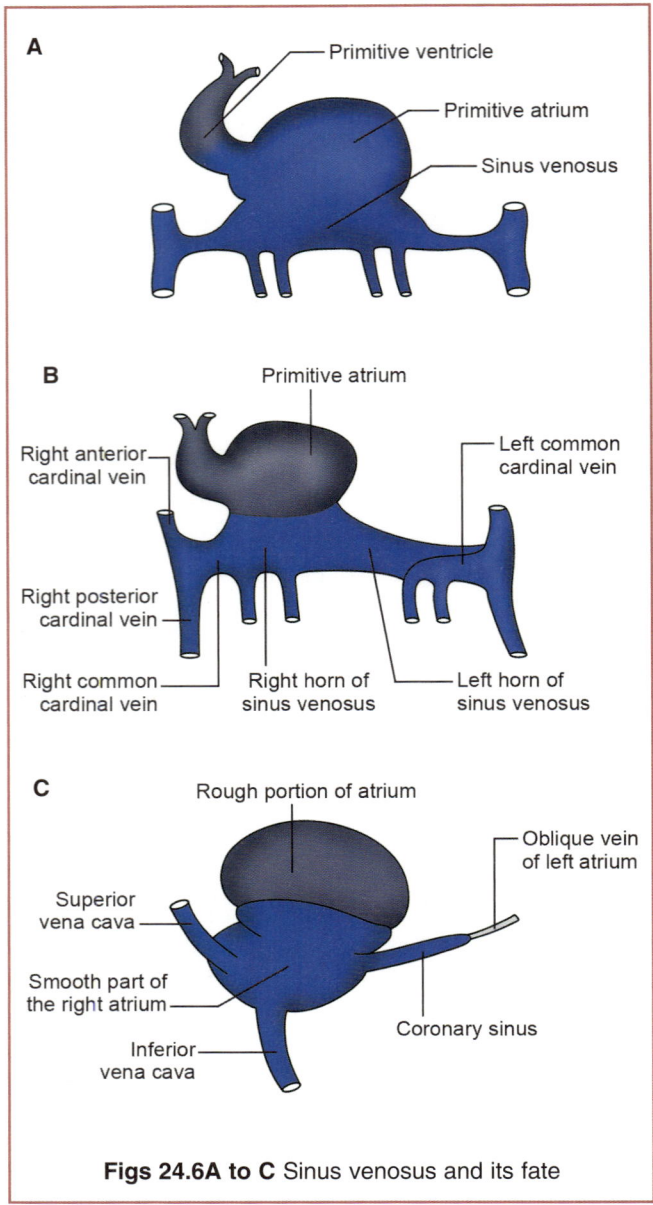

Figs 24.6A to C Sinus venosus and its fate

the tricuspid valve and ventral cusp of the mitral valve divides into ventral and dorsal parts, which fuse to form a common valve with 5 cusps at the single atrio-ventricular canal. This defect is often a feature of Down syndrome.

Tricuspid atresia

The right atrioventricular orifice is closed due to atresia of the tricuspid valve. The blood enters the right ventricle through patent foramen ovale and the interventricular foramen. This will cause enlargement of left ventricle and right ventricle remains small.

Development of interatrial septum

- **Septum primum** (about 32nd day) – A septum arises from the roof and dorsal wall of the primitive atrium (due to the pressure caused by bulbus cordis on primitive atrium) in the midline called septum primum.

- **Foramen primum** – The lower end of the septum primum is concave and growing towards atrioventricular cushion (septum intermedium). The gap between the lower end of the septum primum and atrioventricular cushion is called foramen primum (ostium primum).

- The opening of the single vein can be found in dorsal wall of the left atrium. This vein tap venous plexus in developing lungs

- The lower end of the septum primum grows down to fuse with atrioventricular cushions to obliterate the foramen primum (Figs 24.8A to C).

- Even before the obliteration of foramen primum, the cranial part of the septum primum shows perforation to establish new communication between the two atria.

- This communication is called '**foramen secundum**' (at the end of the 6th week of IUL). Hence septum primum

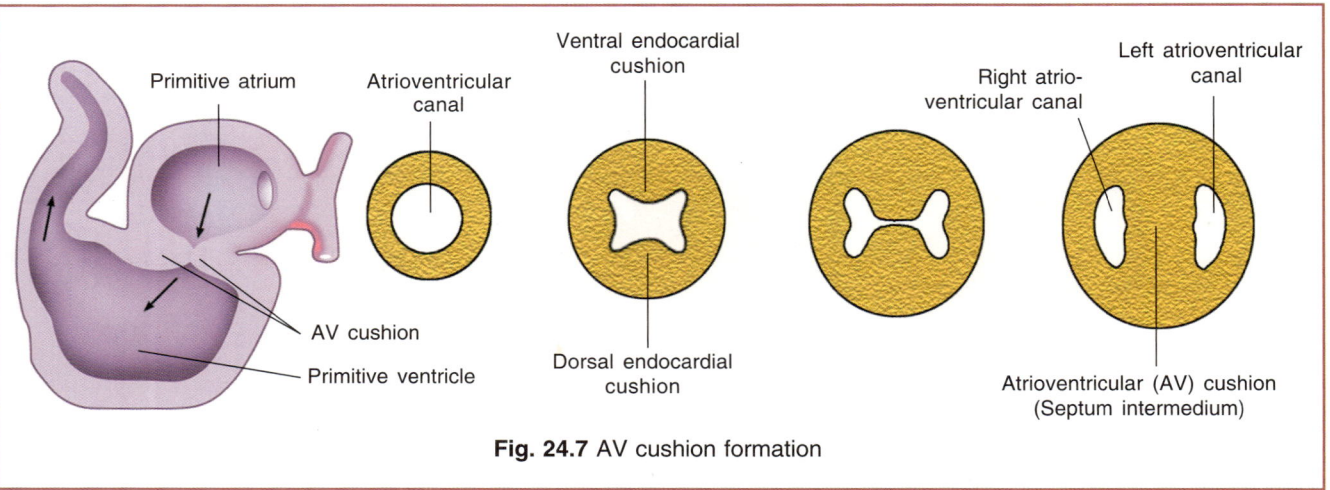

Fig. 24.7 AV cushion formation

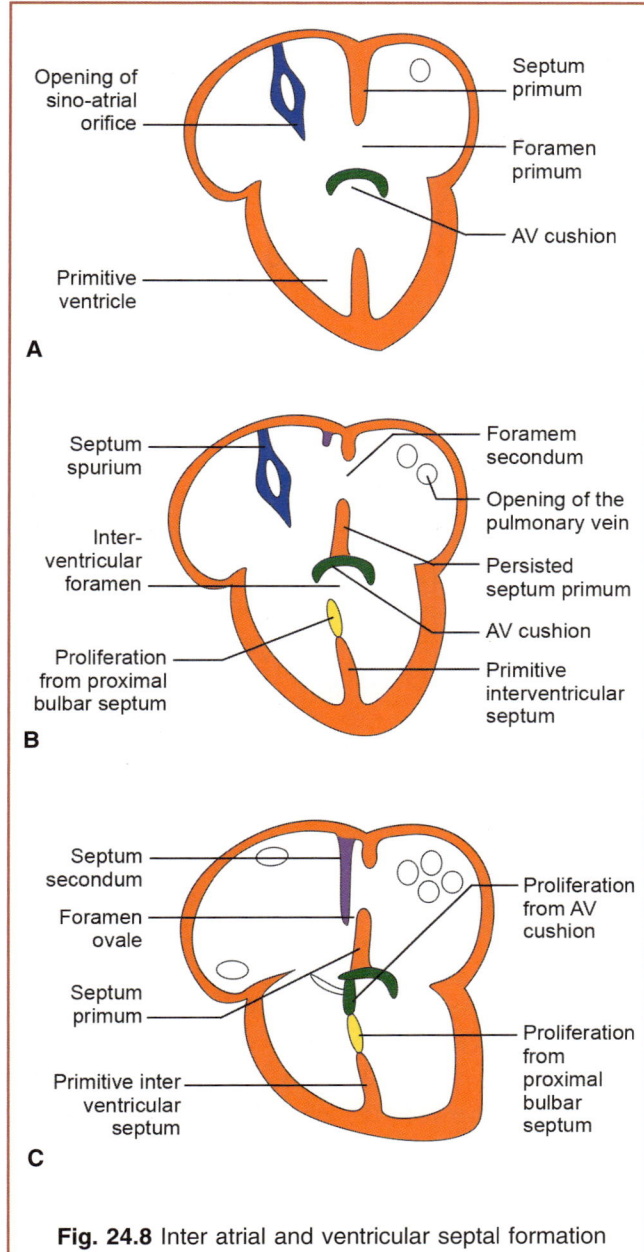

Fig. 24.8 Inter atrial and ventricular septal formation

fails to make a partition between, as it is necessary to have communication between two atria for transferring the oxygenated blood from inferior vena cava to the left atrium.

- **Septum secundum** (during 7th week): It grows downwards from the roof of the atrium to the right side of the septum primum.

- The lower end of septum secundum is free and has a thick edge called 'crescentic margin'

- The ventral end of this crescentic margin reaches the septum intermedium

- The lower part of the septum secundum overlaps the upper end of the septum primum (which is attached to the septum intermedium).

- The valvular space between the two (between lower part of septum secundum and lower remaining part of septum primum) is called '**foramen ovale**'

- The free margin of the septum secundum overrides the orifice of the IVC

- The IVC blood rich in oxygen concentration, bypass the right atrium by directly entering the left atrium through foramen ovale

- For this reason free margin of this septum is called 'crista dividens'

- The upper edge of the septum primum is called 'valve of foramen ovale'

- After birth, owing to the increased pressure in the left atrium (as pulmonary veins bring oxygenated blood to the left atrium), the valve of foramen ovale is pressed against the septum secundum.

- The functional closure takes at birth, but structurally it closes after few days

- About 20% cases, the foramen ovale persists in adult heart (but blood will not mix) and is called 'probe patency of foramen ovale'

- In adult heart septum primum forms a oval depression called 'fossa ovalis'

- The upper, anterior and posterior margins of the fossa is sharp and is called limbus fossa ovalis (annulus ovalis) formed by the lower edge of the septum secundum

Fate of the right and left venous valve

- Left venous valve: eventually fuses with septum secundum

- Right venous valve: It is pushed ventrally and to the right. By superior and inferior limbic bands it is divided into 3 parts and contributes to the formation of

1. Crista terminalis: portion above the superior limbic band along with septum spurium

2. Eustachian valve: portion between superior and inferior limbic band

3. Valve of the coronary sinus: portion below the inferior limbic band

(Look at these structures inter-relations in adult heart)

Development of the left atrium

- During foetal life, left atrium receives one pulmonary vein. This pulmonary vein divides into two branches

S E C T I O N   5

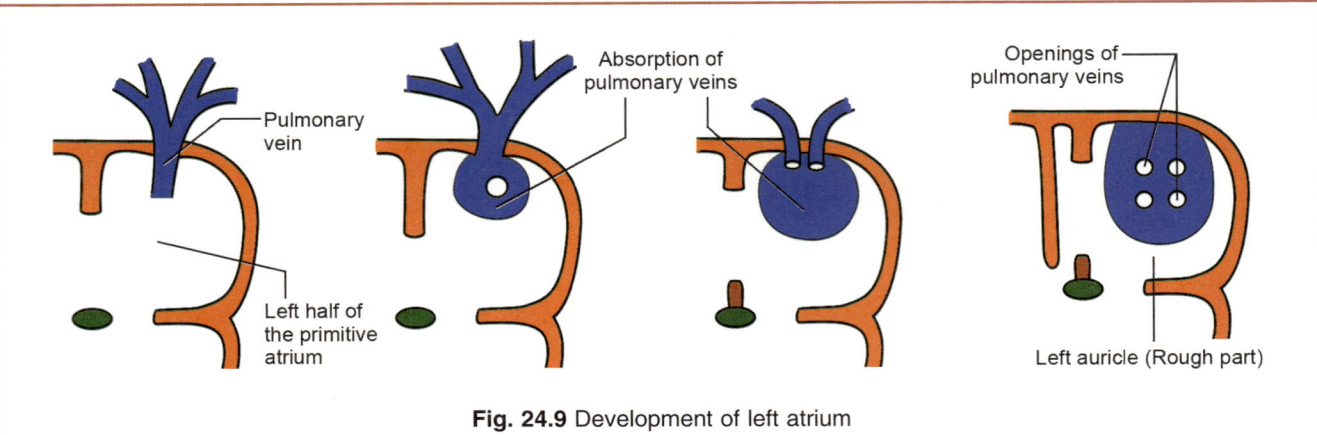

Fig. 24.9 Development of left atrium

for right and left lungs (each of them again divided into two).

- All the four pulmonary veins are absorbed into the posterior wall of the left atrium forming the major smooth part of the left atrium (Fig. 24.9)

- Left auricle (which is rough inside) is developed from left half of the primitive atrium

Summary of the development of the right atrium

1. Posterior smooth part of the right atrium - Absorbed part of the body and right horn of the sinus venosus

2. Anterior rough wall of the right atrium - Right portion of the primitive atrium

3. Interatrial septum – fossa ovalis from septum primum and remaining part of the interatrial septum including limbus fossa ovalis by septum secundum

4. Crista terminalis, valve of IVC and Valve of the coronary sinus by right venous valve

In dextrocardia the heart rotates to the right so that its apex is located in the right 5th intercostal space.

Atrial septal defects (ASD's)

There are 3 types of ASD resulting in left to right shunt

1. **The ostium secundum defect** is the most common congenital defect of the heart.

   - The persistence of foramen secundum is due to excessive resorption of the septum primum or due to failure of development of septum secundum (Fig. 24.10)

   - The shunting of the blood is usually from left to right, hence does not cause cyanosis (usually the right to left shunt causes cyanosis but not left to right (until development of pulmonary

hypertension), however severe pulmonary stenosis with ASD can cause cyanosis).

2. **The ostium primum defect** is due to either failure of septum primum to fuse with endocardial cushions (av cushions) or defect in the endocardial cushions (Fig. 24.11)

3. **Patent foramen ovale:** Failure of septum primum and septum secundum to fuse after birth. It may not have any clinical manifestation and there will not be mixing of blood.

In ASD there is increased load on the right side of the heart leading to progressive enlargement of right atrium, right ventricle and the pulmonary trunk

The disease manifests as fatigue and breathlessness on exertion in the 3rd or 4th decade of life and thereafter Recently, GATA4 and NKX2.5 were reported as the disease genes of atrial septal defect (ASD) but the relationship between the locations of their mutations and phenotypes is not clear.

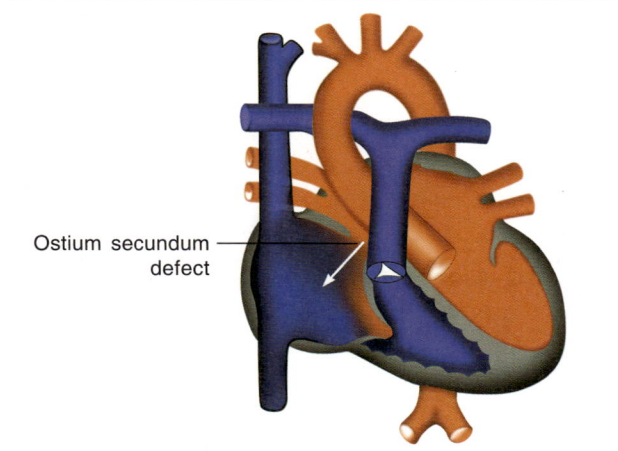

Fig. 24.10 Atrial septal defect—ostium secundum defect

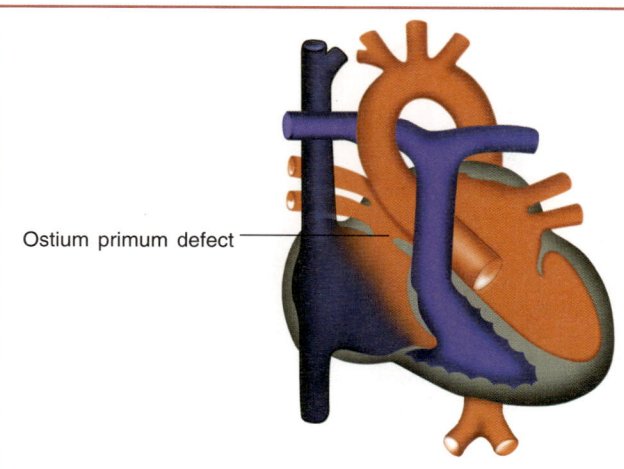

Ostium primum defect

Fig. 24.11 Atrial septal defect—ostium primum defect

Prenatal closure of foramen ovale

Though this is a rare anomaly, any early closure of foramen ovale during prenatal life can cause enlargement of right atrium. The affected baby usually dies after birth. Complete failure of partition of primitive atrium is a rare anomaly and is called Bi-ventricular mono-atrial heart.

CASE -1

A 2-year-old boy was brought to the paediatric clinic by his mother who was concerned about the child's respiratory infection. During the physical examination, a heart murmur was detected. Antibiotics were prescribed for the infection and the child was referred to a pediatric cardiologist.

The cardiologist ordered an ECG and echocardiography. The echocardiogram revealed' a dilated right atrium and ventricle consistent with an ostium secundum atrial septal defect. The defect was surgically closed.

a. What are the normal events in the septation of the primitive atrium?

b. List the various types of atrial septal defect?

Development of the ventricles and their partition

The bulbus cordis gets absorbed into the primitive ventricle forming a bulbo-ventricular cavity. This bulbo-ventricular cavity has a lower dilated portion which communicates with atria and upper conical part which communicate with truncus arteriosus.

The lower dilated part of the bulbo-ventricular cavity gives rise to rough inflowing part of the adult ventricle while the upper conical part forms smooth out flowing

part of the adult ventricle (infundibulum of right ventricle and aortic vestibule in the left ventricle)

Formation of interventricular septum

The ventricular septation takes place at almost same time as atrial septal formation (Fig. 24.12).

- Primitive Interventricular septum - It grows upwards from the floor of the bulbo-ventricular cavity, dividing the dilated part of the bulbo-ventricular cavity into right and left portions (not the upper conical part, which continues with truncus arteriosus). This growth of interventricular septum is a passive process due to dilatation of bulboventricular cavity on each side of the partition

- The upper margin of this septum is concave and free. The posterior portion of this free margin fuses with right edge of the atrio-ventricular cushion (endocardial cushion/septum intermedium) and anterior portion of this free margin fuses with left edge of the atrioventricular cushion.

- The gap between the right and left ventricle above the free margin of the interventricular septum is called 'interventricular foramen'

- This portion is closed by proliferation of tissues from two other sources and in adult heart, this portion forms 'membranous part of the interventricular septum'

- The right and left bulbar ridges appear in the proximal part of the bulbus cordis, fuse with each other to form **proximal bulbar septum**. This proximal bulbar septum grows downwards towards the interventricular septum partially closing interventricular foramen.

- The remaining portion of this foramen is closed by proliferation of tissue from atrioventricular cushions (endocardial cushions/septum intermedium).

- Thus the membranous part of the interventricular septum has an anterior part separating right and left ventricles (interventricular), which is developed from proliferation of tissue from **proximal bulbar septum** and a posterior part which separates right atrium from the left ventricle (atrioventricular), which is developed from proliferation from **AV cushion** (from right edge of the septum intermedium).

Summary of the development of the ventricles

Right ventricle

1. Rough inflowing part is by right part of the primitive ventricle and proximal dilated part of the bulbo-ventricular cavity

SECTION 5

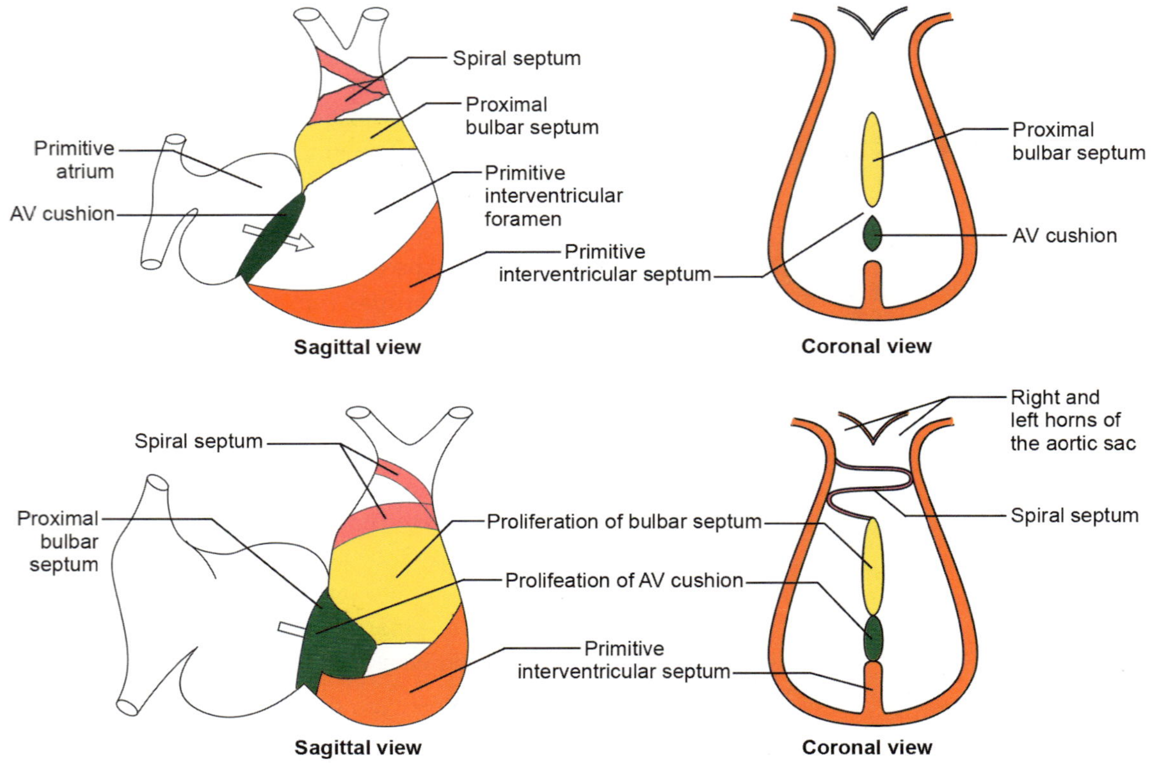

Fig. 24.12 Development of interventricular septum

2. The smooth out flowing part (infundibulum) is by distal conical part of the bulbo-ventricular cavity

Left ventricle

1. Rough inflowing part is by left part of the primitive ventricle

2. The smooth out flowing part (aortic vestibule) is by distal conical part of the bulbo-ventricular cavity

Interventricular septum

1. Lower rough part by primitive interventricular septum

2. Upper membranous part by two sources

   • Anterior inferior part by proliferation of tissue by proximal bulbar septum

   • Posterior superior part by proliferation of tissue by endocardial cushion (septum intermedium)

Ventricular septal defects (VSDs)

Persistent interventricular foramen:
This defect is usually associated with other cardiac anomalies, but it is also possible to have a defect in the membranous part alone. This defect could be due to failure in the contribution from any one or two sources (out of three) involved in interventricular septum. The

blood flow from left to right and then into pulmonary artery. Hence it causes enlargement of right ventricle, pulmonary trunk and pulmonary artery (Fig. 24.13).

Truncus arteriosus and its fate

The upper part of the truncus arteriosus dilates to form aortic sac, which further divides into right and left horns. Each horn of the aortic sac is connected to the corresponding dorsal aortae by six pairs of aortic arch arteries.

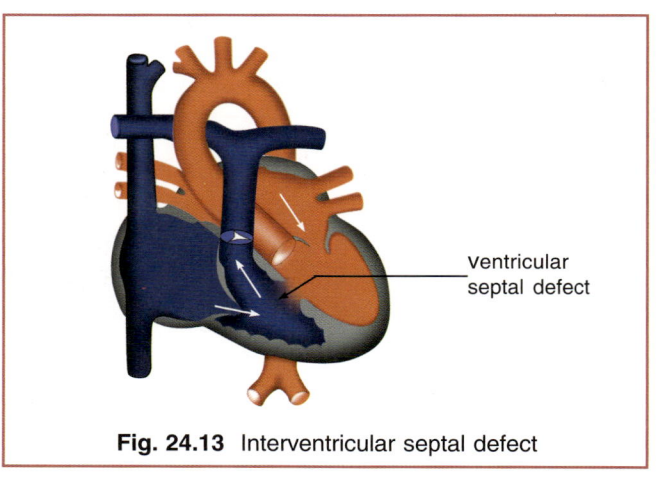

Fig. 24.13 Interventricular septal defect

The truncus arteriosus is internally divided by a spiral-shaped aorticopulmonary septum into two vessels –the ascending aorta and pulmonary trunk (Fig. 24.14).

The upper end of the aorticopulmonary spiral septum fuses with the dorsal wall of the aortic sac between fifth and sixth pairs of the aortic arch arteries.

This will ensure that the pulmonary trunk continues with sixth arch arteries and ascending aorta with upper five pair of aortic arch arteries.

We studied that proximal bulbar septum is formed at the proximal end of the bulbus cordis and contribute to the formation of membranous part of the interventricular septum. Now at the junction of bulbus cordis and truncus arteriosus, a distal bulbar septum is formed. The portion in front of this distal bulbar septum is pulmonary orifice and behind is aortic orifice.

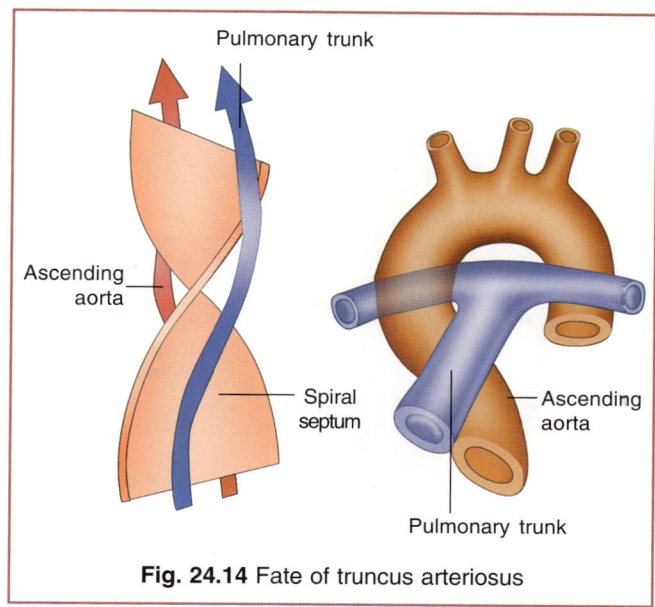

Fig. 24.14 Fate of truncus arteriosus

Pulmonary and aortic valve

At this time, there are four endocardial cushions growing towards the lumen and are named ventral, dorsal, right and left. The distal bulbar septum formed at this site will divide right and left cushions into ventral and dorsal cusps. Thus both pulmonary and aortic orifice are guarded by semilunar valves of 3 cusps (Fig. 24.15)

The lower end of the aorticopulmonary septum continues with distal bulbar septum, which intern continues with proximal bulbar septum. The fusion ensures that the pulmonary orifice is connected to right ventricle and aortic orifice with left ventricle.

Persistent (patent) truncus arteriosus

The truncus arteriosus fails to divide due to defective aorticopulmonary septum or its agenesis. The pulmonary artery arises some distance above the origin of the undivided truncus. It is always accompanied by a defective interventricular septum. The undivided truncus thus overrides both ventricles and receives blood from both sides

Transposition of great vessels (ascending aorta and pulmonary trunk)

The ascending aorta arises from right ventricle and pulmonary trunk from left ventricle. This is due to reverse attachment of lower end of aorticopulmonary septum (Fig. 24.16).

This anomaly can be associated with patent interventricular foramen and is called **Taussig-Bing syndrome.**

Fallot's tetralogy

It is a combination of 4 defects

1. Ventricular septal defect (VSD)

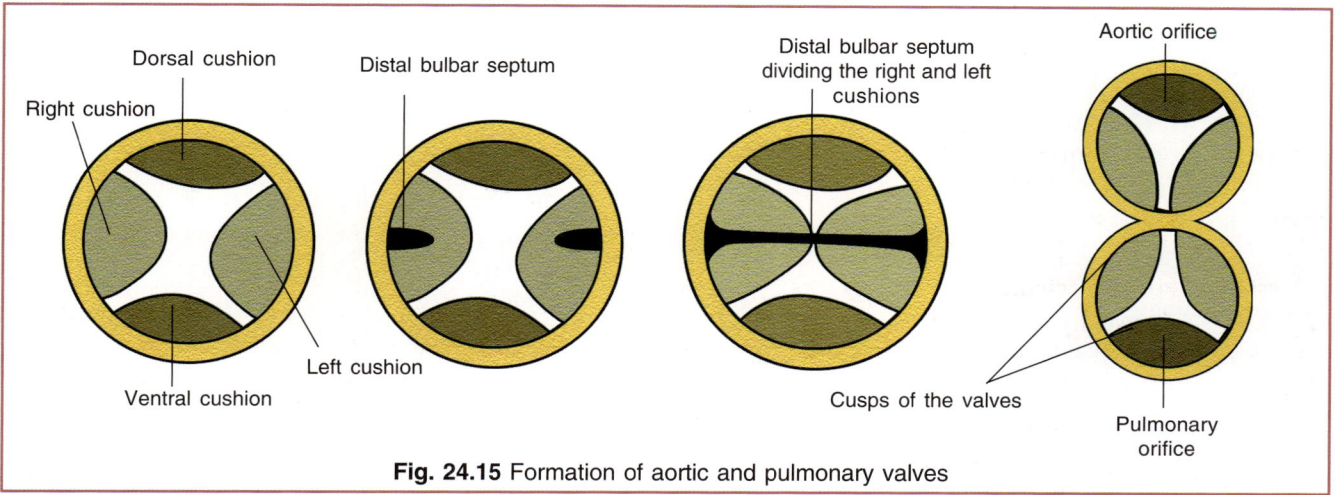

Fig. 24.15 Formation of aortic and pulmonary valves

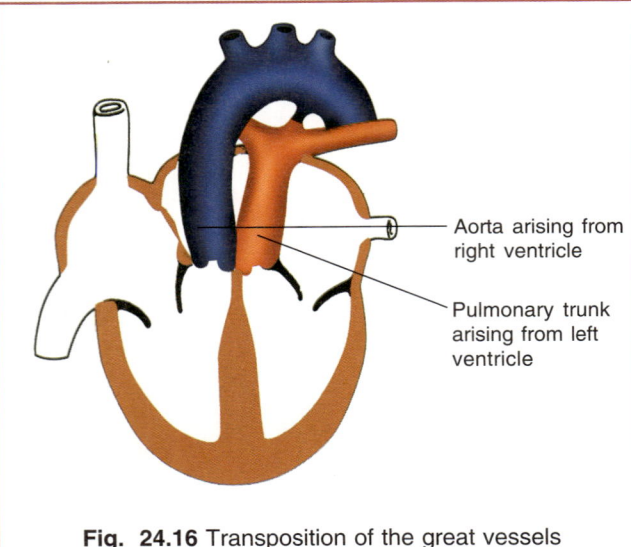

Fig. 24.16 Transposition of the great vessels

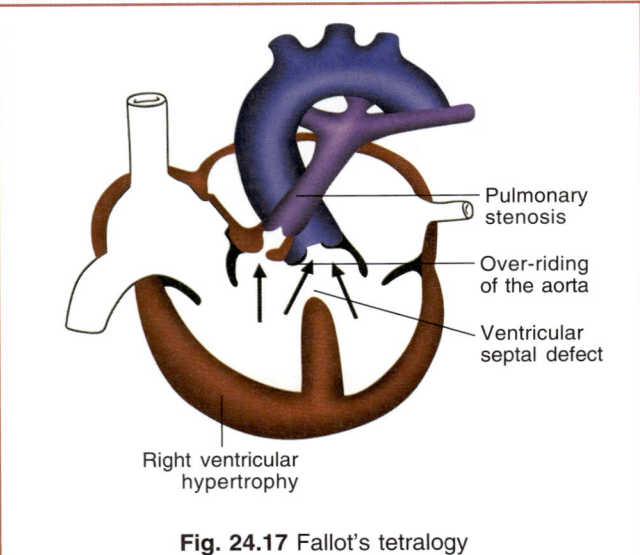

Fig. 24.17 Fallot's tetralogy

2. Over-riding of aorta (ascending aorta having connection to both ventricles)

3. Pulmonary stenosis

4. Right ventricular hypertrophy (Fig. 24.17)

The effects of Fallot's tetralogy are

- The right chambers of the heart enlarge (right ventricular hypertrophy)

- The pulmonary circulation does not receive much blood due to pulmonary stenosis

- The child may have cyanotic spells especially during crying

- There is shortness of breath or dyspnea on exertion, which is relieved by assuming squatting position for few minutes (squatting blocks the venous return and increases the peripheral resistance of arteries so that more blood reaches the lungs

- The growth of the child is retarded due to hypoxia

Acyanotic Heart Disease

is a broad term for any congenital heart defect in which all of the blood returning to the right side of the heart passes through the lungs and pulmonary vasculature in the normal fashion.

- Patent ductus arteriosus (PDA)
- Coarctation of the aorta
- Atrial septal defect (ASD)
- Ventricular septal defect (VSD)
- Aortic stenosis (AS)
- Pulmonary stenosis (PS)

In **cyanotic defects**, a shunt bypasses the lungs and delivers venous (deoxygenated) blood from the right side of the heart into the arterial circulation.

- Tetralogy of Fallot
- Transposition of the great vessels
- Persistent truncus arteriosus

Cardiac shunt

Cardiac shunt is when the blood flow follows a pattern in the heart that deviates from the normal circuit of the circulatory system. It may be described as **right-left, left-to-right or bidirectional**, or as systemic-to-pulmonary or pulmonary-to-systemic.

The direction may be controlled by left and/or right heart pressure, a biological or artificial heart valve or both. The presence of a shunt may also affect left and/or right heart pressure either beneficially or detrimentally.

1. A **left-to-right shunt** is when blood from the left side of the heart goes to the right side of the heart. This can occur either through a hole in the ventricular or atrial septum that divides the left and the right heart or through a hole in the walls of the arteries leaving the heart, called great vessels. Left-to-right shunts occur when the systolic blood pressure in the left side of the heart is higher than the right side of the heart.

   - Patent ductus arteriosus (PDA)
   - Atrial septal defect (ASD)
   - Ventricular septal defect (VSD)
   - Persistent truncus arteriosus

Atrial septal defects and Patent ductus arteriosus are not clinically apparent during childhood. Ventricular septal defects are the most common cardiac congenital defects, but they do not present with early cyanosis

2. A **right-to-left shunt** is a cardiac shunt which allows, or is designed to cause, blood to flow from the right side of the heart to the left side of the heart.
   - Tetralogy of Fallot

3. **No shunt**
   - Coarctation of the aorta
   - Aortic stenosis (AS)
   - Pulmonary stenosis (PS)
   - Transposition of the great vessels

DEVELOPMENT OF AORTIC ARCH ARTERIES

The primitive endothelial heart tubes continue cranially with **ventral aortae**, which is placed ventral to the foregut. Each ventral aorta is connected with corresponding **dorsal aorta** (which are placed dorsal to the foregut) through **first aortic arch artery** which traverses first branchial arch.

The first arch artery formed is connected ventrally to right or left horn of the aortic sac and dorsally to the dorsal aorta. The two dorsal aortae fuse to form single aorta at the level of fourth thoracic segment and extend downwards up to fourth lumbar segment.

Successively 6 arch arteries are formed within the pharyngeal arches, each of them are connected ventrally to respective aortic sac and dorsally to dorsal aorta (Figs 24.18 to 24.20)

Fate of aortic arch arteries
- **First arch artery:**
  Mostly disappears except partly for maxillary artery.

- **Second arch:**
  Mostly regresses except dorsal part for the stapedial artery.

- **Fifth arch artery** Disappears entirely
  The portion of the dorsal aorta, between the attachment of the 3rd and 4th arch artery (ductus caroticus) disappears on both sides. The aortic sac is now connected only with 3rd, 4th and 6th arch arteries. The 3rd and 4th arch artery opens into ventral part and 6th arch artery into the dorsal part of the aortic sac. The truncus arteriosus is divided by the spiral shaped aortico pulmonary septum into ascending aorta and pulmonary trunk. The blood from the pulmonary trunk passes only into the 6th arch artery, while that from the ascending aorta passes into the 3rd and 4th arch artery.

- The portion of the right dorsal aorta, between the attachment of 4th arch artery and the point of fusion between the 2 dorsal aortae disappears.

- Each 6th arch artery gives off an artery to the developing lung bud.

- On right side, portion of the 6th arch artery between this bud and the dorsal aorta disappears

- On the left side it remains patent and forms the **ductus arteriosus**

- These 6th arch artery (ventral part) forms **pulmonary artery**

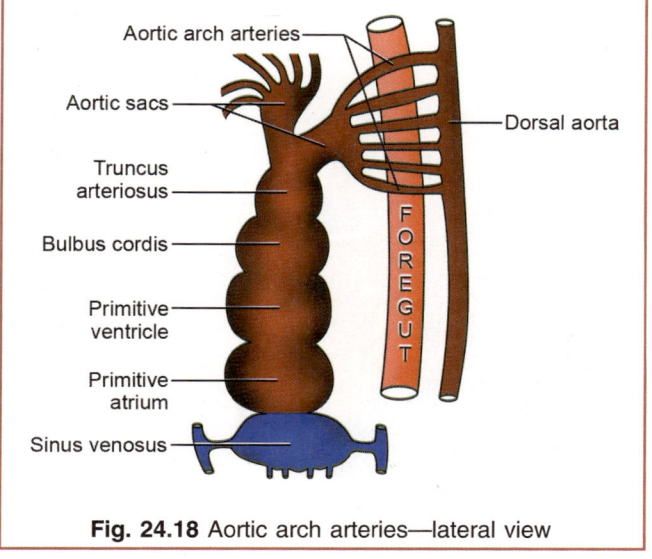

Fig. 24.18 Aortic arch arteries—lateral view

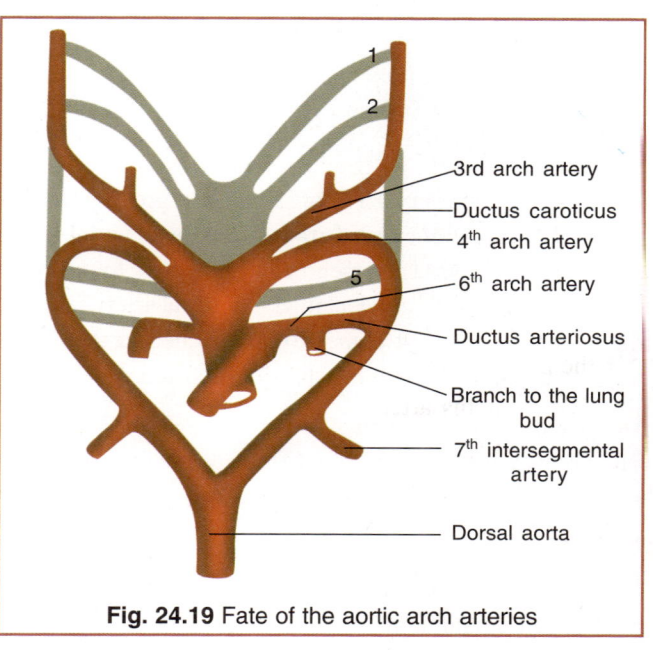

Fig. 24.19 Fate of the aortic arch arteries

S E C T I O N   5

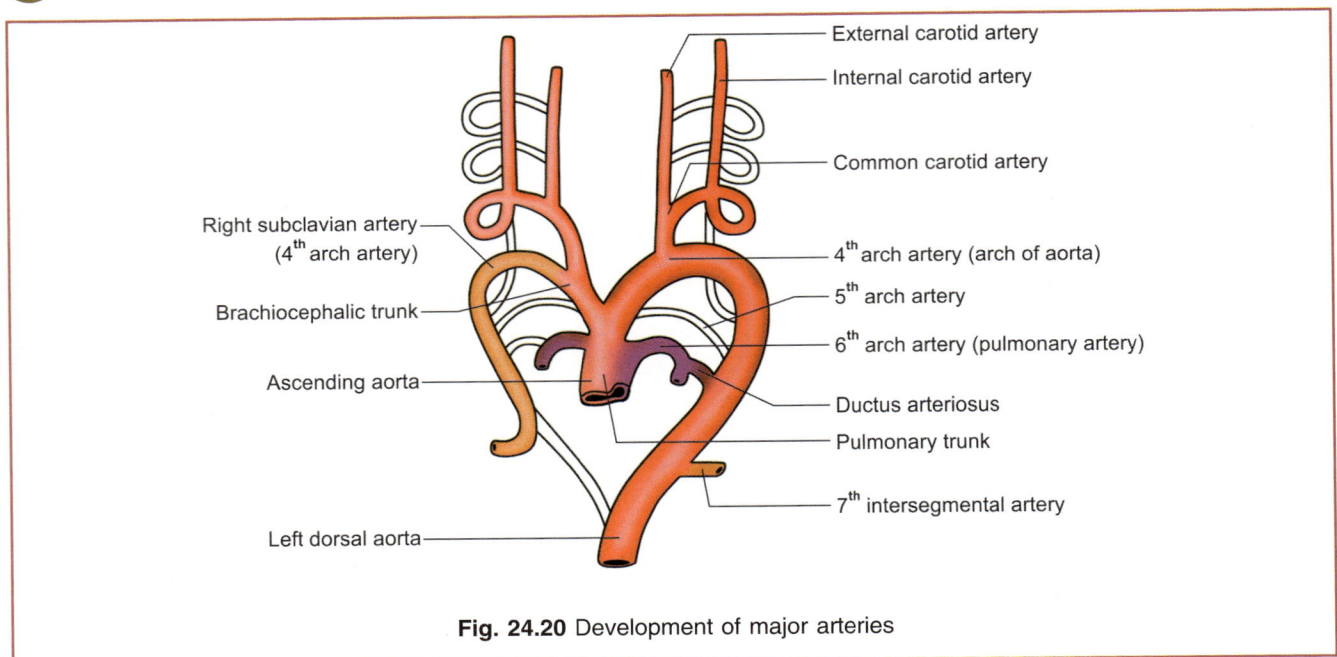

Fig. 24.20 Development of major arteries

- The ductus arteriosus carries most of the blood from the right ventricle to the dorsal aorta. After birth it is obliterated to form **ligamentum arteriosum**

Patent Ductus Arteriosus (PDA)

When the ductus arteriosus remains patent, blood from the aorta flushes through the ductus into the pulmonary artery.

- Overloading of pulmonary circulation results in enlargement of left atrium, left ventricle and ascending aorta.
- PDA is commonly seen in rubella syndrome, which occurs in children whose mother had German measles during pregnancy.
- PDA is more common in females than in males and in population living in high altitudes (Fig. 24.21).

Each 3rd arch artery gives off a bud that grows cranially to form the *external carotid* artery. The dorsal aortae gives off a series of lateral intersegmental branches to the body wall, of which the 7th cervical intersegmental artery supplies the upper limb bud. It comes to be attached to the dorsal aorta near the attachment of the 4th arch artery

Development of Arch of Aorta

The arch of aorta is developed from following sources.

- The ventral part of the aortic sac (Fig. 24.22)
- Its left horn
- The left 4th arch artery
- The left dorsal aorta

Double aortic arches

Due to persistence of the right dorsal aorta distal to the origin of the 7th cervical intersegmental artery. Double aortic arch embraces the trachea and oesophagus (Fig. 24.23).

Right aortic arch

Right dorsal aorta persists below the 7th cervical intersegmental artery and the corresponding portion of the left dorsal aorta disappears

Coarctation of aorta

It is the narrowing of the lumen of the arch of aorta distal to the origin of left subclavian artery. The narrowing is due to abnormality in the tunica media

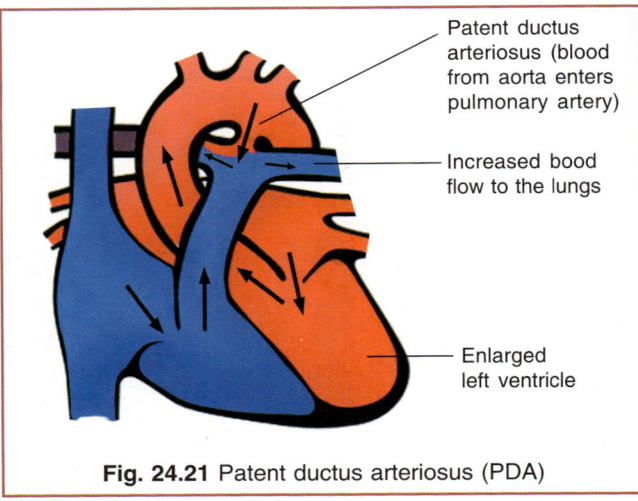

Fig. 24.21 Patent ductus arteriosus (PDA)

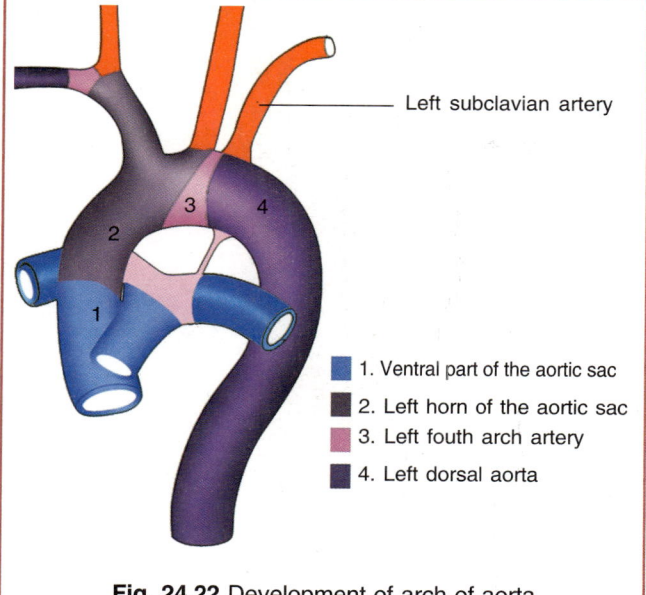

Left subclavian artery

1. Ventral part of the aortic sac
2. Left horn of the aortic sac
3. Left fouth arch artery
4. Left dorsal aorta

Fig. 24.22 Development of arch of aorta

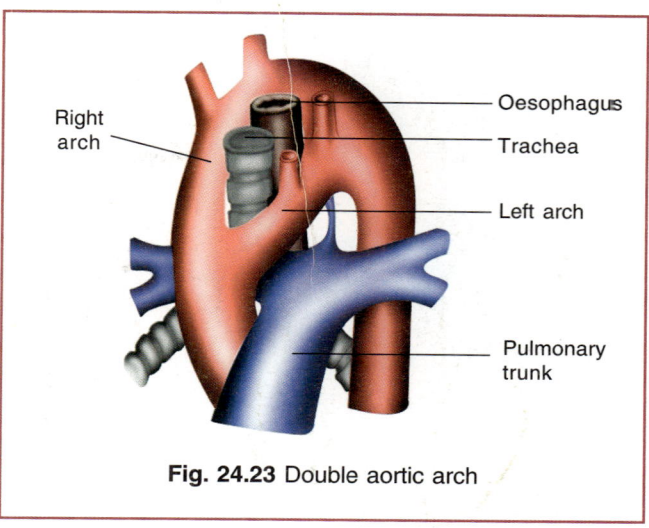

Right arch

Oesophagus

Trachea

Left arch

Pulmonary trunk

Fig. 24.23 Double aortic arch

followed by proliferation of tunica intima. There are 2 types of aortic coarctation – preductal and postductal

1. **Preductal coarctation**

Narrowing occurs proximal to the attachment of the ductus arteriosus. In this case the ductus arteriosus lumen is patent. In this case the descending thoracic aorta receives deoxygenated blood through patent ductus arteriosus (Fig. 24.24)

2. **Postductal coarctation**

Narrowing occurs distal to the attachment of the ductus arteriosus. The ductus arteriosus is usually obliterated. This variety of coarctation is more common and the descending thoracic aorta is filled by a collateral circulation. The blood from the subclavian artery enters the internal thoracic artery and its branches – anterior intercostal arteries (Fig. 24.25). They anastomose with posterior intercostal arteries (reversal blood flow) and the blood enters the thoracic aorta. This can cause dilatation of posterior intercostal arteries, consequently erosion of the lower border of the ribs. This is called 'notching of the ribs' which can be visualized by an X-ray picture (Fig. 24.26). This condition is characterized by reduced blood pressure in the lower limb (femoral) and elevated blood pressure in the upper limb (radial).

CASE - 2

A twenty-three-year-old female visits the hospital with complaints of being easily tired, pain in her lower

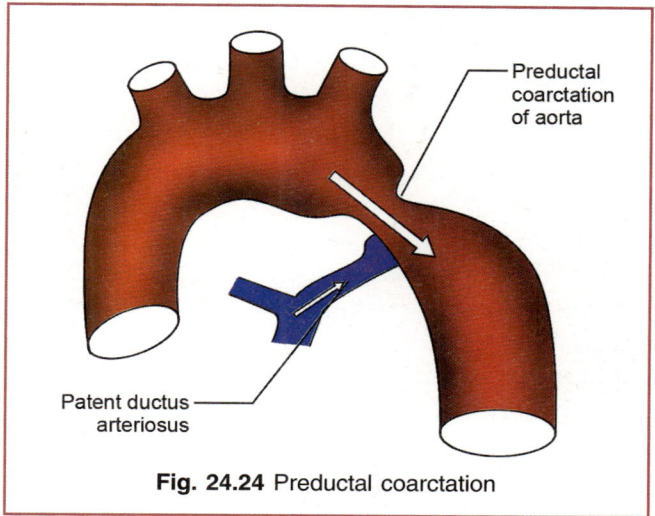

Preductal coarctation of aorta

Patent ductus arteriosus

Fig. 24.24 Preductal coarctation

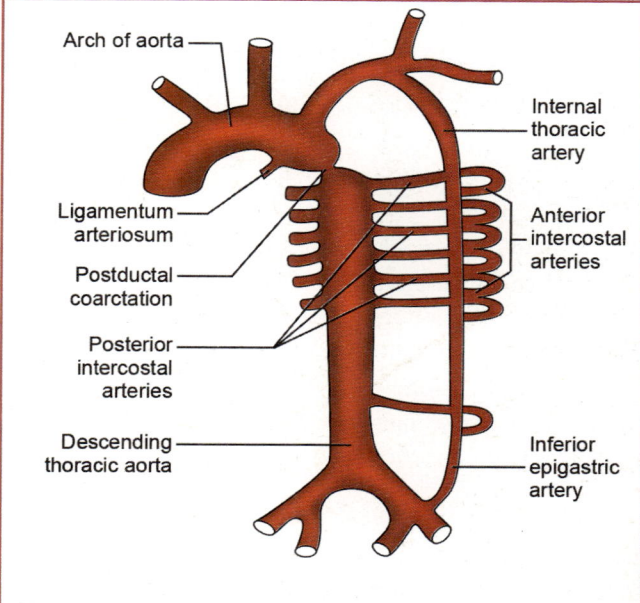

Arch of aorta

Internal thoracic artery

Ligamentum arteriosum

Anterior intercostal arteries

Postductal coarctation

Posterior intercostal arteries

Descending thoracic aorta

Inferior epigastric artery

Fig. 24.25 Postductal coarctation and collateral circulation

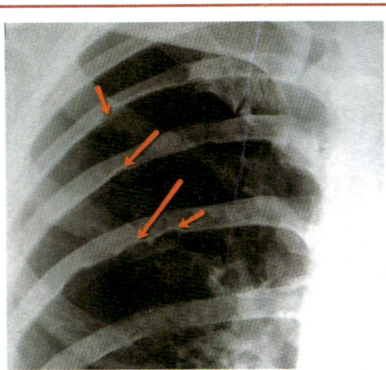

Fig. 24.26 Radiograph showing notching of the ribs in coarctation of aorta

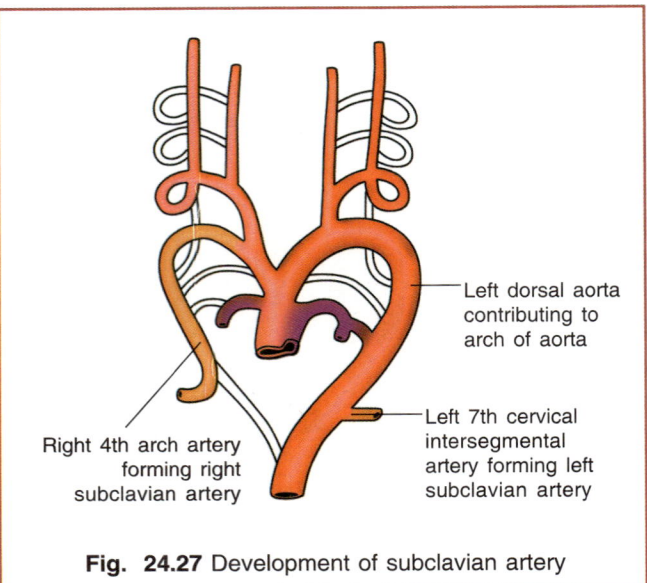

Right 4th arch artery forming right subclavian artery

Left dorsal aorta contributing to arch of aorta

Left 7th cervical intersegmental artery forming left subclavian artery

Fig. 24.27 Development of subclavian artery

extremities with weakness and cold feet, an inability to tolerate vigorous exercise, frequent headaches, and epistaxis (nosebleed). The patient reports these are not new symptoms, but have occurred over a number of years and have recently increased in their incidence.

The physical examination revealed a cool lower extremities with an absence of dorsalis pedis pulses and diminished femoral pulses, the blood pressure in the upper extremities is elevated (190/100), while the blood pressure in the lower extremities is 60/20; a systolic murmur is heard over the 5th left intercostal space which radiates to the interscapular region.

A chest X-ray is performed and significant rib notching is noted along with a visible dilation of the aorta in the region of the aortic knob. The patient is diagnosed with coarctation of the aorta based on physical exam and findings.

a. What is this lesion?
b. Is there a difference in the findings of such a lesion as an adult or as a child?
c. What were the diagnostic clinical features of the case?
d. What single diagnostic finding was found on the chest X-ray?
e. Can you explain why a postductal (inferior) lesion is more compatible with long term survival versus a preductal lesion?
f. What are the treatment options for a patient with this type of lesion?
g. What surgical complications would cause the greatest amount of concern?

Development of brachiocephalic trunk

The right horn of the aortic sac (which is connected with 3rd and 4th aortic arch arteries) forms the brachiocephalic trunk.

Development of descending aorta

The left dorsal aorta below the attachment of the 4th arch artery

Development of subclavian artery

• On *right side* by right 4th arch artery, part of the right dorsal aortae and right 7th cervical intersegmental artery (Fig. 24.27)
• On *left side* entirely by left 7th cervical intersegmental artery

Relation between recurrent laryngeal nerve and 6th arch artery

Initially each recurrent laryngeal nerve winds around the 6th arch artery and then ascends to the larynx. With the degeneration of right 6th arch artery, the right recurrent laryngeal nerve winds around the right 4th artery, which forms the proximal part of the right subclavian artery. Remember 5th arch artery disappears early. On the left side the dorsal part of the 6th artery persists as ductus arteriosus and the left recurrent laryngeal nerve winds around it. The ductus arteriosus forms the ligamentum arteriosum in the adult.

Abnormal origin of the right subclavian artery
• Sometimes the right subclavian artery arises from the junction of the arch of aorta and descending aorta, and courses upwards and to the right behind the trachea and oesophagus (Fig. 24.28).
• This is due to degeneration of the right 4th arch artery, so that the right 7th intersegmental artery and right dorsal aorta caudal to it are continued as right subclavian artery

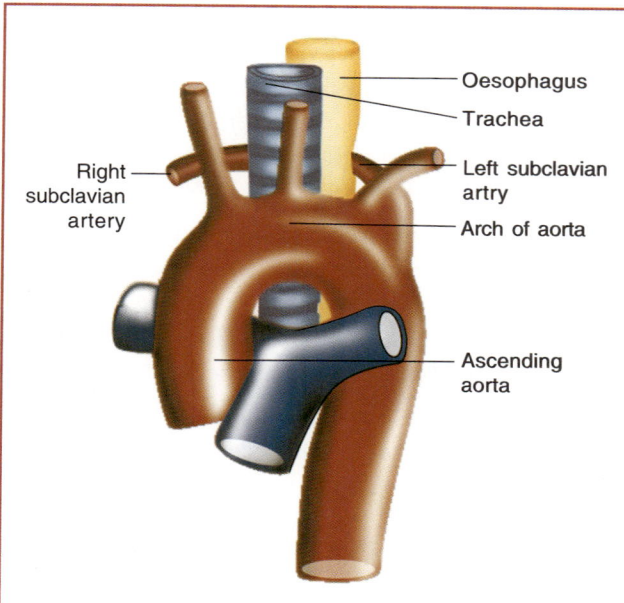

Fig. 24.28 Abnormal origin of the right subclavian artery

- The ventral part of the 3rd arch artery persists as **common carotid artery**
- The dorsal part of the 3rd arch artery and dorsal aorta cephalic to the ductus caroticus forms **internal carotid artery**

Summary of the fate of aortic arch arteries

- **First arch:** Mostly disappears except partly for maxillary artery.
- **Second arch:** Mostly regresses except dorsal parts or the stapedial artery.
- **Third arch:** Ventral part forms common carotid artery dorsal part forms stem of internal carotid artery.
- **Fourth arch:** Right side it forms proximal part of right subclavian artery left side it persists as part of arch of aorta.
- **Fifth arch:** Disappears entirely.
- **Sixth arch:** On right side the ventral part persists as right pulmonary artery dorsal part disappears. On the left side the ventral part forms the left pulmonary artery and the dorsal part persist as ductus arteriosus in fetal life and ligamentum arteriosum after birth.

DEVELOPMENT OF MAJOR VEINS

Development of the superior vena cava

The anterior cardinal vein brings blood from head end of the embryo while posterior cardinal vein from caudal end. The anterior and posterior cardinal veins of the two sides join to form **common cardinal vein (duct of Cuvier)** on each side and opens into corresponding horns of the sinus venosus. The venous blood from the upper limb will drain into anterior cardinal vein through subclavian vein (Fig. 24.29).

Now the two anterior cardinal veins are inter-connected by a transverse anastomosis. This communication is established proximal to the junction of anterior cardinal vein with subclavian vein. The part of the left cardinal vein caudal to this anastomosis regresses and also major part of the left common cardinal vein (except for its caudal end where it opens into left horn of the sinus venosus). The body and left horn of the sinus venosus forms **coronary**

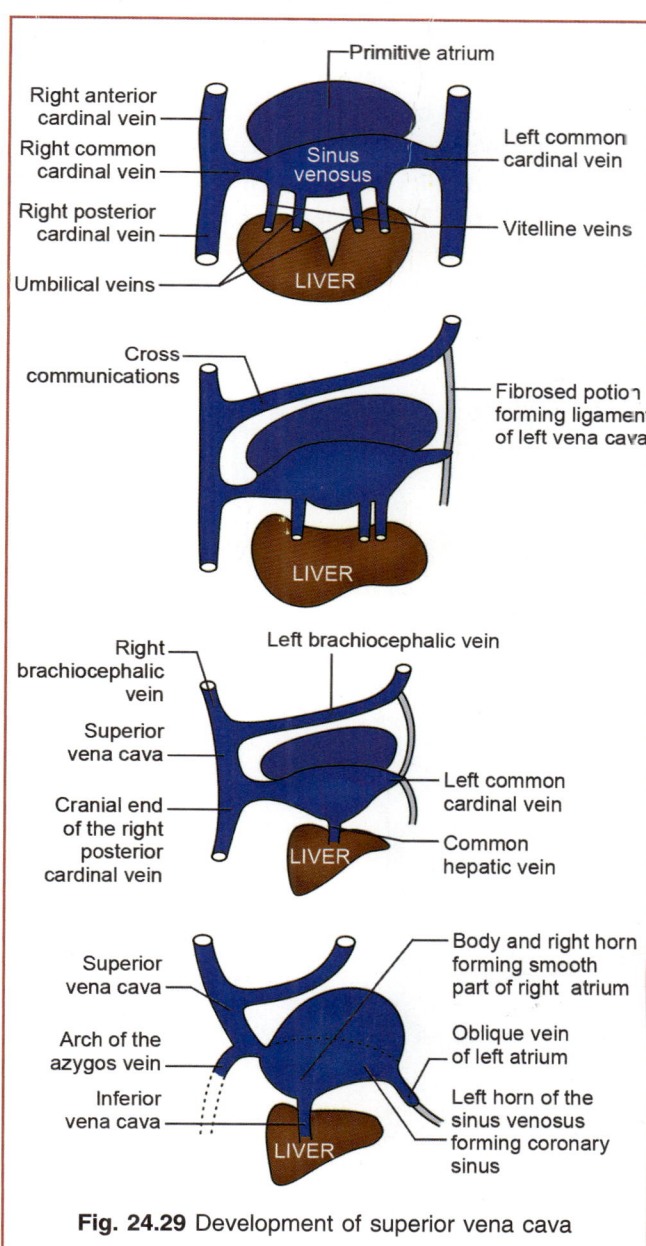

Fig. 24.29 Development of superior vena cava

sinus while this persistent terminal end of the left common cardinal vein forms **oblique vein of left atrium** (of Marshall)

The superior vena cava is developed from
1. The Right anterior cardinal vein (caudal to the transverse anastomosis)
2. The Right common cardinal vein

The transverse anastomosis between the two anterior cardinal veins contributes to the development of left brachiocephalic vein. In adult, note that left brachiocephalic vein is oblique in course, passing in front of the branches of arch of aorta.

Development of the inferior vena cava (Fig. 24.30)

- The lower (caudal) ends of the **posterior cardinal vein** receive blood from developing lower limb and pelvis. The caudal part of the right and left posterior cardinal veins are interconnected by a transverse anastomosis.
- The **subcardinal veins** are formed in relation to the mesonephros. The upper and lower ends of the subcardinal veins are connected to respective posterior cardinal veins. These subcardinal veins bring blood from developing kidney (renal veins). At this level the right and left subcardinal veins are also connected by a transverse anastomosis. The cranial end of the right vein is connected to right hepatocardiac channel (Figs 24.30A to D).

- The **supracardinal veins** (thoracolumbar veins) are formed parallel to subcardinal veins. These supracardinal veins also connect cranially and caudally with posterior cardinal veins. Each supracardinal veins also connect to respective subcardinal vein just below the renal veins.

- The major part of these longitudinal venous channels disappear and the adult form is achieved like this

The **inferior vena cava** is developed from following sources

1. The lower end of the right posterior cardinal vein

2. The lower part of the right supracardinal vein (between its junction with the posterior cardinal vein, and supra cardinal and subcardinal anastomosis)

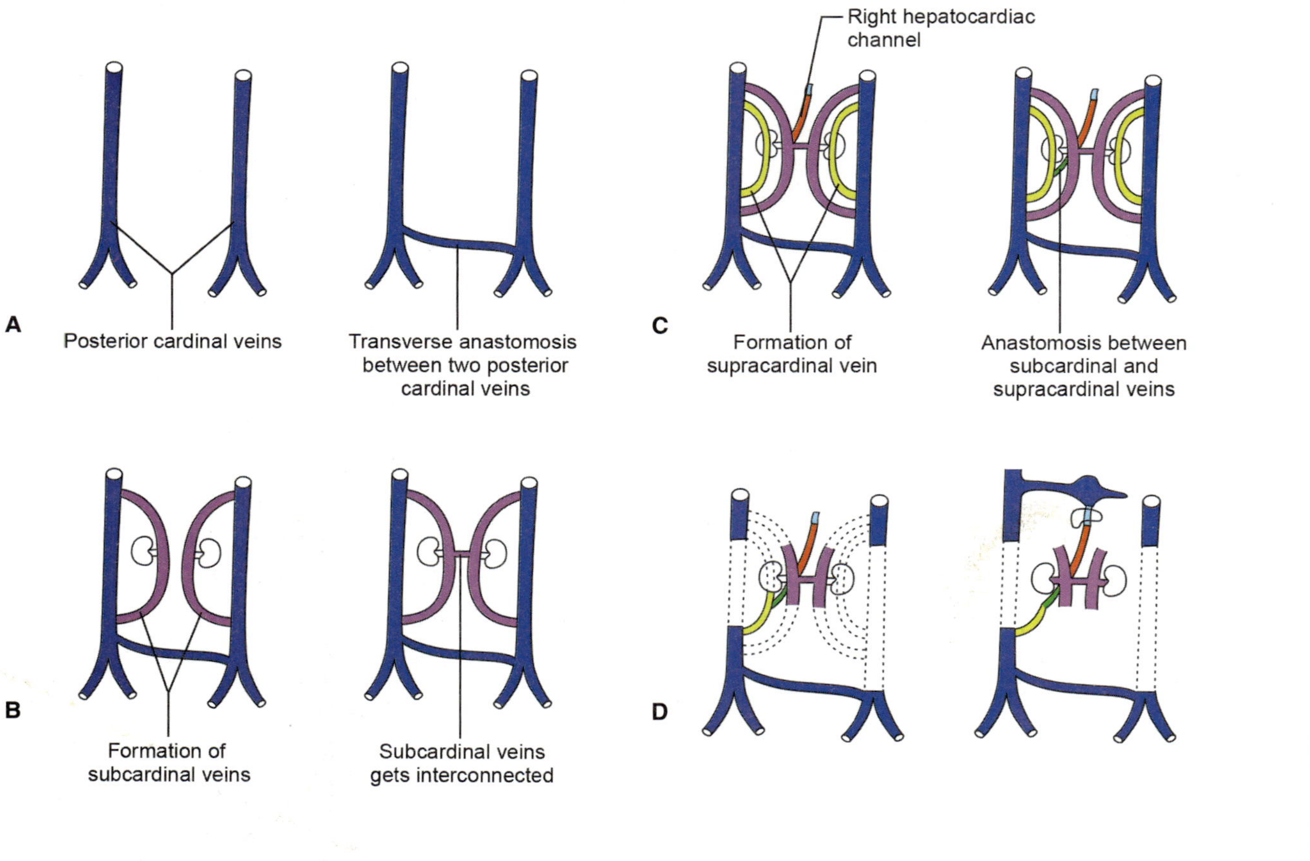

A Posterior cardinal veins   Transverse anastomosis between two posterior cardinal veins

C Right hepatocardiac channel   Formation of supracardinal vein   Anastomosis between subcardinal and supracardinal veins

B Formation of subcardinal veins   Subcardinal veins gets interconnected

D

Fig. 24.30A to D Development of inferior vena cava

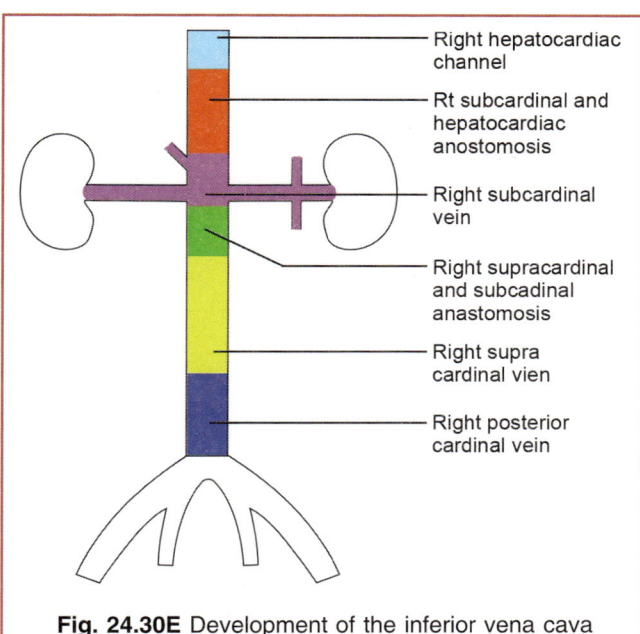

Right hepatocardiac channel

Rt subcardinal and hepatocardiac anostomosis

Right subcardinal vein

Right supracardinal and subcadinal anastomosis

Right supra cardinal vien

Right posterior cardinal vein

Fig. 24.30E Development of the inferior vena cava

3. The anastomosis between right supracardinal and right subcardinal veins

4. A small portion of the right subcardinal vein

5. The anastomosis between right subcardinal vein and right hepatocardiac channel

6. The right hepato cardiac channel (the terminal ends of the vitelline veins opening into the sinus venosus forms hepato cardiac channel and with regression of the left horn of the sinus venosus, the left hepato cardiac channel disappears and right hepato cardiac channel contributes to the development of cranial most part of the inferior vena cava (Fig. 24.30C).

Hepatocardiac channel

The hepatic bud grows into the septum transversum (unsplit intra embryonic mesoderm) to form the liver. The umbilical and vitelline veins open into the sinus venosus and the terminal part of these veins are traversing the septum transversum. These vessels break down to form sinusoids of the liver. These sinusoids of the liver will open into sinus vensosus through small persistant terminal part of the vitelline veins. These are called **right and left hepato-cardiac channel**. With regression of the left horn of the sinus venosus, the left hepato cardiac channel disappears. All the blood from vitelline and umbilical veins will flow pass through right hepato cardiac channel (Fig. 24.31).

With the regression of the right umbilical vein, the oxygenated blood from the placenta will reach the liver through left umbilical vein. Within the developing liver a vascular channel is formed between left umbilical vein and right hepatocardiac channel to facilitate the blood flow. This vascular passage is called **ductus venosus.**

Development of the portal vein

We have studied the fate of terminal part of the vitelline veins traversing the septum transversum. The portion of the right and left vitelline veins outside the developing liver contribute to the formation of portal vein (Figs 24.32A to D)

The right and left vitelline vein ascends on either side of the midgut (future duodenum). The right and left vitelline veins are connected to each other by 3 transverse anastomosis, of which the upper and lower anastomosis is ventral to the duodenum, while the middle anastomosis is

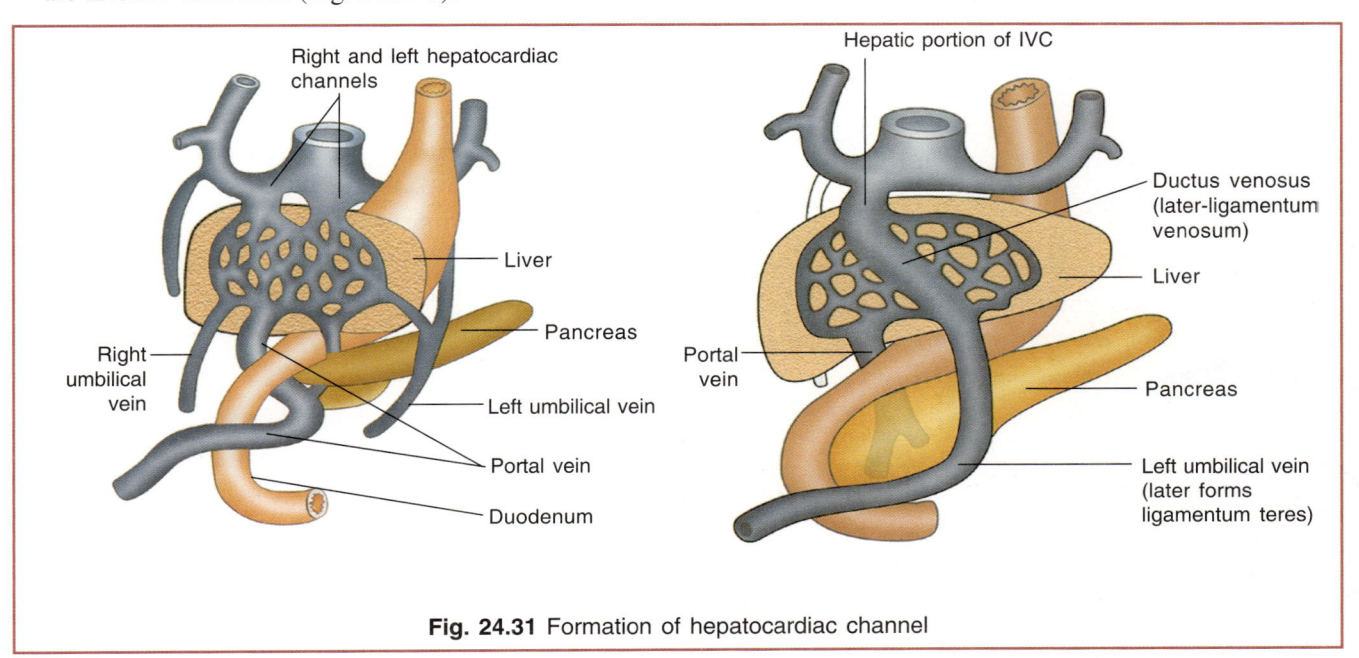

Right and left hepatocardiac channels

Liver

Pancreas

Right umbilical vein

Left umbilical vein

Portal vein

Duodenum

Hepatic portion of IVC

Ductus venosus (later-ligamentum venosum)

Liver

Portal vein

Pancreas

Left umbilical vein (later forms ligamentum teres)

Fig. 24.31 Formation of hepatocardiac channel

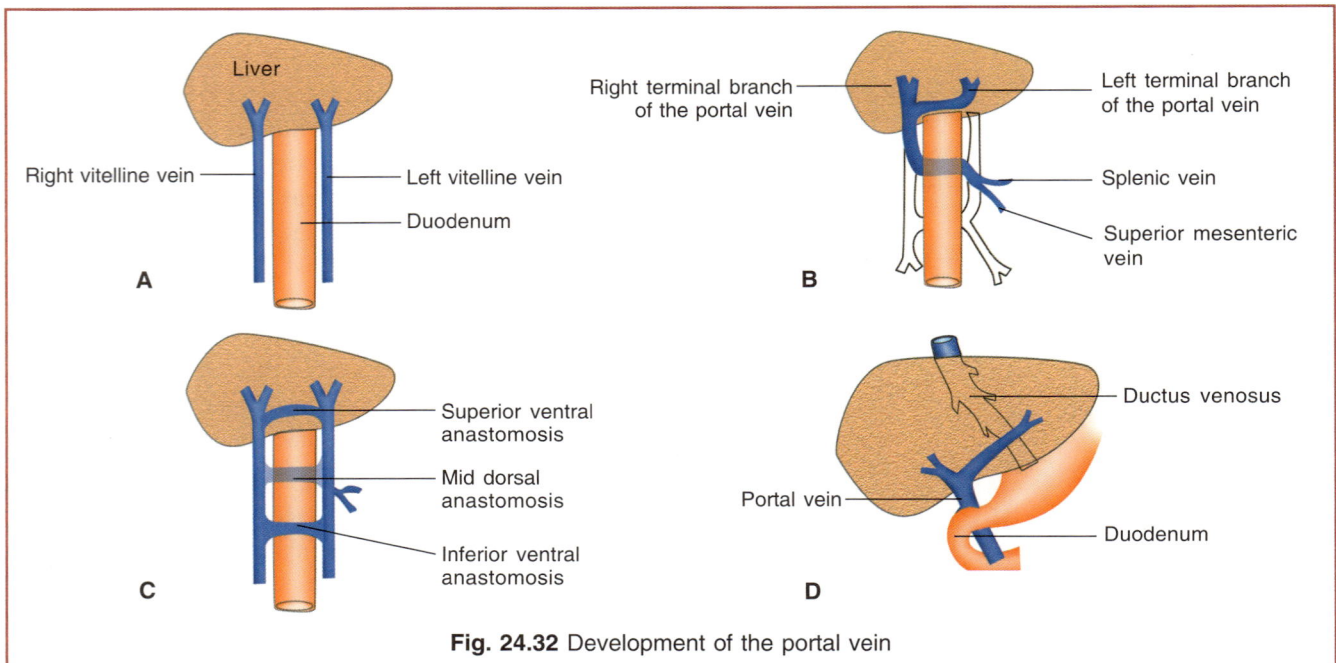

Fig. 24.32 Development of the portal vein

dorsal. The superior mesenteric and splenic veins join left vitelline vein, little caudal to the lower dorsal anastomosis. With the disappearance of some part of the vitelline vein, the adult portal vein is developed from following sources

1. The left vitelline vein between the entry of superior mesenteric vein and splenic vein (infraduodenal part of the portal vein)
2. Dorsal anastomosis between right and left vitelline vein (retroduodenal part of the portal vein)
3. Upper part of the right vitelline vein (supraduodenal part of the portal vein)

The left terminal branch of the portal vein is formed by the cranial ventral anastomosis and also by a small portion of the left vitelline vein

The short right terminal branch of the left portal vein is developed from upper part of the right vitelline vein.

The left umbilical vein is now opening into the left terminal branch of the portal vein, while ductus venosus (within the liver) connects the left terminal branch of the portal vein into the right hepatocardiac channel (inferior vena cava). Later the left umbilical vein forms **ligamentum teres** and ductus venosus is fibrosed to form **ligamentum venosum.**

CIRCULATION BEFORE AND AFTER BIRTH

Foetal circulation

- During foetal life, the oxygenated blood (about 80% saturated) reaches the foetus from the placenta by left umbilical vein.

- This umbilical vein ends in developing liver, where most of its blood enters ductus venosus and then into the inferior vena cava (short-circuiting the liver).

- But small amount of blood from umbilical vein enters the liver sinusoids and mixes with blood from portal circulation (vitelline veins which form portal vein also end in liver sinusoids), which accounts for the enlargement of the liver in foetal life and in the new born. Hence blood from the liver sinusoids also enters inferior vena cava, which opens into the right atrium (Fig. 24.33).

- A sphincter in the ductus venosus near the entrance of the umbilical vein regulates flow of umbilical blood through the liver sinusoids. When this sphincter relaxes, the more oxygenated blood from the umbilical vein enters inferior vena cava. When the sphincter constricts, the blood entering inferior vena cava is less oxygenated (venous blood from the lower limb ascending through inferior vena cava). The sphincter of the ductus venosus prevents the overloading of the heart. It is said that the sphincter action is due to uterine contraction.

- Hence the blood in the terminal part of the inferior vena cava entering right atrium is mixed (oxygenated blood from umbilical vein and less oxygenated blood from lower limb passing through inferior vena cava).

- From the right atrium most of the blood enters the left atrium through foramen ovale. The blood flow is guided by valve of the inferior vena cava.

SECTION 5

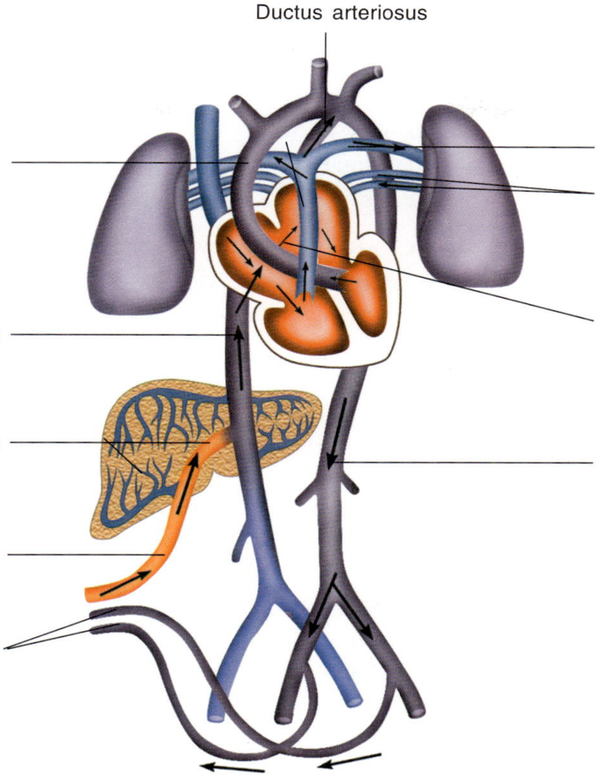

Fig. 24.33 Foetal circulation

- A small amount of the blood, which does not enter left atrium mixes with deoxygenated blood entering the right atrium from superior vena cava.

- The blood that has entered left atrium mixes with small amount of desaturated blood returning from the lung via pulmonary veins.

- From the left atrium, the blood enters left ventricle and then into ascending and arch of aorta. This blood is more oxygenated and supplies vital organs like brain (through carotid arteries) and musculature of heart (coronary arteries), which are vulnerable to the oxygen lack.

- The less oxygenated blood from the right atrium enters the right ventricle and then into the pulmonary trunk.

- From the pulmonary trunk, small amount of blood enters the lung through right and left branches of the pulmonary artery, but major amount of blood enters the distal part of the arch of the aorta through ductus arteriosus.

- The arch of aorta carrying more oxygenated blood and ductus arteriosus carrying less oxygenated blood get mixed at the distal end of the arch of aorta.

- After coursing through the descending aorta, blood enters the umbilical arteries and finally reaches placenta. The oxygen saturation in the umbilical arteries is about 58%.

The oxygenated blood from the placenta passing through umbilical vein into various organs of the foetus, get mixed with desaturated blood. The mixing occur in the following places

a. In the liver – by small amount of blood returning from portal system (vitelline veins)

b. In the inferior vena cava – by venous blood returning from lower limbs, kidneys, pelvis

c. In the right atrium - by venous blood returning from head and upper limb through superior vena cava

d. In the left atrium - by venous blood returning from lungs through pulmonary veins

e. At the entrance of the ductus arteriosus into the aorta by venous blood from pulmonary trunk

S E C T I O N   5

Circulatory changes at birth

1. Closure of the umbilical arteries

The umbilical arteries are closed immediately after birth, ensuring that no blood is permitted after birth to leave the foetus. After 2 to 3 months, the umbilical arteries fibrose to form **medial umbilical ligaments,** but its proximal part remains patent forming superior vesical arteries.

2. Closure of the umbilical vein and ductus venosus

It occurs shortly after the closure of umbilical arteries. Hence blood from the placenta may enter the newborn for some time after birth. The umbilical vein gets obliterated to form ligamentum teres, which occupies a fissure in the liver. The ductus venosus (the vascular channel connecting umbilical vein to right hepatocardiac channel), is also obliterated and forms ligamentum venosum.

3. Closure of the ductus arteriosus

It is closed immediately after birth under the influence of bradykinin, a substance released from the lung during initial inflation. Closure of the ductus arteriosus after birth is by high oxygen tension, and by the administration of prostaglandin inhibitor substance. The patency of the ductus arteriosus is maintained by low oxygen tension of foetal blood and by prostaglandin E2. In adult the obliterated ductus arteriosus forms ligamentum arteriosum.

4. Closure of the foramen ovale

With functioning of the lungs after birth, more amount of blood rushes into the left atrium, which raises the pressure inside the left atrium. The septum primum is mechanically pushed towards the septum secundum to obliterate the foramen ovale. The anatomical closure of this foramen may take one year. In about 20% of the individuals, the foramen may remain patent without mixing of the blood (probe patent foramen ovale). Crying by the baby creates a shunt from right to left, which may cause cyanotic episodes in the newborn.

DEVELOPMENT OF RESPIRATORY SYSTEM

- The lung buds (respiratory diverticulum) grows from the ventral wall of the foregut (endoderm) during 4th week of development (Fig. 24.34).

- Hence lining epithelium of the larynx, trachea, bronchi, bronchiole and alveoli of the lung are endodermal in origin. However the cartilages, musculature and connective tissues of the respiratory tract are derived from splanchnopleuric mesoderm surrounding the foregut.

- When the lung bud grows downwards it communicates with foregut. Now right and left tracheoesophageal ridges appear separating it from the foregut.

- Gradually, these ridges fuse to form tracheoesophageal septum, thus that part of the foregut is divided into dorsal part forming oesophagus and ventral part trachea and lung buds.

- **Larynx:** The lining epithelium of the larynx is endodermal in origin from proximal part of the respiratory diverticulum. This diverticulum where it communicates with foregut forms laryngeal orifice/inlet. The cartilages and muscles are derived from fourth and sixth cartilage.

- The lower end of the lung bud during separation from foregut becomes bifid and are called bronchial buds

- The proximal part of the lung bud forms larynx and trachea

- At the beginning of the 5th week each bronchial bud enlarges to form right and left main bronchi

- These growing lung bud invaginates into peri-cardioperitoneal canals (part of intraembryonic coelom) on each side

- With this the pericardial and peritoneal cavities are separated by pleuropericardial and pleuroperitoneal folds

- The splanchnopleuric layer of mesoderm of the coelomic cavity forms visceral pleura outside the lung, while somatopleuric layer forms parietal pleura (lining the body wall)

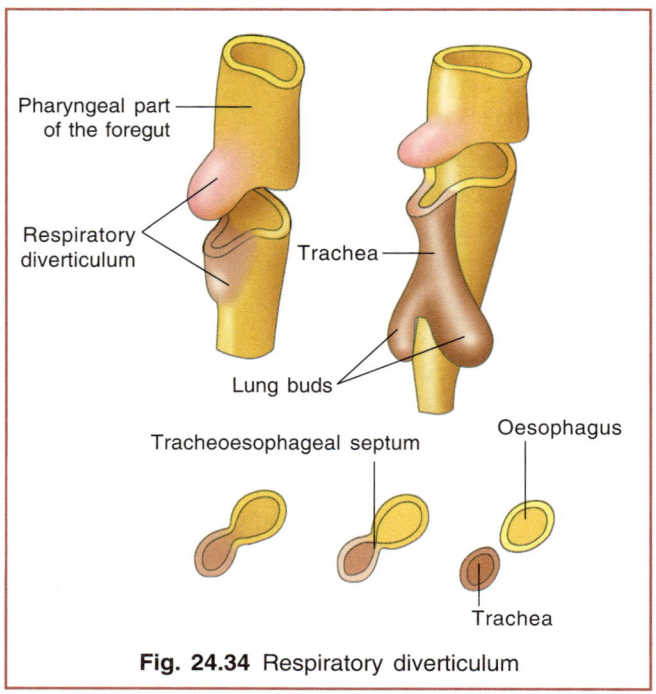

Fig. 24.34 Respiratory diverticulum

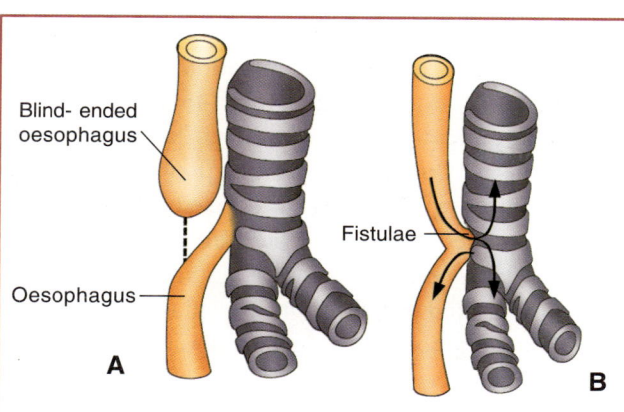

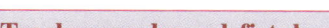

Fig. 24.35 Tracheo-oesophageal fistulae

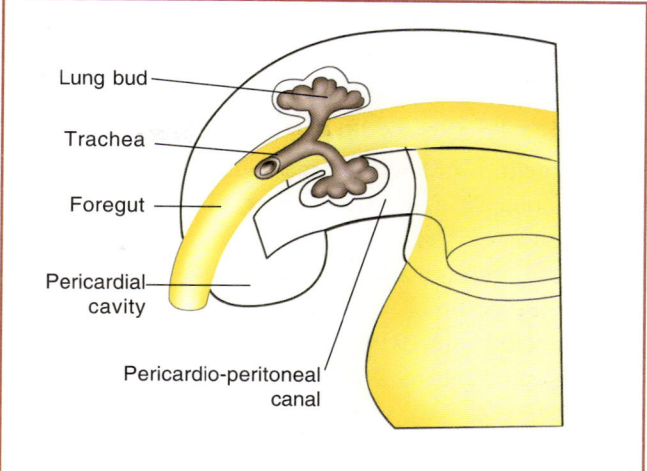

Fig. 24.36 Development of lung buds into the pericardio-peritoneal canal

Tracheoesophageal fistula

- The abnormal partition of the oesophagus and trachea can cause oesophageal atresia with or without tracheoesophageal fistulas (TEF)
- The complication of tracheoesophageal fistula is 'hydramnia' (excess of amniotic fluid). The amniotic fluid will not enter into the stomach. The amniotic fluid and gastric contents can enter the trachea through fistula and cause pneumonia
- The infants born with tracheoesophageal fistula will choke with first feed.
- In 90% of the tracheoesophageal fistula, the upper portion of the oesophagus ends in a blind pouch and lower portion forms a fistula with the trachea (Fig. 24.35A)
- 'H' type of trachea-oesophageal fistula-In this case the oesophagus communicates with trachea without obliteration of its lumen (Fig. 24.35B)
- Isolated cases where the upper portion of the oesophagus communicates with trachea while lower portion is a blind segment

Maturation of the lungs

The maturation of the lungs is divided into four periods.

1. Pseudoglandular period (between 5th and 16th week of development): The lung buds branch repeatedly up to terminal bronchiole (Fig. 24.36)

2. Canalicular period (between 16th week and 26th week of development): During this period, the terminal bronchiole divides into respiratory bronchioles, which further divides into alveolar ducts

3. Terminal sac period (between 26th week to birth): From the alveolar ducts, primitive alveoli are formed and they establish close contact with capillaries. During the 7th month, sufficient numbers of capillaries are present to ensure adequate gas exchange, hence the premature infant will able to survive.

4. Alveolar period (8 months to childhood): The alveoli mature and are contact with endothelium of the capillaries. During the last two months of prenatal period and also for several years after birth, the cells lining the alveoli become thinner (type I alveolar epithelial cells) and surrounding capillaries invaginate into these alveolar sacs. Mature alveoli are not present before birth. At the end of 6th month of intrauterine life, **type II alveolar epithelial cells** are formed (under the influence of fibroblast-pneumocyte factor/FPF, produced by the lung fibroblasts). These cells secrete a phospholipid-rich fluid called surfactant, which is required to reduce the surface tension. The amount of surfactant in the fluid increases, particularly during the last 2 weeks before birth.

The foetal breathing movements cause aspiration of amniotic fluid, which is necessary for lung development and also to condition the respiratory muscles.

The urine liberated from the foetal kidney maintains the volume of amniotic fluid, which is required for development of lung. Hence renal agenesis affect branching of bronchial tree in lung causing pulmonary hypoplasia (Potter's syndrome).

When the respiration begins at birth, most of the fluid inside the lung is absorbed by blood and lymph capillaries except surfactant which remains deposited over the alveolar cell membrane. When the air enters the alveoli during first breath, the surfactant layer prevents collapsing of the alveoli during expiration.

Growth of the lung after birth is due to an increase in the number of respiratory bronchioles and alveoli and not to an increase in the size of the alveoli. New alveoli are formed during the first 10 years of postnatal life.

In premature infants, the inadequate surfactant can cause collapse of lung during expiration. This is called respiratory distress syndrome (RDS). This is the common cause of death in the premature infant. Now there are artificial surfactant and also treatment of premature babies with glucocorticoids to stimulate surfactant production to tackle these problems.

Other anomalies of lungs

1. The apex of the right lung may be a separate lobe, divided by a pleural fold with azygos vein. The medial part of the divided apex is called lobe of the azygos vein

2. Congenital cysts of lung – These are formed by dilation of terminal or larger bronchi. These cysts give a 'honeycomb' appearance on radiograph.

The fetal adrenal gland consists of an inner active fetal zone and an outer dormant adult zone. The fetal zone produces mainly androgens in concert with the placenta. The outer zone is dormant during early fetal life and produces only small amounts of cortisol. Late in gestation, the production of cortisol gradually increases, and is thought to be responsible for fetal lung maturation (stimulates surfactant production). The secretion of cortisol from the adult zone of the adrenal cortex is controlled by ACTH and CRH from both the fetal pituitary and the placenta. Interestingly, CRH secretion from the placenta is upregulated by cortisol. Therefore, in late gestation, cortisol secretion from the adult zone of the fetal adrenal cortex is augmented by high placental CRH secretion. In summary, both maternal and fetal cortisol help to accelerate fetal lung maturation by stimulating surfactant production. The lecithin-sphingomyelin ratio is a marker of fetal lung maturity. Values above 1.9 are indicative of mature fetal lungs. Phospholipids including dipalmitoylphosphatidylcholine, are a major component of pulmonary surfactant. The level of phosphatidylcholine (also called lecithin) is measured in amniotic fluid in order to gauge fetal lung maturity. When the lecithin sphingomyelin (LIS) ratio in amniotic fluid is -2, the fetal lung is considered mature, meaning that it is producing adequate surfactant to avoid neonatal respiratory distress syndrome after birth.

CASE - 3

During a routine physical examination, the physician noted that a 13-year-old boy, had a long continuous heart murmur at the second intercostal space near the left sternal border. A systolic thrill was also noted in the same region. When questioned, the patient's mother recalled that the boy had periods of cyanosis and breathlessness as an infant, but that his previous pediatrician said that the murmur and the symptoms were nothing to be concerned about. She also mentioned that he tires easily during physical activity. Chest X-rays and Doppler ultrasound were ordered. The radiographs indicated slight left ventricular hypertrophy, and ultrasound revealed a patent ductus arteriosus. A surgery is planned to ligate the ductus arteriosus. The surgery resulted in successful ligation of the ductus arteriosus; however, later the boy experienced hoarseness when speaking. Laryngoscopy revealed paralysis of the left vocal fold.

a. What is the ductus arteriosus, and where is it located?

b. What is the prenatal function of the ductus arteriosus, and what usually happens to it after birth?

c. What are the eventual consequences if the ductus arteriosus is not closed? Should ES's first pediatrician have been concerned?

d. What likely caused paralysis of the left vocal fold?

e. Why would Doppler ultrasound be used to diagnose a patent ductus arteriosus?

Solutions to the Clinical case studies

Case-1

   a. Refer text
   b. Refer text

Case-2

a. A narrowing of the arch of aorta usually found immediately near the attachment of the ligamentum arteriosum, distal to the left subclavian artery.

b. The most frequently occurring lesions are those which occur as an adult. These lesions are found in the postductal region of the aorta and the patients are frequently asymptomatic presenting only with headaches and epistaxis. The average lifespan for a patient with this type of lesion is 30–40 years.

c. The most important clinical finding was the difference in blood pressure in the upper versus lower extremity. This presented as diminished pulse in the lower

SECTION 5

extremities, coolness, fatigue and pain in the lower extremities (subsequent to anaerobic metabolism and lactic acid buildup). The higher blood pressure in the upper extremities was evident not only by the blood pressure itself, but also by the headaches and nosebleeds. The systolic murmur indicates a fluid overload or, in this case, stricture of the aorta and an inability to completely eject the volume through the aorta.

d. Post coarctation dilation was seen in the region of the aortic knob. There was also rib notching, which reflects the erosion of bone by intercostal arteries that have become dilated and tortuous by the great volume of blood they are carrying as collateral blood flow.

e. A postductal lesion allows good collateral circulation from proximal to distal portions of the aorta via the anterior intercostals from internal thoracic artery anastomosing with posterior intercostal branches of descending aorta.

A preductal lesion presents a life threatening situation early in infancy. The distal aorta is initially filled via a patent ductus arteriosus, but as the ductus closes blood flow to the distal aorta diminishes, and the infant's survival may be threatened.

f. Surgical intervention, which includes resection of the coarctation and end-to-end anastomosis, patch aortoplasty or a bypass with a prosthetic graft. The treatment of choice for this patient would most likely be a bypass with a prosthetic graft.

g. Significant hemorrhage secondary to damage to the dilated intercostal arteries. Because it is necessary to clamp the aorta for the procedure, paraplegia may result from diminished blood flow to the spinal cord.

Case-3

a. The ductus arteriosus is a foetal shunt between the pulmonary artery and the arch of the aorta.

b. In the foetus, the ductus arteriosus allows oxygenated blood returning to the heart from the placenta to bypass the uninflated lungs and enter the systemic circulation. Following birth (usually within a few days), the ductus arteriosus functionally closes off and forms a fibrous cord called the ligamentum arteriosum. Complete anatomic closure of the ductus arteriosus may take up to 6 weeks. If the ductus arteriosus remains open, it forms a left-to-right shunt which carries some blood from the left side of the heart into the pulmonary trunk.

c. Initial consequences of a patent ductus arteriosus include cardiac failure and pulmonary edema in infants

(accounting for the cyanosis and breathlessness experienced by the boy); however, a patent ductus arteriosus is often compatible with survival to adulthood. Cardiac failure (which may be the reason for the slight left ventricular hypertrophy observed in this case) and bacterial endocarditis are common complications. If left untreated, pulmonary hypertension develops, resulting in hypertrophy of the right ventricle and eventually in a reversal of flow (to right-to-left), leading to cyanosis, clubbing of fingers and toes, and polycythemia due to systemic circulation of large amounts of deoxygenated blood, as well as right heart failure.

d. Paralysis of the left vocal fold resulted from damage to the left recurrent laryngeal nerve, which loops under the arch of the aorta adjacent to the ligamentum arteriosum (ductus arteriosus) after leaving the vagus nerve. The left recurrent laryngeal nerve innervates the muscles of the left larynx (the right recurrent laryngeal nerve, which loops similarly under the right subclavian artery), with the exception of the left cricothyroid muscle, supplied by the external laryngeal nerve (branch of the vagus). Surgeons must take great care in identifying and protecting the left recurrent laryngeal nerve when performing procedures in the region of the aortic arch.

e. Doppler ultrasound permits the visualization of blood flow and can thus be used to identify a patent ductus arteriosus. This technique is preferable to traditional angiography, which may also be used, because it is noninvasive, involves no radiation, and is fairly inexpensive.

MCQs

1. A persistent portion of the septum primum acts as a valve for the interatrial communication during fetal life and postnatally becomes fused to septum secundum in order to close
   A. Foramen magnum
   B. Foramen ovale
   C. Foramen lacerum
   D. Foramen rotundum

2. Once the infant is delivered and its first breath, which structure immediately closes to block the right-to-left shunt?
   A. Allantois
   B. Ductus arteriosus
   C. Ductus venosus
   D. Foramen ovale

3. Physical examination of a 5-year-old child reveals a heart murmur. An echocardiogram shows an ostium primum type of atrial septal defect. This defect results from failure of the
   A. Ostium primum to form within the septum primum
   B. Ostium secundum to form within the septum primum
   C. Septum primum to fuse with the endocardial cushions
   D. Septum primum to fuse with the septum secundum

4. Which of the following statements is most correct with respect to the development of interatrial septum?
   A. Foramen secundum appears in septum secundum
   B. Foramen primum is closed when septum secundum reaches endocardial cushions
   C. The abnormal flow of blood is from right to left
   D. Complete and timely closure of the endocardial cushions is essential

5. A new born baby is known to have multiple cardiac anomalies. An echocardiogram shows a ventricular septal defect, hypertrophy of the right ventricle, pulmonary stenosis and an overriding aorta. Which of the following embryologic defect underlies this condition?
   A. Fallot's tetralogy
   B. Patent ductus arteriosus
   C. Interatrial septal defect
   D. Mitral stenosis

6. A newborn baby is cyanotic at birth. As the child grows older, the parents notice that he is always squatting. The X-ray film of the chest shows an enlarged boot-shaped heart that is consistent with right ventricular hypertrophy. The echocardiogram revealed ventricular septal defect. Which of the following other defects would most likely have been noted?
   A. Overriding pulmonary artery
   B. Left ventricular hypertrophy
   C. Atrial septal defect
   D. Pulmonary stenosis

7. A 36-year-old woman with a history of type 2 diabetes mellitus gives birth to a term male infant. Immediately after birth, the infant is noted to be cyanotic and tachypneic. His hypoxemia quickly worsens over minutes, and he is taken to cardiac catheterization, where a balloon is guided to perforate the atrial septum. He is also given an infusion of prostaglandin El. The infant's hypoxia stabilizes, and he is later taken for definitive, corrective surgery. Which of the following is the underlying pathophysiology of this infant's hypoxemia?
   A. Coarctation of the aorta
   B. Concomitant ventricular septal defect
   C. Delayed closure of the ductus arteriosus
   D. Failure of the aorticopulmonary septum to spiral

8. A newborn baby develops a bluish color when crying. Which of the following congenital defects may be the cause of the cyanosis?
   A. ASD-septum secundum type
   B. Persistent truncus arteriosus
   C. Primum type atrial septal defect
   D. Patent truncus arteriosus

9. An autopsy of an infant who died with multiple congenital anomalies reveals a malformed heart. The aorta arises from right ventricle. The pulmonary artery overrides ventricular septal defect. Which of the following terms best describes this infant's heart?
   A. ASD
   B. Right ventricular hypertrophy
   C. Taussig-Bing malformation
   D. Tetralogy of Fallot

10. A neonate born 3 hours ago is having difficulty in breathing. The baby was born prematurely at 28 weeks gestation. He is tachypneic and is using his accessory muscles to breathe with nasal flaring and grunting. The baby's heart rate is 120/mm. blood pressure is 100/60mm Hg, and respiratory rate is 55/mm. Analysis of amniotic fluid reveals a lecithin:sphingomyelin ratio of 0.9. What is this baby's lung lacking?
    A. Elasatse
    B. Angiotensin-converting enzyme
    C. Dipalmitoyl phosphatidylcholine/surfactants
    D. Collagen

11. Six-hour-old baby boy who was born full-term and without complications now presents with cyanosis and dyspnea. Physical examination reveals absent breath sounds on the left with bowel sounds present in the left hemithorax. Heart sounds are distant on the left but heard well on the right. An X-ray film of the chest confirms the presence of bowel loops in the chest. These findings can all be explained by failed development of a single part of a specific structure. Which of the following is the most likely structure that has failed to develop properly?
    A. Midgut loop
    B. Mesencephalon
    C. Bulbus cordis
    D. Pleuroperitoneal folds

12. A 6-year-old boy who was born prematurely brought to his pediatrician because his mother says that he tires easily. She also says that he has had several respiratory infections. On examination, the boy is noted to be below the fifth percentile in height: jugular venous pressure is elevated; lips are slightly cyanotic: and a continuous machine-like murmur is heard over the left upper sternal border. The congenital anomaly responsible for these signs and symptoms produces which of the following patterns of blood flow in fetal life?

   A. It shunts blood from the inferior vena cava to the aorta
   B. It shunts blood from the left pulmonary artery to the aorta
   C. It shunts blood from the left ventricle to the right ventricle
   D. It shunts blood from the portal vein to the inferior vena cava

13. A term infant is born after an uncomplicated pregnancy to a 35-year-old woman. On cutting the umbilical cord, the physician notes an abnormality' that leads him to consult a pediatric cardiologist. Which of the following abnormalities did this physician most likely observe?

   A. Single umbilical vein
   B. Single umbilical artery
   C. Single allantoic duct
   D. Two umbilical arteries

14. A baby was observed at birth to be non-cyanotic. The mother was known to have been infected with rubella during pregnancy. On physical examination, the patient is found to have a continuous murmur that is present in both systole and diastole. The patient also has digital cyanosis. Which of the following is the most likely congenital anomaly?

   A. Patent ductus arteriosus
   B. Tetralogy of Fallot
   C. Transposition of the great vessels
   D. Ventricular septal defect

15. A new born infant displays wheezing respiration, which is aggravated when she was fed, flexes her neck and cries. Radio imaging studies of her chest revealed double aortic arches compressing her trachea and esophagus. This rare developmental defect results from

   A. Persistence of the right dorsal aorta distal to the origin of the 7th cervical intersegmental artery
   B. Ductus caroticus fails to disappear
   C. Fifth pair of aortic arch artery fails to disappear
   D. Degeneration of right fourth arch artery

16. A pediatrician is called in to evaluate an infant who has not been able to swallow at all since birth. His mother reports that every time she tries to breastfeed him the infant chokes and coughs. The mother denies any use of alcohol or drugs during pregnancy. She also denies any history of sexually transmitted diseases. She says that her pregnancy and delivery were uneventful, but remembers the obstetrician being concerned about excess amniotic fluid seen on her ultrasound. Which of the following is most likely to be seen on the infants X-ray of the chest?

   A. Air in the stomach
   B. Herniation of the stomach, spleen and intestines
   C. Lung hypoplasia
   D. Pleural effusion

17. The heart of an embryo first begins beating at which of the following ages?
   A. 2 weeks
   B. 3weeks
   C. 4 weeks
   D. 6 weeks

18. In the developing fetus, which of the following provides a bypass from portal circulation?
   A. Ductus venosus
   B. Ductus arteriosus
   C. Foramen ovale
   D. Umbilical vein

19. Which of the following is a remnant of a structure that allowed bypass from pulmonary circulation in the developing fetus?
   A. Ligamentum teres
   B. Ligamentum venosum
   C. Ductus arteriousus
   D. Ligamentum arteriosum

20. A 3-day-old girl is brought to the pediatric clinic because of breathing difficulties and poor feeding. She coughs, chokes, and spits up milk very soon after beginning to suckle. Physical examination and radiographs reveal the presence of the most common type of tracheo-oesophageal fistula. The infant's defect likely resulted from
   A. Failure of the buccopharyngeal membrane to rupture
   B. Failure of the tracheoesophageal ridges to fuse
   C. Incomplete recanalization of the larynx
   D. Patent thyroglossal duct

21. An autopsy is performed on a man who died of an unknown cause. The pathologist discovers that the

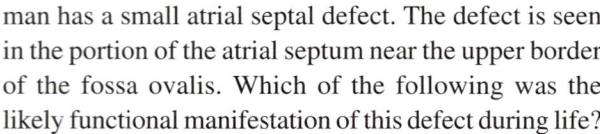

man has a small atrial septal defect. The defect is seen in the portion of the atrial septum near the upper border of the fossa ovalis. Which of the following was the likely functional manifestation of this defect during life?

A. No cyanosis occurred prenatally or postnatally
B. Postnatal cyanosis due to a shunt of blood from the left atrium to the right atrium
C. Postnatal cyanosis due to a shunt of blood from the right atrium to the left atrium
D. Prenatal cyanosis due to a shunt of blood from the right atrium to the left atrium

22. A woman comes to the physician for a prenatal visit. Examination reveals that her uterus is considerably larger than her gestational age would predict. An ultrasound examination is ordered and it reveals that she has polyhydramnios. Which of the following congenital defects of the foetus would be most likely to be associated with this abnormality?

A. Atrial septal defect
B. Esophageal atresia
C. Lung hypoplasia
D. Meckel's diverticulum

23. A patient is complaining of difficulty swallowing. A barium contrast X-ray shows a constriction of the esophagus at the level of the third thoracic vertebra. An aortogram shows that the patient has a double aortic arch. Which of the following developmental abnormalities explains this finding?

A. Abnormal persistence of the right dorsal aorta
B. Abnormal persistence of the right fourth aortic arch
C. Abnormal persistence of the right seventh intersegmental artery
D. Abnormal persistence of the right sixth aortic arch

24. While many congenital cardiac defects can be discovered and monitored before birth, others present in a delayed fashion. Pediatric clinics often see patients who present with early cyanosis, which is later found to exist in the context of a congenital heart defect.

Which of the following is the most common cause of cyanosis within the first few weeks of life?

A. Atrial septal defect
B. Patent ductus arteriosus
C. Tetralogy of Fallot
D. Ventricular septal defect

Answer to the MCQs

1. B
2. D
3. C
4. D
5. A
6. D
7. D
8. B
9. C
10. C
11. D
12. B
13. B
14. A
15. A
16. A
17. C
18. A
19. B
20. B
21. A
22. B
23. A
24. C

SECTION 5

Major questions

1. Define a typical intercostal space. Name its contents. Describe the course, branches, distribution and applied anatomy of a typical intercostal nerve

2. Define 'bronchopulmonary segments'. Name the bronchopulmonary segments of the right and left lung. Discuss their applied aspects

3. Describe the pleura under – parts of parietal pleura, pleural reflection, nerve supply to the pleura, pleural recesses and their applied aspects

4. Draw a neat labeled diagram of medial surface of right/ left lung

5. Describe the right atrium under-external features, internal features, development and its anomalies

6. Describe the right ventricle under-external features, internal features, development and its anomalies

7. Describe the blood supply of the heart in detail. Discuss its applied anatomy

8. Describe the nerve supply of the heart and trace the pain pathway in angina and discuss the areas of referred pain

9. Describe the arch of aorta under-extent, relations, branches, development and applied anatomy

10. Describe the oesophagus under-parts, major relations, lymphatic drainage, microscopic structure and applied anatomy

Short notes

1. External intercostal muscle

2. Internal thoracic artery

3. Apex of the lung

4. Root of the lung

5. Hilum of the lung

6. Costodiaphragmatic recess

7. Pericardial sinuses

8. Bronchopulmonary segments

9. Lymphatic drainage of the lung and its clinical significance

10. Phrenic nerve and its applied anatomy

11. Right coronary artery

12. Left coronary artery

13. Cardiac plexus

14. Coronary sinus

15. Coronary sulcus

16. Interventricular septum

17. Ligamentum arteriosum

18. Azygos vein

19. Thoracic duct

20. Normal constrictions of oesophagus

21. Patent ductus arteriosus

22. Fallot's tetralogy

23. Sinus venosus and its fate

24. Fourth arch artery

25. Development of interatrial septum and its defects

26. Development of interventricular septum and its defects

27. Trachea

28. Microscopic structure of trachea

29. Greater and lesser splanchnic nerves

Objective Structured Practical Examination/ Spotters/Must Identify Structures

UPPER LIMB

1. Identification of Pectoralis major/minor muscle, its nerve supply or actions
2. Identification of serratus anterior muscle, its nerve supply or effect of its nerve injury or root value of the nerve supplying it
3. Identification of axillary nerve passing through quadrangular space, its root value or naming the muscles supplied by it or naming the artery accompanying it
4. Identification of deltoid muscle, its nerve supply or actions
5. Identification of supraspinatus, its insertion or nerve supply or action
6. Identification of axillary artery, naming its branches (any 2)
7. Identification of radial nerve (at lower triangular space), its root value or naming the artery accompanying it in this area
8. Identification of musculocutaneous nerve, its root value or naming the muscles supplied by it
9. Identification of biceps brachii, its insertion or nerve supply or actions
10. Identification of brachial artery, naming it's any 2 branches or level of termination or terminal branches
11. Identification of ulnar nerve behind the medial epicondyle, its root value or naming the clinical condition resulting from its injury
12. Identification of radial nerve in the spiral groove, naming its cutaneous branches in this area or effect of its injury in this area.
13. Identification of triceps muscle, its insertion, nerve supply or action
14. Identification of brachialis, its insertion, nerve supply or action
15. Identification of cephalic vein (anywhere in its course) and its termination
16. Identification of median cubital vein, its clinical significance
17. Identification of bicipital aponeurosis, its superficial and deep relations
18. Identification of median nerve in the cubital fossa or in the forearm, its root value or effect of lesion or naming the muscles supplied by it in the forearm

19. Identification of radial nerve in the cubital fossa, its root value or effect of injury at this area.
20. Identification of pronator teres, its nerve supply or action
21. Identification of radial or ulnar artery in the cubital fossa or in the forearm
22. Identification of brachioradialis muscle, its nerve supply or action
23. Identification of flexor digitorum profundus or superficilais, nerve supply, insertion
24. Identification of flexor retinaculum, naming the structure passing superficial or deep to it
25. Identification of superficial palmar arch, its formation or completion or branches
26. Identification of median nerve or ulnar nerve in the forearm, naming the muscles supplied by it in this region
27. Identification of median nerve or ulnar nerve in the hand, naming the muscles supplied by it in this region or its cutaneous distribution in the hand
28. Identification of lumbricals, its nerve supply and actions
29. Identification of adductor pollicis brevis, its nerve supply and action
30. Identification of supinator muscle, its nerve supply and action
31. Identification of extensor retinaculum, structure passing superficial or deep to it or attachment
32. Identification of first dorsal interossei muscle, its nerve supply and actions
33. Cutaneous nerve supply to any finger marked
34. Lymphatic drainage of thumb or little finger
35. Identification of anatomical snuff box, naming the carpal bone present in its floor or artery present in its floor
36. Identification of right or left clavicle, its unique features or identifying its medial or lateral end, naming the bone it articulates with
37. Identification of coracoid process of scapula, what type of epiphysis, does it belongs? Or naming the muscles attached to it
38. Naming the muscles attached to supraglenoid or infraglenoid tubercles
39. Naming the nerves in contact with the humerus and their effect of injury

40. Identification of lesser or greater tubercles of humerus and structure attached to it
41. Identification of surgical neck of the humerus, naming the structures encircling it
42. Identification of radial groove, naming the structure related to it
43. Identification of medial epicondyle, naming the structure passing behind it
44. Identification of capitulum or trochlea and their specific articulations
45. Identification of tuberosity of radius, naming the muscle attached to it
46. Identification of tuberosity of ulna, naming the muscle attached to it
47. Identification of radial notch of the ulna and naming the bone articulating with it or naming what type of joint is it
48. Identification of styloid process of ulna, naming the tendon passing just behind it
49. Identification of head of the ulna and its articulations
50. Identification of dorsal tubercle of the radius, its immediate medial and lateral relations
51. Naming the bones articulating with lower end of the radius
52. Identification of all carpal bones in articulated hand or in a radiograph.
53. Identification of hook of the hamate or pisiform bone, structure attached to it.

LOWER LIMB

1. Identification of ligamentum patellae, its lower attachment
2. Identification of tibial or fibular collateral ligaments of knee joint
3. Identification of medial or lateral menisci, what type of tissue it is made up of?
4. Identification of anterior or posterior cruciate ligaments, in what position of the knee they get stretched?
5. Identification of tibilais anterior, its insertion, nerve supply or actions
6. Identification of extensor retinaculum of the ankle, naming the structure passing superficial or deep to it
7. Identification of deep peroneal nerve, naming the muscles supplied by it or effect of its injury
8. Identification of popliteal artery, its terminal branches
9. Identification of popliteal muscle, its nerve supply, action
10. Identification of tendocalcaneus, its insertion, action
11. Identification of soleus muscle, its nerve supply

12. Identification of tibialis posterior muscle, its insertion, nerve supply and actions
13. Identification of common peroneal nerve its effect of lesion or naming its cutaneous branches
14. Identification of tibial nerve in the popliteal fossa, naming any muscles supplied by it
15. Identification of dorsalis pedis artery, its formation or continuation
16. Identification of peroneus longus or bevis, insertion, nerve supply and actions
17. Identification of superficial peroneal nerve. Naming the muscles supplied by it
18. Cutaneous innervations to dorsum of the foot
19. Lymphatic drainage from great toe or little toe
20. Identification of right or left hip bone
21. Identification of anterior superior iliac spine, naming the structures attached to it
22. Identification of tubercle of the iliac crest, its vertebral level
23. Identification of ischial spine, structure related or attached
24. Identification of ischial tuberosity, naming the muscles attached to it
25. Identification of greater trochanter of the femur, specific attachment
26. Naming the chief artery supplying the neck of the femur
27. Identification of lesser trochanter, naming the structure attached to it
28. Identification of adductor tubercle of femur and structure attached to it
29. Identification of intercondylar area of the tibia, naming the structure attached to it in anterior to posterior direction
30. Identification of tibial tuberosity and structure attached to it
31. Naming the structure attached to a groove on the posterior aspect of the medial condyle of tibia (for semimembranosus)
32. Naming the muscles attached to upper part of the medial surface of the tibia
33. Naming the bone articulating with the under surface of the tibia
34. Identification of medial malleolus, naming the structure attached to it
35. Naming the tendon related just behind the medial malleolus of the tibia
36. Naming the ligament attached to the head of the fibula
37. Naming the structure encircling the neck of the fibula and effect of its injury

SECTION 5

38. Identification of median crest of the fibula, naming the structure related to them
39. Identification of lateral malleolus, naming the ligament attached to it or naming the bone articulating with it
40. Identification of talus, naming the bones articulating with it (specific)
41. Identification of sustantaculum tali, structure attached to it or name the structure passing below it
42. Identification of tuberosity of navicular bone, structure attached to it
43. Identification of medial mallelous and structure attached to it
44. Naming the tendon passing through the groove on the plantar surface of the cuboid bone

THORAX

1. Identification of internal thoracic artery, its origin or terminal branches or naming it's any 2 branches
2. Identification of external intercostal muscle, its nerve supply and action
3. Identification of intercostal nerve, naming the structures supplied by it
4. Identification of posterior intercostal artery, its origin
5. Identification of structures at the hilum of the lung (bronchus, pulmonary artery, vein)
6. Identification of transverse or oblique fissure of the lung, their surface marking
7. Identification of lingula and naming the broncho-pulmonary segments present in it
8. Identification of major impression on medial surface of right (superior vena cava, arch of the azygos vein, inferior vena cava, cardiac impression) or left (arch of the aorta, descending aorta) lung
9. Identification of apex of the heart, its surface marking or what chamber of the heart does it belongs
10. Identification of interior of the right atrium, naming the openings (tributaries) present in it
11. Identification of crista terminalis, its development or naming the structure present in its upper part
12. Identification of fossa ovalis or limbus fossa ovalis, its development
13. Identification of anterior papillary muscles in the right ventricle, naming the structure connected to its base

14. Identification of septomarginal trabaculae, naming what part of conducting system passes through it?
15. Identification of interior of the left atrium, its posterior relations or name the vessels opening into it
16. Identification of pulmonary trunk & its development
17. Identification of ascending aorta, naming the arteries arising from it or its development
18. Identification of right coronary artery, naming its branches or naming the parts of the conducting system supplied by it
19. Identification of posterior interventricular artery, naming the vein accompanying it
20. Identification of circumflex artery, its origin or any 2 branches or area supplied by it
21. Identification of LAD, naming the vein accompanying it or naming it's any 2 branches or area supplied by it
22. Identification of coronary sinus, where does it terminate? or its tributaries or development
23. Identification of arch of the aorta, naming its branches or its development
24. Identification of ligamentum arteriosum, its embryological basis or naming the nerve winding around it
25. Identification of descending thoracic aorta, naming it's any 2 branches
26. Identification of azygos vein its termination or any 2 tributaries
27. Identification of oesophagus, its normal constrictions
28. Identification of thoracic duct, its termination
29. Identification of thoracic part of the sympathetic chain

OSTEOLOGY

1. Naming the structure posterior to manubrium sterni
2. Identification of sternal angle, its significance
3. Naming the structures related to neck of the first rib
4. Naming the structure related to the groove on the upper surface of the first rib or structure attached to the scalene tubercle
5. Identification of typical rib, its specific articulation, naming the structure traversing the costal groove
6. Identification of 12th rib, giving reasons for your identification
7. Identification of typical thoracic vertebra, giving specific reason for identification or naming its parts

Index